# ESSENTIALS OF COMPUTERS FOR NURSES

# NOTICE

Medicine is an ever-changing science. As new research and clinical experience broaden our knowledge, changes in treatment and drug therapy are required. The authors and the publisher of this work have checked with sources believed to be reliable in their efforts to provide information that is complete and generally in accord with the standards accepted at the time of publication. However, in view of the possibility of human error or changes in medical sciences, neither the editors nor the publisher nor any other party who has been involved in the preparation or publication of this work warrants that the information contained herein is in every respect accurate or complete, and they are not responsible for any errors or omissions or for the results obtained from use of such information. Readers are encouraged to confirm the information contained herein with other sources. For example and in particular, readers are advised to check the product information sheet included in the package of each drug they plan to administer to be certain that the information contained in this book is accurate and that changes have not been made in the recommended dose or in the contraindications for administration. This recommendation is of particular importance in connection with new or infrequently used drugs.

# ESSENTIALS OF COMPUTERS FOR NURSES

• • • • • • • • • • • • • • • • • • • • • • • • •

## SECOND EDITION

**VIRGINIA K. SABA**
**R.N., Ed.D., F.A.A.N., F.A.C.M.I.**
Georgetown University School of Nursing
Washington, D.C.

**KATHLEEN A. McCORMICK**
**R.N., Ph.D., F.A.A.N., F.A.C.M.I.**
Senior Science Adviser
Center for Information Technology
Agency for Health Care Policy and Research
Public Health Service, D.H.H.S.
Rockville, Maryland

**McGRAW-HILL**
*Health Professions Division*

New York   St. Louis   San Francisco
Auckland   Bogotá   Caracas   Lisbon
London   Madrid   Mexico City   Milan
Montreal   New Delhi   San Juan
Singapore   Sydney   Tokyo   Toronto

# McGraw-Hill

*A Division of The McGraw·Hill Companies*

## ESSENTIALS OF COMPUTERS FOR NURSES

234567890 DOCDOC 9876

ISBN 0-07-105418-9

This book was set in New Century Schoolbook
by V&M Graphics, Inc.
The editors were Gail Gavert and Lester A. Sheinis;
the production supervisor was Clare B. Stanley;
the text and cover designer was Karen K. Quigley;
the indexer was Geraldine Beckford.
R. R. Donnelley & Sons Company was printer and binder.

This book is printed on acid-free paper.

**Library of Congress Cataloging-in-Publication Data**

Saba, Virginia K.
   Essentials of computers for nurses / Virginia K. Saba,
Kathleen A. McCormick.
      p.  cm.
   Includes bibliographical references and index.
   ISBN 0-07-105418-9
   1. Nursing—Data processing. 2. Computers. 3. Information
storage and retrieval systems—Nursing. I. McCormick, Kathleen
Ann. II. Title.
   [DNLM: 1. Computers—nurses' instruction. 2. Automatic Data
Processing—nurses' instruction. 3. Nursing. WY 26.5 S113e 1995]
RT50.5.S23 1995
610.73´0285—dc20
DNLM/DLC
for Library of Congress                     95-6198

This book was written by Kathleen A. McCormick in her private capacity.
No official support or endorsement by the Department of Health and Human
Services, the Public Health Service, or the Agency for Health Care Policy and
Research is intended or should be inferred.

# CONTENTS

# FOREWORD

• • • • • • • • • • • • • • • • • • • • • • • • • •

The computer revolution is rapid and ongoing. It has impacted on the expansion of knowledge in health care and information management. The great strides in and amplification of information management are occurring because it has now been demonstrated that the use of computers in health care can increase the quality, effectiveness, and efficiency of documenting practice; improve administration in many health care settings; and broaden the education of professionals as well as the conduct of research. And there is movement in this revolution toward an electronic superhighway as a national information infrastructure. These new, and other, innovative movements are described in this second edition of *Essentials of Computers for Nurses*.

To many consumers of health care services, the technology seems linked directly to escalating health care costs. But the computer technology is described in several applications in this book as a means of providing care more effectively and efficiently at affordable costs. The use of computers in nursing is described by the authors as essential to improve health and the quality of care through effective documentation and record keeping.

When the first Nursing Information Systems Conference was held at the University of Illinois in Chicago, in June 1977, the concept of information system use in nursing was in its infancy. With nurturing and development, many of the concepts envisioned at that time have become realities for nurses and nursing.

In this new edition of *Essentials of Computers for Nurses*, those historical developments are highlighted, and the advances in computer technology presented. The application sections have been updated to include many new advanced usages of computers, such as in critical paths and outcomes management. The state of the science of nursing vocabulary is presented from both national and international perspectives. This new edition, therefore, should be useful to nursing in all English-speaking countries until the book is translated into other languages.

Like all sciences, nursing information science is not complete. In this book, the authors have defined areas where further research and application studies are needed. Among these, research on the Nursing Minimum Data Set (NMDS) should figure predominantly if nurses are to contribute to the development of the computer-based health care record. The NMDS was designed to be appropriate for use in any setting where nursing care is provided. This book is designed to serve as a textbook in nursing educational programs. Its objectives will have been achieved if students come to appreciate the place of computers for nurses and identify some of the factors—economic, political, professional—that will advance the profession of nursing as nurses participate in information science.

Harriet H. Werley, Ph.D., R.N., F.A.A.N., F.A.C.M.I.
Distinguished Professor
School of Nursing
The University of Wisconsin–Milwaukee
Milwaukee, Wisconsin

# PREFACE

•••••••••••••••••••••••••••

This second edition of *Essentials of Computers for Nurses* is a comprehensive text on computer technology for nurses and other health professionals. There are so many new essentials of computers for nurses that we have selectively described only those applications that have had sustained usage in nursing. It includes issues and trends in the field—such as the electronic information superhighway, computer-based patient record, data standards and nomenclatures—as well as how the new technology is impacting on health policy.

The text provides an update of computer history as it impacts on the nursing profession. It highlights the milestones of nursing informatics and new applications in nursing practice, education, research, administration, community health, and intensive care. Information on new computer technologies that entered the market since the first edition is also covered.

In this revision, we made a concerted effort to direct students and readers to new national resources that update the state of the science. Because there are so many corporate mergers and so many new companies enter this market, we tried to instruct the readers about "where to seek current information." We omitted many of the applications and examples from the first edition; thus, this book has less chance of becoming outdated before it is printed.

The book consists of four parts. The first part provides historical perspectives of the computer and nursing. In the second part, an overview of computer hardware including microcomputers (personal computers), on-line networks, software, database management systems, and data processing provides state-of-the-art information. The third part focuses on computer systems and gives a current review of nursing and other health care systems, including a description of the status of the computer-based patient record system. Another chapter focuses on implementing systems as well as on the upgrading and reengineering of existing nursing information systems.

The fourth part focuses on computer applications in nursing administration, practice, education, and research, including computer applications in intensive care, community health, and home health. The former chapter on prospective payment has been replaced with a new chapter on the integration of guidelines, outcomes, critical paths, and benchmark or profiles into information systems. The chapter on community and home health systems highlights the Home Health Care Classification (HHCC) System. This new system is being used for assessing and documenting home health care using its unique HHCC vocabulary.

Many parts of the text have been expanded to incorporate what we currently know about the important advances in computer technology in nursing informatics internationally. We believe that this book will be especially useful to those nurses who contribute to such advancements in Australia, Belgium, Canada, Denmark, Sweden, the United Kingdom, and other countries with whom we network to share our applications in nursing informatics.

In a recent paper to the British Library, Dr. Donald Lindberg, Director, National Library of Medicine, made the statement that, by the year 2000, those health providers who are illiterate in information systems and computer technology will be likened to the reading illiterate at the turn of the twentieth century. Another futurist mentions that the information area is doubling every six months. Other futurists describe the new libraries as libraries without walls. The electronic information superhighway has been described as an "infobahn" with no speed limits. We are all entering an educational framework of lifelong learning because we can no longer learn everything we need to know for our careers in structured and "brief" formal educational programs.

The future is exciting and challenging. Students, faculty, practitioners, and other nurses who wish to avoid becoming the illiterate of the new century are invited to read this book and learn of nursing's proud contributions in nursing informatics—information science, computer science, and nursing science. We need to become articulate spokespersons of the contributions of nursing informatics to health care and of the need for nursing data, information, and knowledge in our profession.

Virginia K. Saba, R.N., Ed.D., F.A.A.N., F.A.C.M.I.
Kathleen A. McCormick, R.N., Ph.D., F.A.A.N., F.A.C.M.I.

# ACKNOWLEDGMENTS

● ● ● ● ● ● ● ● ● ● ● ● ● ● ● ● ● ● ● ● ● ● ● ● ●

This book took a great deal of effort to research, write, and compile. There are obviously many people whose contributions we wish to acknowledge. No book of this magnitude could have been completed without an editor who believed that the authors could accomplish this task. We wish to thank Gail Gavert for her patience, perseverance, and dedication to this book. The final product is an effort of the editorial team headed by Lester A. Sheinis at McGraw-Hill.

We also wish to thank Helen Foerst who reviewed numerous drafts of these chapters. Her many instructive and helpful comments and criticisms influenced the final manuscript. Barbara and Eugene Levine contributed by reading the chapters for clarity and consistency. Additionally, Nursing Informatics Experts (Judith Ronald, Dorothy Pocklington, and Mary Anne Schroeder) contributed their time by reviewing and commenting on specific topics, as well as Dr. Alan Zuckerman on the state of the art of computers.

There are several persons who contributed significantly to this edition. Kathy Milholland, who also authored Chapter 11, was prompt with her chapter and revisions when requested. Joan Burggraf Riley authored Chapter 14 and shared her innovative approach to and practical experience in teaching nursing informatics and technologies.

We are grateful to Lois Colliani and the staff of the National Library of Medicine for their comments on the Research Applications. The contributions of the National Library of Medicine to knowledge resources in health care are continuously being added to information science and are building the new library without walls in our future.

We are grateful to Andrew McLaughlin who prepared the final version using computer programs that resembled professional copyediting techniques, to Charles Morris for his graphical illustrations, and to Dolores Reinertson for the many textual tables she prepared.

To the hundreds of participants in Virginia's and Kathleen's lectures who have listened, read, and commented on parts of this book, we acknowledge their contributions.

Family and personal friends also contributed toward the production of the book. We are grateful to Dr. Faye G. Abdellah who inspired us and believed in this book from the beginning. Also, we thank our families and friends who provided emotional support.

Because of the length of time Kathleen spent in Virginia's library, there were many weekends that Francis, Sr., Francis, Jr., and Christopher McCormick went without Mom. We thank you for giving of your time so that we could complete this book.

To Christopher, especially, who was in the formative years of 3 to 7, we hope that you have learned something about the perseverance required to complete a task. To Ellen Berman, author and friend, who knows the dedication required to complete a book, we thank you for being Kathleen's backup Mom and for providing so much support.

# HISTORICAL PERSPECTIVES OF THE COMPUTER AND NURSING

# 1

• • • • • • • • • • • • • • • • • • • • • •

# HISTORICAL PERSPECTIVES OF NURSING AND COMPUTERS

## OBJECTIVES

- Describe the historical perspectives of nursing and computers.
- Describe early computer-based nursing applications in hospitals, community health agencies, education, and research.
- List the milestones of computers in nursing and nursing informatics.

The computer, a powerful technological tool, has transformed the nursing profession. Today computers are essential equipment in hospitals, community health agencies, academic institutions, research centers, and other settings where nurses function. Computers are vital tools of the nursing profession, making nursing part of the technological revolution.

Today nurses are concerned not only with computers, computer technology, and computer systems but also with nursing information systems (NISs) and nursing informatics. "Nursing informatics" has emerged as a new term to describe the use of computer technology in nursing and NISs. Nursing informatics encompasses computer technology that enables nurses to manage society's health care needs more efficiently and effectively. At the same time, it makes nurses more accountable. As in all fields of health care, efficiency, effectiveness, and accountability depend largely on how well computers are understood and used.

Computers are used to manage information in patient care, monitor the quality of care, and evaluate the nursing process. NISs are also being used to manage planning, budgeting, and policy making for nursing services. Moreover, computer applications are being used to enhance nursing education with new media modalities. Computers are providing students with computer-based literature, information, and knowledge databases. They are converting libraries into information centers without walls. Computers are also being used to support nursing research, test new systems, design new knowledge databases, and address the changing role of nursing in the health care industry.

This textbook provides an overview of what a computer is and how it functions. It describes computer applications for nursing and discusses how computers affect the nursing profession. It also discusses NISs and nursing informatics, terms that are used interchangeably here.

This chapter provides an overview of the historical perspectives of nursing and computers by describing five time periods and five nursing components. It highlights how early computer-based nursing applications in hospitals, community health agencies, ambulatory care centers, educational institutions, and research centers set the stage for today's NISs. It describes the major milestones that influenced the introduction of computers into the nursing profession.

The chapter is divided into three sections:

- Historical perspectives of nursing and computers
- Early computer-based nursing applications
- Landmark events in nursing and computers

## HISTORICAL PERSPECTIVES OF NURSING AND COMPUTERS

Computer technology was introduced into nursing in response to the need to keep the field abreast of changing and developing technologies in the health industry and in nursing practice. It can be analyzed in three ways: (1) according to five time periods: prior to the 1960s, the 1960s, the 1970s, the 1980s, and the 1990s, (2) according to four major nursing areas: nursing administration, nursing practice, nursing education, and nursing research, and (3) from the perspective of nursing standards and legislation that affected the nursing profession and its need for technology.

For nursing to enter the computer age, the profession had to review, revise, and update practice standards so that they could be implemented in computer systems; develop a variety of materials that could be computerized, such as the nursing minimum data set, standardized nursing vocabularies, and nursing care planning protocols; and design several computer instruments to support the use of the new technology. A brief discussion of the historical perspectives of nursing and computers in five time periods follows.

## Five Time Periods

### Prior to the 1960s

Beginning in the 1950s, as the computer industry grew, the use of computers in the health care industry grew. In the early days of this evolving field a few professionals formed a cadre of pioneers using computers for health care. During this period the nursing profession was expanding and undergoing major changes. The image of nursing was improving, nursing practices and services were expanding in scope and complexity, and the number of nurses was increasing. These events and initiatives created an incentive to bring computers into the profession.

Computers were initially used in hospitals and community health agencies for basic business office functions. Early computer equipment used punched cards to store data and computer programs and employed card readers and sorters to prepare the data for processing. Very early electronic computers were essentially large calculating machines that were linked together and operated by paper tape and that used teletypewriters to print their output. As the technology advanced, the equipment improved.

### 1960s

During the 1960s, as the computer began to be used in the health care setting, critical questions such as "Why computers?" and "What should be computerized?" were asked. Nursing practice standards were reviewed, and nursing resources were analyzed. Studies were conducted to determine which aspects of nursing should be automated and how computer technology could be utilized effectively in the health care industry. The hospital nursing station was viewed as the hub of communications and the most appropriate site for the development of computer applications.

During this period, computers improved and technology advanced. Health care facilities grew. The introduction of cathode ray tube (CRT) terminals, on-line data communication, and real-time processing added other essential dimensions to computer systems, making them more accessible and "user-friendly."

Hospital information systems (HISs) were developed primarily to process financial transactions and serve as billing and accounting systems. At that time a few HISs emerged that could document and process medical orders; these systems also offered selected patient and nursing care activities. Vendors were beginning to enter the field and market software applications to automate various hospital functions; however, because of the limitations of the technology, the lack of standardization, and the diversity of paper-based patient care records, progress was slow.

## 1970s

The introduction of computers into nursing was inevitable as technology advanced and nurses began to recognize the value of the computer to their profession. During this decade giant steps were taken in both dimensions: nursing and computers. Nurses began to recognize the computer's potential for improving the documentation of nursing practice and the quality of patient care. Nurses began to pioneer the use of the computer for the repetitive aspects of managing patient care. They assisted in the design and development of nursing applications for larger HISs. Nursing applications began to influence the way in which patient care in hospitals, community health agencies, and ambulatory care settings was documented. Further, nurses were instrumental in designing computer applications to support nursing education and research.

Computer applications for financial and management functions and patient care information systems were seen as cost-saving technologies. As a result, a few mainframe hospital information systems (HISs) were designed and developed, many of which became the forerunners of the HISs of today. Most of the early systems were funded by contracts or grants from federal agencies: the National Center for Health Services Research (NCHSR) and the Division of Nursing (DN), U.S. Department of Health, Education, and Welfare (National Center for Health Services Research, 1980).

During this period several state and large local health departments, visiting nurse associations (VNAs), voluntary agencies, and other community health agencies developed or contracted for their own computerized management information systems (MISs) to administer community health, public health, and home health nursing services. Generally, public health MISs provided statistical information required by local, state, and federal agencies for the allocation of program funds, whereas home health services and VNAs provided billing and other financial information needed for reimbursement for patient services by Medicare, Medicaid, and other third-party payers.

## 1980s

During the 1980s the field of informatics advanced in the health care industry and nursing. Nursing informatics became an accepted specialty, and many nursing experts entered the field. Technology challenged creative professionals. The use of computers in nursing became revolutionary. As computer systems were implemented in health care settings, the use of the "man-machine" became critical to their successful implementation. The needs of nursing took on a cause-and-effect modality. That is, as the new computer technologies emerged, computer system configurations changed and computer architecture advanced; thus the need for computer software programs for nursing had to be identified. It became apparent that the nursing profession needed to revise and update its practice standards, develop data standards, and develop taxonomies and classification schemes, including a unified language, so that the new standards could be implemented in computer-based patient record systems.

NISs emerged to document several aspects of patient records, including order/entry results reporting systems that emulated the Kardex, documentation of the nursing process, and medical and nursing orders. Vital signs systems with graphic summaries and displays emerged for critical care systems, along with narrative nursing notes that could be captured on word-processing packages. Computerized discharge planning summaries were developed and used as referrals to skilled nursing facilities, home health agencies, and ambulatory care centers. These summaries were made available to patients.

In the 1980s the introduction of the microcomputer (personal computer) made computers accessible, affordable, and usable by nurses. Microcomputers brought computing power to the workplace for practicing nurses. The introduction of user-friendly software packages allowed nurses to create their own applications. Further, microcomputers began to be used as terminals for the existing mainframe systems. This innovation made systems more usable, since microcomputers could be used not only as terminals to communicate with the mainframe computer but also for other applications in hospital units.

## 1990s

Beginning in the 1990s, technology became an integral part of health care settings, nursing practice, and the nursing profession. Several professional organizations expanded their programs and developed initiatives to address informatics. Policies and legislation were introduced to facilitate the promotion and enhancement of computer technology.

The nursing profession became actively involved in the promotion of nursing informatics. Nursing informatics was approved by the American Nurses Association (ANA) in 1992 as a nursing specialty. The demand for nursing informatics expertise increased greatly. Evidence of that growth can be found in the variety of organizations that have developed guidelines and mandated the information needed for clinical nursing practice and the quality of patient care.

Nursing issues began to emerge in several areas. Issues involving the documentation of nursing practice, including the need for computer-based nursing practice standards, data standards, nursing minimum data sets, and national databases, emerged. Another issue was the need for a unified nursing language, including nomenclatures, vocabularies, taxonomies, and classification schemes. The use of innovative technologies for all levels of nursing education also emerged. The need to enhance nursing research by identifying knowledge representation, design of decision support, and expert systems using aggregated data was still another issue.

The 1990s brought computers to the bedside and to all the settings where nurses practice. Workstations and local area networks (LANs) were developed for hospital nursing units. Information and knowledge data-bases were integrated into bedside systems. The Internet began to be used for high performance computing and communication (HPCC) "information highway" networks. The Internet also began to be used to communicate the computer-based patient record (CPR) across facilities and settings and over time. It became the means for communicating on-line services and resources to the nursing community.

By the year 2000, it is predicted that clinical information systems that integrate hospital information, patient information, and nursing informa-tion will be the information management systems (technological tools) used to process an ever-increasing amount of complex patient data. Fur-ther, clinical HISs will be individualized and become patient-specific in-formation systems that will be stored on a "smart card" and considered a patient's lifelong health record.

## Four Major Nursing Areas

The second area that addresses the historical perspectives of nursing and computers focuses on the four major nursing areas: nursing administra-tion, nursing practice, nursing education, and nursing research.

### Nursing Administration

Nursing administration in hospitals emerged with the introduction of nursing departments and the expansion of patient care services. The need for complex computations in hospital nursing service departments to determine resource requirements prompted the use of the computer. In the early 1920s studies showed that the ratio of staff nurses to patients varied greatly among hospitals (Roberts, 1954). From the 1930s through the 1960s nurse staffing was based on the ratio of patients to personnel and the number of nursing care hours needed per patient per day. These figures were determined by staffing studies that used time-and-motion methods (Aydelotte, 1973).

Nursing administrative activities in nursing departments also ad-vanced as nurses became qualified. In the 1950s federal funds became available for graduate nursing education with a major in nursing admin-istration. This led to a redefinition of the nursing administrator's role in hospital nursing departments. It also led to studies and a recognition of the need for nursing data to evaluate nursing management activities such as personnel management, nurse staffing, quality assurance, and an array of other new functions, all of which required computer-based applications.

### Nursing Practice

The need for computers in nursing arose as nursing practice increased in scope and complexity. Over 100 years ago nursing theory began with Florence Nightingale's six canons. Her *Notes on Nursing: What It Is, and*

*What It Is Not* alluded to the need for a computing device. Nightingale described the need for nurses to record manually "the proper use of fresh air, light, warmth, cleanliness, quiet, and the proper selection and administration of diet" (Nightingale, 1946, p. 6). She stated that the purpose of documenting such observations was to collect, store, and retrieve data so that patient care could be managed intelligently (Seymer, 1954).

Until the 1930s nursing notes on patient care generally focused on the medical diagnosis and medical record. In 1937 Henderson recommended that nurses write nursing care plans as a tool for planning, providing, and communicating patient care (Harmer and Henderson, 1939; Henderson, 1964). By 1960, a century after Florence Nightingale wrote on the six canons of nursing, assessment of nursing practice had become part of the patient's record. Three schemes were available for documenting patient care: "21 nursing problems" for assessing patient needs developed by Abdellah and associates (1960), "14 major activities" for categorizing nursing care identified by Henderson (1964), and Orem's "7 components" of universal self-care (1971).

Between the 1960s and the 1970s, as early computer systems were being developed, "studies of the nursing unit" were conducted to determine which aspects of nursing should be computerized in a hospital setting. Nursing practice standards were reviewed. Nursing resources were analyzed, and studies were conducted to determine how computer technology could be utilized effectively. Similar studies were conducted outside hospitals.

Beginning in the 1970s, as computer technology became part of the profession, many changes occurred in nursing practice. Nurses developed theories, methods, and frameworks to assess patients' needs, determine care requirements, and document plans of care. As professional nursing became a science, clinical practice standards changed and several nursing classification schemes (vocabularies) were developed that documented nursing practice in different health care settings.

In 1973 the initial list of nursing diagnoses was developed. This list of "37 nursing diagnoses" was critical for assessing health conditions that required nursing interventions (Gebbie, 1975). The list of nursing diagnosis labels was expanded to "50 nursing diagnoses" in 1982 and to "114 diagnostic categories" in 1992 (Kim et al., 1984; North American Nursing Diagnosis Associations, 1992).

In 1976 a list of 49 nursing problems was developed to describe conditions addressed by community health nurses. The Community Health Nursing Problem Scheme was revised, expanded, and finalized in 1986. The resulting product is now called the Omaha System and currently consists of "44 Client Problems" and "63 Intervention Labels" (Martin and Sheets, 1992; Visiting Nurse Association of Omaha, 1986).

In 1991 the Saba Home Health Care Classification (HHCC) (Nursing Diagnoses and Interventions) was developed to document nursing processes in home health care. This HHCC is structured and organized according to "20 Home Health Components" and currently consists of two schemes: HHCC of Nursing Diagnoses, which consists of "145 Home Health Nursing Diagnoses" with "3 Expected Outcomes/Goals" that are used as modifiers, and the HHCC of Nursing Interventions, which currently consists of "160 Home Health Nursing Interventions" with "4 Types of Intervention Actions" that are used as modifiers (Saba, 1992).

In 1992 another scheme for documenting nursing practice in hospitals was introduced: the Nursing Intervention Classification (NIC). It currently consists of "336 nursing intervention labels" with definitions and related activities (McCloskey and Bulechek, 1992).

In 1993 the International Council of Nurses (ICN) introduced the International Classification of Nursing Practice (ICNP). It consists of three alphabetized lists of existing labels or nomenclatures for (1) nursing diagnoses/problems, (2) nursing interventions, and (3) outcomes. The nomenclatures were collected from the United States, Canada, and several European countries (International Council of Nurses, 1993).

All of these systems are continually being expanded and updated. New terms are being added and deleted.

### Nursing Education

Nursing education began to use computers as educational programs developed and grew. Formal education was suggested by Florence Nightingale, and her concepts have influenced nursing education over the years (Nightingale, 1946). In the early 1900s, as the number of hospitals increased, schools of nursing were established in hospitals. Training nursing students in hospitals was viewed as an economical way of staffing hospitals. The students cared for the sick under a physician's supervision (Lysault, 1973).

During and after the 1950s, federal funds supported the introduction of new types of educational nursing programs. Two-year community college and junior college programs were introduced, replacing many hospital schools of nursing (Montag, 1954). Graduate programs were initiated, making it possible for nurses to obtain master's and doctoral degrees with a specialization in education, research, administration, supervision, or advanced clinical practice.

Like other major areas of the nursing profession, nursing education began to use computers as educational programs advanced and grew. As schools of nursing expanded and the number of student nurses increased, there was an urgent need for computers to assist in the management of schools and student records. In addition, there was a need to use computer technology to assist students in the educational process. Thus, in nursing education the computer has become an essential tool that supports both the management and the teaching of students.

## Nursing Research

Nursing research also provided the impetus to use the computer to analyze nursing data. Statistical analyses were first performed by Florence Nightingale, who was involved not only in nursing education and practice but also in nursing statistics and health services research (Werley, 1981). Nightingale manually collected and analyzed pertinent information because she recognized the need for solid nursing data to improve the health care delivery system of her day.

The emphasis on nursing research did not advance until 1955, when the Public Health Service Act was passed. That legislation provided funds for nursing research through grants to educational and health care institutions and individuals. As a result of federal funding, nurses started to conduct research to investigate nursing problems. Research began to be conducted to improve nursing practice, determine the supply and requirements of nurses, highlight staffing needs, develop educational standards, and determine the direction of nursing education (Gortner and Nahm, 1977; Vreeland, 1964).

The use of computers for processing nursing research study data allowed new correlations and interpretations to be made. The information derived from computer processing of research data led to changes in the practice of nursing. As computer technology advanced, the time needed for processing research and survey data decreased and analytic techniques improved, resulting in more reliable and usable findings.

Databases to support nursing research also emerged, including bibliographic retrieval systems for nursing literature and other literature that contained relevant content, such as drug data. Further, plans for an electronic library were developed to employ technological advances in information management and the communication of electronic databases.

## Nursing Standards and Legislation

The third perspective that is significant is that of nursing standards and legislation. These two areas have affected the nursing profession and its need for technology.

### Nursing Standards

In 1951 the standards for nursing practice imposed by hospital organizations were formalized when the Joint Commission on Accreditation of Hospitals (JCAH) was established. The JCAH stressed the need for adequate records on patients in hospitals and set standards for the documentation of medical records by nurses (Namdi and Hutelmyer, 1970).

Between the 1960s and the 1970s hospital staffing began to change as nursing practice models were introduced. Different types of staffing studies were conducted, using innovative engineering methods that focused on four major techniques: (1) time and task frequency, (2) work sampling, (3) observation, and (4) self-reporting of nursing activities. These studies produced patient classification/acuity methods as a means of determining staffing requirements that were based on resource use instead of the ratio of beds to staff members. Generally, they characterized a patient in terms of acuity of illness or ability for self-care. Other studies were conducted that attempted to measure the quality and outcome of care. Tools were developed, such as questionnaires, that measured the degree of patient satisfaction. Several of these new methods were computerized.

***JCAH Nursing Standards*** In the 1970s the JCAH, which considered nursing notes to be legal documents, recommended that the nursing process be used as the framework for documenting nursing care (Joint Commission on Accreditation of Hospitals, 1970). Thus, in the 1980s computer systems emerged that were designed to improve the efficiency of patient care and the accuracy of resource use. Even though these systems varied, they streamlined the process and met the JCAH accreditation standards.

In 1981 the JCAH also recommended that hospitals classify patients by using a reliable method for allocating nursing staffing that was more equitable than the traditional ratio of nurses to patients. The need for the computer became apparent as the requirements for nursing resources became more complex and the volume of data increased. The computer was needed to process acuity schemes, analyze workload data, and measure quality indicators. As a result, many computerized patient classification/acuity instruments were developed that measured nursing care to determine nursing resources (Alward, 1983; Joint Commission on Accreditation of Hospitals, 1981).

In 1990 the Joint Commission on Accreditation of Health Care Organizations (JCAHO) advocated the continuation of acuity systems to determine resource use as well as plans for documenting nursing care (Joint Commission on Accreditation of Health Care Organizations, 1994). The commission also initiated a major effort to redesign the JCAHO accreditation process. As a result, the 1994 JCAHO *Accreditation Manual for Hospitals* contains many changes. It includes a new chapter, "The Management of Information," that addresses information management processes for meeting the needs of a health care facility. The new standards outline what a patient record should contain, what data should be collected, and how the information in the database should be organized (Corum, 1993). It also includes standards for assessing quality of care to address not only "what is done" but also "how it is done." These new standards are affecting the systems that are used and the way data are collected.

***ANA Nursing Practice and Data Standards*** The ANA also has been involved in establishing nursing "practice" standards. In 1980 the ANA defined the nature and scope of nursing practice in *Nursing: A Social*

*Policy Statement*, using the nursing process as a framework. The ANA also recommended the development of a patient classification/acuity system for nurse staffing (American Nurses Association, 1980).

In 1982 the ANA formed the Steering Committee on Classification of Nursing Practice, which began to develop strategies to identify and classify the phenomena of nursing practice. In 1991 the ANA revised its *Standards for Clinical Nursing Practice*, using the nursing process as its conceptual framework (American Nurses Association, 1991).

In 1989 the ANA assumed the responsibility for developing nursing databases to measure and describe the cost and quality of nursing services. This activity was assigned to the ANA Cabinet on Nursing Practice, which in 1990 formed the ANA Steering Committee on Databases to Support Nursing Practice to carry out this charge. This committee was mandated to (1) support activities related to nursing classification schemes, uniform data elements, data sets, and databases, (2) develop standardized national data sets for clinical nursing practice, and (3) coordinate efforts related to the development of computer-based databases for nursing practice standards, data standards, and payment reform.

In 1990 the ANA House of Delegates recognized the nursing minimum data set (NMDS) as the minimum data elements that should be included in any paper-based or computer-based patient record. The NMDS became the umbrella for four classification schemes that the committee "recognized" in 1992. The committee determined that the four schemes not only were the most complete and mature classification systems available for nursing practice but also met its criteria for a unified nursing language system (UNLS). The schemes include (1) North American Nursing Diagnosis Association (NANDA), Taxonomy I of Nursing Diagnoses, (2) Visiting Nurse Association of Omaha, Community Health Problem and Intervention System, (3) Saba, HHCC (Nursing Diagnoses and Interventions), and (4) University of Iowa, Nursing Interventions Classification (NIC) (Lang et al., in press). These schemes are described in Chap. 7.

## Legislative Influences

At the federal level, several pieces of legislation have been enacted during the past 50 years that have significantly influenced the introduction of the computer into nursing. These acts stimulated the growth and advancement of the nursing profession. Computer technology developed and supported this growth and development through the development of nursing information systems, the measurement of quality of care, and reimbursement for patient care services. Other legislation has also influenced this trend. The following acts are probably the most significant.

The initial **Nurse Training Act of 1943** (PL 74-78) established the U.S. Cadet Nurse Corps. Enactment was delegated to the United States Public Health Service (US PHS) and was designed to ensure an adequate supply of nurses during World War II not only for the military but also for civilian hospitals on the home front. This legislation began the trend toward expanding schools of nursing and increasing the number of nurses.

The **Health Amendments Act of 1956** (PL-911) established trainee-ships for professional nurses. Title II of this act provided additional funds for professional nurses, including public health nurses, to obtain graduate education (advanced training) in the areas of teaching, administration, and supervision. The act increased the supply and expanded the managerial skills of nurse administrators and supervisors. It also increased the number of graduate programs in schools of nursing and the supply of graduate nurses.

The **Nurse Training Act of 1964** (PL 88-581), Title VIII Nurse Training Amendment to the Public Health Service Act, was also responsible for an increase in the number of schools of nursing and the number of nurses. This legislation, administered by the Division of Nursing, US PHS, Department of Health and Human Services (DHHS), was funded for 3-year intervals, has been periodically revised, and is still enacted by Congress (its most recent passage was in 1992). It provided extensive financial support to both institutions and students for nursing education. It also mandated various projects for determining requirements and projecting the supply of nurses.

The **Social Security Amendments of 1965, Medicare and Medicaid** (PL 89-97), were enacted to improve and increase health services to the aged and indigent. These amendments provided reimbursement for the cost of health care services for eligible persons over age 65 and for certain low-income persons. This legislation promoted the development of community and home health information systems to document care in order to provide the data needed for reimbursement for services and health care.

Another important piece of legislation was the **Quality Assurance Program of 1972** (PL 92-603), which established Professional Standards Review Organizations (PSROs) to evaluate and monitor health care. The first step in implementing this legislation was the collection and analysis of data on quality of care.

The **National Health Planning and Resources Development Act of 1974** (PL 93-641) established health planning agencies throughout the nation with authorization to establish planning methods and criteria. It mandated the creation of the National Health Planning Information Center (NHPIC), which contained a nursing component (Saba and Skapik, 1979). NHPIC housed a reference collection and a computerized database with literature on health planning methodologies and health resources, including personnel, facility, and cost studies. The NHPIC database is now part of the MEDLARS (**Med**ical **L**iterature and **A**nalysis **R**etrieval **S**ystem) as the Health Planning and Admin (Health Planning and Administration) on-line database.

In 1974 the **Health Services Research, Health Statistics, and Medical Libraries Act** (PL 93-353) was passed. This law mandated that the National Center for Health Services Research (NCHSR) undertake research activities covering all aspects of health services in this country. NCHSR supported numerous grants and contracts that focused on technological solutions to the health care problems facing the nation. Its program initiated projects that used computer technology to develop innovations in health care systems. Several projects have focused on the development of computer-based information systems to support the needs not only of health care administrators but also of the providers of patient care.

In 1983 the passage of the **Social Security Amendments** (PL 98-21) mandated under Medicare Part A a prospective payment system (PPS) commonly known as diagnosis related groups (DRGs). This system replaced the retrospective cost-based reimbursement system. This new system of payment for in-hospital Medicare and Medicaid patient services was based on 467 DRGs. PPS required that patients' diagnoses and charges for services, including nursing, be integrated with medical record data for billing, general ledger, and cost accounting purposes. Such integration required a cost accounting computer system.

The **Omnibus Budget Reconciliation Act of 1987** (PL 100-203) contained many provisions that affected the Medicare program. This law mandated that plans of care be included as part of the clinical record. The **Omnibus Budget Reconciliation Act of 1989** (PL 101-239) required that the Department of Health and Human Services (HHS) conduct research on the outcomes of health care services and procedures. As a result of this act, in December 1989, the NCHSR was renamed and reestablished as the Agency for Health Care Policy and Research (AHCPR).

AHCPR is the organization in the federal government that is the focal point for research on medical effectiveness and health services. The purpose of the agency is to enhance the quality, appropriateness, and effectiveness of health care services and improve access to that care. The agency is mandated not only to carry out its original activities but also to develop standards for clinical databases, clinical practice guidelines, and quality outcomes in order to improve the quality, appropriateness, and effectiveness of health care services through a broad program of scientific research and information dissemination (Agency for Health Care Policy and Research, 1990, 1992).

The **Health Security Act of 1993,** which was proposed but not passed, was intended to simplify and streamline the health care system and lower costs by using technology to free doctors and nurses from paperwork. It recommended a single standardized reimbursement claims form that could be completed in a computer and transmitted automatically on high-speed computer and communication network highways. The 1993 Agenda for Health Care Reform proposed new methods for monitoring quality and tracking health care that required a variety of analytic and data collection skills that would be facilitated by the computer (White House Domestic Policy Council, 1993).

Other relevant legislation has been passed by Congress to improve health care and health services. All these laws require accurate data collection and analysis, making the computer an essential tool for their implementation. The relevant legislation that has influenced computer use in nursing is listed in Table 1.1.

### Historical Summary

Changes in the nursing profession since Florence Nightingale's time have dealt primarily with redefining nursing practice, managing nursing services, advancing nursing education, and planning nursing research. Expansion in all health fields made it necessary for nurses to study and use technological advances that affect the delivery of care. The computer is the only tool that can manage the complexity and volume of the data being collected to implement such change.

Computers emerged during the last four decades in the health care industry. Hospitals began to use computers to update paper-based patient records. Computer systems in health care settings provided the information management capabilities needed to assess, document, process, and communicate patient care. As a result, the "man-machine" interaction of nursing and computers became a new and lasting symbiotic relationship (Blum, 1990; Collen, 1994; Kemeny, 1972).

**TABLE 1.1**     LEGISLATION THAT INFLUENCED COMPUTER USE IN NURSING

| Legislation and Year | Public Law |
| --- | --- |
| Nurse Training Act of 1943 | 78–74 |
| Health Amendments Act of 1956 | 84–911 |
| Nurse Training Act of 1964 | 88–581 |
| Social Security Amendments of 1965<br>Medicare and Medicaid | 89–97 |
| Quality Assurance Program of 1972<br>Professional Standards Review Organizations (PSROs) | 92–603 |
| National Health Planning and Resources Devemopment Act of 1974 | 93–641 |
| Health Services Research, Health Statistics, and Medical Libraries Act of 1974 | 93–353 |
| Social Security Amendments of 1983<br>Prospective Payment System (PPS) and Diagnosis Related Groups (DRGs) | 98–21 |
| Omnibus Budget Reconciliation Act of 1987 | 100–203 |
| Omnibus Budget Reconciliation Act of 1989 | 101–239 |
| High Performance Computing Act of 1991 | 102–194 |
| Health Security Act of 1993 | Not adopted |

# EARLY COMPUTER-BASED NURSING APPLICATIONS

Several computer-based nursing applications were developed before the mid-1970s as part of larger HISs, and many of them still exist. Each in its own way developed different nursing applications to improve the documentation of nursing practice and manage patient care. The applications were designed for hospitals, ambulatory care settings, and community health agencies. Additionally, several significant nursing projects were conducted to improve nursing care documentation methodologies that in turn could be computerized. The major nursing applications that influenced the industry are subsystems or components of early HISs, ambulatory care systems, and community health systems that are described below. Special projects that influenced the design of nursing information systems are also highlighted:

- Early hospital information systems
- Early ambulatory care information systems
- Early community health nursing information management systems
- Early computer-focused nursing projects

## Early Hospital Information Systems

Early HISs were designed for mainframe computers that could support hundreds of CRTs in nursing units and other departments where data were entered and/or received. The CRTs were primarily dumb terminals through which data were input either on a keyboard or via a video screen activated by a light pen. Many of these systems were developed and tested on one nursing unit before being implemented throughout a hospital, revised, or discontinued.

### Technicon Medical Information System

In 1973 the Technicon Medical Information System (TMIS), now called TDS by the Health Care Systems Corp., was developed at El Camino Hospital in Mountain View, California. TMIS is considered the oldest hospital/patient information system. In 1965 this hospitalwide computer system was initiated by the Lockheed Missiles and Space Company to make its communication technology available to hospitals (Hodge, 1990).

The original TMIS managed all patient information during a hospital stay. It consisted of nursing care protocols generated from patients' medical diagnoses and predicted outcome measures that were used as guides to record patients' problems and care plans. Thousands of nursing care protocols were developed for the original system. This system was housed in a mainframe computer that supported a large number of CRTs on the nursing units. The CRTs were dumb terminals that could be activated by a light pen and were connected to the mainframe (Cook and Mayers, 1981; Cook and McDowell, 1975; Mayers, 1974).

In 1975 the TMIS was installed at the Clinical Center of the National Institutes of Health (NIH) in Bethesda, Maryland, where patient care functions were expanded to encompass extensive research protocols. The nursing care protocols were revised and designed to document plans of care by using the nursing process and nursing diagnosis. The NIH nursing care planning information system follows the nursing process by using 13 patient care needs based on Maslow's hierarchy of needs to assess patients. It then identifies the appropriate diagnoses that nurses are licensed to treat. The nursing diagnoses are further divided into expected outcomes and nursing actions with data points to determine the progress or point of expected achievement (McNeely, 1983; Romano et al., 1982).

The current TDS, now almost 29 years old, still has one of the most advanced user functions at the nurses' station. Recently, the system has been revised and its hardware architecture and software have been upgraded. For example, at NIH, the original CRTs have been upgraded to "mouse"-activated microcomputers with video screens that are more user-friendly.

### Burroughs/Medi-Data HIS
Another early hospital information system was the Burroughs/Medi-Data HIS which was developed in the 1970s at Charlotte Memorial Hospital in Charlotte, North Carolina. This system was designed to provide more accurate information, faster communication, and standardized patient care documentation. The initial system consisted of the diagnosis and other pertinent information on a patient, and a care plan containing physicians' and nurses' orders. The nursing portion of the system consisted of a database of 200 symptoms or conditions requiring nursing action, called "initiators of care," that were activated through a CRT. As a result, it became possible to devise a standardized care plan to document patient care. The computer system generated summary reports and care plans for each shift (Smith, 1974; Somers, 1971).

### Problem-Oriented Medical Information System
The Problem-Oriented Medical Information System (PROMIS) was in the forefront of patient care data handling. PROMIS was in development at the Medical Center Hospital of Vermont in Burlington, Vermont, as early as 1968. Its goal was to create a computerized problem-oriented medical record (POMR) (Weed, 1969). The major purpose was to establish a system that collected, stored, and processed all relevant medical information on a patient and provided feedback to providers of care as a means of evaluating the care given. PROMIS incorporated the four phases of medical care: collection of information (database), development of a problem list, development of a plan of action, and follow-up for each problem (progress notes) (Giebnik and Hurst, 1975; Lindberg, 1977).

PROMIS also incorporated video displays for nursing, called "frames," that consisted of nursing care protocols for a patient's specific disease or medical condition. The frames helped nurses formulate SOAP plans for patient care (subjective symptoms, objective signs, assessment, and plans) on the CRTs, which were activated with a light pen. Thus, a computerized method of planning and documenting patient care using the POMR structure with SOAP notes was developed (Gane, 1972; McNeill, 1979; Pryor et al., 1985). PROMIS was developed and tested for nearly 4 years on a gynecology ward and for 6 months on a medical ward. It was then redesigned and used on a medical ward for approximately 3 years. However, federal funding was halted in 1981–1982, and the research on and development of the PROMIS system ceased. It has reappeared in new concepts of knowledge coupling (Weed, 1991).

## Health Evaluation Logical Processing System

The Health Evaluation Logical Processing (HELP) System developed at the Latter-Day Saints Hospital in Salt Lake City, Utah, is another system that originated in the late 1960s. It was under development for over 20 years. The basic goal was to create an integrated computer-based patient care record system and a knowledge base. HELP was designed to meet the medical, clinical, administrative, decision-making, teaching, and research goals of the hospital. To achieve those goals, a large number of sets of applications for data acquisition and decision support logic in clinical environments focusing on critical and/or intensive care were developed. Nursing was involved in its order/entry results review applications (Pryor, 1992).

## Decentralized Hospital Computer Program

Another pioneer in the field of hospital information systems was the Department of Veterans Affairs. In the 1970s the Veterans Administration (VA) began to develop a clinical computing system known as the Decentralized Hospital Computer Program (DHCP). The VA developed the system over the course of a decade, and it was implemented in more than 170 medical centers by the late 1980s. The VA's DHCP consists of three modules that focus on (1) system/database management, (2) administrative management, and (3) clinical management. As part of the clinical management module, the VA launched the Clinical Record Project, which includes a nursing subsystem. The VA is still committed to developing its own state-of-the-art system (Andrews and Beauchamp, 1989; Dayhoff et al., 1990).

## Tri-Service Medical Information System

The U.S. Department of Defense (DOD) began contracting for the development of a clinical information system in the mid-1970s. The system, which originally was known as the Tri-Service Medical Information System (TRIMIS) and is now called the Composite Health Care System (CHCS), has taken over a decade to design, develop, and be implemented. In the mid-1980s TRIMIS completed the design specifications; however, when the contract was awarded, it had been reorganized as CHCS. In the early 1990s the system began to be tested in military health care facilities and settings around the country (Committee on Armed Services, 1990).

The design of the system required that multiple task forces be assembled to develop its specifications, including a group for the design of the nursing activities. In September 1982, the Tri-Service Nursing Requirements Committee was appointed to explore computer support for nursing activities for the system. The specific task identified by the committee was the design requirements for nursing management and hospital nursing records, with the goal of improved patient care. The result was a nursing information system that identified the design specifications for nursing patient care and unit management as well as the nursing administration of inpatient, outpatient, and operating room areas (Rieder and Norton, 1984).

## Other Early Hospital Information Systems

Several other early systems were developed to capture nursing data. The **Texas Institute for Rehabilitation and Research**, Houston, hospital data management system focused on the individual patient care process and used CRTs connected to the hospital's computer (Cornell and Carrick, 1973; Giebnik and Hurst, 1975; Valbona and Spencer, 1974). The **Institute of Living** in Hartford, Connecticut, developed the first real-time computerized psychiatric information system designed to facilitate patient care (Lindberg, 1977). The system provided an integrated patient record that included nurses' progress notes and other pertinent information.

## Early Ambulatory Care Information Systems

### Computer-Stored Ambulatory Record System

The earliest computerized ambulatory care information system was the Computer-Stored Ambulatory Record system (COSTAR). It was developed between 1968 and 1978 at Massachusetts General Hospital's (MGH) Laboratory of Computer Science for ambulatory patients served by the prepaid Harvard Community Health Plan. The purpose of COSTAR was to computerize medical records so that patient care encounter data could be integrated to meet providers' medical, financial, and administrative needs. The initial system used precoded encounter forms that all health care providers, including nurses, had to complete manually and that were later keyed into the computer in batches. A standardized dictionary was developed to provide uniform documentation. The system provided selected portions of the patient's medical record, producing various quality controls essential for patient management (Barnett, 1976).

COSTAR was upgraded to be an on-line system allowing interaction between the users (nurses) and a mainframe computer at MGH's com-

---

puter laboratory. The on-line system allowed retrieval of patient information via the CRT. COSTAR is still available and has been adapted to run
on minicomputers and/or microcomputers.

## The Medical Record System

The Medical Record (TMR) System began in 1968 at Duke University
Medical Center's Department of Community Health Services in Durham,
North Carolina. The goal was to replace paper charts with computerized
records for the practicing physician. TMR initially focused on capturing
patient histories and physical examinations in a prenatal clinic. It was
later designed to meet the needs of ambulatory care practice and the clinical requirement for a primary care record. TMR was finally designed to
cover all the activities of an HIS in order to satisfy managerial, patient
care, and research needs in inpatient and outpatient settings. It was
designed to permit nurses and other health care providers to enter data
directly into the database during the process of patient care (Pryor, 1992).

## Indian Health Service System

Another pioneering system was the Indian Health Service System designed
by the Bell Aerospace Company for the Papagoe Indian reservation in
Tucson, Arizona. This system was designed to provide centralized lifelong
surveillance and document and communicate the health care services,
status, and conditions of all Papagoe reservation residents who received
health care services. It provided a centralized database that contained
medical summaries and information on patients, including all health care
services received (inpatient, outpatient, and community health nursing).
All health care providers, including nurses, use a computer terminal to
access patient files. For example, through the use of an on-line terminal in
the office or car, a community health nurse can obtain the latest health
care information before visiting a patient in the home. This system still
exists, but the software continues to be revised and the hardware upgraded (Brown et al., 1971; Giebnik and Hurst, 1975.)

# Early Community Health Nursing
# Information Management Systems

## Statewide Systems

One of this nation's first statewide computer-based community health
information systems was begun in 1970 by the New Jersey State Department of Health. This agency developed, tested, and implemented a home
health management information system for community nursing service
agencies. The major goals of the system were to (1) help community health
care agencies make more effective use of their limited resources,
(2) reduce the difficulty of providing information to organizations, and (3)
find improved data handling methods for those agencies. The system con-

sisted of precoded paper forms that were batch processed by computer, producing reports designed to facilitate state reporting requirements and assist community health nursing directors in managing their agencies. Because the processing of forms was slow, tedious, and costly and could not be done on-line, the system was abandoned in the late 1970s (Saba and Levine, 1981).

In 1973 another statewide system, the Nursing Information System for Public Health Nursing, was initiated by the Florida Department of Health and Rehabilitative Services. The goal was to produce accurate, timely, and comprehensive information about the work performed by public health nurses. The system was designed to create a statistical database that could provide information to improve management, report costs, and justify public health activities. The system went through several revisions, beginning with a batch-processing paper system and moving to an on-line transmission of data that is still used today.

## Early Computer-Focused Nursing Projects

Several computer-focused nursing projects and other activities were funded by the Division of Nursing (DN), U.S. Public Health Service (PHS), Department of Health, Education, and Welfare (DHEW) to help community health nursing agencies develop computer-based information systems. Each of these projects advanced the documentation requirements for the different health care settings and influenced the development of today's systems (Saba, 1981b, 1982).

### Community Health Nursing Projects

In 1971 the **Rockland County Project** was conducted by the Rockland County Health Department in New York. It attempted to computerize patients' progress by using innovative methodology designed for the public health setting. The project represented one of the first attempts to computerize care in that setting (Rockland County Health Department, 1971).

The **Buffalo Project** constituted another attempt to computerize patient care needs. The project, "Systematic Nursing Assessment," attempted to develop a standardized tool that could be computerized to assist nurses in their assessment of patients' needs and then be used for making decisions about patient care. The project was conducted by the State University of New York at Buffalo's School of Nursing (Taylor and Johnson, 1974).

In the early 1970s the **Philadelphia Project** attempted to develop a system that could be used to plan and evaluate community health nursing (CHN) services. It was conducted by a VNA (Community Nursing Services of Philadelphia, 1976).

Another **CHN Project** was initiated in 1975 to develop a problem classification scheme for community health/public health nursing by the

VNA of Omaha, Nebraska. Its goal was to design a system for document-ing nursing services and develop a methodology for computerization. The project produced a problem classification scheme consisting of 49 problem labels categorized into four domains that were potentially amenable to nursing interventions. Each problem was identified by a cluster of signs and symptoms. The project was continued over the next 18 years and is still in operation (Simmons, 1982; Visiting Nurse Association of Omaha, 1986).

### Hospital Nursing Projects

In 1977 another project was initiated by the DN, PHS to determine the **Effects of the Computerized Problem-Oriented Record** (COPR) on the nursing components of patient care. This project was conducted by the Department of Nursing of the Medical Center Hospital of Vermont in Burlington. It identified the differences in recording nursing care under the computerized system and under the manual problem-oriented system. No conclusions, however, could be drawn because of the inadequate length of time during which the system was operational. Nevertheless, the project's three data collection instruments—record review, time sampling, and nurse satisfaction—were used by other researchers to evaluate other hos-pital information systems (Hanchett, 1981).

## Educational Applications

During the 1960s special-purpose computerized information systems were developed in educational institutions. Computer-based education (CBE), which encompassed computer-assisted instruction (CAI) and computer-managed instruction (CMI), became popular on college campuses. Systems were designed to computerize and individualize student instruction while serving a large number of students simultaneously on-line in a classroom.

   **Programmed Logic for Automatic Teaching Operation** (PLATO) was the first on-line CBE system to be developed. It was designed so that students could use a CRT to interact with the computer in the classroom. Many nursing courses were adapted for PLATO, which became an excel-lent tool for teaching drill and practice courses. PLATO individualized the learning process, provided instant feedback on student progress, and tracked student progress for the faculty (Bitzer and Boudreaux, 1968).

   In the 1980s, as the technology advanced and with the introduction of the microcomputer, CAI programs were developed as applications for indi-vidual microcomputers. They were less expensive and easier to imple-ment. Schools of nursing could purchase their own CAI programs and did not have to subscribe to an on-line transmission service. As a result, PLATO was no longer in demand, and CAI and interactive video (IV) pro-grams emerged as stand-alone microcomputer applications. CBE materi-als continued to be developed, and their use affected nursing education.

## Research Applications

The earliest computer system designed to support nursing research was the development in the late 1950s and early 1960s of the computerized document retrieval system MEDLARS by the National Library of Medicine (NLM).

In 1972, MEDLARS was advanced to an on-line system and MEDLINE became the first of several MEDLARS databases to become available on-line nationwide. As a result, on-line computerized searches of the medical and nursing literature became possible (National Library of Medicine, 1986). MEDLARS used the computer to index the medical literature and produce *Index Medicus*. In 1965 "Special List Nursing," a special file in the MEDLARS database, was established. This file indexed the nursing periodical literature and prepared the *International Nursing Index* for publication by the American Journal of Nursing Company (American Journal of Nursing, 1992; Saba, 1981a).

During this period several other indexes of relevant nursing literature were computerized as bibliographic retrieval systems. The major ones include the Cumulative Index to Nursing and Allied Health Literature (CINAHL) developed by the Seventh-Day Adventist Association in Glendale, California; the Educational Resources Information Center (ERIC) of nursing education literature; the SOCIAL SCI for the Social SciSearch Citation Index; and Dissertation Abstracts (Saba et al., 1989).

During the late 1980s and early 1990s researchers began to gain access to on-line "public use" federal databases consisting of aggregated data. Databases such as the Health Care Financing Administration (HCFA) database, the Medicare and Medicaid claims database, and the Uniform Clinical Data Set (UCDS) became available. Even though nursing information was not an integral part of these databases, some inferences on nursing care could be made from other patient data contained in them. Knowledge databases that focused on a specific topic or disease condition were developed and could be remotely accessed on-line, such as a drug database, a clinical condition cancer database, such as the PDQ (Physician Data Query), and diagnostic and clinical care protocol database systems such as DxPlain and RECONSIDER.

In the 1980s other computer applications for conducting research were introduced as the technology advanced. The Sigma Theta Tau International Honor Society of Nursing planned and developed an electronic library to provide on-line access to nursing information and research literature. In the 1990s several other on-line electronic databases were created by nursing organizations, such as AJN Network, ANA*NET, and E.T. NET (Saba, 1995).

During that time several statistical software computer packages, such as SAS (Statistical Analysis System) and SPSS (Statistical Package for the Social Sciences), became available for research applications; these packages could statistically process and analyze data on a mainframe, minicomputer, or microcomputer. Several packages also became available for the personal computer (PC), using the Microsoft Windows operating system, which not only provided a graphic interface but were user-friendly.

## LANDMARK EVENTS IN NURSING AND COMPUTERS

Computers were introduced into the nursing profession over 30 years ago. The major milestones of nursing are interwoven with the advancement of computer technology, the increased need for nursing data, the development of nursing applications, and changes that made the nursing profession an autonomous discipline. The major developments in the use of computers and nursing and in the introduction of nursing informatics are described below chronologically, by program effort, or by organizational initiative. The major efforts are categorized as follows and outlined in Table 1.3 (pp. 38–41):

- Early conferences
- Special-interest and working groups
- Academic events
- American Nurses Association initiatives
- National League for Nursing initiatives
- International events
- Educational resources
- Collaborative events

### Early Conferences

Early conferences on computers and nursing were conducted as computerized systems were introduced into the health care industry. These conferences were designed to teach nurses about computer systems and computer data. They were conducted so that nurses could learn about state-of-the-art nursing information systems.

#### Invitational Conferences
In 1973 the first invitational conference was held on computerized management information systems (MISs) for public health/community health agencies (PH/CHAs). It was designed to help agency administrators address their reporting requirements for reimbursement for Medicare and Medicaid home health services. This initial national conference was followed by five workshops held around the country, culminating in a state-of-the-art national conference in 1976. The workshops and conferences were designed to teach public and community health nurses how to investigate, initiate, and implement computerized MISs. The workshops yielded

guidelines and demonstrated how computer systems could be used for statistical reporting, cost analysis, and agency administration. This effort was funded by the Division of Nursing, US PHS, DHEW under the auspices of the National League for Nursing (NLN) (National League for Nursing, 1974, 1975, 1976, 1978).

In 1977 the first Invitational Research Conference focused on state-of-the-art NISs and the use of computer technology in the delivery of patient care. This conference highlighted computer applications in documenting all aspects of nursing care, including care plans, elements of the nursing process, and nursing notes. It provided current information on computer applications that were being developed not only in hospitals but also in other health care settings. This conference was sponsored by the University of Illinois's College of Nursing in Chicago (Werley and Grier, 1981).

The first computer conference for military nurses was held in 1979. A TRIMIS conference was held to introduce military nurses to the emerging role of computers in health care and nursing. It was conducted by the TRIMIS Army Nurse Consultant Team at Walter Reed Hospital in Washington, D.C. The Army Nurse Corps was committed to educating nurses about computers and conducted several workshops in the United States and abroad on this topic. The most recent was held in 1993, when the Army Nurse Corps conducted the Postgraduate Short Course on Computer Applications in Nursing.

As interest in computers increased, the first NIH National Nursing Conference was conducted in 1981. It is considered a critical event in the field. It was a 1-day conference that focused on state-of-the-art computers and nursing and was attended by more than 700 nurse administrators, practitioners, clinicians, researchers, and educators. The Nursing Department of the Clinical Center, NIH, hosted this conference in collaboration with the Division of Nursing of the US PHS and the Army Nurse TRIMIS–ARMY Nurse Consultant team. The NIH conference held a second National Nursing Conference on Computers in 1982 and a third in 1984 (National Institutes of Health, 1983, 1984).

### SCAMC

A focus on nursing was introduced in the Annual Symposium on Computer Applications in Medical Care (SCAMC) at the fifth symposium in 1981. Papers that dealt with nursing information systems and the nursing aspects of computer technology were presented in four nursing sessions by pioneers in the field. The symposium offered technical sessions, demonstrations, workshops, tutorials, hands-on experience, poster sessions, and exhibits of systems for the health care industry. SCAMC gave nurses an opportunity to learn how computer applications could affect patient care (Heffernan, 1981).

SCAMC, now sponsored by the American Medical Informatics Association (AMIA), continues to include nursing papers, presentations, and sessions in its annual SCAMC symposia, which are still conducted. SCAMC continues to offer nursing tutorials and workshops for novice and advanced nursing informaticians.

## Special-Interest and Working Groups

In 1981 the first special interest group, Computers in Nursing (SIG-CIN), was formed. It convened at the fifth annual SCAMC to hold the first nursing sessions and became an informal group that met at annual SCAMC meetings. The group had an executive board, published an annual newsletter, and provided mailing lists of members for local groups. The SIG-CIN was responsible for designing the nursing tract for SCMC. The group also conducted a business meeting and hosted a reception at the annual SCAMC symposium.

SIG-CIN was dissolved in 1991 with the formation of the AMIA's Nursing Informatics Working Group. This group has essentially the same mission as the SIG-CIN: to promote the advancement of nursing informatics within the larger multidisciplinary context of health informatics. The new group holds its annual business meeting and reception at the SCAMC symposium, which it cosponsors.

### Study Group

In 1982 a study group on NISs was convened at the University Hospitals of Cleveland, Ohio, to discuss issues and describe categories of data needed for NISs. It identified the functions, structures, and components needed for NISs and the specific applications that had to be developed, such as resource allocation and patient care management. The meeting was funded by the NCHSR (Kiley et al., 1983; Study Group on Nursing Information Systems, 1983).

### Academic Events

Educational strategies to make nurses computer-literate were initiated in the 1970s. Several universities started to hold conferences as part of their continuing education programs. Hospitals and national associations initiated workshops as forums for teaching the state of the art, and computer conferences provided other forums for learning. Also, as nurses became computer-literate, they began to present papers, conduct workshops, demonstrate applications, and describe their research. In the 1980s formal academic courses were introduced into schools of nursing, and in the 1990s graduate programs at the master's and doctoral levels were established.

### Workshops and Institutes

In 1980 the first university-based workshop on computer use in health care was conducted by the University of Akron School of Nursing in Ohio.

It was a 1-week course designed to orient nurses to all aspects of computer applications in nursing. Several nurses with expertise in computer technology constituted the faculty and presented various computer applications in nursing. In the early 1980s other workshops were conducted by many universities. In general, they focused on computers and nursing. Boston University conducted two such workshops in 1982 and 1984; the University of Texas at Austin conducted one in 1983.

### University Conferences

In 1982 a series of annual conferences was initiated at the New Jersey State University College of Nursing at Rutgers. The major focus of its Annual National Computer Conference was to educate nurses on computer applications and nursing informatics for the development and uses of existing software, to share experiences, and to prevent "reinventing the wheel." Since then, Rutgers has continued to conduct an annual conference. Rutgers also compiled key papers presented at these conferences and published a book on computer applications in nursing education and practice (Arnold and Pearson, 1992).

In 1985 the Annual New York University Medical Center Seminar was started, with a focus on computers and nursing practice. It targets nurses who want to learn state-of-the-art applications for clinical nursing practice. The seminars also include exhibits by vendors of hospital and nursing information systems.

The first microcomputer seminar was convened in 1984 by the University of California at San Francisco. It was a 1-week microcomputer seminar that included hands-on experience with generic microcomputer software applications. Other universities conducted similar workshops. In 1986, a 1-week Microcomputer Institute for Nurses was conducted and co-sponsored by the faculty at two university schools of nursing: Georgetown University in Washington, D.C., and the University of Southwestern Louisiana in Lafayette. The purpose of the course was to give nurses in service and academic settings an overview of microcomputers, including hands-on experience with several generic microcomputer software packages.

Between 1985 and 1990 the Southern Regional Education Board (SREB) administered by the Southern Council on Collegiate Regional Education (SCCREN) was awarded a grant by the DN, PHS. Through this grant, the "SREB Continuing Nursing Education in Computer Technology Project," SREB conducted over 40 basic workshops, 3 regional conferences, and 12 seminars for nurse educators in 15 states. The workshops were conducted at universities in the south to help nurse educators become competent in the use of computers. SREB also promoted the integration of computers into the nursing curriculum (Aiken, 1990; Mikan, 1992).

In 1989 the Nurse Scholars Program, which is sponsored by the HBO and HealthQuest Company in Atlanta, Georgia, was begun. It is a 1-week program that is conducted annually and is designed to help nurses evaluate, select, and use health care information systems. Scholars are expected to share this knowledge with the nursing community. This program gives nursing educators the opportunity to gain a comprehensive understanding of automated health care information systems and the hospital technology expected in the year 2000 (Skiba et al., 1992).

In 1991 a summer institute in nursing and health care informatics was first conducted by the University of Maryland's School of Nursing in Baltimore. It is a 1-week program focusing on nursing informatics, the effect of information technology on nursing practice, the selection and evaluation of information systems, and strategies for implementing a system. This institute is conducted annually.

## Academic Courses and Programs

Several university schools of nursing initiated courses on computer technology at the graduate and undergraduate levels. The first university to offer an undergraduate elective course was the State University of New York at Buffalo in 1977. In the early 1980s a three-credit course was offered at the NIH in Bethesda, Maryland, as part of its educational program. In the mid-1980s the School of Nursing at Georgetown University began to offer graduate and undergraduate elective courses on the essentials of computers for nurses.

During this period many literacy programs were sponsored by continuing education departments in colleges and universities nationwide. Special courses, workshops, and meetings were offered to introduce nurses to computers and computing.

In the late 1980s and early 1990s universities began to educate nurses in computer applications in nursing, NISs, and nursing informatics at the graduate level. The University of Maryland and the University of Utah began to offer graduate degrees in nursing informatics. The University of Maryland initiated the first doctorate nursing informatics program in 1992 and now offers a doctorate to nurses specializing in nursing informatics.

Many other universities offer academic courses in computer applications in nursing. Some schools have made such a course a requirement for a graduate degree in nursing administration. Others offer it as an elective at the graduate level and still others are integrating computer concepts into graduate-level nursing courses. Generally, these courses are offered at universities where nursing informatics pioneers and experts are faculty members, such as Georgetown University, Washington, D.C.; the University of New York at Buffalo; the University of California at San Francisco; Case Western Reserve in Cleveland, Ohio; George Mason University in Fairfax, Virginia; the University of Texas at Austin; and the University of Maryland, Baltimore, Maryland.

# American Nurses Association Initiatives

During the 1980s the ANA got involved in the promotion of computer technology for nursing practice and launched many initiatives. In 1984 the ANA formed the Council on Computer Applications in Nursing (CCAN). In 1986 the ANA passed a resolution urging that the organization assume a leadership role and encourage the development and implementation of NISs to improve patient care and provide essential data to nurses, the nursing profession, and other professionals in the health care field.

In 1990 a resolution was passed advocating that the ANA establish national nursing databases to support clinical nursing practice and establish standards for NISs to develop comprehensive payment systems for nursing practice. As a result of the resolution, the Steering Committee on National Databases to Support Clinical Nursing Practice was formed. In 1990 the ANA House of Delegates recognized the NMDS as the minimum data elements that should be included in any paper-based or computer-based patient record. In 1992 the ANA passed another resolution that supported the involvement of nursing in CPRs.

## ANA Council on Computer Applications in Nursing

Since its formation, the ANA CCAN has been active in promoting computer technology in nursing, including the development of computer-based nursing materials. It has published a newsletter, several monographs, and other materials critical to advancing this field. Beginning in 1986, it became involved in conducting a demonstration theater and software exchange at the biennial ANA conventions, and it has given several awards for excellence in the field. Its major activities are shown in Table 1.2.

## ANA Steering Committee on Databases to Support Nursing Practice

In 1990 the ANA established the Steering Committee on Databases to Support Nursing Practice. This committee was directed to propose policy and program initiatives regarding nursing classification schemes, uniform nursing data sets, and the inclusion of nursing data elements in national databases; build national data sets and coordinate initiatives in this regard; and provide advice on the process so that the profession could recognize vocabularies and taxonomies (Lang et al., 1995).

### Unified Nursing Language System

An initiative being supported by the ANA Database Steering Committee is the promotion of the Unified Nursing Language System (UNLS). The UNLS was initiated in 1992 with the submission of four nursing taxonomies approved by the ANA Steering Committee on Databases to the National

**TABLE 1.2**   ANA COUNCIL ON COMPUTER APPLICATIONS IN NURSING
(CCAN) PUBLICATIONS, ACTIVITIES, AND AWARDS

**Monographs**
- 1988   Computer Design Criteria for Systems That Support the Nursing Process
- 1987   Computers in Nursing Education
- 1991   Computers in Nursing Research: A Theoretical Perspective
- 1993   Next-Generation Nursing Information Systems
- 1994   Computers in Nursing Management

**Directory**
- 1987   Computer Nurse Directory, 1st ed.
- 1991   Second Computer Nurse Directory, 2d ed.

**Newsletter**
- 1986   Input/Output, 1st ed.
- 1992   Input/Output, last ed.

**Demonstration Theater and Software Exchange**
- 1986, 1988, 1990, 1992, 1994   ANA Biennial Conferences

**Awards: Computer Nurse of the Year Award**
- 1988   Harriet H. Werley, PhD, RN, FAAN, FACMI
- 1990   Virginia K. Saba, EdD, RN, FAAN, FACMI
- 1992   Kathleen A. McCormick, PhD, RN, FAAN, FACMI

Library of Medicine for inclusion in the Unified Medical Language System
that was introduced in 1986 (Humphreys and Lindberg, 1992; McCormick
et al., 1994).

### Recognized Nomenclatures

The ANA Database Steering Committee also "recognized" four nomencla-
tures/classification schemes as meeting the criteria for creating a nursing
language. These schemes are also considered acceptable nursing data standards for documenting nursing care in NISs and CPR systems. They
include the (1) North American Nursing Diagnosis Association (NANDA)
Taxonomy I Revised of Nursing Diagnoses (North American Nursing Diagnosis Association, 1990), (2) the Visiting Nurse Association of Omaha
Community Health Problem and Intervention System, (3) the Saba Home
Health Care Classification (HHCC) of Nursing Diagnoses and Interventions, and (4) the University of Iowa Classification of Nursing Interventions (NIC). These schemes are described in Chap. 7.

### Nursing Informatics Specialty

In January 1992 the ANA designated nursing informatics as a nursing
specialty and defined it. The CCAN established a subcommittee to develop
the requirements for a certification program to credential a new nursing
specialist called an "informatics nurse specialist." The process includes the
development of a scope of practice, guidelines, and standards as well as

the actual questions for the credentialing examination which is scheduled to be offered in 1995 (American Nurses Association, 1994; Council on Computer Applications in Nursing, 1992).

## National League for Nursing Initiatives

The NLN promotes educational initiatives for nursing informatics. In 1985 it formed the National Forum on Computers in Health Care and Nursing, which in 1989 was renamed the Council on Nursing Informatics. The NLN also passed resolutions supporting computer technology in nursing. In 1987 the NLN passed a resolution recommending the inclusion of computer technology in nursing education. In 1991 it passed another resolution that recommended that computer technology in nursing become a part of the educational accreditation criteria for schools of nursing.

The NLN hosts the NLN Council for Nursing Informatics at its conferences and at several other educational conferences annually. The NLN Council for Nursing Informatics has published several documents that focus on the educational criteria for integrating nursing informatics into nursing curricula and into books and education materials. In 1987 the NLN published its first document on nursing and computers: *Guidelines for Basic Computer Education in Nursing* (Ronald and Skiba, 1987).

## International Events

### Working Groups

In 1981 the IMIA formed Working Group 8 on nursing informatics. It included representatives from 25 countries, including the United States. This working group met at the IMIA MEDINFO meetings that are held every 3 years and also began to sponsor its own international symposia on "Nursing Uses of Computers and Information Sciences."

In 1982 Working Group 8, now called the Special Interest Group— Nursing Informatics, conducted its first international meeting for nurses and professionals interested in this field. The meeting was designed to assist in the worldwide development of computers in nursing. The event started with an open forum in London, followed by a postconference closed workshop for the working group in Harrogate, Yorkshire. The working group held intensive discussions to describe the state of the art in computers in nursing and attempted to predict future needs. The group's postconference deliberations were published later (Scholes et al., 1983).

Working Group 8 has held subsequent meetings in (1) 1985 in Calgary, Alberta, Canada (Hannah et al., 1985), (2) 1988 in Dublin, Ireland (Daly and Hannah, 1988), (3) 1991 in Melbourne, Australia (Hovenga et al., 1991), (4) 1994 in San Antonio, Texas (Grobe and Pluyter-Wenting, 1994), and (5) 1997 in Stockholm, Sweden. The meetings followed a similar format; that is, an open meeting was followed by an invitational workshop with a working group selected to address a specific critical issue and prepare a publication on that topic.

## Special Meeting

In 1987 the IMIA Working Group 8: Task Force on Education convened in Sweden under the auspices of the Stockholm County Council. The group defined the critical competencies needed to guide the preparation and education of nurses for their roles in informatics. Nursing computer competency, defined as "having sufficient knowledge, judgment, skill, or strength," was identified as the major criterion for the skills that should be taught and emphasized in an educational program designed to teach computer technology in nursing (Peterson and Gerdin-Jelger, 1988). The task force was a working group.

## International Conferences

In 1983, for the first time, a large international group of nurses participated in two 1-day nursing sessions at the Fourth World Congress on Medical Informatics, MEDINFO 1983, held in Amsterdam. On the first day scientific papers on computer applications in nursing were presented; the second day consisted of seminars focusing on nursing systems. This conference, sponsored by the IMIA, is held every 3 years (Fokkens, 1983; Van Bemmel et al., 1983).

Subsequent international conferences sponsored by IMIA continued to include a nursing tract and several nursing functions. They were held as follows: MEDINFO 1986 in Washington, D.C.; MEDINFO 1989 in Singapore; MEDINFO 1992 in Geneva, Switzerland; and MEDINFO 1995 in Vancouver, British Columbia, Canada.

## International Initiatives

Several international initiatives have taken place. Some have already been described; however, two organizations that are involved in initiatives deserve special attention. They are the World Health Organization (WHO) and the International Council of Nurses (ICN).

## World Health Organization

The WHO is involved in the promotion of informatics around the world. In 1989 the ANA submitted to the WHO an "International Classification of Nursing Diagnosis" for inclusion in the *10th Revision of the International Classification of Diseases and Health-Related Conditions (ICD-10)*. This classification was a coded version of *NANDA Taxonomy I: Revised* (Fitzpatrick et al., 1989; World Health Organization, 1992a). The classification was not submitted to the WHO review and voting process primarily because it had not received approval from the international nursing community. However, it was presented in 1989 at the ICN Quadrennial Congress in Seoul, Korea, for review by its member organizations at their regional meetings. WHO plans to present the nursing classification for a vote at its General Assembly when it is certain that it has the support of the international nursing community.

The WHO World Health Assembly (WHA) passed a resolution (WHA 42-27) recommending "strengthening nursing and midwifery in support of strategies for Health for ALL (HFA)." The resolution included several recommendations, one of which requested the Director-General to "promote and support the training of nursing/midwifery in . . . the development of information systems" (World Health Organization, 1992b, p. 1).

As a result of this resolution, a WHO workshop on nursing informatics was held in October–November 1991 at the WHO Regional Offices for the Americas/Pan American Sanitary Bureau in Washington, D.C. The major purpose of the workshop was to highlight the status of nursing informatics at various levels around the world: national, regional, and global. The workshop was also designed to educate its participants on the principles, development, and uses of nursing management information systems, focusing on system design and hardware and software requirements.

In September 1992, as a follow-up to the WHO workshop, a Work Group on Nursing Management Information Systems was convened in Geneva. The work group focused on WHO activities related to health information systems. It identified the major constraints inhibiting the collection of data needed for human resource management. The work group also believed that nurses, the chief providers of primary health care, have the professional responsibility to ensure that basic health care needs in the community are met and to monitor the quality and effectiveness of care. The work group stated that "management information is necessary to ensure the right persons for the right jobs and in the right places at the right times, all within budgetary constraints" (World Health Organization, 1993). The participants in these two workshops included representatives from professional nursing organizations, representatives from four WHO regions, and other experts in nursing informatics, midwifery, and human resource planning.

### International Council of Nurses
In 1991 the ICN initiated a project to develop the International Classification of Nursing Practice (ICNP). The major objective was to establish a common language for nursing practice to improve communication among nurses and between nurses and other health care providers. The ICNP project emerged from an initiative of the ICN Council of Representatives at the quadrennial meeting in Seoul, Korea, in 1989, where the Professional Services Committee agreed that it would develop a common language and classification for the international nursing community. The ICNP was presented at the 1993 ICN Congress in Madrid, Spain, and is being reviewed and expanded by other countries around the world (International Council of Nurses, 1993).

## Educational Resources

In 1984 the first nursing journal in the field, *Computers in Nursing*, was published. This journal, which began in 1982 at the School of Nursing of the University of Texas at Austin as a newsletter, now has an editorial staff of eight experts in the field of computers and nursing. It is the only nursing journal that focuses on nursing informatics and computer applications in nursing.

The *Directory of Educational Software for Nursing* was introduced as a handout at a workshop at Computers in Health Care 84: A Symposium and Exhibition, which was held in Sacramento, California (Bolwell, 1984–1993). The original directory contained brief descriptions of 52 CAI tools from a collection of software demonstrated at the symposium. The directory is updated and published annually and provides information on the majority of microcomputer programs including CAI and IV software programs, that are available to the nursing community.

In 1986 the *Nurse Educator's Microworld* was also introduced by Bolwell to give nurse educators using or planning to use a microcomputer a comprehensive source of information on software programs. It is a newsletter that provides periodic information on the field of nursing.

Information from numerous journal articles, books, trade journals, and papers from proceedings of computer conferences also provide state-of-the-art information for this specialty. Books on computers in health care did not appear until 1977. From 1977 to 1983 only six books were published in this area (Pocklington and Guttman, 1984). Since then, many textbooks have offered comprehensive information about computers and nursing, nursing informatics, and nursing applications.

## Educational Resource Centers

Schools of nursing have established computer resource centers to support the introduction of computer technology in their educational programs. Several centers have been established through grant funds from the Helene Fuld Institute. A computer resource center generally consists of a laboratory with microcomputers for teaching nurses about generic software packages and/or other nursing software that can be demonstrated on that equipment. These centers also have interactive video equipment for running both CAI and IAV software. More recently many microcomputer laboratories have installed LANs that link microcomputers together. Additionally, they have installed modems that allow on-line access from remote faculty offices, student rooms, and classrooms.

## Educational Software

Several organizations have begun to develop not only CAI but also IAV software. Early in the development of educational media, several publishing companies began to develop CAI and IAV software; however, as the industry evolved, these activities were transferred to private vendors, and organizations emerged that are specifically dedicated to these activities. These organizations are involved in the development and dissemination of multi-media educational technologies that include CAI and IAV software programs.

### Educational Library

In 1992 and 1993 the Sigma Theta Tau International Honor Society of Nursing, Virginia Henderson International Nursing Library (INL), initiated an electronic library. The INL consists of a collection of electronic databases and knowledge resources, including an on-line network. An on-line communication network was created not only to transmit its on-line journal but also to share research information with the nursing community (Graves, 1994; Hudgings, 1992).

### Educational Networks

The AJN Network is an on-line service created by the American Journal of Nursing Company (AJN). AJN created this new computer network as an on-line service to provide and offer formal and informal continuing educational services to nurses. Another on-line network is ANA*NET, which was initiated by the ANA. It consists of public and private databases compiled to assist ANA staff and state nursing associations by providing instant access to information that addresses their information needs. E.T. Net (**E**ducational **T**echnology **N**etwork) is another nursing network developed by the NLM. It is an on-line computer conference network that links developers and users of interactive technology in health care education. It is also a bulletin board system that electronically links developers and users of interactive educational materials.

Other on-line electronic systems have been created, including the electronic accreditation software program developed by the NLN. This will result in an on-line nationwide NLN accreditation database that is available to the nursing community. Computer-based testing for the registered nurse examination, NCLEX-RN, is now being administered on-line nationwide.

## Collaborative Events

Several collaborative events took place in the late 1980s and early 1990s that advanced the field of computers in nursing. These initiatives consisted of conferences and projects that recommended computer technology as a means of enhancing the nursing profession. Other events continue to occur as technology becomes an integral part of nursing programs, conferences, and media.

In 1985 the **First Invitational Nursing Minimum Data Set** Conference was held in Chicago (Werley and Lang, 1988). A follow-up task force to the conference met later in the year and finalized the NMDS. The NMDS consists of 16 data elements that provide the basis for the nursing component of the computer-based patient record. In 1990 the NMDS was approved by the ANA as the standard data set structure for automating nursing practice and the development of a national database.

In 1986 **National Commission on Nursing Implementation Project** (NCNIP) Work Group II, Research and Development, advocated that NISs track care. In 1989 NCNIP conducted an invitational conference in collaboration with the ANA CCAN and the NLN Nursing Informatics Forum and selected NIS vendors. The major purpose was to outline for the industry the nursing perspective on state of the art of information systems. The conference was attended by developers and vendors, nurse purchasers, and users of NISs interested in planning collaborative efforts in the design and development of future NISs. This project culminated in a 1993 report on the next generation of NISs (Zielstorff et al., 1993).

In 1987 Sigma Theta Tau International conducted a survey of interest and needs for an **Electronic Nursing Library and Resource Center**. The results of this survey led to the establishment of the International Nursing Library, which later was named after Virginia Henderson. Sigma Theta Tau developed a strategic plan for an electronic library, including plans to develop several knowledge databases that would support nurse researchers. The electronic networks were intended to be used to communicate with nurse researchers around the world.

The **Secretary's Commission on Nursing Shortage** in its 1988 final report stated that the federal government should sponsor further research and encourage health care delivery organizations to develop and use automated information systems and other new labor-saving technologies to better support nurses and other health professionals (Office of the Secretary, 1988).

The **Priority Expert Panel E: Nursing Informatics Task Force** initiated in 1988 by the National Center for Nursing Research (NCNR), now the National Institute for Nursing Research (NINR), was one of a series of expert panels established by the NCNR to develop a national nursing research agenda. This initiative began with a conference designed to develop broad priorities for the NCNR. This was followed by the establishment of Priority Expert Panel E, which was charged with setting priorities for research topics (National Institutes of Health, 1992). This group met periodically and deliberated over a 2-year period. The panel "was committed to maintaining the clinical perspective, assessing needs for research that would bear directly on improving patient care" (NCNR Priority Expert Panel, 1993, p. 12). The panel produced a report that outlined six program goals, each with a series of recommendations for research. The major landmark events in computers in nursing are listed in Table 1.3.

**TABLE 1-3**   LANDMARK EVENTS IN COMPUTERS AND NURSING

| Year | Title | Sponsor | Site |
| --- | --- | --- | --- |
| 1973 | First Invitational Conference on Management Information Systems for Public/Community Health Agencies | NLN, Division of Nursing, U.S. Public Health Service | Fairfax, VA |
| 1974–1975 | Five Workshops on Management Information Systems for Public/Community Health Agencies | NLN, Division of Nursing, U.S. Public Health Service | Nationwide |
| 1976 | State of the Art Conference in Management for Public/Community Health Agencies | NLN, Division of Nursing, U.S. Public Health Service | Washington, DC |
| 1977 | First Research Conference on Nursing Information Systems | University of Illinois College of Nursing | Chicago, IL |
| 1977 | First Undergraduate Academic Course on Computers and Nursing | State University of New York at Buffalo | Buffalo, NY |
| 1979 | First Military Conference on Computers in Nursing | TRIMIS Army Nurse Consultant Team, Walter Reed Hospital | Washington, DC |
| 1980 | First Workshop on Computer Usage in Health Care | University of Akron School of Nursing, Continuing Education Department | Akron, OH |
| 1981 | Special-Interest Group: Computers in Nursing (SIG-CIN)* | SCAMC Event* | Washington, DC |
| 1981 | First National Conference on Computer Technology and Nursing | NIH Clinical Center, TRIMIS Army Nurse Consultant Team, and Division of Nursing, US PHS | Bethesda, MD |
| 1981 | First Nursing Session at Fifth Annual Symposium on Computer Applications in Medical Care (SCAMC-5)* | SCAMC, Inc.* | Washington, DC |
| 1982 | Study Group on Nursing Information Systems | University Hospitals of Cleveland, Case Western Reserve University, National Center for Health Services Research, US PHS | Cleveland, OH |
| 1982 | First Annual National Computer Conference | Rutgers, State University, College of Nursing | Newark, NJ |

|  |  |  |
|------|-------|----------|
| 1982 | First International Meeting: Working Conference on Nursing Uses and Computers on Nursing[†] | Working Group, International Medical Informatics Association (IMIA)[†] | London and Harrogate, Yorkshire, England |
| 1982 | Second National Conference on Computer Technology and Nursing | NIH Clinical Center, TRIMIS Army Nurse Consultant Team, and Division of Nursing, US PHS | Bethesda, MD |
| 1982 | First newsletter: *Computers in Nursing* | School of Nursing, University of Texas at Austin | Austin, TX |
| 1983 | First MEDINFO-83: Fourth World Congress on Medical Informatics[‡] | International Medical Informatics Association (IMIA)[‡] | Amsterdam, Holland |
| 1983 | Third National Conference on Computer Technology and Nursing | NIH Clinical Center, TRIMIS Army Nurse Consultant Team, and Division of Nursing, US PHS | Bethesda, MD |
| 1983 | Second Annual Joint Congress and Conference | American Association of Medical Informatics (AIMA) | San Francisco, CA, and Baltimore, MD |
| 1983 | Newsletter: *Computers in Nursing* | Lippincott | Philadelphia, PA |
| 1983 | Fourth National Conference on Computer Technology and Nursing | NIH Clinical Center, TRIMIS Army Nurse Consultant Team, and Division of Nursing, US PHS | Bethesda, MD |
| 1984 | First Microcomputer Seminar | University of California at San Francisco | San Francisco, CA |
| 1984 | First nursing computer journal: *Computers in Nursing* | Lippincott | Philadelphia, PA |
| 1984 | Council on Computer Application in Nursing (CCAN) | American Nursing Association (ANA) | Kansas City, MO |
| 1984 | Annual Directory of Educational Software for Nursing | Christine Bolwell and National League for Nursing | New York, NY |
| 1985 | National Forum on Computers in Health Care and Nursing | National League for Nursing (NLN) | New York, NY |
| 1985 | Annual Seminar on Computers and Nursing Practice | New York University Medical Center | New York, NY |
| 1985 | Nursing Minimum Data Set Conference | University of Illinois School of Nursing | Chicago, Il |
| 1985–1990 | Continuing Nursing Education in Computer Technology Project | Southern Regional Education Board (SREB) | Atlanta, GA |

39

**TABLE 1-3** LANDMARK EVENTS IN COMPUTERS AND NURSING *(continued)*

| Year | Title | Sponsor | Site |
|---|---|---|---|
| 1986 | Microcomputer Institute for Nurses | Georgetown University and University of Southwestern Louisiana | Washington, DC, and Lafayette, LA |
| 1987 | Working Group and Task Force on Education | IMIA Working Group 8 | Stockholm, Sweden |
| 1987 | Survey on Electronic Nursing Library and Resources Center | Sigma Theta Tau International | Indianapolis, IN |
| 1988 | Recommendation No. 3: Support Automated Information Systems | Secretary's Commission on Nursing Shortage | Washington, DC |
| 1988 | Priority Expert Panel E: Nursing Informatics Task Force | National Center for Nursing Research (NCNR) | Bethesda, MD |
| 1989 | First nurse scholars program | HBO and HealthQuest Corp. | Atlanta, GA |
| 1989 | Invitational Conference on State-of-the-Art of Information Systems | National Commission of Nursing Implementation Project (NCNIP) | Orlando, FL |
| 1990 | ANA Steering Committee on Databases to Support Nursing Practice | American Nurses Association | Washington, DC |
| 1991 | Nursing Informatics Working Group 8 | AMIA/SCAMC Event* | Washington, DC |
| 1991 | International Classification of Nursing Practice (ICNP) | International Council of Nurses (ICN) | Geneva, Switzerland |
| 1991 | WHO Workshop on Nursing Informatics | World Health Organization (WHO) | Washington, DC |
| 1991 | First summer institute in nursing and health care informatics | University of Maryland School of Nursing | Baltimore, MD |
| 1991 | First doctor of philosophy, nursing informatics program | University of Maryland School of Nursing | Baltimore, MD |
| 1992 | Education Technology Network (E.T. Net) | National Library of Medicine, US PHS | Rockville, MD |

| 1992 | WHO Workshop on Nursing Management Information Systems | World Health Organization (WHO) | Geneva, Switzerland |
| 1992 | Unified Nursing Language System (UNLS) | ANA and National Library of Medicine | Washington, DC |
| 1992 | ANA Nursing Informatics Specialty | American Nurses Association | Washington, DC |
| 1992 | Virginia Henderson International Nursing Library (INL) | Sigma Theta Tau International Honor Society | Indianapolis, IN |
| 1993 | ANA Recognized Four Nursing Taxonomies | American Nurses Association Database Steering Committee | Washington, DC |
| 1993 | Electronic Library | Sigma Theta Tau International Honor Society | Indianapolis, IN |
| 1993 | AJN Network On-Line | American Journal of Nursing Company | New York, NY |
| 1993 | ANA*NET On-Line | American Nurses Association | Washington, DC |
| 1993 | ANC Postgraduate Course: Computer Applications for Nursing | Army Nurse Corps (ANC) | Washington, DC |
| 1994 | NCLEX-RN On-Line | National Council Licensure Examination for Registered Nurses | New York, NY |

*AMIA/SCAMC conducted an annual symposium on computer applications in medical care in cooperation with numerous professional societies, governmental units, universities, and health care organizations, including the American Nurses Association (ANA) and the National League for Nursing (NLN).

†Working Group 8 Nursing Informatics international conferences conducted every 3 years: 1985—Calgary, Alberta, Canada; 1988—Dublin, Ireland; 1991—Melbourne, Australia; 1994—San Antonio, Texas; 1997—Stockholm, Sweden.

‡MEDINFO conducted by IMIA every 3 years: 1983—MEDINFO, Amsterdam, Holland; 1986—MEDINFO, Washington, DC; 1989—Singapore; 1992—Geneva, Switzerland; 1995—Vancouver, British Columbia, Canada.

## SUMMARY

This chapter described the historical perspectives of nursing and the computer, the developments of computer applications in nursing, and the milestones that influenced the introduction of computers into the nursing profession. It described advances in five time periods—prior to the 1960s, the 1960s, the 1970s, the 1980s, and the 1990s—and in four nursing areas: nursing practice, nursing service, nursing education, and nursing research. The chapter also discussed legislation that affected the nursing profession and its need for technology.

Computer applications in nursing and early computerized information systems were described. These systems are considered to be the forerunners of systems that are still used in hospitals. In community health, several projects were described because of their influence on today's systems. Additionally, computer applications that support nursing education and research were highlighted.

The last section focused on landmark events in nursing and computers, including major milestones in national and international conferences, symposia, workshops, and organizational initiatives that contributed to the computer literacy of nurses. The success of these conferences and the appearance of a nursing journal on this topic demonstrated the intense interest nurses had in learning more about computers. These advances confirmed the status of computers as a new specialty in the nursing profession.

## REFERENCES

Abdellah, F., Beland, I., Martin, A., and Matheney, R. (1960). *Patient-Centered Approaches to Nursing*. New York: Macmillan.

Agency for Health Care Policy and Research. (1990). *AHCPR: Purpose and Programs* (DHHS Publication No. OM90-0096). Rockville, MD: PHS, US DHHS.

Agency for Health Care Policy and Research. (1992). *AHCPR Fact Sheet*. Rockville, MD.

Aiken, E. (1990). *Continuing Nursing Education in Computer Technology: A Regional Experience* (Grant No. DlONU24198). Atlanta, GA: Southern Regional Education Board.

Alward, R. R. (1983). Patient classification systems: The ideal vs. reality. *Journal of Nursing Administration, 13*(2), 14–19.

American Journal of Nursing. (1975–1992). *International Nursing Index*. New York.

American Nurses Association. (1980). *Nursing: A Social Policy Statement*. Kansas City, MO.

American Nurses Association. (1991). *Standards for Clinical Nursing Practice*. Kansas City, MO.

American Nurses Association. (1994). *Scope of Practice for Nursing Informatics*. Washington, DC.

Andrews R. D., and Beauchamp, C. (1989). A clinical database management system for improved integration of the Veterans Affairs hospital information system. *Journal of Medical Systems, 13,* 309–320.

Arnold, J. M., and Pearson, G. A. (1992). *Computer Applications in Nursing Education and Practice.* New York: National League for Nursing (Publication No. 14-2406).

Aydelotte, M. (1973). *Nursing Staffing Methodology: A Review and Critique of Selected Literature* (DHEW Dec-NU [NIH] 73-433). Washington, DC: U.S. Government Printing Office.

Barnett, O. G. (1976). *Computer-Stored Ambulatory Record (COSTAR)* (DHEW Publication No. HRA 76-3145). Rockville, MD: National Center for Health Services Research, PHS, US DHEW.

Bitzer, M. D., and Boudreaux, M. C. (1969). Using a computer to teach nursing. *Nursing Forum, 8*(3), 234–254.

Blum, B. I. (1990). Medical informatics in the United States, 1950–1975. In B. Blum and K. Duncan (Eds.), *A History of Medical Informatics* (pp. xvii–xxx). Reading, MA: Addison-Wesley.

Bolwell, C. (1984–1993). *Directory of Educational Software for Nursing* (Pub. No. 41-2279). New York: National League for Nursing Press.

Brown, V. B., Mason, W. B., and Kaczmarski, M. (1971). A computerized health information service. *Nursing Outlook, 19*(3), 158–161.

Collen, M. F. (1994). The origins of informatics. *Journal of the American Medical Informatics Association, 1*(2), 91–107.

Committee on Armed Services. (1990). *Defense's Acquisition of the Composite Health Care System.* Washington, DC: U.S. House of Representatives, GAO (T-IMTEC-90-04).

Community Nursing Services of Philadelphia. (1976). *Development of a Computerized Record System to Store and Summarize Information Relevant to Administration, Evaluation and Planning of Nursing Services* (Contract No. 1-NU-241271). Washington, DC: Division of Nursing, HRA, US DHEW.

Cook, M., and Mayers, M. (1981). Computer-assisted data base for nursing research. In H. Werley and M. Grier (Eds.), *Nursing Information Systems* (pp. 149–156). New York: Springer.

Cook, M., and McDowell, W. (1975). Changing to an automated information system. *American Journal of Nursing, 75*(1), 46–51.

Cornell, S. A., and Carrick, A. G. (1973). Computerized schedules and care plans. *Nursing Outlook, 21*(12), 781–789.

Corum, W. (1993). JCAHO's new information management standards. *Healthcare Informatics, 10*(8), 20–21.

Council on Computer Applications in Nursing. (1992). *Report on the Designation of Nursing Informatics as a Nursing Specialty.* Washington, DC.

Daly, N., and Hannah, K. J. (Eds.). (1988). *Proceedings of Nursing and Computers: Third International Symposium on Nursing Use of Computers and Information Science.* Washington, DC: Mosby.

Dayhoff, R. E., Maloney, D. L., and Kuzman, P. M. (1990). Examination of architecture to allow integration of image data with hospital information systems. In R. A. Miller (Ed.), *Proceedings of the Fourteenth Symposium on Computer Applications in Medical Care* (pp. 694–698). Washington, DC: IEEE Computer Society Press.

Fitzpatrick, J. J., Kerr, M. E., Saba, V. K., et al. (1989). Translating nursing diagnosis into ICD code. *Nursing Outlook, 89*(4), 493–495.

Fokkens, O. (Ed.). (1983). *MEDINFO 83 Seminars.* Amsterdam: North-Holland.

Gane, D. (1972). The computer in nursing. In J. Hurst and H. Walker (Eds.), *The Problem-Oriented System* (pp. 251–257). New York: Medcom Press.

Gebbie, K. M. (Ed.). (1975). *Summary of the Second National Conference: Classification of Nursing Diagnoses.* St. Louis: National Group for Classification of Nursing Diagnoses.

Geibnik, G. A., and Hurst, L. L. (1975). *Computer Projects in Health Care.* Ann Arbor, MI: Health Administration Press.

Gortner, S. R., and Nahm, M. H. (1977). An overview of nursing research in the United States. *Nursing Research, 26*(1), 10–33.

Graves, J. R., (1994). Updates: Virginia Henderson International Nursing Library. *Reflections, 20*(3), 39.

Grobe, S., and Pluyter-Wenting, E. (1994). *Nursing Informatics: An International Overview for Nursing in a Technological Era.* Amsterdam: Elsevier.

Hanchett, E. S. (1981). Appropriateness of nursing care. In H. Werley and M. Grier (Eds.), *Nursing Information Systems* (pp. 235–242). New York: Springer.

Hannah, K. J., Guillemin, E. C., and Conklin, D. N. (1985). *Nursing Uses of Computers and Information Science: Proceeding of the IFIP-IMIA International Symposium on Nursing Uses of Computers and Information Science.* Amsterdam: North-Holland.

Harmer, B., and Henderson, V. (1939). *Textbook of the Principles and Practice of Nursing* (4th ed.). New York: Macmillan.

Heffernan, S. (Ed.). (1981). *Proceedings: The Fifth Annual Symposium on Computer Applications on Medical Care.* New York: IEEE Computer Society Press.

Henderson, V. (1964). The nature of nursing. *American Journal of Nursing, 64*(8), 62–68.

Hodge, M. H. (1990). History of the TDS Medical Information System. In B. I. Blum and K. Duncan (Eds.), *A History of Medical Informatics* (pp. 328–344). Reading, MA: Addison-Wesley.

Hovenga, E. J. S., Hannah, K. J., McCormick, K. A., and Ronald, J. S. (1991). *Nursing Informatics '91: Proceedings of the Fourth International Conference on Nursing Use of Computers and Information Science.* Amsterdam: North-Holland.

Hudgings, C. (1992). The Virginia Henderson International Nursing Library: Improving access to nursing research databases. In J. M. Arnold and G. A. Pearson (Eds.), *Computer Applications in Nursing Education and Practice* (pp. 3–8). New York: National League for Nursing (Publication No. 14-2406).

Humphreys, B. L., and Lindberg, D. A. B. (1992). The unified medical language system project: A distributed experiment in improving access to biomedical information. In K. C. Lun, P. DeGoulet, T. E. Piemme, and O. Rienhoff (Eds.), *MEDINFO 92* (pp. 1496–1500). Amsterdam: North-Holland.

International Council of Nurses. (1993). *Nursing's Next Advance: An International Classification for Nursing Practice (ICNP): A Working Paper.* Geneva, Switzerland.

Joint Commission on Accreditation of Health Care Organizations (1994). *Accreditation Manual for Hospitals.* Oakbrook Terrace, IL.

Joint Commission on Accreditation of Hospitals. (1970). *Accreditation Manual for Hospitals.* Chicago.

Joint Commission on Accreditation of Hospitals. (1981). *Accreditation Manual for Hospitals*. Chicago.

Kemeny, J. G. (1972). *Man and the Computer*. New York: Scribner.

Kiley, M., Holleran, E. J., and Weston, J. L., et al. (1983). Computerized nursing information systems (NIS). *Nursing Management, 14*(7), 26–29.

Kim, M. J., McFarland, G. K., and McLane, A. M. (Eds.). (1984). *Classification and Nursing Diagnoses: Proceedings of the Fifth National Conference*. St. Louis: Mosby.

Lang, N. M, Hudgings, C., Jacox, A., et al. (1995). Toward a national database for nursing practice. In *Database Steering Committee: An Emerging Framework for the Profession: Data System Advances for Clinical Nursing Practice*. Washington, DC: American Nurses Association.

Lindberg, D. (1977). *The Growth of Medical Information Systems in the United States*. Lexington, MA: Lexington Books.

Lysaught, J. P. (1973). *From Abstract into Action*. New York: McGraw-Hill.

Martin, K. S., and Scheet, N. J. (1992). *The Omaha System: Applications for Community Health Nursing*. Philadelphia: Saunders.

Mayers, M. (1974). *Standard Nursing Care Plans*. Palo Alto, CA: K.P. Co. Medical Systems.

McCloskey, J. C., and Bulechek, G. M. (Eds.). (1992). *Nursing Interventions Classification (NIC): Iowa Intervention Project*. St. Louis: Mosby.

McCormick, K. A., Lang, N., and Zielstorff, R. (1994). Toward standard classification schemes for nursing language: Recommendations of the American Nurses Association Steering Committee on Databases to Support Clinical Nursing Practice. *Journal of the American Medical Informatics Association*, 1, 421–427.

McNeely, L. D. (1983). Preparation and data base development. In National Institutes of Health: *1st National Conference: Computer Technology and Nursing* (pp. 17–25) (NIH Pub. 83-2142). Bethesda, MD: NIH, PHS, US DHHS.

McNeill, D. G. (1979). Developing the complete computer-based information system. *Journal of Nursing Administration, 9*(12), 34–46.

Mikan, K. J. (1992). Implementation process for computer-supported education. In J. M. Arnold and G. A. Pearson (Eds.), *Computer Applications in Nursing Education and Practice* (pp. 191–199). New York: National League for Nursing (Publication No. 14-2406).

Montag, M. (1954). Experimental programs in nursing education. *Nursing Outlook, 2*(12), 620–621.

Namdi, M. F., and Hutelmyer, C. M. (1970). A study of the effectiveness of an assessment tool in the identification of nursing care problems. *Nursing Research, 19*(4), 354–358.

National Center for Health Services Research (1980). *Computer Applications in Health Care* (NCHSR Research Report Series, DHHS Pub. No. 80-3251). Hyattsville, MD.

National Institutes of Health. (1983). *1st National Conference: Computer Technology and Nursing* (NIH Pub. 83-2142). Bethesda, MD: NIH, PHS, US DHHS.

National Institutes of Health. (1984). *2nd National Conference: Computer Technology and Nursing* (NIH Pub. 84-2623). Bethesda, MD: NIH, PHS, US DHHS.

National Institutes of Health. (1992). *Patient Outcomes Research: Examining the Effectiveness of Nursing Practice* (NIH Pub. No. 93-3411). Bethesda, MD: NIH, PHS, US DHHS.

National League for Nursing. (1974). *Management Information Systems for Public Health / Community Health Agencies: Report of the Conference.* New York.

National League for Nursing. (1975). *Management Information Systems for Public Health / Community Health Agencies: Workshop Papers.* New York.

National League for Nursing. (1976). *State of the Art in Management Information Systems for Public Health / Community Health Agencies: Report of a Conference.* New York.

National League for Nursing. (1978). *Selected Management Information Systems for Public Health / Community Health Agencies.* New York.

National Library of Medicine. (1986). *Building and Organizing the Library's Collection: Report of Panel 1.* Bethesda, MD: NIH, PHS, US DHHS.

NCNR Priority Expert Panel on Nursing Informatics. (1993). *Nursing Informatics: Enhancing Patient Care* (NIH Publication No. 93-2419). Bethesda, MD: National Center for Nursing Research, NIH, PHS, US DHHS.

Nightingale, F. (1946). *Notes on Nursing, What It Is and What It Is Not* (facsimile of 1859 edition). Philadelphia: Lippincott.

North American Nursing Diagnosis Association. (1990). *Taxonomy I Revised— 1990.* St. Louis.

North American Nursing Diagnosis Association. (1992). *NANDA: Nursing Diagnosis: Definitions and Classifications.* St. Louis.

Office of the Secretary. (1988). *Secretary's Commission on Nursing: Final Report* (Vol. 1). Washington, DC: US DHHS.

Orem, D. E. (1971). *Nursing: Concepts in Practice.* New York: McGraw-Hill.

Peterson, H. E., and Gerdin-Jelger, U. (Eds.). (1988). *Preparing Nurses for Using Information Systems: Recommended Informatics Competencies* (Pub. No. 14-2234). New York: National League for Nursing.

Pocklington, D. B., and Guttman, L. (1984). *Nursing Reference for Computer Literature.* Philadelphia: Lippincott.

Pryor, A. T. (1992). Current state of computer-based record systems. In M. J. Ball and M. F. Collen (Eds.), *Aspects of the Computer-Based Patient Record* (pp. 67–82). New York: Springer-Verlag.

Pryor, T. A., Califf, R. M., Harrell, F. E., et al. (1985). Clinical data bases. *Medical Care, 23*(5), 623–647.

Rieder, K. A. and Norton, D. A. (1984). An integrated nursing information system: A planning model. *Computers in Nursing, 2*(3), 73–79.

Roberts, M. (1954). *American Nursing: History and Interpretation.* New York: Macmillan.

Rockland County Health Department. (1971). *Rockland County Pilot Study: Nursing Care of the Sick* (Contract No. H 108-67-35). Washington, DC: Division of Nursing, HRA, US DHEW.

Romano, C., McCormick, K., and McNeely, L. (1982). Nursing documentation: A model for a computerized data base. *Advances in Nursing Science, 4,* 43–56.

Ronald, J. S., and Skiba, D. J. (1987). *Guidelines for Basic Computer Education in Nursing.* New York: National League for Nursing.

Saba, V. K. (1995). A new nursing vision: The information highway. *Nursing Leadership Forum, 1*(2), 44–51.

Saba, V. K. (1981a). A comparative study of document retrieval system of nursing interest (Dissertation No. 8124656). *Dissertation Abstracts International, 42*(5), 1837 A.

Saba, V. K. (1981b). How computers influence nursing activities in community health. In National Institutes of Health, *1st National Conference: Computer Technology and Nursing* (pp. 7–12). Bethesda, MD: NIH, PHS, US DHEW.

Saba, V. K. (1982). The computer in public health: Today and tomorrow. *Nursing Outlook, 30*(9), 510–514.

Saba, V. K. (1992). The classification of home health care nursing diagnoses and interventions. *CARING Magazine, 11*(3), 50–57.

Saba, V. K., and Levine, E. (1981). Patient care module in community health nursing. In H. Werley and M. Grier (Eds.), *Nursing Information Systems* (pp. 243–262). New York: Springer.

Saba, V. K., Oatway, D. M., and Rieder, K. A. (1989). How to use nursing information sources. *Nursing Outlook, 37*(4), 189–195.

Saba, V. K., and Skapik, K. (1979). Nursing information center. *American Journal of Nursing, 79*(1), 86–87.

Scholes, M., Bryant, Y., and Barber, B. (Eds.). (1983). *The Impact of Computers on Nursing: An International Review*. Amsterdam: North-Holland.

Seymer, L. R. (1954). *Selected Writings of Florence Nightingale*. New York: Macmillan.

Simmons, D. A. (1982). Computer implementation in ambulatory care: A community health model. In NIH, *2d National Conference: Computer Technology in Nursing* (pp. 19–23). Bethesda, MD: NIH, PHS, US DHEW.

Skiba, D. J., Ronald, J. S., and Simpson, R. L. (1992). HealthQuest/HBO Nurse Scholars Program: A corporate partnership with nursing education. In J. M. Arnold and G. A. Pearson (Eds.), *Computer Applications in Nursing Education and Practice* (pp. 227–235). New York: National League for Nursing (Publication No. 14-2406).

Smith, E. J. (1974). The computers and nursing practice. *Supervisor Nurse, 5*(9), 55–62.

Somers, J. (1971). A computerized nursing care system. *Hospitals, 45*(8), 93–100.

Study Group on Nursing Information Systems. (1983). Special report: Computerized nursing information systems: An urgent need. *Research in Nursing and Health, 6*(3), 101–105.

Taylor, D. B., and Johnson, O. H. (1974). *Systematic Nursing Assessment: A Step toward Automation* (DHEW Publication No. 7417). Washington, DC: U.S. Government Printing Office.

Valbona, C., and Spencer, W. A. (1974). Texas Institute for Research and Rehabilitation Hospital computer system (Houston). In M. Collen (Ed.), *Hospital Computer Systems* (pp. 662–700). New York: John Wiley.

Van Bemmel, J. H., Ball, M. S., and Wigertz, O. (Eds.). (1983). *Medinfo 83* (Vols. 1–2). Amsterdam: North-Holland.

Visiting Nurse Association of Omaha. (1986). *Client Management Information System for Community Health Nursing Agencies*. Rockville, MD: Division of Nursing, BHP, HRSA, PHS, US DHHS. (NTIS Pub. HRP-0907023).

Vreeland, E. M. (1964). Trends in nursing education reflected in the federal medical services. *Military Medicine, 129*(5), 415–422.

Weed, L. (1991). *Knowledge Coupling: New Premises and New Tools for Medical Care and Education*. New York: Springer.

Weed, L. (1969). *Medical Records, Medical Education and Patient Care*. Cleveland: Case Western Reserve University Press.

Werley, H. (1981). Nursing data accumulation: Historical perspective. In H. Werley and M. Grier (Eds.), *Nursing Information Systems* (pp. 1–10). New York: Springer.

Werley, H., and Grier, M. (Eds.). (1981). *Nursing Information Systems*. New York: Springer.

Werley, H., and Lang, N. M. (Eds.). (1988). *Identification of the Nursing Minimum Data Set*. New York: Springer.

White House Domestic Policy Council. (1993). *The Clinton Blueprint: The President's Health Security Plan*. Washington, DC: White House.

World Health Organization. (1992a). *International Statistical Classification of Diseases and Health Related Problems: Tenth Revision* (ICD-10). Geneva, Switzerland: WHO.

World Health Organization. (1992b). *Report of a WHO Workshop on "Nursing Informatics."* Geneva, Switzerland: WHO.

World Health Organization. (1993). *Report of a Nursing Management Information System*. Geneva, Switzerland: WHO.

Zielstorff, R. D., Hudgings, C. I., and Grobe, S. J. (1993). *Nursing Information Systems: Essential Characteristics for Professional Practice*. Washington, DC: American Nurses Association.

## BIBLIOGRAPHY

Austin, C. J. (1979). *Information Systems for Hospital Administration*. Ann Arbor, MI: Health Administration Press.

Ball, M. (1973). Fifteen hospital information systems available. In M. Ball (Ed.), *How to Select a Computerized Hospital Information System* (pp. 10–27). Basel, Switzerland: S. Karger.

Ball, M. (1974). Medical data processing in the United States. *Hospital Finance Management, 28*(1), 10–30.

Ball, M. J., and Hannah, K. J. (1984). *Using Computers in Nursing*. Reston, VA: Reston Publishing.

Blum, B. (1982). *Proceedings: The Sixth Annual Symposium on Computer Applications in Medical Care*. New York: IEEE Computer Society Press.

Blum, B. I. (Ed.). (1982). *Computers and Medicine: Information Systems for Patient Care*. New York: Springer-Verlag.

Bridgman, M. (1953). *Collegiate Education for Nursing*. New York: Russell Sage Foundation.

Bronzino, J. D. (1982). *Computer Applications for Patient Care*. Reading, MA: Addison-Wesley.

Brown, E. L. (1948). *Nursing for the Future*. New York: Russell Sage Foundation.

Bullough, B., and Bullough, V. (1966). *Issues on Nursing*. New York: Springer.

Cohen, G. (Ed.). (1984). *Proceedings: The Eighth Annual Symposium on Computer Applications in Medical Care*. New York: IEEE Computer Society Press.

Collen, M. F. (1983). General requirements for clinical departmental systems. In J. H. Van Bemmel, M. J. Ball, and O. Wigertz (Eds.), *MEDINFO 83* (pp. 736–739). Amsterdam: North-Holland.

Collen, M. F. (Ed.). (1974). *Hospital Computer Systems*. New York: John Wiley.

Cornell, S., and Bush, F. (1971). Systems approach to nursing care plans. *American Journal of Nursing, 71*(7), 1376–1378.

Dayhoff, R. E. (Ed.). (1983). *Proceedings: The Seventh Annual Symposium on Computer Applications in Medical Care.* New York: IEEE Computer Society Press.

Dick, R. S., and Steen, E. B. (Eds.). (1991). *The Computer-Based Patient Record: An Essential Technology for Health Care.* Washington, DC: National Academy Press.

Donnelley, G. F., Mangel, A., and Sutterley, D. C. (1980). *The Nursing System: Issues, Ethics, and Politics.* New York: John Wiley.

Edmunds, L. (1983). Making the most of a message function for nursing services. In R. Dayhoff (Ed.), *Proceedings: The Seventh Annual Symposium on Computer Applications in Medical Care* (pp. 511–513). New York: IEEE Computer Society Press.

Federal Security Agency. (1950). *The United States Cadet Nurse Corps.* Washington, DC: U.S. Government Printing Office.

Fedorowicz, J. (1983). Will your computer meet your case-mix information needs? *Nursing and Health Care, 4*(9), 493–497.

Fiddleman, R. H., and Kerlin, B. D. (1980). *Preliminary Assessment of COSTAR V at the North (San Diego) County Health Services Project* (Grant No. CS-D-000001-03-0). McLean, VA: MITRE Corporation.

Flynn, J. B., Foerst, H., and Heffron, P. B. (1984). Nursing: Past and present. In J. B. McCann/Flynn and P. B. Heffron (Eds.), *Nursing: From Concept to Practice* (pp. 31–88). Bowie, MD: Robert J. Brady.

Fordyce, E. M. (1984). Theorists in nursing. In J. B. McCann/Flynn and P. B. Heffron (Eds.), *Nursing: From Concept to Practice* (pp. 237–258). Bowie, MD: Robert J. Brady.

Gebbie, K. M. (Ed.). (1976). *Summary of the Second National Conference: Classification of Nursing Diagnoses.* St. Louis: National Group for Classification of Nursing Diagnoses.

Goldmark, J. (1923). *Nursing and Nursing Education in the United States.* New York: Macmillan.

Gordon, M. (1981). Identifying data through the nursing diagnosis approach. In H. Werley and M. Grier (Eds.), *Nursing Information Systems* (pp. 32–35). New York: Springer.

Grobe, S. J. (1984). *Computer Primer and Resource Guide for Nurses.* Philadelphia: Lippincott.

Hannah, K. J. (1976). The computer and nursing practice. *Nursing Outlook, 24*(9), 555–558.

Health Care Financing Administration (HCFA). (1983). *HCFA Legislative Summary: Prospective Payment Revision: Title VI of the Social Security Amendment* (PL 98-21, No. 381-858:343). Washington, DC: U.S. Government Printing Office.

Henderson, V. (1966). *The Nature of Nursing.* New York: Macmillan.

Henderson, V. (1973). On nursing care plans and their history. *Nursing Outlook, 21*(6), 378–379.

Henderson, V., and Nite, G. (1978). *Principles and Practice of Nursing* (6th ed.). New York: Macmillan.

Hope, G. S. (1984). Delivery system and nursing in the 21st century. In J. M. Virgo (Ed.), *Health Care: An International Perspective* (pp. 215–224). Edwardsville, IL: International Health Economics and Management Institute.

Hudgings, C. (1991). An international nursing library: Worldwide access to nursing research databases. In E. S. Hovenga, K. J. Hannah, K. A. McCormick, and J. S. Ronald (Eds.), *Nursing Informatics '91* (pp. 780–784). New York: Springer-Verlag.

Kalish, P. A., and Kalish, B. J. (1977). *Federal Influence and Impact on Nursing* (NTIS Publication No. HRP-0900636). Annandale, VA: National Technical Information Service.

Kerlin, B., and Greene, P. (1981). *COSTAR: An Overview and Annotated Bibliography* (Contract No. 233-79-3201). McLean, VA: MITRE Corporation.

Lun, K. C., DeGoulet, P., Piemme, T. E., and Rienhoff, O. (Eds.). *MEDINFO 92* (pp. 1496–1500). Amsterdam: North-Holland.

Mayers, M. G. (1972). *A Systematic Approach to the Nursing Care Plan.* New York: Appleton-Century-Crofts.

McCann/Flynn, J. B., and Heffron, P. B. (Eds.). (1984). *Nursing: From Concept to Practice.* Bowie, MD: Robert J. Brady.

McCloskey, J. (1981). Nursing care plans and problem-oriented health records. In H. Werley and M. Grier (Eds.), *Nursing Information Systems* (pp. 119–126). New York: Springer.

McDonald, C. J., and Barnett, G. O. (1990). Medical-record systems. In E. H. Shortliffe and L. E. Perreault (Eds.), *Medical Informatics: Computer Applications in Health Care* (pp. 181–218). Reading, MA: Addison-Wesley.

McFarland, G. K., Leonard, H. S., and Morris, M. M. (1984). *Nursing Leadership and Management: Contemporary Strategies.* New York: John Wiley.

Medical Information Resources Management Office. (1991). *Decentralized Hospital Computer Program.* Salt Lake City, UT: Department of Veterans Affairs, Veterans Health Administration.

Naisbitt, J. (1982). *Megatrends: Ten New Directions Transforming Our Lives.* New York: Warner Books.

National Center for Health Services Research. (1976). *The Program in Health Services Research* (DHEW Publication No. [HRA] 78-3136). Hyattsville, MD.

National Center for Health Services Research. (1979). *Automation of the Problem-Oriented Medical Record* (NCHSR Research Summary Series, DHEW Publication No. HRA 77-31770). Rockville, MD.

National League for Nursing Education. (1937). *A Study of Nursing Services in Fifty Selected Hospitals.* New York.

National Library of Medicine. (1981). *MEDLARS: The Computerized Literature Retrieval Services of the National Library of Medicine* (NIH Brochure Pub. No. 83-1286). Bethesda, MD.

National Library of Medicine. (1986). *Report of Panel 4: Long Range Plan: Medical Informatics.* Rockville, MD: NIH, PHS, DHHS.

New Jersey State Department of Health. (1969). *Study of Home Health Agencies in New Jersey* (Contract No. 1-NU-04147). Hyattsville, MD: Division of Nursing, HRA, US DHEW.

Office of Technology Assessment. (1983). *Diagnoses Related Groups (DRGs) and the Medical Program: The Implications for Medical Technology* (Technical Memorandum OTA-TM-H-17). Washington, DC: U.S. Congress, Office of Technology Assessment.

Pritchard, K. (1982). Computers 3: Possible applications in nursing. *Nursing Times, 78*(8), 465–466.

Pritchard, K. (1982). Computers 4: Implication of computerization. *Nursing Times, 78*(8), 491–492.

Randall, A. M. (1984). Surviving the '80's and beyond: Strategic planning for health care data processing. In J. M. Virgo (Ed.), *Health Care: An Interna-*

*tional Perspective* (pp. 115–132). Edwardsville, IL: International Health Economics and Management Institute.

Rogers, M. E. (1970). *An Introduction to the Theoretical Basis of Nursing*. Philadelphia: Davis.

Rosenberg, M., and Carriker, D. (1966). Automating nurses' notes. *American Journal of Nursing*, 66(5), 1021–1023.

Roy, C. (1975). A diagnostic classification system for nursing. *Nursing Outlook*, 23(2), 90–94.

Stewart, I. M. (1943). *The Education of Nurses: Historical Foundations and Modern Trends*. New York: Macmillan.

Stratman, W. C. (1979). *A Demonstration of PROMIS* (NCHSR Research Summary Series, DHEW Pub. No. [PHS] 79-3247). Hyattsville, MD: National Center for Health Services.

Sweeney, M. A., and Olivieri, P. (1981). *An Introduction to Nursing Research*. Philadelphia: Lippincott.

Veazie, S., and Dankmyer, T. (1977). HISs, MISs and DBMSs: Sorting out the letters. *Hospitals*, 51(20), 80–84.

Virgo, J. M. (Ed.). (1984). *Health Care: An International Perspective*. Edwardsville, IL: International Health Economics and Management Institute.

Wesseling, E. (1972). Automating the nursing history and care plan. *Journal of Nursing Administration*, 2(3), 34–38.

Young, D. A. (1984). Prospective payment assessment commission: Mandate, structure and relationships. *Nursing Economics, 2*, 309–311.

Yura, H., and Walsh, M. B. (1973). *The Nursing Process: Assessing, Planning, Implementing, Evaluating* (2d ed.). New York: Appleton-Century-Crofts.

Zielstorff, R. D. (Ed.). (1980). *Computers in Nursing*. Wakefield, MA: Nursing Resources.

# *2*

• • • • • • • • • • • • • • • • • • • • • • •

# HISTORICAL PERSPECTIVES OF THE COMPUTER

## OBJECTIVES

- Discuss early computer developments.
- Describe future computer developments.
- Describe the development of the microcomputer.
- Identify five computer generations.
- Discuss the growth of the computer industry.

The computer, like the nursing profession, has a history that spans several centuries. People have used devices for counting since the beginning of recorded history. Many people, mostly working independently, helped translate the concept of the computer into reality. It took a long time for the first computer to emerge; however, since its appearance, computer development and use have grown with extraordinary speed and revolutionary effects.

This chapter covers the earliest known computing devices as well as the latest computers. The history of the computer can be described by referring to two series of events: the early development of a number of calculating devices and the recent technological contributions that influenced the development of today's computers. A brief description of computer generations, the microcomputer revolution, and the phenomenal growth of the computer industry follows. This chapter discusses the following major topics:

- Early computer developments
- Advanced computer developments
- Microcomputer developments
- Computer generations
- Computer industry growth

## EARLY COMPUTER DEVELOPMENTS

Significant early computer developments primarily involved computing devices (Table 2.1). The major devices that influenced the development of the modern computer include the following:

- Abacus
- Napier's "bones" rods
- Pascal's Pascaline
- Leibniz's calculator
- Jacquard's loom
- Babbage's analytical engine
- Hollerith's tabulator

### Abacus

People have used devices for counting and computing since the beginning of recorded history. The abacus, derived from the Greek *abox*, meaning a "board," has been used for centuries, appearing in Egypt and China as early as 5000 B.C. It is a device in which numbers are represented by beads that are fixed on a frame with a crossbar and are used for addition and subtraction. It is the first calculating machine and the earliest computing device (Fig. 2.1).

**TABLE 2.1**    EARLY COMPUTER DEVELOPMENTS

| Inventor | Invention | Year |
|---|---|---|
| Abacus | First computing device | 5000 B.C. |
| Napier's "bones" rods | Computing device to multiply and divide | 1617 |
| Pascal's Pascaline | First mechanical calculator to add and subtract | 1642 |
| Leibniz's calculator | First mechanical calculator to multiply and divide | 1694 |
| Jacquard's loom | First automatic weaving machine with punched paper cards | 1804 |
| Babbage's analytical engine | First design for a modern computer | 1834 |
| Hollerith's tabulator | First electric tabulator | 1889 |

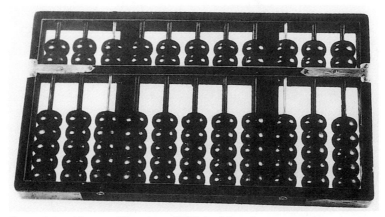

**Figure 2.1**   Abacus. (Courtesy IBM Archives.)

## Calculators

It was not until the 1600s, just before the industrial revolution, that a number of other computing devices appeared. The first calculator, Napier's "bones" rods, invented by John Napier (1550–1617), was an ingenious multiplication system using numbered white rods that when arranged side by side could be manipulated to multiply numbers (Fig. 2.2).

In 1642 Blaise Pascal (1623–1662) of France invented the first mechanical calculator, the Pascaline. His ingenious device consisted of numbered dials, using the decimal system, that were turned to the appropriate numbers for addition and subtraction. It was the forerunner of the modern adding machine. In 1694 Gottfried von Leibniz (1646–1716) of Germany invented a hand-cranked calculator that improved on Pascal's machine. The Leibniz calculator not only could add and subtract but also could multiply, divide, and take square roots (Fig. 2.3).

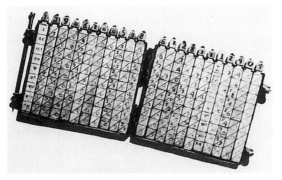

**Figure 2.2**   Napier's "bones" rods. (Courtesy IBM Archives.)

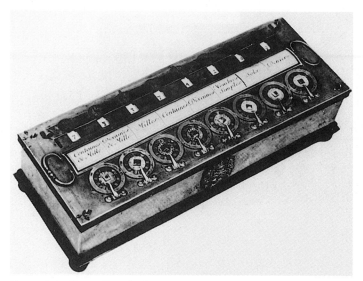

**Figure 2.3**　Pascal's calculator. (Courtesy IBM Archives.)

## Jacquard's Loom

In 1804 Joseph M. Jacquard of France designed an automatic weaving loom for the textile industry. This was the first programming device that could automatically control weaving looms. It used heavy paper cards pre-punched with holes representing coded information, which were linked in a series to control the patterns to be woven. These coded cards were the forerunner of the punched cards used in the computer industry (Fig. 2.4).

## Babbage's Analytical Engine

Charles Babbage (1791–1871) of England, known as the "father" of the modern computer, made significant advances in the history of computing. In 1812 he conceived his difference engine to mechanize algebraic functions. In 1834 he designed another machine, the analytical engine, which was based on the first model. This steam-powered machine was designed to carry out all kinds of mathematical computations and included the five basic components—input, processor, control, storage, and output—found in today's computers. Known as Babbage's folly, it was never built. Babbage was about 100 years ahead of his time.

In 1842 Augusta Ada Byron, the Countess of Lovelace and Babbage's friend, translated his paper on the analytical engine. She enhanced Babbage's folly by describing a computer program using the binary numbering system instead of the decimal numbering system to "code" his machine. She is considered the first computer programmer (Fig. 2.5).

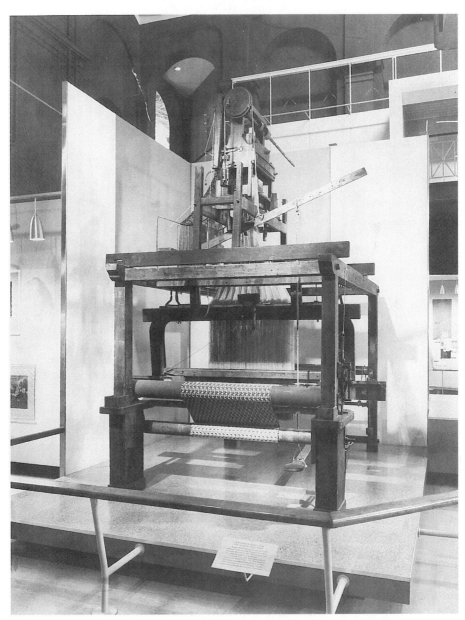

**Figure 2.4**   Jacquard's loom. (Smithsonian Institution Photo No. 45599.)

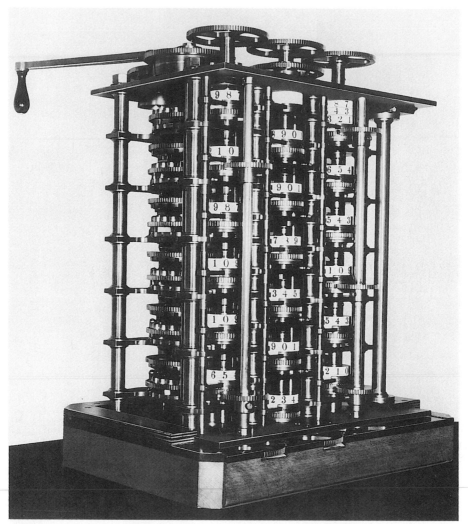

**Figure 2.5**   Babbage's difference machine (engine). (Courtesy IBM Archives.)

## Hollerith's Tabulator

In 1889 Herman Hollerith (1860–1926), an employee at the U.S. Census Bureau, invented an electrical tabulator and sorter that could read and sort holes that coded data on punched cards. Hollerith borrowed the concept from Jacquard's weaving loom cards. The Hollerith machine tripled the speed of processing for the 1890 U.S. Census. Later, Hollerith improved his punched card and designed 80-column, 12-row punched cards that were used in the computer industry as input and storage media for both data and computer programs for many years. He left his position at

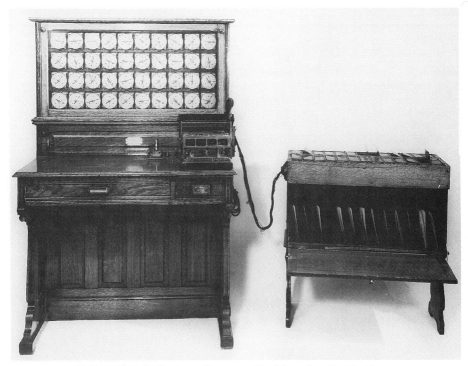

**Figure 2.6**    Hollerith's tabulator and sorter. (Smithsonian Institution
Photo No. 64563.)

the Census Bureau to establish his own tabulating company, which in
1924 became known as International Business Machines (IBM). Little of
significance occurred between Hollerith's inventions and World War II,
which generated a new impetus to increase computing power (Fig. 2.6).

## ADVANCED COMPUTER DEVELOPMENTS

The development of today's computer spans a very short period compared
with the centuries that led up to its creation. World War II probably had
the greatest impact because it speeded research and development. Many
scientists in the United States, Great Britain, and Germany contributed
to technological advancements that influenced computer design and ush-
ered in more reliance on the computer. This period is sometimes called the
second industrial revolution.

In the United States the first large-scale computers were conceived
and built as university projects sponsored by the military, which needed a
way to perform rapid calculations for ballistics and other military requirements. The major developmental designs that represent recent computer
history are shown in Table 2.2 and described in this chapter.

**TABLE 2.2**     ADVANCED COMPUTER DEVELOPMENTS

| Inventor | Invention | Year |
|---|---|---|
| Atanasoff and Berry | ABC: first digital computer | 1942 |
| Aiken | Mark I: first large-scale digital computer | 1944 |
| Echert and Mauchley | ENIAC: first electronic general-purpose computer | 1946 |
| Von Newman | Stored program concept | 1945 |
| Maurice Wilkes | EDVAC: experimental computer | 1949 |
| Echert and Mauchley | EDSAC: experimental computer | 1951 |
| MIT | WHIRLWIND I: experimental computer | 1952 |
| Echert and Mauchley | UNIVAC I: first commercial mainframe computer | 1951 |
| DEC (Digital Equipment Corp.) | PDP-8: first minicomputer | 1965 |
| Altair 8800 | First microcomputer: personal computer | 1975 |
| Seymour Cray | Cray I: first supercomputer | 1976 |

The next major developments that affected the design of the modern computer include the following:

- ABC
- Mark I
- ENIAC
- Stored program concept
- EDSAC, EDVAC, WHIRLWIND I
- UNIVAC I
- PDP-8
- Cray-I
- Altair-8800

## ABC

In 1942 Dr. John Atanasoff and his assistant, Clifford Berry, built the first electronic digital computer, the ABC (Atanasoff-Berry Computer), at Iowa State College. This single-purpose machine composed of vacuum tubes, capacitors, and punched cards was designed to solve large equations and perform complex mathematical calculations for Atanasoff's students.

## Mark I

In 1944 Professor Howard Aiken, a Harvard University engineer, with the aid of IBM, built the first large-scale automatic electronic computer, the Mark I. It was an electronic calculating device designed to solve mathematical problems. It was the largest machine ever built to incorporate the ideas of Charles Babbage. At Harvard the Mark I was used for several years to calculate ballistic tables for the U.S. Navy (Fig. 2.7).

## ENIAC

The Mark I was followed in 1946 by the ENIAC (**E**lectronic **N**umerical **I**ntegrator **a**nd **C**alculator) built by Presper Eckert, Jr., and Dr. John Mauchly at the University of Pennsylvania. This first general-purpose electronic digital computer weighed 30 tons, contained 18,000 vacuum tubes, and occupied over 15,000 square feet. It was built to assist the U.S. Army. It used decimal numbers and did not store computer programs; each job had to be wired separately.

## Stored Program Concept

It was not until later in 1945 that Dr. John Von Newmann, a mathematician at the Institute for Advanced Studies at Princeton, New Jersey, originated the stored program concept. He stated that the computer could store both numbers (data) and operating instructions (programs) and that

**Figure 2.7**   Harvard's Mark I. (Courtesy IBM Archives.)

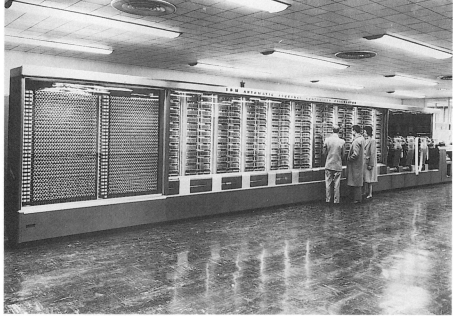

the data could be automatically processed. He also recommended that the computer use the binary (2 numbers) instead of the decimal (10 numbers) system to process data. Von Newmann's principles led to the development of today's computers.

## EDSAC, EDVAC, WHIRLWIND I

As a result of Von Newmann's recommendations, three computers were built between 1947 and 1951 that incorporated the stored program concept and used binary numbers. Even though these computers were experimental, they established the basic architecture for today's computers. In 1949 the first electronic computer was developed outside the United States by Maurice Wilkes of Cambridge University, Great Britain: the EDSAC (**E**lectronic **D**elay **S**torage **A**utomatic **C**alculator). In 1951 the second electronic computer was developed in the United States for the U.S. Army at the Aberdeen Proving Grounds in Maryland by Echert and Mauchley: the EDVAC (**E**lectronic **D**iscrete **V**ariable **A**utomatic **C**omputer). The third, WHIRLWIND I, was built at the Massachusetts Institute of Technology in Cambridge. This computer not only processed data but also was used to design several hardware and software innovations, such as magnetic core memory.

## UNIVAC I

In 1951 UNIVAC I (**Univ**ersal **A**utomatic **C**omputer) was also produced by Eckert and Mauchley, who had left the university to work for the Remington Rand Corporation. It incorporated the stored program concept and used the binary number system. The UNIVAC I consisted of 5,000 vacuum tubes and required a great deal of electric power. It generated a lot of heat, necessitating air-conditioning, and, because of its size, it was expensive to manufacture. It became the first commercially available electronic computer and the first computer to be used by large governmental agencies. Thus, UNIVAC I initiated the computer age and the five computer generations.

## PDP-8

In 1965 the Digital Equipment Corporation (DEC), one of the largest companies in this field, introduced a small, inexpensive computer called a minicomputer. Even though it was no larger than a medium-size file cabinet, it functioned like a larger computer and cost less. The PDP-8 was one of the most popular items in the DEC minicomputer series. During this time IBM introduced its family concept of computers, offering scientific and business applications to large and small organizations; one of these machines was a minicomputer (Fig. 2.8).

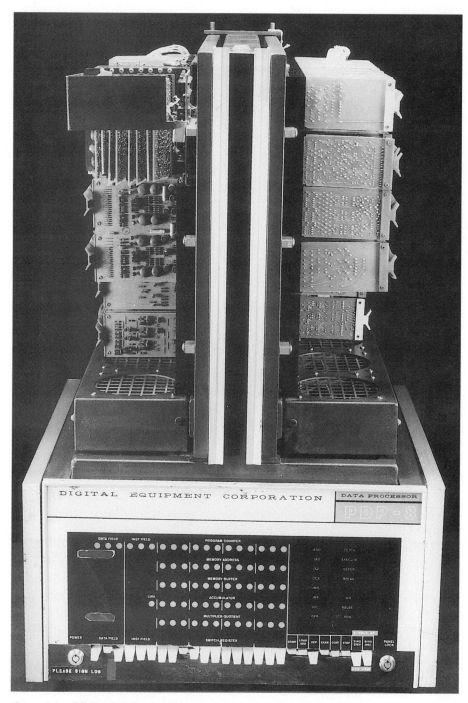

**Figure 2.8** PDP-8 DEC minicomputer. (Smithsonian Institution Photo No. 90-5950.)

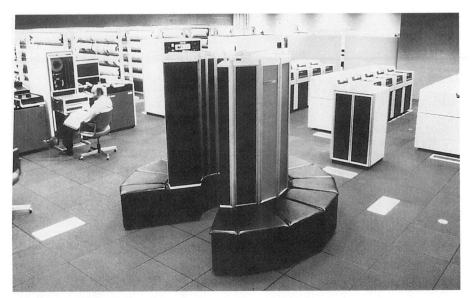

**Figure 2.9**   Cray-I computer installation. (Smithsonian Institution Photo No. 89-20457.)

## Cray-I

In 1976 Seymour Cray developed a large and very fast scientific computer, the Cray-I supercomputer. As the first commercial supercomputer, it could perform millions of calculations per second and process huge amounts of data. Several supercomputers were built for solving lengthy and complex mathematics and engineering problems. They were used by engineers, the scientific community, and the federal government for research on nuclear, space, and other complex problems (Fig. 2.9).

## Altair-8800

The first microcomputer to enter the computer field was offered as a do-it-yourself computer kit for hobbyists. In the January 1975 issue of *Popular Electronics*, it was promoted in an advertisement under the name MITS Altair-8800 and was considered the first commercially available micro-computer (Fig. 2.10).

## MICROCOMPUTER DEVELOPMENTS

Early microcomputers, or personal computers (PCs), were considered single-user machines, whereas mainframes and minicomputers were designed for multiple users. By 1977 several major microcomputer manufacturers had begun to enter the field and produce assembled computers.

In 1977 the first "ready-to-use" microcomputer was the Apple II, developed by Steve Jobs and Steve Wozniack. It had a disk drive using an 8-in. magnetic disk, which became a standard for the early commercial personal computer industry. Tandy Radio Shack's TRS-80 Model 1 and the Commodore PET (Personal Electronic Transactor) were also produced and sold as fully assembled microcomputers. Each brand had a stored memory with tape or disk drives, a keyboard, and a printer (Table 2.3).

By 1981 the microcomputer had begun to have a great impact on the home, school, and business environments. In that year IBM entered the microcomputer field with its PC (personal computer) (Fig. 2.11). Also during that year, the "first portable computer" was introduced by Adam Osborne, the Osborne I (Fig. 2.12). Several different PC clones were also introduced and functioned almost identically to the IBM PC. The IBM clones, such as the Compaq, were generally less expensive than IBM PCs.

In 1983 the first touch screen microcomputer was introduced by Hewlett-Packard. In 1984 the Apple Macintosh introduced the "mouse" to activate and digitize different data items, which were illustrated by icons on the monitor. During this time Kurzweil also introduced the voice synthesizer as another method of activating the microcomputer. In 1984 the introduction of shared data and data communication made it possible for the first local area network (LAN) to be introduced. The LAN advanced the microcomputer from a single-user device to one that could accept multiple users. In the mid-1980s CD-ROM (compact disk read-only memory)

**Figure 2.10**   Altair-8800 microcomputer. (Smithsonian Institution Photo No. 88-19284.)

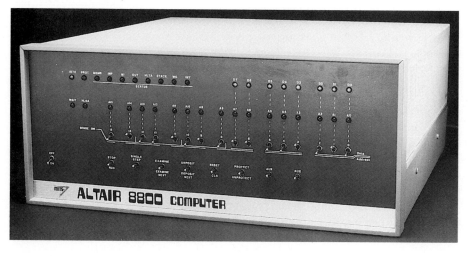

**TABLE 2.3**   MICROCOMPUTER HARDWARE DEVELOPMENTS

| Inventor | Invention | Year |
|---|---|---|
| Ted Hoff | Microprocessor on a chip | 1971 |
| Altair-8800 | Hobbyist do-it-yourself kit: first microcomputer | 1975 |
| IBM | Laser printer | 1975 |
| Steve Jobs and Steve Wozniack | Apple II computer: first assembled microcomputer | 1977 |
| Commodore | PET: fully assembled computer | 1977 |
| Charles Tandy | Radio Shack: TRS-80, Model 1 | 1977 |
| Shugart Assoc. | Floppy diskette, 5¼ in. | 1978 |
| Seagate Tech. | Hard disk (Winchester) | 1980 |
| IBM | IBM PC (personal computer) | 1981 |
| Adam Osborne | Osborne I: first portable computer | 1981 |
| Sony | First interactive video system | 1982 |
| Compaq | First IBM PC clone | 1983 |
| Hewlett-Packard | First touch screen PC | 1983 |
| Kurzweil | Voice synthesizer | 1983 |
| Apple Computer | Macintosh (mouse-driven) | 1984 |
| Magnetic disk | PC floppy diskette 3½ in. | 1984 |
| Data Communication Network | Local area networks | 1984 |
| Optical Disc Corp. | First optical videodisk | 1984 |
| Optical Disc Corp. | Compact disk read-only memory CD-ROM optical storage | 1984 1985 |
| NEC/Zenith | Early laptop computers | 1986 |
| IBM | Info Window touch screen display system | 1986 |
| Pioneer | First CD-ROM disk drives | 1988 |
| Apple | Newton MessagePad computer | 1993 |
| IBM | ThinkPad | 1993 |
| Hewlett-Packard | Palmtop computer | 1993 |
| Dauphin Technology | Pen-based hand-held computer | 1993 |

emerged as an optical storage device. CD-ROM disks are used to store large volumes of data such as encyclopedias, dictionaries, and software libraries. They are used interactively, making these databases available to PC users. CD-ROM has the same format as audio compact disks. By the early 1990s CD-ROM multimedia microcomputer systems became commercially available.

In the late 1980s, as the microcomputer grew more powerful, portable microcomputers became smaller and more compact. In the late 1980s and

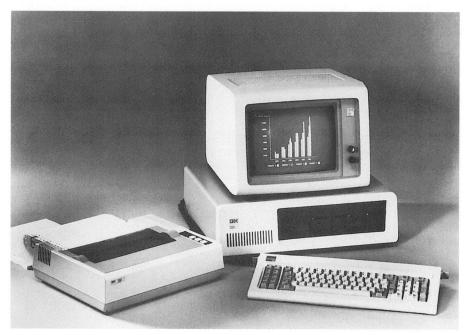

**Figure 2.11**   Personal computer. (Courtesy IBM Archive.)

early 1990s the introduction of laptop and notebook computers made it possible for a microcomputer to be placed in a briefcase. These computers weigh approximately 4 pounds and are the size of the standard piece of paper (8½ by 11 in.).

In 1993 several different versions of notebook, hand-held, pen-based computers emerged. Several notebook computers emerged, including the IBM ThinkPad, NEC Notebook, and Toshiba Dynapad. Hewlett-Packard introduced the Palmtop Computer, and Dauphin Technology introduced its pen-based hand-held computer; the Apple Newton, a MessagePad computer, was also introduced.

The Newton is a "personal digital assistant" that serves as a digital scratch pad, address book, fax machine, and hand-held portable computer. It combines computing power with handwriting recognition and communications capability. This new computer offers a new concept for data processing and storage. It encompasses a new approach to computing technology by using an object-oriented operating system. It has no disk drives, file structures, or directories, yet it interfaces with the large Apple models. The Apple Newton weighs under 1 pound; it is battery-powered and pocket-sized.

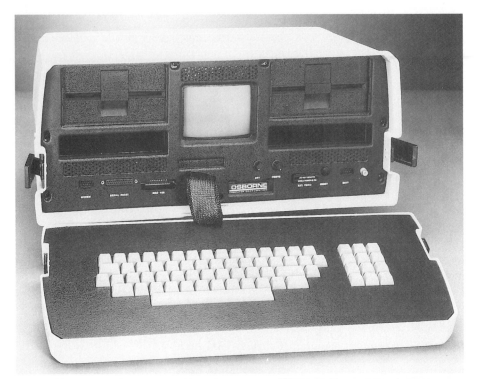

**Figure 2.12**    Osborne portable microcomputer. (Smithsonian Institution Photo No. 86-13443.)

Several hand-held computers are pen-based, paperless, and portable. They are creating a new size of computer and offering a new approach for microcomputer users. These computers are replacing the notepads carried by health professionals and will provide endless applications for tomorrow's users.

## Microcomputer Hardware

Microcomputers led to the creation of many new input, output, and storage media and devices (see Chap. 3 for further details).

### Input Devices

Input devices included tape and disk drives, keyboards that were changed in composition, and printers ranging from dot matrix to laser printers. Floppy disks, also called diskettes, were gradually reduced in size from 8 in. to the standard 5¼ in. or 3½ in. As diskettes shrunk in size, they increased in storage capacity. The 5¼-in. diskettes ranged in storage from 360 thousand bytes (K) to 1.2 million bytes (MB), and the 3½-in. ranged from 720K to 1.44MB.

## Main Memory

The main memory capacity of the initial microcomputers was very small and was measured in bytes (characters). In the mid-1980s, as microprocessor chips increased in capacity, main memory also increased in capacity from 4K to 640K and then to the 1MB, 2MB, 8MB, and even 16MB range. This new capacity equaled and even surpassed that of many of the earlier minicomputers and mainframe computers.

## Storage Media

Early microcomputers used the magnetic disks that continue to be the preferred media for secondary storage. They include both floppy disks and hard disks. Floppy disks provide off-line storage, and hard disks provide on-line storage. Hard disks are generally permanently installed in the microcomputer. As the technology advanced, the number of hard disks that could be installed in a microcomputer increased in number and storage capacity. Thus, early hard disks that stored 64K expanded to hard disks that could store from 20MB to over 500MB. Hard disks continue to expand in storage capacity, and microcomputers can also be enhanced with external hard disks.

# Microcomputer Software

As the microcomputer advanced, computer programs (software) were developed specifically to make single-user microcomputers user-friendly (Table 2.4) (see Chap. 4 for further details).

## High-Level Languages

The first high-level language for the microprocessor was BASIC (**B**eginners **A**ll-Purpose **S**ymbolic **I**nstruction **C**ode), which was developed at Dartmouth as an easy-to-learn high-level language. It was adapted by Paul Allen and Bill Gates to become Microsoft BASIC, the first programming language specifically designed for the microcomputer. It was followed by several other high-level languages that were adapted for the microcomputer, such as MUMPS.

## Operating Systems

The development and introduction of an operating system (OS) led to the use of a control unit for the microcomputer. An operating system is a set of computer programs that provide the user with control of the computer's resources. The operating system is essential for the computer to function.

In 1976 the first operating system, the CP/M (central program for microprocessors), was introduced by Gary Kidall and was then used in many computers. Apple Corporation developed its own operating system, which was inherent only in Apple computers. In 1980 Bill Gates of Microsoft introduced another operating system, the Microsoft Disk Operating

**TABLE 2.4**     MICROCOMPUTER SOFTWARE DEVELOPMENTS

| Inventor | Invention | Year |
|---|---|---|
| Nolan Bushnell | Atari video game | 1972 |
| Paul Allen | Microsoft: BASIC interpreter | 1975 |
| Bill Gates and Gary Kidall | CP/M operating system | 1976 |
| Don Bricklin and Bob Frankston | VisiCalc: spreadsheet package | 1979 |
| Paul Lutus | AppleWriter: word processing | 1979 |
| Rob Barnaby | WordStar: word processing | 1979 |
| Bill Gates | MS-DOS: microsoft disk operating system | 1980 |
| Wayne Ratliff and Ashton-Tate | dBASE II: database package | 1981 |
| Jonathan Sachs and Michell Kapor | Lotus 1-2-3: spreadsheet package | 1982 |
| WordPerfect | WordPerfect: word processing | 1984 |
| Microsoft (MS) | MS Windows: operating system, keyboard version | 1985 |
| Aldus | PageMaker: desktop publishing | 1986 |
| Microsoft (MS) | MS Windows: operating system, mouse version | 1990 |
| Microsoft (MS) | MS Windows/NT: operating system | 1994 |
| IBM | OS/2 Version 2: operating system | 1994 |
| Apple/IBM | Power PC: operating system | 1994 |
| Sun Microsystems | Solaris Unix: operating system | 1994 |

System (MS-DOS). MS-DOS was adopted in 1981 by IBM for its first personal computer (IBM PC). MS-DOS has gone through several versions, has constantly been enhanced, and has persisted for several years as the most widely used operating system for the IBM PC and its clones. MS-DOS is a separate software package that is provided with the purchase of an IBM PC or clone.

In 1985 Bill Gates introduced a new operating system called Microsoft Windows to run on PCs with MS-DOS. It was designed to provide a graphical interface with the existing MS-DOS. It was introduced as a keyboard version but was enhanced in 1990, when it appeared with a mouse version. (A mouse is a hand-held device that moves the cursor on the screen.) Microsoft Windows makes the PC more accessible and powerful. In this environment keystrokes, mouse actions, and commands are achieved by pressing a shortcut key or selecting a macro name. MS Windows gives the appearance of an Apple Macintosh to the IBM PC or any other computer that uses it as an OS. It can do this because it is a shell, a program that uses icons (graphic symbols) to illustrate and send commands, for example, a "file cabinet" to represent graphically the use of the "file manager." Windows also manages other software packages specifically developed to run under it. It is considered more user-friendly than MS-DOS.

In the early 1990s several other new operating systems with enhanced capabilities emerged for the PC. Microsoft Windows introduced its version, the "newest technology Microsoft Windows," or MS-Windows/NT. This new operating system is similar to the new operating system introduced by IBM, the PC Operating System Version 2 (OS/2). Still another operating system was introduced by Apple Corporation, the Power PC, along with a version of UNIX, Solaris Unix, used in minicomputers, introduced by Sun Microsystems for microcomputer workstations.

These new operating systems all offer several advanced features: (1) multiuser, multitasking processing, (2) a built-in graphical interface, (3) built-in networking capability, and (4) the ability to run applications developed for different operating systems. These multitasking and multiuser operating systems make it possible to share processing resources with LANs and facilitate communications between LAN terminals and/or workstations.

## Software Packages

The use of an operating system makes it possible for ready-to-use software packages to be run on the microcomputer. Generally, software packages are generic; that is, they are standardized computer programs designed for a specific type of process, not for a specific application or user. For example, word processing, spreadsheets, and database management are the major types of software packages available for microcomputer users.

In 1979 Dan Bricklin and Bob Frankston introduced VisiCalc, the first ready-to-use, user-friendly computer program. It was considered the first software package. VisiCalc was designed for "number crunching" and could generate any type of spreadsheet, for example, one that could be used for financial management. In 1979 word-processing software packages were introduced to prepare written documents and reports. The two major word-processing software packages were AppleWriter introduced by Paul Lutus and WordStar introduced by Rob Barnaby.

During the 1980s several other types of specialized software packages emerged. In 1982 Wayne Ratliff introduced a database management package, dBASE II, that was designed to organize large files of data. In 1982 Michell Kapor introduced a friendlier spreadsheet package, Lotus 1-2-3, that quickly replaced VisiCalc. WordPerfect was introduced in around 1984; it quickly replaced WordStar and has become the word-processing software package of choice for preparing documents. During the 1980s other software packages were introduced in the field as new types or enhancements of other types. Some of the newer packages introduced in the field include Microsoft Word for word processing, QuattroPro as a spreadsheet,

Paradox for database management, Harvard Graphics for graphic displays, and PageMaker for desktop publishing.

## Communication Networks

The introduction of communication networks emerged as computer technology advanced. The original on-line communication networks were analog systems that used telephone communication lines, whereas today networks are using fiber-optic digital communication systems. In the 1970s, the early networks communicated by using telephone lines. They were used primarily by commercial vendors that offered on-line services, such as CompuServe. During the 1970s, fiber-optic digital networks also began to be used to communicate and transmit data. The Advanced Research Projects Agency Network (ARPANET), designed by the Department of Defense, was created to link major research centers that conducted military research; this required high-speed computing power. In the 1980s ARPANET was replaced by the National Science Foundation Network (NSFNET), which also linked supercomputers in large research centers and universities with one another.

### Internet

In the 1990s on-line digital networks expanded radically. As a result, a nationwide system of linked supercomputers was created: Internet. Internet is a network of networks that not only provides on-line communication services to other users and networks on the network but also offers them the resources of the network. It offers communication services, transfer of data text files, E-mail, bulletin boards, and a multitude of other on-line services and resources. Internet is being used by federal agencies, universities, and organizations as an information-sharing network.

The story of microcomputer history is ongoing, fluctuating almost daily. The microcomputer industry has one major feature: It will persist and will always be changing. New hardware architecture, software platforms, and communication technologies will make microcomputers more powerful in the future. The main effect of the microcomputer is to make the computer available to everyone in the home, linking its users with millions of others around the world.

## COMPUTER GENERATIONS

The history of the computer would be incomplete without a description of computer generations. Beginning in the 1940s, each generation of computers represented advances in electronic components. Generally, these components (or logic circuits) were replaced by devices that improved the computer's processing power. An overview depicts the rapid changes that

**TABLE 2.5**    COMPUTER GENERATIONS

| Generation | Electronic Component | Years |
|---|---|---|
| First | Vacuum tubes (1951–1958) | 1950s |
| Second | Transistors (1959–1963) | Early 1960s |
| Third | Integrated circuit (1964–1970) and/or Large-scale integrated circuit | Late 1960s |
| Fourth | Microprocessor | 1971–present |
| Fifth | Microprocessor on a chip | 1975–present |

have occurred in recent computer history. There are many opinions regarding the number and dates of the computer generations, but most authorities agree that there have been five generations (Table 2.5). Computer generations are usually defined according to their electronic components. They include the following:

- First generation: vacuum tubes
- Second generation: transistors
- Third generation: integrated circuits (ICs) and large-scale integrated circuits (LSICs)
- Fourth generation: microprocessors
- Fifth generation: microprocessor on a chip and integrated processor on a chip

## First Generation

### Vacuum Tubes

The first generation of commercial computers emerged in the 1950s (1951–1958). Their logic devices consisted of vacuum tubes that resembled electric light bulbs. These computers generated a great deal of heat and thus required air-conditioning, had limited storage capacity, and primarily used punched cards and magnetic drums for storage (Fig. 2.13).

The first-generation computers were programmed by writing machine language using binary digits (0s and 1s), which was tedious. Commodore Grace Hopper of the U.S. Navy, along with her research computer staff at Harvard, developed the first language-translator program, which she called a compiler. It was a set of programs that could translate code and/or symbolic languages into machine language. She coined the term "debug" when she had to remove a moth from the processing unit (Fig. 2.14).

During this generation Sperry Rand Corporation produced the first commercial computer: UNIVAC I. Several other computer companies—IBM, RCA, Burroughs, National Cash Register, and Honeywell—also entered the field, developing alternative versions of the first-generation computer.

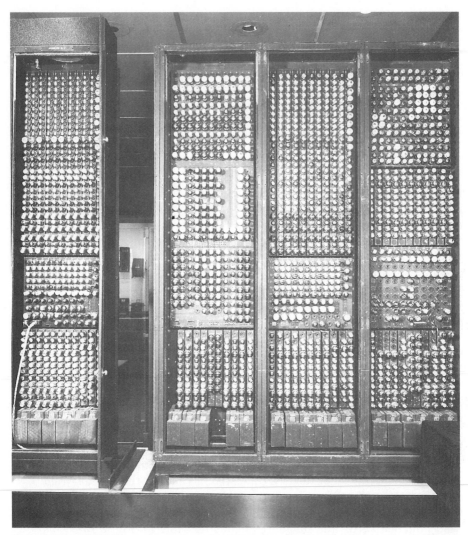

**Figure 2.13**   ENIAC vacuum tubes. (Smithsonian Institution Photo No. 61799-A.)

## Second Generation

### Transistors

Second-generation computers prevailed in the early 1960s (1959–1963). They were characterized by the use of transistors, which were developed by Bell Laboratories to replace vacuum tubes. Transistors were smaller, faster, and more flexible and reliable than vacuum tubes. Furthermore, they required less electric power, generated less heat, and were cheaper to produce.

Transistors increased the speed and storage capacity of second-generation computers, which used magnetic core storage, magnetic tapes, and disks for input, output, and secondary storage. Because of their characteristics, second-generation computers were advertised as being more reliable and having a larger memory. These computers were programmed using advances in software development, including a mnemonic code for assembly languages, low-level languages, and early high-level programming languages. The first high-level programming languages were FORTRAN (**For**mula **Tran**slator) for engineers and COBOL (**C**ommon **B**usiness-**O**riented **L**anguage) for business programmers.

## Third Generation

### Integrated Circuits

Third-generation computers were introduced in the mid-1960s (1964–1970). They were characterized by integrated circuits (ICs), which were electronic transistor circuits etched onto small silicon wafers. A generation breakthrough, they replaced transistors. ICs lasted longer because they did not require fragile wires like those used in transistors. They were

**Figure 2.14**   Grace Hopper and colleagues at the UNIVAC. (Smithsonian Institution Photo No. 83-4878.)

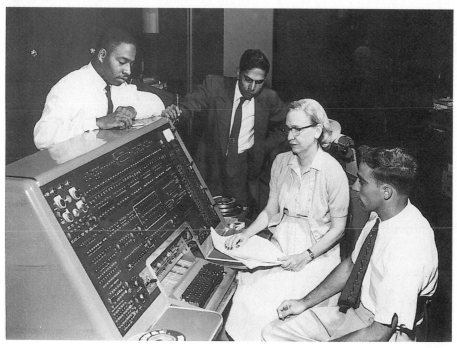

faster, more reliable, and more compact. Because of their size, they required less electric power, generated less heat, and were cheaper to produce. ICs led to the production of faster, more reliable, and more efficient computers, with increased storage capacity and processing speed.

Third-generation computers used magnetic disks for input, output, and secondary storage. Many new high-level programming languages were developed during this period. The first "operating system," CP/M, which made it possible to process more than one computer program at a time (multiprogramming), was introduced. The operating system also made it possible to communicate with the mainframe computer via on-line terminals. As a result, many users at different locations could access the computer at one time.

### Large-Scale Integrated Circuits

Computer experts differ on when the third generation of computers ended and the fourth generation began. However, some experts include the introduction of large-scale integrated circuits (LSICs) in the third generation, and others consider them to be part of the fourth generation. LSICs were microminiaturized circuits that were chemically etched on silicon chips; they are commonly known as chips.

LSICs contained advanced circuitry and were extremely sophisticated. Computers using these chips had increased storage capacity, reliability, and durability and had the processing speed of mainframes and minicomputers. They could store large amounts of data in auxiliary storage devices. Also, advances in data communication allowed these computers to communicate electronically with each other, be accessed by users via terminals at remote sites, and be shared (timesharing) by multiple users employing telephone lines or other communication methods that involved integrated software.

In this generation spectacular growth was also seen in the development of minicomputers. IBM introduced its concept of a family of computers, one of which was a minicomputer, offering scientific and business applications to large and small organizations.

## Fourth Generation

### Microprocessor

In 1971 the introduction of the microprocessor started the fourth generation of computers. This invention was considered evolutionary rather than revolutionary. The first microprocessor, the Intel 4004, was developed by Ted Hoff of Intel, a company founded by Robert Noyce. It was a single silicon chip, approximately ⅙ in. long and ⅛ in. wide, that contained 2,250 microminiaturized transistor circuits. The microprocessor is the heart and brains of the microcomputer. It contains the computing power needed to process hundreds of instructions and tell other components of the system what to do.

# Fifth Generation

### Microprocessor on a Chip

The first microprocessor on a chip is considered to have started the fifth generation. Ted Hoff conceptualized that a microprocessor could contain the arithmetic and logic circuitry needed for computer computations and that these circuits could be packed onto one chip, resulting in a single programmable microprocessor called a microprocessor on a chip. This chip contains the arithmetic logic unit (ALU) that performs the calculations and logical decisions needed to process data and the control unit that organizes the work. Together, they contain the components of a computer's central processing unit (CPU); when combined with a memory chip, they became a "microcomputer" (Figs. 2.15 and 2.16).

### Microprocessor Developments

Microprocessors (chips) doubled in processing capability with each technological advance. They advanced from processing one word, or 8 bits (characters), to 16 bits (two words), 32 bits (four words), and 64 bits (eight words) at a time. The early microcomputers developed by Radio Shack used the Z-80 microprocessor chip to process 8 bits (one word), whereas the early IBM PCs and IBM clones used the Intel 8086, 8088, and 80286 microprocessor chips to process 16 bits (two words). As the Intel chips advanced, the 80386, 80486, and pentium (80586) microprocessor chips processed 32 bits and 64 bits. The Motorola 68000 microprocessor was also introduced to process 32 bits for Apple Macintosh and Radio Shack TRS-80 computers. Their newer 68020, 68030, and 68040 microprocessors (chips) followed and were used for the Apple Macintosh, the NeXT computer, and the Hewlett-Packard workstation (Table 2.6). The newest 64-bit Power PC is being used in both IBM and Apple Macintosh microcomputers.

**Figure 2.15**    Chip configuration. (Smithsonian Institution Photo No. 77-6966.)

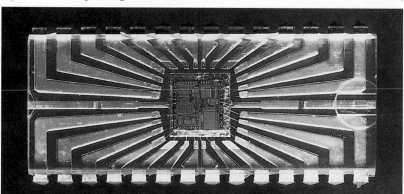

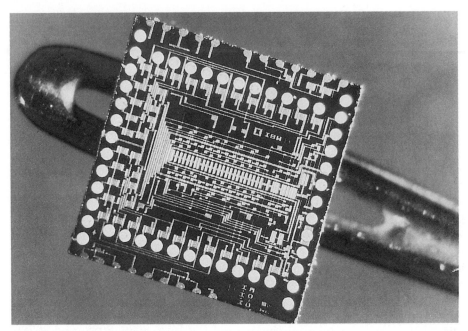

**Figure 2.16**   Integrated circuit chip. (Courtesy IBM Archives.)

## Processors on a Chip

There are essentially two types of microprocessors on a chip. The initial "complex instruction set computing" (CISC) processor on a chip processes data one instruction at a time. The newer type is the "reduced instruction set computer" (RISC) processor on a chip; it is smaller, faster, and more powerful. It altered CISC processing from one instruction to sets of multiple instructions. This new capability makes it possible not only to reduce and simplify the number of instructions needed to process a program but also to increase the processing speed. Thus, the RISC chip is changing the processing capabilities of microcomputers; however, it requires a more

**TABLE 2.6**   COMPARISON OF MAJOR MICROPROCESSORS

| Company | Operating System | Microprocessor | Word Size |
|---|---|---|---|
| Intel | CP/M: Radio Shack | Z-80 | 4–8 bits |
| Intel | IBM: MS-DOS PC | 8086/88 | 8–16 bits |
| Intel | IBM: MS-DOS PC | 80286 | 16 bits |
| Intel | IBM: MS-DOS PC | 80386 | 16–32 bits |
| Intel | IBM: MS-DOS PC | 80486 | 32 bits |
| Intel | IBM: PS/2, Model 80 | Pentium (80586) | 64 bits |
| Motorola | Apple: Macintosh | 68000 | 32 bits |
| Motorola | Apple; NeXT | 68020/30/40 | 32 bits |
| Motorola | IBM PC and Apple Macintosh | Power PC | 64 bits |

complex computer that is easier to program but harder and more costly to build. The RISC processor on a chip offers many new features and functions for newer computers.

# New Technologies

Advances in computer technology continue to emerge and are considered as enhancing the fifth generation. These advances include optical computing, gigachips with billions of transistors, superconductivity to develop resistance-free states, nanotechnology, molecular conductivity, virtual reality, and high-speed performance computing using the Internet. The new technologies are being viewed as key innovations for the biomedical sciences.

### Virtual Reality

Virtual reality is an emerging technology that depicts three-dimensional reality. It requires not only advanced hardware headsets to view actual images on some type of video display but also special software that simulates actual situations or environments. A digitized human is now being used to depict humans in virtual reality simulations.

### Internet

The Internet has been expanded to create an invisible electronic information highway. It is a network of networks, linking millions of users around the world. Internet not only offers services such as E-mail, bulletin boards, and the transfer of data files using a file transfer protocol (FTP) but also provides linkages to on-line resources around the world. It allows hospitals, clinics, doctors' offices, and universities as well as health care providers, educators, researchers, and other users to share and communicate health care data.

### Software Advances

Computer advances have also emerged that are (1) emulating aspects of human thought or artificial intelligence, (2) solving complex problems by using expert systems and neural networks, (3) processing the English language by using natural language programs, and (4) performing high-speed processing by using parallel processing platforms. The majority of expert systems are based on deductive reasoning; given a large body of facts, the expert system works through it by following a set of prescribed rules.

More recently, computer scientists have been trying to equip expert systems with the power to reason inductively. These new systems, using natural language programs, and/or neural networks, are designed to generate probabilities in order to produce realistic guesses. When "what if–then" questions that represent basic rules are used, programs can be applied to specific problems with known answers, so that the results can be checked and the software modified accordingly.

Since 1990 Americans and Japanese have been competing to achieve the goals outlined as characteristic of the next generation. They are continuing to research new types of computer hardware architecture and software for tomorrow's computers. Despite these activities, there is still much discussion on what the next generation of computers will look like and when it will appear.

## COMPUTER INDUSTRY GROWTH

The growth of the computer industry has been revolutionary. In the early 1950s, when computers were commercially introduced, only a few large-scale models existed. However, by the mid-1950s almost 1,000 computers, primarily owned by the federal government, were in existence and by 1958 approximately 2,550 computers were being used in the United States. By the mid-1960s an estimated 18,200 large general-purpose computers were functioning.

By 1970 an estimated 100,000 computers were in operation, and in 1976, more than 20 years after the introduction of computers, the number had increased to 220,000. By 1980 an estimated 500,000 microcomputers existed. In 1981 an estimated 313,000 microcomputers were sold, and the number jumped into the millions by 1983.

With the use of the microprocessor in various games, automobiles, and appliances, the total number of computers grew to over 100 million in 1986. It is estimated that this number increased to 1.1 billion in 1991 and 2.2 billion in 1992. In 1990 there were more than 10,000 companies in the computer industry, compared with approximately a dozen companies in the 1960s. In 1993, 328,000 customers signed up for on-line computer services, bringing the number of homes reached by on-line services to 3.9 million. Today microcomputers not only are used for business, scientific, and medical applications but have become common household items.

## SUMMARY

This chapter provided an overview of the historical development of the computer. It described the many people and inventions that led to the creation of modern computers: mainframes, supercomputers, minicomputers, and microcomputers.

Early computer developments began with several computing devices: the abacus, Napier's "bones" rods, Pascal's Pascaline, Leibniz's calculator, Jacquard's loom, Babbage's analytical engine, and Hollerith's tabulator and sorter. Recent computer developments began during World War II to assist the military. The first electronic computer was the Mark I, followed by the ENIAC. The introduction of the stored program concept and the use of the binary number system led to the development of the EDSAC, EDVAC, and WHIRLWIND I, which were used to test and perfect these concepts and led to the production of the first commercial computer (UNIVAC I), the first minicomputer (PDP-8), the first supercomputer (Cray-I), and the first microcomputer (Altair).

The next section described the growth of the microcomputer, including an overview of microcomputer hardware and software developments. The five generations in the computer age were also discussed: vacuum tubes, transistors, integrated circuits, microprocessors, and the microprocessor on a chip. The introduction of the microprocessor on a chip revolutionized the computer industry and made possible the microcomputer. The chapter concluded with a description of new technologies, including a brief overview of the growth of the computer industry.

## BIBLIOGRAPHY

Abelson, P., and Hammond, A. (1977, Mar. 18). The electronics revolution. *Science*, 1087–1091.

The age of miracle chips. (1978, Feb. 20). *Time*, 44–45.

Bernstein, J. (1976, Feb. 15). When the computer procreates. *New York Times Magazine*, 34–38.

Boraiko, A. (1982). The chip: Electronic minimarvel that is changing your life. *National Geographic*, 162(4), 421–458.

Brookshear, J. G. (1991). *Computer Science: An Overview* (3d ed.). New York: Benjamin/Cummings.

Bylinsky, G. (1975, Nov.). Here comes the second computer revolution. *Fortune*, 92, 134–138, 182, 184.

Capron, H. L. (1990). *Computers: Tools for the Information Age* (2d ed.). Menlo Park, CA: Benjamin/Cummings.

Capron, H. L., and Williams, B. K. (1990). *Computers and Data Processing* (2d ed.). Menlo Park, CA: Benjamin/Cummings.

Covert, C. (1983). Chip shots: A brief history of the indispensable silicon chip. *TWA Ambassador, 16*(1), 102–106.

Davis, M. (1983). The chip at 35. *Personal Computing, 8*(7), 127–131.

Denning, P. J. (1971). Third generation computer systems. *Computer Survey, 3*(4), 176–213.

Editors of Time-Life Books. (1987). *Revolution in Science.* Alexandria, VA: Time-Life Books.

Editors of Time-Life Books. (1988). *The Chipmakers.* Alexandria, VA: Time-Life Books.

Editors of Time-Life Books. (1989). *Personal Computer.* Alexandria, VA: Time-Life Books.

Editors of Time-Life Books. (1989). *Understanding Computers: Illustrated Chronology and Index.* Alexandria, VA: Time-Life Books.

Enlander, D. (1980). *Computers in Medicine: An Introduction.* St. Louis: Mosby.

Frederick, O. (1983, Jan. 3). The computer moves in. *Time,* 14–24.

Golden, F. (1983, Jan. 3). Big dimwits and little geniuses. *Time,* 30–32.

Graham, N. (1986). *The Mind Tool: Computers and Their Impact on Society* (4th ed.). New York: West.

Hart, A. (1992). *Knowledge Acquisition for Expert Systems* (2d ed.). New York: McGraw-Hill.

Hopper, G. M., and Mandell, S. L. (1987). *Understanding Computers* (2d ed.). New York: West.

Hutchinson, S. E., and Sawyer, S. C. (1988). *Computers: The User Perspective* (2d ed.). Boston: Irwin.

Institute of New Generation Computer Technology. (1983). Outline of research and development plans for fifth-generation computer systems. *Byte, 5*(46), 396–401.

International Business Machines. (1974). *More about Computers.* Armonk, NY: IBM.

Libes, S. (1983). Editor's page. *Microsystems, 4*(5), 8–9.

Machine of the year: The computer moves in. (1983, Jan. 3). *Time, 121*(1), 13–40.

Mandell, S. L. (1985). *Introduction to Computers Using the IBM PC.* New York: West.

Mandell, S. L. (1986). *Computers and Data Processing Today: With Basic* (2d ed.). New York: West.

Maynard, M. M. (1983). UNIVAC I. In A. Ralston and E. D. Reilly, Jr. (Eds.), *Encyclopedia of computer science and engineering* (2d ed.) (pp. 1546–1547). New York: Van Nostrand Reinhold.

McKeown, P. G. (1986). *Living with Computers.* New York: Harcourt Brace Jovanovich.

McLeod, R., Jr., and Forkner, I. (1982). *Computerized Business Information System: An Introduction to Data Processing.* New York: John Wiley.

Pfaffenberger, B. (1991). *Que's Computer User's Dictionary.* Carmel, IN: Que Corp.

Pylyshyn, Z. W. (Ed.). (1970). *Perspectives on the Computer Revolution.* Englewood Cliffs, NJ: Prentice-Hall.

Popyk, M. K. (1988). *Up and Running! Microcomputer Applications.* New York: Addison-Wesley.

Ralston, A., and Reilly, E. D., Jr. (Eds.). (1983). *Encyclopedia of Computer Science and Engineering* (2d ed.). New York: Van Nostrand Reinhold.

Randell, B. (1983). Digital computers: History: Origins. In A. Ralston and E. D. Reilly, Jr. (Eds.), *Encyclopedia of Computer Science and Engineering* (2d ed.) (pp. 532–535). New York: Van Nostrand Reinhold.

Reid, T. R. (1982, July 25). Birth of a new idea. *Washington Post,* B1, B5.

Rosen, S. (1969). Electronic computers: A historical survey. *Computer Survey, 1*(1), 7–36.

Rosen, S. (1983). Digital computers: History: Contemporary and future. In A. Ralston and E. D. Reilly, Jr. (Eds.), *Encyclopedia of Computer Science and Engineering* (2d ed.) (pp. 540–554). New York: Van Nostrand Reinhold.

Roth, A. D. (1983). Japanese fifth generation initiative: How will it impact the U.S. Government. *Computer News, 2*(6), 1, 14–15.

Rowan, H. (1980, Mar. 16). High industry productivity. *Washington Post,* G1–G2.

Sanders, D. H. (1970). *Computers and Management.* New York: McGraw-Hill.

Schnaidt, P. (1990). *LAN Tutorial with Glossary of Terms.* New York: Miller Freeman.

Schrage, M. (1983, Jan. 1). Xerox scientist to head supercomputer effort. *Washington Post,* C7.

Science: The numbers game. (1978, Feb. 20). *Time,* 54–58.

Shaw, M (1983). Ada. In A. Ralston and E. D. Reilly, Jr. (Eds.), *Encyclopedia of Computer Science and Engineering* (2d ed.) (pp. 8–11). New York: Van Nostrand Reinhold.

Shelly, G. B., and Cashman, T. J. (1984). *Computer Fundamentals for an Information Age.* Brea, CA: Anaheim.

Shore, J. (1989). *Using Computers in Business.* Carmel, IN: Que Corp.

Stern, R. A., and Stern, N. (1982). *An Introduction to Computers and Information Processing.* New York: John Wiley.

Sullivan, D. R., Lewis, T. G., and Cook, C. R. (1985). *Computing Today: Microcomputer Concepts and Applications.* Boston: Houghton Mifflin.

Sullivan, D. R., Lewis, T. G., and Cook, C. R. (1986). *Using Computers Today.* Boston: Houghton Mifflin.

Vacroux, A. G. (1975). Microcomputers. *Science America, 232*(5), 32–40.

Wilkes, M. V. (1983). Babbage, Charles. In A. Ralston and E. D. Reilly, Jr. (Eds.), *Encyclopedia of Computer Science and Engineering* (2d ed.) (pp. 157–158). New York: Van Nostrand Reinhold.

Wilkes, M. V. (1983). Digital computers: History: Early. In A. Ralston and E. D. Reilly, Jr. (Eds.), *Encyclopedia of Computer Science and Engineering* (2d ed.) (pp. 535–540). New York: Van Nostrand Reinhold.

Williams, M. R. (1985). *A History of Computer Technology.* Englewood Cliffs, NJ: Prentice-Hall.

Yau, S. S., and Brasch, F. M. (1983). Computer circuiting. In A. Ralston and E. D. Reilly, Jr. (Eds.), *Encyclopedia of Computer Science and Engineering* (2d ed.) (pp. 306–317). New York: Van Nostrand Reinhold.

# THE COMPUTER

# 3

· · · · · · · · · · · · · · · · · · · · · · · ·

# COMPUTER HARDWARE

## OBJECTIVES

- Define and describe a computer.
- Describe computer classes and types.
- Describe four functional components of a computer.
- Identify computer devices and media.
- Describe computer communications.

The "computer age" has evolved from electronic calculators to programmable information-processing machines to new tools that are used in all areas of people's lives. Today, in the health care industry and especially in the nursing profession, computers are used to process data for patient care. Computers serve as tools for a variety of nursing activities.

Computer hardware refers to a computer's physical components: the machine itself, the parts one can see and touch. The computer consists of many different component parts, including external or peripheral devices that enable it to process data. To understand how a computer processes data, it is necessary to examine the component parts and devices of computer hardware.

This chapter covers various aspects of computer hardware: classes, characteristics, and types. It also highlights the functional components of

the computer and describes the devices and media that are used to communicate, store, and process data. It includes the following major categories:

- Definition of a computer
- Computer classes
- Computer types
- Computer functional components
- Computer communications

## DEFINITION OF A COMPUTER

The computer is an electronic information-processing machine that
processes data under the direction of stored sequences of instructions (programs). It uses various input and output devices to communicate with the
user. In essence, it is a machine that accepts data as input, stores data in
a structured form, processes data by performing arithmetic and logical
operations, and generates the results as output.

A computer is generally described in terms of several major characteristics—automatic, electronic, general-purpose—and in terms of speed, reliability, and storage capacity. A computer is "automatic" because it is
self-instructed; that is, it automatically processes data by using programs
called software. A computer is "electronic" because it uses microelectronic
components etched on silicon chips for its circuitry. This means that
its basic building blocks are microminiaturized. A computer is "general-
purpose" because the user can program it to process all types of problems
and can solve any problem that can be broken down into a set of logical
sequential instructions. A computer is also characterized by its "speed"
and split-second processing of large amounts of data, its "reliability"
resulting from the silicon circuitry, and its ability to "store" large amounts
of data that can be retrieved quickly.

A computer is also described by its architecture: the design of the individual hardware components and the microprocessor used. The hardware
platform refers to the standard of the specific hardware as characterized
by the manufacturer of the computer, such as IBM, Apple Corporation, or
Hewlett-Packard.

## COMPUTER CLASSES

Three broad classes of computers exist:

- Analog
- Digital
- Hybrid

## Analog Computer

An analog computer operates on continuous physical or electrical magnitudes, measuring ongoing continuous quantities such as voltage, current, temperature, and pressure. Selected physiological monitoring equipment that accepts continuous signals is also an analog computer. An analog computer handles data in continuously variable quantities rather than digitizing the data or transforming them into discrete digital representations.

## Digital Computer

A digital computer, by contrast, operates on discrete discontinuous numerical digits, using the binary numbering system. It represents data by using discrete values for all data and instructions that are represented by numbers, letters, and symbols. The data are coded by using combinations of machine-readable binary digits (1s or 0s) that signify on and off impulses. A digital computer solves problems by performing arithmetic calculations and logical comparisons on data in digital form. Because most computers used in the health care industry are digital, aside from various types of physiological monitoring equipment, this book focuses on digital computers unless otherwise specified.

## Hybrid Computer

A hybrid computer, as its name implies, contains features of both the analog computer and the digital computer. It is used for specific applications such as complex signal processing. It is also found in some monitoring equipment that converts analog signals to digital ones for data processing.

## COMPUTER TYPES

Four basic types of computers exist. These types were developed as the computer industry evolved, and each was developed for a different purpose. The basic types of computers are supercomputers, mainframes, minicomputers, and microcomputers. These computers differ in size, composition, memory and storage capacity, processing time, and cost. They generally have had different applications and are found in many different areas of the health care industry.

## Supercomputers

The largest type of computer is the supercomputer. A supercomputer is a computation-oriented computer that is specially designed for scientific applications requiring large amounts of calculations. It is extremely large, fast, and expensive. The supercomputer is designed primarily for the analysis of scientific and engineering problems and tasks requiring extensive computational manipulations and calculations. It is used primarily in areas such as defense and weaponry, weather forecasting, and scientific research. The supercomputer is also providing a new source of power for the high-performance computing and communication (HPCC) environment.

## Mainframes

The mainframe computer is the fastest, largest, and one of the most expensive types of computer used for processing, storing, and retrieving data. It is a large multiuser central computer that meets the transactional computing needs of a large organization. A mainframe can process millions of instructions per second and access billions (gigabytes) of characters of data. A mainframe computer serves a large number (hundreds) of users via input/output terminals that can be located close to (local) or far from (remote) the central computer. The users are connected to the central computer on-line through a communication network.

A mainframe is composed of a central console, on-line cathode ray tube (CRT) terminals used as input devices, and a central processing unit (CPU) with main memory (primary storage), secondary storage (auxiliary memory), and on-line printers used as output devices. The console is a terminal used by an operator to run the CPU. CRT terminals are used to display the data being transmitted to the CPU for processing and/or to a printer to produce a hard copy of the information processed by the computer.

A mainframe has an extremely large memory and fast operating and processing times and can process several functions at one time (multiprocessing). The secondary storage uses storage devices that are directly accessible to the main memory. The CPU and secondary storage devices are usually located together in a specially designed room equipped with temperature and humidity controls that is separate from the input/output terminals (Fig. 3.1).

Mainframes are used for efficient management of data. They are used to collect, store, and process extensive amounts of data from many sources to provide timely information for decision making. They simplify data processing, improve performance, and reduce the cost of data processing. Mainframes are found in large health care facilities, generally hospitals, state health departments, and community health agencies. They are used for processing in large-scale integrated hospital information systems.

## Minicomputers

A minicomputer is a smaller version of the mainframe. This term also refers to a multiuser central computer that meets the computing needs of a small organization. A minicomputer is composed of essentially the same

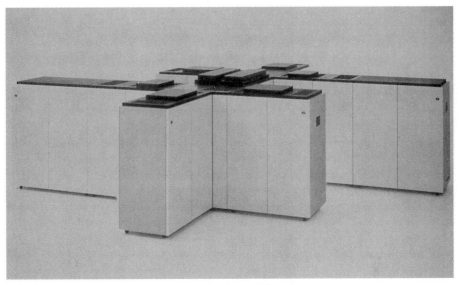

**Figure 3.1**   Mainframe computer. (Courtesy IBM.)

hardware as a mainframe but is smaller and weighs much less; it can be placed on a desk or in the corner of a room. Unlike a mainframe, it does not require a special air-conditioned facility. The minicomputer traditionally serves a smaller number of local and remote terminals, has less memory and secondary storage, and has slower operating and processing speeds than the mainframe. Because it costs less than a mainframe, a large number of users can afford to purchase a minicomputer outright (Fig. 3.2).

Minicomputers are found in many medium-size hospitals and community health agencies. They are used for similar applications as mainframes, but on a smaller scale. However, in hospitals they are generally found in specialty departments, such as the laboratory, pharmacy, or nursing department, and are programmed to process the operations of the specific specialty. Today the distinctions between mainframes and minicomputers are diminishing.

## Microcomputers

The microcomputer is the newest and smallest type of computer. It is called a personal, a desktop, or a home computer. With the introduction of the microprocessor on a chip, the microcomputer became a reality and has made computer power accessible to most providers in the health care industry. Early microcomputers were designed to be operated by one user and to process one "job" (computer program) at a time. The early microcomputer can be identified by its small main memory capacity (512K). However, beginning

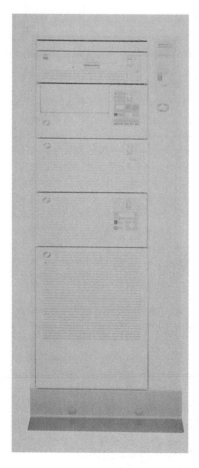

**Figure 3.2**   Minicomputer. (Courtesy IBM.)

in the mid-1980s, as newer microcomputer models emerged, they became available with several megabytes (MB) of random access memory (RAM) ranging from 1, 2, 4, and 8MB to 16MB RAM and are continuing to expand.

The technology is changing so fast that microcomputers are performing like minicomputers and even mainframes. A microcomputer functions in a way similar to that of larger computers; however, it is housed in one location, and its hardware components are different. Instead of having multiple hardware parts in different locations, a microcomputer is assembled as a complete desktop or portable system that contains all the components needed for it to function. A microcomputer includes (1) a video display terminal, (2) a keyboard, (3) a disk drive(s), and (4) a CPU.

The video display terminal (VDT) replaced the CRT vacuum tube with a solid-state display screen that uses semiconductor technology. The video screen allows the user to view the input/output, and input devices such as the light pen and the mouse (a hand-held device that moves the cursor) use the video screen to input data and send commands to the CPU. Still other media, such as scanners, compact disks, and voice synthesizers, are also used for input. The keyboard, which resembles that of a typewriter, can be used to input data. Disk drives are used as input and output devices. They allow magnetized media that represent data to be transferred from floppy disks (diskettes) to the CPU and vice versa. The CPU, the internal component of a microcomputer, consists of a microprocessor on a chip (Fig. 3.3). It is often referred to as the "brain" of the computer and directly or indirectly controls every function performed by the computer. It also controls secondary storage on internal hard disks. The printer is an output device and is considered optional equipment.

Microcomputers are being used in all areas of the health care industry, even those formerly associated with minicomputers or mainframes. Hospital nursing departments are using microcomputers to process specific applications such as patient classification, nurse staffing and scheduling, and personnel management. Microcomputers, or personal computers (PCs),

**Figure 3.3** Microprocessor on a chip. (Courtesy IBM.)

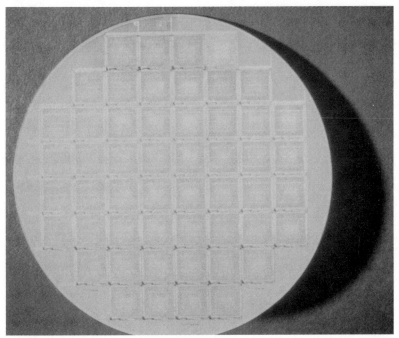

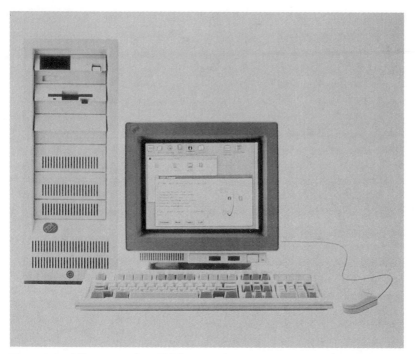

**Figure 3.4**   Microcomputer: IBM personal computer. (Courtesy IBM.)

are also found in educational and research settings, where they are used for a multitude of special educational and scientific applications (Fig. 3.4).

## Microcomputer Sizes

Microcomputers are also available as portable, laptop, and notebook computers. The portable and laptop versions vary in size, but all are smaller than a standard desktop microcomputer. A notebook microcomputer is generally 8½ by 11 in. and weighs approximately 4 pounds. Even though they are smaller than the standard desktop microcomputer, many have as much memory, storage capacity, and processing capabilities as a standard desktop.

Recently, an even smaller microcomputer was introduced: the hand-held computer. This computer is offered by several manufacturers as a smaller version of a portable computer; however, others, such as the Apple Newton, are being introduced using pen-based technology. The Newton MessagePad is not only a computer but also a personal digital assistant that can read handwriting. It is pocket-sized, weighs less than a pound, runs on four AAA batteries, and fits in the palm of the hand. Still other manufacturers are developing other types of hand-held, pen-based computers offering different and newer processing concepts and technologies.

## COMPUTER FUNCTIONAL COMPONENTS

A computer has four functional components that are necessary to process information. These component parts, which are illustrated in Fig. 3.5, are basic to all computer systems and are not limited to any single computer manufacturer. They include (1) the input unit, (2) the CPU, which consists of the control unit, arithmetic logic unit (ALU), and main memory, (3) secondary storage unit, and (4) output unit.

   This section presents a brief overview of these four functional components, including the various computer hardware devices and the media that implement them. These components include the following:

- Input unit
- Central processing unit
- Secondary storage unit
- Output unit

**Figure 3.5**   Four functional components of the computer.

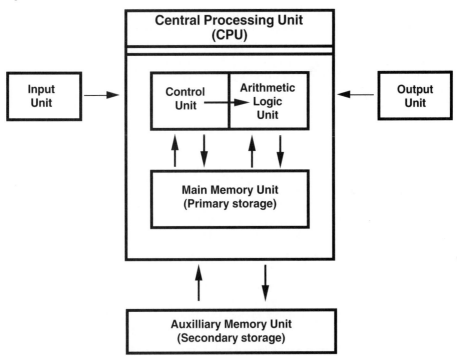

## Input Unit

The input unit acts as a "reception desk," accepting data and instructions and translating them into binary digits (machine language) to be input into the computer's memory in the CPU. Several kinds of input devices and media are used to input data. They include a variety of devices that are part of the computer terminal, such as the keyboard, display monitor, mouse (device), and light pen/touch screen; media that are used to read or sense data, such as optical character recognition (OCR) and magnetic-ink character recognition (MICR); and other, newer technological advances, such as a voice synthesizer and compact disks (CDs). Many of these input devices are also used as output or storage devices or media. They include

- Terminals
- Keyboards
- Monitors
- Mouse
- Light pen/touch screens
- Optical character recognition

- Magnetic-ink character recognition
- Voice synthesizers
- Imaging
- Magnetic storage media
- Optical Disks

### Terminal

A terminal is a device that is used to communicate with a computer's CPU. It consists of a keyboard, an input/output monitor, and a device to communicate with the CPU when it is linked to another computer and/or a mainframe (Fig. 3.6).

Mainframes and minicomputers primarily use CRT terminals to translate input data and instructions into machine language, using binary code. Early computers used CRTs to communicate and transmit data from a remote site to a central mainframe connected directly through telephone lines or via modems used as interface devices. Other communication media, such as cable, microwave, and even satellite, are also used. Microcomputers used as terminals, by contrast, employ VDTs with solid-state screens to display data and are replacing CRTs.

There are primarily three different types of terminals: dumb, smart, and intelligent (microcomputers). Dumb terminals are used to transmit keyed data to and from the computer without processing the data in any way. They enter and display data (input/output). Smart terminals store, edit, and minimally process data before transmitting the data to the computer, enabling a user to edit the data according to predefined rules. They are used to receive and display output data, and some can be programmed to perform computer processing tasks. Intelligent terminals and microcomputers are also being used to communicate with mainframe computers and with each other in local area networks (LANs). They can be programmed to

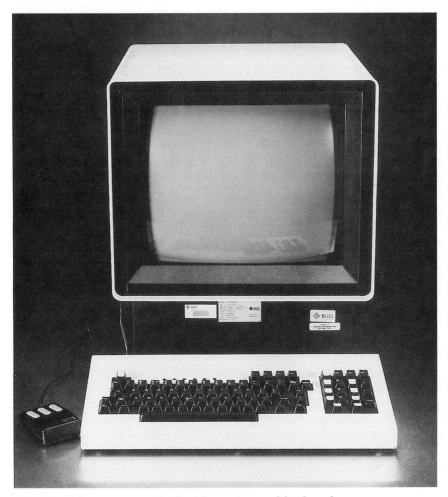

**Figure 3.6** Computer terminal with monitor and keyboard. (Smithsonian Institution Photo No. 91-14954.)

perform processing functions and used to process computer programs other than the specific application of the computer system. Even though they are more expensive, they offer additional processing capabilities.

Terminals are also used for teleprocessing, which involves using a computer through one or more on-line communication links. In teleprocessing, terminals are located in many different places and are connected to a central computer by a communication network, usually through modems. The computer is shared by several different users; this is called timesharing.

Teleprocessing has been used in small hospitals and community health agencies that cannot afford a mainframe or minicomputer system.

These agencies generally contract with a vendor or service bureau and timeshare their on-line computer services. Computer use by each terminal operator is tracked by the CPU, and the users are billed accordingly. This timesharing method makes major computer resources available to users with a moderate budget.

## Keyboard

The keyboard is the most common input device. It is a component of a terminal that is connected to a monitor. There are several different types of keyboards; however, regardless of type, they all have similar sections of keys: (1) typewriter keys, (2) function keys, (3) a numeric keypad, (4) cursor keys, (5) toggle keys, and (6) special operations keys.

The typewriter key section is the largest and contains keys that follow the standard QWERTY arrangement. (This term represents the first six letters in the first alphabetic row.) The function keys F1–F12 are software-specific; that is, they are programmable because their function is dependent on the software program being processed. For example, F10 is used to retrieve a file in one word-processing package and to save in another. Generally, a software package provides a template for the function keys that defines how those keys are used for that specific package. Three other keys on the keyboard are labeled "Shift," "Ctrl," and "Alt." They are used in combination with the function keys to carry out other commands.

The numeric keypad is a second set of numeric keys that are arranged differently from those that accompany the alphabetic keys. The numeric keypad is a separate rectangular calculator-type section that enables the user to enter numeric data more efficiently. The section can be converted to represent other keys, including moving the cursor in four directions, by turning on the Num Lock key. The four cursor keys are used to direct the position of the pointer on the display monitor. They control the movement up ($\uparrow$), down ($\downarrow$), right ($\rightarrow$), and left ($\leftarrow$) over the display screen. The toggle keys have a dual purpose. When a toggle key is pressed once, the function is "on"; when it is pressed a second time, the function is "off." The major toggle keys include "Num Lock," "Caps Lock," "Scroll Lock," and "Insert/Typeover."

There are also special operations keys that are unique to the microcomputer and are used to make the keyboard easy to manipulate. The Home and End keys bring the cursor to the beginning or end of a document, Print Screen prints the screen display, Esc (Escape) interrupts or cancels a function, a Tab key moves the cursor to predetermined set tabs, the Del key deletes text, a space bar and an Enter ($\dashv$) key are provided to insert spaces, and there are several other keys with symbols that are useful in preparing a document or doing a mathematical calculation.

## Monitor

The monitor is a display screen component of a terminal that allows the user to view the computer input: information- and data-processing actions. The

VDT uses a solid-state monitor and is replacing the CRT as an input/ output device. VDT terminals are associated primarily with microcomputers. Monitors, regardless of type, are available in a variety of shapes and sizes.

The resolution or clarity of the monitor screen is related to the number of dots (pixels) on the screen. The most common and least expensive monitor has a black-and-white or monochrome display; color monitors (super VGA color) cost more but allow for a variety of colors for both the foreground and the background. The average monitor represents half a standard page (8½ by 11 in.) with 26 lines down and 80 characters across. Most monitors allow for scrolling; the user can scroll up and down and right and left, displaying different portions of a document.

The most recent technological enhancements allow users to divide the screen into several smaller windows or frames that display different sections of the program being run. Windows are display screens that are divided into sections that resemble windowpanes. This option makes it possible to view data from different parts of the file at one time and can also show several programs or files that are running at the same time. Another new feature is the use of small pictures on the screen that represent various types of functions and applications; these pictures are called icons. An icon is a graphic representation of an object, concept, function, or message. The combination of windows and icons is making video display screens and software programs more user-friendly.

### Mouse

The mouse was introduced for the microcomputer as a new type of input device to replace the arrow keys on the keyboard. It is a hand-manipulated mechanical device that electronically instructs the cursor to move across the video display screen. It resembles a bar of soap with a tail. As the user slides the mouse across a desktop pad or moves a ball, the cursor (a pointer) moves across the screen. The user "clicks" a mouse button in front and on top of the device to instruct the pointer to (1) select an icon or button, (2) activate the process, and (3) implement a function. The mouse is becoming the most common input device for microcomputers.

### Light Pen/Touch Screen

A light pen is a photosensitive device that responds to light images when it is placed against a VDT screen. When the pen comes in contact with the display screen, it highlights the item and sends data to the computer. Touch screens are used as input by accepting data that a user touches on the screen. Sensors on the screen pinpoint the location touched and activate a function.

### Optical Character Recognition

OCR is a specialized computer input medium that allows the computer to read data directly from a form or document. An electronic optical scanning device, a wand reader, or a bar code reader reads special marks, bar codes, numbers, letters, or characters. This device converts the optical marks, characters, and bar codes into electrical signals that become computer input.

OCR-readable codes include those outlined in areas on the answer sheet of the nursing state board examinations. The bar codes called Universal Product Code symbols (zebra-striped bars) are another example. Ten bars, about 1 in. long, that signify different numbers are used to code groceries or medical items. When read with a special scanning device, they can become input in some hospital inventory systems.

### Magnetic-Ink Character Recognition

MICR is another medium for reading characters by computer. Here the characters are made of magnetized particles printed on paper. An MICR reader can examine the shape of the magnetic-ink characters and convert them into binary code for the computer. The most common example of MICR is the magnetized characters printed on bank checks.

### Voice Synthesizer

A voice synthesizer allows users to input data into the computer by speaking into a connected microphone. Also known as a speech synthesizer, it digitizes the sound for processing by the CPU. Although automatic recognition of the human voice has not been perfected, voice input is used in situations that require only a few spoken words and is becoming a common medium for all computer systems.

### Imaging

Several different types of image input devices transform images from various types of graphics into a digital form the computer can accept and represent on the screen and then process. Many types of graphic images on paper, such as x-rays, can be scanned as computer input and/or digitized for computer use.

### Magnetic Storage Media

Various types of magnetic media used primarily for secondary storage or auxiliary memory are also used as input. They include magnetic tape, cassette tape, magnetic disks, floppy disks, and hard disks (see the discussion on storage units, below). When used as input, these media require a tape or disk drive to read and write data as input/output media.

### Optical Disks

Optical disk technology refers to a "family" that involves both optical and magnetic disk systems. It includes compact disk read-only memory that is used as computer storage. A CD-ROM is a round, metal-coated plastic disk on which digital information is stored. A digital CD-ROM has a large storage capacity, quick retrieval speed, and durability. CD-ROMs are used to store and retrieve full text efforts such as encyclopedias, dictionaries, textbooks, bibliographic products, clinical practice guidelines and standards, and alerting products.

CD-ROMS are being used for the storage of complex digitized images and photos as well as audio and sound. They are read by using a CD-ROM disk drive, which is a new optional component of desktop microcomputers. The newer CD-ROMs and CD-ROM disk drives are converting desktop microcomputers into multimedia computer systems. They are offering new media sources of information.

***Laser Disks***   Optical disks also include laser videodisk technology, which is used to store video and sound images for interactive video software programs. These interactive videodisk systems require a microcomputer, an interactive videodisk player, and a software program to control the relationships between the software program and the visual and sound clips on the interactive videodisk. The information is retrieved from the videodisk by the reflection from the surface of a small laser beam as the disk rotates rapidly. Laser CD-ROMs are used for interactive video software programs developed for educational purposes.

## Central Processing Unit

The CPU controls, directs, and supervises the entire computer system and is the "heart" and/or "brain" of the computer. It contains the electronic components essential for computer operation, including the following:

- Control unit
- Arithmetic logic unit
- Main memory unit

### Control Unit

The control unit monitors all computer system activities. Its major component is the operating system, which is responsible for directing its own resources and the operations of the computer. The operating system is the major software program for the control unit, a set of internal computer programs in the CPU responsible for directing, coordinating, and supervising computer instructions. The control unit converts all computer languages into machine language (binary form), which is the only language a computer understands.

This unit controls the machine's input/output devices, controls the movement of data to and from the main memory, schedules and performs the instructions of software programs, and performs all data-processing operations, including output. It is analogous to a telephone exchange that uses controlling instruments to ring phones and connect and disconnect circuits. The master control program, also called the operating system, not only manages the computer's internal functions but also allows the user to control many computer operations.

### Arithmetic Logic Unit

The ALU, the "workhorse" of the computer, is the simplest component to understand. It is a set of internal programs in the CPU that is responsible for performing arithmetic calculations and logical operations and comparisons as directed by the control unit or operating system. The arithmetic calculations include addition, subtraction, multiplication, and division.

The logical operations can be reduced to three basic comparisons: (1) equal to, (2) less than, and (3) greater than. The logic unit compares the values of data being processed and is based on the true-false propositions set forth by George Boole, the founder of Boolean algebra. In 1854 Boole developed sets of algebralike symbols and rules or truth tables to facilitate the description of logical functions. Boole's rules for manipulating true-false propositions rely on the logical connectives "and," "or," and "and not" (Fig. 3.7).

The computer performs several basic comparisons or combinations of comparisons to process data. For example, the question of whether a patient's temperature is within the normal range illustrates three major comparisons (as shown at the top of page 103):

---

**The "AND" Function**

| | | |
|---|---|---|
| True (1) and True (1) | = | True (1) |
| True (1) and False (0) | = | False (0) |
| False (0) and True (1) | = | False (0) |
| False (0) and False (0) | = | False (0) |

**The "OR" Function**

| | | |
|---|---|---|
| True (1) or True (1) | = | True (1) |
| True (1) or False (0) | = | True (1) |
| False (0) or True (1) | = | True (1) |
| False (0) or False (0) | = | False (1) |

**The "NOT" Function**

| | | |
|---|---|---|
| True (1) not False (1) | = | True (1) |
| False (1) not True (0) | = | False (0) |

**Figure 3.7** Boolean true-false propositions.

1. Equal to (=): a comparison in which one data element is equal to another data element. (The patient's temperature is normal at 98.6°F or equal to 98.6°F.)

2. Less than (<): a comparison in which one data element is less than another. (The patient's temperature is subnormal at 95.2°F or less than 98.6°F.)

3. Greater than (>): a comparison in which one data element is greater than another. (The patient's temperature is elevated at 101.8°F or greater than 98.6°F.)

## Main Memory Unit

The main memory unit, also called primary storage, stores computer software, data, and instructions that the computer processes. Memory is logically organized and arranged so that stored data and instructions can be located and accessed easily. It uses specific addresses, similar to those used in a post office, to store and locate data. Every coded character that is stored has its own address (mailbox). The addresses do not move, but data and instructions change from address to address.

*Memory Size* The size of main memory continues to increase. Main memory size is generally expressed in terms of the size, in thousands of bytes of memory, of the main memory chips in the CPU. The size of main memory varies among mainframes, minicomputers, and microcomputers. However, this determines what data and instructions can be stored and processed. A mainframe generally has at least 2,048K of main memory. However, whereas the first microcomputers used 64K chips and later models progressed to 640K chips, today a microcomputer has at least 4 to 8MB and can have even 16 or 32MB of memory.

The size of main memory influences which computer programs can be processed and the amount of data that can be stored. These components have to be compatible; that is, a computer program cannot require more memory than the computer has. For example, a computer program requiring 1,024K of memory cannot be loaded on a machine with 512K of memory. Even though the computer may have millions of bytes of data on-line in secondary storage, the size of the main memory controls what and how much data can be processed at one time.

*Memory Words* The processing power of main memory also is described by the number of words the memory can process at one time. A word consists of 8 bits, or 1 byte. A word is what is transferred from memory to ALU. A mainframe generally transfers at least 32 bits (four words) at a time, making it four times as fast as a machine processing 8-bit words and twice as fast as a microcomputer processing 16-bit words. Some machines now process 64 bits (eight words), which continues to increase the capabilities of memory. The processing power of microcomputers is increasing and catching up with that of the mainframes.

***Memory Speed***   Another characteristic of main memory is its speed. Each computer has a clock that controls and executes a processing operation cycle. Early computers processed data in milliseconds and then microseconds, and today data are processed in nanoseconds and even picoseconds (trillionths of a second). Early computers operated at speeds of 1 MHz (one megahertz) of processing power, or 1-million processing cycles per second, whereas the newest models operate at speeds of 10, 16, 25, 33, 46, and 66 MHz and are continuing to increase in speed.

***Memory Media***   The main memory in most computers consists of electronic components: thousands of microminiaturized circuits etched on tiny silicon chips that are only several square millimeters in size. The chip, which has revolutionized the computer industry, is compact, extremely reliable, and long-lasting. It uses little electricity and is relatively inexpensive to produce. The number of circuits etched on a chip continues to increase, decreasing computer size and increasing computer power.

Early microcomputers used the Intel 8086 or 8088 chip, which was replaced by the faster and more powerful 80286, 80386, 80486, and Pentium (80586) chips. Other computers used the Motorola 6800, 68020, 68030, 68040, and the new Power PC chip. The capacity of chips continues to expand. Traditionally a chip was designed to process one instruction at a time; however, the newest RISC (**r**educed **i**nstruction **s**et **c**omputer) processor on a chip is designed to process a set of instructions simultaneously. This new technological advance will allow computers to be smaller yet have greater processing power.

The electronic circuits in memory, or "logic gates," can sense the absence or presence of electronic impulses that represent data stored in memory. Absence (off) is represented by the binary digit 0, and presence (on) by the binary digit 1. The 0 or 1 is called a bit, which is the accepted abbreviation for **bi**nary **d**igit. (The binary numbering system uses a base of 2, unlike the decimal numbering system, which uses a base of 10.)

A unique 8-bit coding scheme called the American Standard Code for Information Interchange (ASCII) combines 8 binary digits into 1 byte (character); this is similar to combining letters to make a word. The ASCII code is used to translate all characters—letters, numbers, and symbols—into machine language using binary code (Fig. 3.8).

***Memory Types***   Memory has two types of storage: read-only memory (ROM) and random access memory (RAM).

**READ-ONLY MEMORY:**   Read-only memory refers to the permanent storage of programs and data. This means that data and programs can be read but not written on or altered. ROM generally contains the programs, called firmware, used by the control unit of the CPU to oversee the computer's functions. In microcomputers this also may include the software programs used to translate the computer's high-level programming languages

| ASCII Character | Binary | ASCII Character | Binary |
|---|---|---|---|
| 0 | 0011 0000 | M | 0100 1101 |
| 1 | 0011 0001 | N | 0100 1110 |
| 2 | 0011 0010 | O | 0100 1111 |
| 3 | 0011 0011 | P | 0101 0000 |
| 4 | 0011 0100 | Q | 0101 0001 |
| 5 | 0011 0101 | R | 0101 0010 |
| 6 | 0011 0110 | S | 0101 0011 |
| 7 | 0011 0111 | T | 0101 0100 |
| 8 | 0011 1000 | U | 0101 0101 |
| 9 | 0011 1001 | V | 0101 0110 |
| A | 0100 0001 | W | 0101 0111 |
| B | 0100 0010 | X | 0101 1000 |
| C | 0100 0011 | Y | 0101 1001 |
| D | 0100 0100 | Z | 0101 1010 |
| E | 0100 0101 | $ | 0010 0100 |
| F | 0100 0110 | * | 0010 1010 |
| G | 0100 0111 | ? | 0011 1111 |
| H | 0100 1000 | : | 0011 1010 |
| I | 0100 1001 | # | 0010 0011 |
| J | 0100 1010 | @ | 0100 0000 |
| K | 0100 1011 | ; | 0010 1100 |
| L | 0100 1100 | BLANK | 0010 0000 |

**Figure 3.8** ASCII codes.

into machine language (binary code). ROM storage is not erased when the computer is turned off. ROM is analogous to a phonograph record that one can play but not change. ROM is generally developed by computer manufacturers.

*RANDOM ACCESS MEMORY:* Random access memory refers to working memory that is used for primary storage. It is volatile and is used as temporary storage. RAM can be accessed, used, changed, and written on repeatedly. It contains data and instructions that are stored and processed by computer programs called applications programs. RAM is the work area available to the user for all processing applications, the user's computer desktop. The computer programs, which are not permanent, are read or written by a user and may be altered. RAM is lost if and when the power is turned off in a microcomputer, unlike ROM, which is not lost.

## Storage Units

The storage unit, also called secondary memory, is used to expand the main memory capacity of a computer system because main memory has limited storage capacity. Secondary storage is separate from main memory and can be on-line or off-line. If it is on-line, the computer has immediate access; that is, it can read and retrieve data that are stored on magnetic disks. If the storage is off-line, the computer must wait until a computer operator loads a magnetic tape or inserts a magnetic disk containing the data needed for processing into a read/write disk drive.

Secondary storage is measured by the number of bytes of storage capacity of the storage device. A byte is 8 bits, or one character (letter, number, or symbol). Storage capacities are expressed in thousand of bytes. Thus, 1K refers to 1,000 kilobytes, which signifies $2^{10}$ or 1,024 bytes. The following terms are used:

- 1,000 bytes (actually 1,024) = 1K (1 kilobyte)
- 1,000,000 bytes = 1MB (1 million bytes, or 1 megabyte)
- 1,000,000,000 bytes = 1GB (1 billion bytes, or 1 gigabyte)
- 1,000,000,000,000 bytes = 1TB (1 trillion bytes, or 1 terabyte)

The common types of secondary storage or auxiliary memory include the following:

- Magnetic disks/magnetic tapes
- Floppy disks/diskettes
- Hard disks
- Optical disks

### Magnetic Disks/Magnetic Tapes

Magnetic disks and magnetic tapes are used both as secondary storage or auxiliary memory and as input/output media in mainframes, minicomputers, and microcomputers. Magnetic disks and magnetic tapes make it possible for computers to store large volumes of data at a relatively low cost.

When data are recorded onto magnetic disks and magnetic tapes by a computer, they are converted into magnetized spots representing machine-readable binary code. They are read or written through special input devices called disk drives or tape drives. These devices contain a read/write head that can sense, interpret, and convert the magnetized spots into electronic impulses the computer can understand (Fig. 3.9).

*Magnetic Tapes* Magnetic tape is used as storage in mainframes and minicomputers. A magnetic tape resembles a ½-in. reel of film. Magnetic tapes are used primarily in mainframe computer systems to store data that are not essential for daily system operation, such as the records of discharged patients, and can be stored in an off-line mode. Magnetic tapes are stored on shelves and mounted onto devices called magnetic tape drives when needed as computer input.

*Magnetic Disks* Magnetic disks make it possible for on-line interactive information computer systems in large health care facilities to store and process large volumes of data. Magnetic disks resemble metal platters and

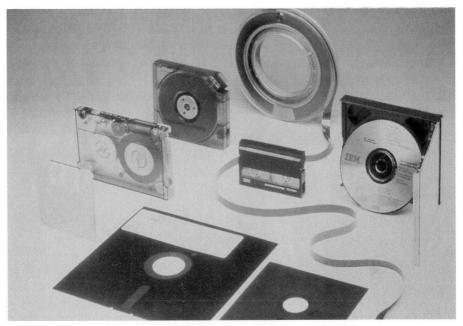

**Figure 3.9**   Magnetic tape, magnetic disk, and floppy disk. (Courtesy IBM.)

are used as on-line storage. Generally, a stack of 8 or 10 record-album-size disks, all connected and enclosed in what resembles a large cake dish, is assembled in a disk pack. Magnetic disks are installed permanently or mounted as needed onto magnetic disk drives. They are connected together and to the mainframe computer to provide on-line access. Magnetic disks make it possible for multiple users to have direct access to the computer system.

### Floppy Disks/Diskettes
A floppy disk, commonly called a diskette, is another form of secondary storage or auxiliary memory. It also is used as an input/output medium. Floppy disks are primarily used by microcomputers. Data are read to and written from disk drives in the same manner as they are with magnetic tapes and magnetic disks. As a floppy diskette turns, a read/write head transfers electronic impulses between the diskette and the memory. Each diskette has a disk window that exposes the area on the magnetic surface where the data can be retrieved or stored. A write-protect notch is also cut on the side of the jacket to prevent the head from writing on the disk.

***Tracks and Sectors*** A floppy disk or diskette, which resembles a 45-rpm record, is a flexible Mylar oxide-coated disk that is thinly covered with magnetic spots. Diskettes are available in 5¼- and 3½-in. sizes. The latter are newer and are becoming the industry standard; they are encased in a hard plastic case that is sturdy and easy to store. A 5¼-in. diskette can hold 360K to 1MB of data, and a 3½-in. disk can hold 720 K to 1.44 MB of data. Each floppy disk is sectioned into 9 to 15 concentric rings or tracks, and each track is sectioned into 40 to 48 or 80 to 96 sectors. Sectors store the smallest unit of data, whereas tracks and sectors are used to provide the addresses of fields of data.

Floppy disks are available in various formats—single- or double-sided and single- or double-density—which influence the number of characters they can store. The procedure for marking the tracks and sectors is called formatting; this initializes the size and number of sectors on the disk and is essential for preparing a disk for use.

### Hard Disks

The hard disk, originally called a "Winchester," is another form of secondary storage and an input/output medium. It is a hard metal recordlike platter produced for permanent installation in microcomputers. The installation of hard disks has dramatically increased the on-line auxiliary storage capacity of microcomputers. Microcomputers can have an almost unlimited number of hard disks on-line and off-line as secondary storage.

Unlike a floppy disk, a hard disk is rigid and generally is encased in a nonremovable sealed container. Its storage capacity is many times (a 20 to 40 multiple) that of a floppy disk, and it has a much faster access speed than does a floppy disk. It comes in various sizes, depending on the desired storage capacity and requirements, ranging from 10MB to 40MB in older microcomputers to 100MB to 500MB and over of storage in newer machines. It is the most reliable mass secondary storage for some minicomputers and microcomputers and is becoming the preferred storage medium (Fig. 3.10).

### Optical Disks

Optical laser disks are also used for storage. Optical media use a laser beam to read and digitize analog data from an optical disk. Optical disk and storage units are generally connected to the computer as on-line storage devices. A new type of optical disk storage device is the "jukebox" robotic mechanism. It consists of approximately 50 double-sided optical WORM (**w**rite **o**nce **r**ead **m**any) disks that are linked together. Much as music jukeboxes played records, it automatically loads a requested disk and then spins it for information retrieval.

Another version of optical disk storage is CD-ROM. CD-ROM is read by a CD-ROM disk drive, which is an option on multimedia computers. CD-ROMs are used to digitize not only read-only data but also other media, such as audio and images. These innovations are making multimedia computers easy to use and will replace interactive laser video computer systems.

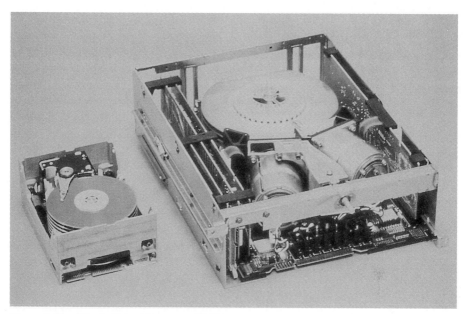

**Figure 3.10**   Hard disk. (Courtesy IBM.)

## Output Unit

The fourth functional component of a computer is the output unit, which is the reverse of the input unit. It generally provides a hard copy (paper) of the information produced by the computer system. The output is the final product of the data processed by the computer. The output unit can also transmit data to secondary storage and to other computers.

   Several different output devices and media can be present, but most input and secondary storage devices are also used as output. They include the following:

- Video display terminals
- Printers
- Microfilm/microfiche

- Graphics/images
- Magnetic media
- Voice output

### Video Display Terminals

A VDT screen, also called a monitor, is the most common output unit. Formerly called a CRT terminal because of its internal construction (vacuum tubes), it allows a user to view an exact replica of the printed output on the screen. This terminal displays the data-processing actions and allows the user to modify drafts without having to produce printed output.

Other variations of computer terminals also can be considered output devices. They include portable, notebook, and hand-held computer terminals and produce output that is displayed on the video screen or printed on paper.

## Printers

The printer, the most important output device, converts information produced by the computer system into printed form, rendering data in the binary code into readable English. The major types of printed output include printed hard copy (paper), microfilm (microfiche), photographs, and graphic copy. Printed paper copy, known as "hard copy," is output produced on paper, in contrast to "soft copy," which refers to what is displayed on the video display screen. Paper copy is printed by four common types of printers: dot matrix, daisy wheel, inkjet, and laser.

***Dot Matrix Printer*** Dot matrix printers are the most common and least expensive impact printers. They are "character printers" that use small wires to produce characters composed from series of dots. A dot matrix printer is more flexible than the individual character types in that combinations of dots can form a wider variety of characters as well as graphics. Dot matrix printers print one character at a time or, in the case of a line printer, one line of characters at a time. The printer's speed is generally measured by the number of characters or lines it can print per minute.

***Daisy Wheel Printer*** The daisy wheel is a character printer that resembles a typewriter, printing one character at a time. It is an impact printer that uses a typewriter ball such as a daisy wheel to strike the paper and produces letter-quality output. Its speed is measured by the number of characters it prints per second. This type of printer is generally slower and costs less than a line printer.

***Inkjet Printer/Plotter*** An inkjet printer and plotter is a nonimpact printer. Nonimpact printers can print at very high speeds and produce graphic displays. The inkjet printer fires small bursts of ink onto the paper, and the plotter places two-dimensional patterns such as graphs on paper. These printers have the flexibility of dot matrix printers and operate more quietly. They can be adapted for color printing. They produce near-laser results and are cheaper than laser printers.

***Laser Printer*** A laser printer is a nonimpact printer that uses a laser beam. Laser printers offer a substantial increase in output quality over many other printers. A laser printer's engine is composed of an integrated system of electronic and chemical parts that work together with optical processes to produce a printed image. Laser printers generally use fonts or printing typefaces as their printing elements, making documents look typeset. They are also used for printing graphic images and illustrations.

## Microfilm/Microfiche

Microfilm and microfiche are output media. The computer output on microfilm (COM) is output photographed from a special high-resolution display, producing a microfilm that contains miniaturized photographs on a film strip. The COM can also produce small photographs on a 4-by-6-in. film sheet known as a microfiche. A microfiche saves space, since one sheet can store from 100 to 200 pages of filmed output.

## Graphics/Images

Graphics are another form of output. The most common graphic displays are those produced from a graphic software package on a CRT terminal designed to display graphic as well as alphanumeric data. They generally include line, bar, or pie chart graphs. Graphs can be printed as hard copy by using a dot matrix printer with graphic capability (Figs. 3.11 to 3.13). Graphics, such as colored maps and charts, can also be displayed. Inkjet printers can produce graphic images in many colors. Plotters are used for drawing hard copy maps and charts. Most plotters use mechanical pens to produce color graphics.

## Magnetic Media

All magnetic media used for secondary storage (magnetic tape, cassette tape, magnetic disks, floppy disks, and hard disks) also act as output. These media, like input, use tape or disk drives to read and write and produce computer data (see the discussion on storage units above, for a complete description).

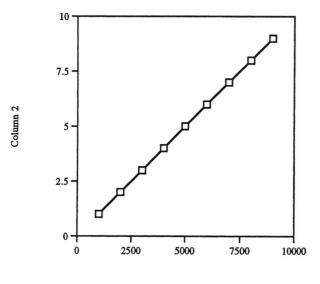

**Figure 3.11**
Graphic line chart.

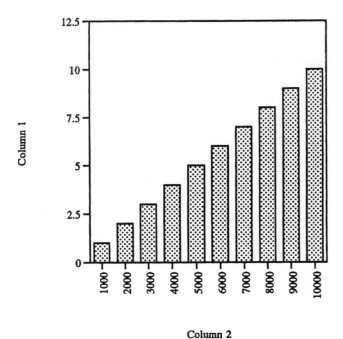

**Figure 3.12**   Graphic bar chart.

**Figure 3.13**   Graphic pie chart.

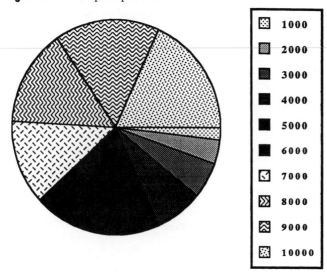

## Voice Output

Voice output devices, sometimes called voice synthesizers, are available to vocalize data stored in main memory. It is easier for a computer system to produce voice output than to accept voice input. Voice output is commonly used today in telephone banking and often is used for short responses by companies offering telephone support.

# Computer Communications

The merger of communications and computers began with the use of communication lines such as telephone, microwave or cable, and satellite systems to transmit data signals. Communication devices are essential to computer networks. They include the following:

- Modems
- Local area networks
- Wide area networks
- Internet

## Modems

The modem is a communication device that is used to connect a terminal with a mainframe or another computer. A modem (**mo**dulating and **dem**odulating device) translates digital data into analog signals for transmission over telephone lines to the computer system, which also uses a modem to convert the incoming analog signals back to their original digital form for input into the computer. Modems connect users at remote computers via telephone lines to another computer in another location. If one dials the remote computer's modem, data can be sent to and received from remote sources. Modems facilitate the function of modulating and demodulating input and output devices. Modems are also described by the rate of communication transmission or line transfer, called the baud rate.

Fax modems are a new feature for microcomputers. A fax modem can be used to send and receive faxes of text and/or graphics, view them on the display screen, and/or print them out as hard copy. Computer programs for fax modem communication can save faxes as data files for editing and storage. They also can save the graphics and images using OCR technology and convert them into text files for storage.

## Local Area Networks

A local area network is a communication network that allows users to share hardware, software, and data. It generally links two or more computers in one location in a linear or circular arrangement for sharing data. A LAN, which resembles a telephone network, is designed to transmit information within a limited geographic area such as a room, office, or building or within a specified radius. A LAN enables the sharing of information and computer resources. Specifically, it is used to (1) link workstations (computers that sit in the network) together to share databases and files, (2) access larger remote computers to process data, (3) move large data files between mainframes, minicomputers, and/or microcomputers, and (4) exchange data files with others in the network.

Before the development of LANs, data were shared and accessed via direct connection, as terminals were cabled to the mainframe or central computer, where all data and programs were stored. This type of communication network had a configuration that limited access to mainframe computers to dedicated users. However, today's LANs make it possible for individual microcomputer or workstation users to communicate and to share data, programs, and resources such as laser printers and high-speed capacity storage devices.

A LAN requires specific hardware and software to function. The hardware is represented by the type of wiring used, whereas the software refers to the communication program used to support the hardware. LANs consist of workstations connected by coaxial cable, optical fiber, or standard telephone lines. The topology of a LAN, in addition to the communication cable that connects the workstations and/or peripherals (input and output devices), includes a special internal computer circuitry unit, an operating system that controls the resources and data, and a software program to transmit data from one computer to another. The three most common types of LANs are

- Star networks
- Ring networks
- Bus networks

***Star Networks*** A star network has a centralized topology. In this configuration all workstations, which are referred to as nodes in the network, share a single high-speed cable and a single centralized file server or network server. The file server stores data and transmits them to other workstations on the network. It is usually a microcomputer with a large-capacity hard disk that stores shared data centrally and manages access to the data, including routing all programming instructions.

The main advantage of the star network is that several users can use the workstations on the LAN and access the file server at one time. In this configuration, a LAN can also support a print server. The print server connects the LAN to a shared printer with a memory buffer that accepts files and stores them in a printing queue (Fig. 3.14).

***Ring Networks*** A ring network has a decentralized network topology. A network cable connects nodes and circulates from node to node (computer to computer) in a closed ring-shaped LAN. Data storage and access are distributed among the workstations on the LAN. Each workstation (node) stores different software programs that can be accessed by any authorized

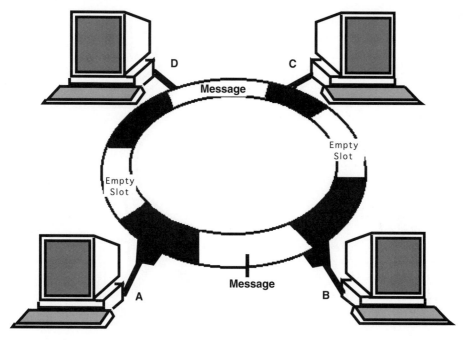

**Figure 3.14**   Star LAN.

workstation as needed. A ring network does not require a file server to control its activity. When one workstation needs data from another one, the data are passed along the ring (Fig. 3.15).

***Bus Networks*** A bus network also has a decentralized topology. It consists of a number of microcomputers connected by a single cable or optical fiber. The microcomputers share data by using the communication line, or bus line. There is no host computer. The bus network is configured so that if one workstation fails, it does not affect the entire network. A bus network is linear instead of ring-shaped (Fig. 3.16).

Several computer companies offer LANs. Ethernet generally refers to the cabling arrangement for the bus topology; "token ring," provided by IBM, is used for a ring network. LANs produced by different companies require different software programs to manage the LANs, the cabling, and the transmission medium; however, Novell Netware is a program designed for several LAN configurations.

### Wide Area Networks

A wide area network (WAN) is a communication network that is similar to a LAN but spans a large geographic area. It is used to link health care facilities in remote areas to one another and/or to a main health care

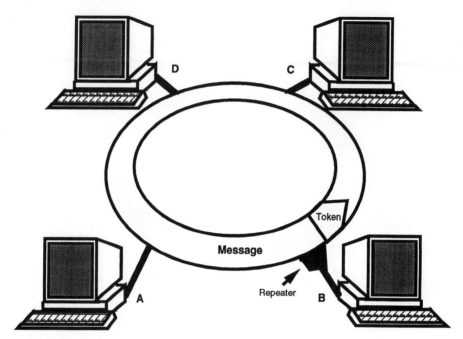

**Figure 3.15**   Ring LAN.

**Figure 3.16**   Bus LAN.

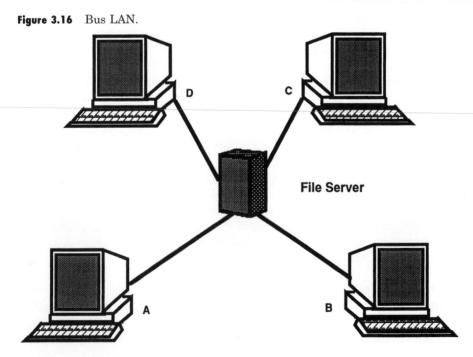

facility that serves as the host computer system. WANs are found in large cities, where they link the units of a large health care system together, such as local health departments and the state health department. WANs also are found in rural areas, where small hospitals are linked to large city hospitals that serve as backup and provide consultative services.

### Internet

The Internet is the world's largest collection of computer networks, linking millions of local networks together. It is an invisible electronic information highway that is used to communicate, transmit, and retrieve digital computer data via fiber-optic lines. It is somewhat similar to telephone networks that use on-line analog (sound wave signals) communication. Internet is in essence a "free" worldwide electronic communication network that is not controlled by a single organization or country, although several commercial "outernets" charge for incoming and outgoing services. Internet not only provides different services and/or applications but also offers different tools or protocols ("road maps") to connect with other local networks anywhere in the world.

The Internet requires a computer and a communication software program to connect directly to a local network "node," which in turn facilitates the interaction between the user's computer via Telnet and other local networks on the Internet highway. The local network node can also act as a "host" server for resources the local network may offer. It requires a computer, a modem, and computer communication software. The Internet provides several major services, including (1) communication services such as electronic mail and bulletin boards, (2) file transfer protocols, and (3) tools and protocols for traveling on the Internet, such as Gopher, MOSAIC, and World Wide Web (WWW).

***Electronic Mailboxes***   Electronic mailboxes (E-mail) are used to send messages (letters, memos, and reports) to another person or group. This is a one-to-one communication, with one user sending a message to one user or to many users individually on the network, each of whom receives the messages individually. Messages can be stored and forwarded without the receiver having to be present. Mailboxes can be used to upload (send) work from a home office to an office computer and download (receive) files. E-mail is used to transmit letters and other messages via data communications channels, combining the features of telephone calls and conventional mail.

***Electronic Bulletin Boards***   Electronic bulletin boards are different from E-mail in that the messages are open to everyone on the system. Bulletin boards are used to post messages and transmit articles, memos, notices, and/or other information that must be shared with all the users of the system or a particular subgroup. Bulletin boards are used by professional organizations to communicate news items instead of mailing the information.

*File Transfer Protocol*  A file transfer protocol (FTP) allows a user on a host computer to access and/or transfer files to and from another host over a network. It is a service that is available on the Internet and any other communication network that has the ability to transmit digital data. The use of fiber-optic communication lines makes it possible to transmit digital data, files, and databases.

*Tools and Protocols*  The Internet also makes available several tools or protocols to travel on the information highway and link other local networks. They include (1) Gopher, which allows the transmission of text-based information, (2) MOSAIC, which allows "browsing" and transmission of graphic and sound information, and (3) WWW, which also allows browsing and the transmission of text, audio, graphics, and images. The Internet is expanding rapidly and continuing to grow as fast as local network resources are created, services are expanded, and tools and protocols are developed.

### Telenet

Telenet is another public telecommunication network used by commercial vendors to communicate on-line with their users. Telenet uses telephone lines as its on-line communication network for offering on-line services and resources such as CompuServe and Prodigy. It traditionally has been used for on-line telephone access to large databases such as MEDLINE at the National Library of Medicine. Telenet was the major public communication service for on-line communication until the Internet emerged.

## SUMMARY

This chapter described hardware, which consists of all the tangible parts of a computer. It also described computer classes, characteristics, and types. The computer classes are analog, digital, and hybrid. The computer characteristics were defined as automatic, electronic, general-purpose, and digital. The computer types are supercomputers, mainframes, minicomputers, and microcomputers.

The chapter outlined the four major functional components of a computer: input units, central processing unit (consisting of the operating system, the arithmetic logic unit, and main memory), secondary storage (an extension of main memory), and output unit. The input unit acts as the "reception desk," the CPU runs the computer, and the output unit produces printed material.

Different devices and media were described in detail, including the most common input devices: terminals and keyboards. The two different types of main memory—ROM (read-only memory) and RAM (random access memory)—were discussed. ROM is used for permanent storage, and RAM is used for temporary storage. The major secondary storage devices were highlighted, including magnetic tapes, magnetic disks, floppy disks (diskettes), and hard disks. Finally, output unit devices and media were reviewed. They include not only VDTs but also various types of printers, microfilm, microfiche, graphics and images, voice output, and magnetic media. Computer communication devices were described, including terminals, modems, and local area networks.

## BIBLIOGRAPHY

Bonner, P. (1983, Nov.). Hard disks made easy. *Personal Computing,* 66–73.

Boraiko, A. A. (1982). The chip: Electronic minimarvel that is changing your life. *National Geographic, 162*(4), 421–458.

Brookshear, J. G. (1991). *Computer Science: An Overview* (3d ed.). New York: Benjamin/Cummings.

Capron, H. L. (1990). *Computers. Tools for the Information Age* (2d ed.). Menlo Park, CA: Benjamin/Cummings.

Capron, H. L., and Williams, B. K. (1984). *Computer and Data Processing* (2d ed.). Menlo Park, CA: Benjamin/Cummings.

Dern, D. P. (1993). *The Internet Guide for New Users.* New York: McGraw-Hill.

DeVoney, C. (1986). *Using PC DOS.* Indianapolis, IN: Que Corp.

Doletta, T. A. (1983). Terminals. In A. Ralston and E. D. Reilly, Jr. (Eds.), *Encyclopedia of Computer Science and Engineering* (2d ed.) (pp. 1489–1495). New York: Van Nostrand Reinhold.

Editors of Time-Life Books. (1985). *Understanding Computers: Computer Basics.* Alexandria, VA: Time-Life Books.

Editors of Time-Life Books. (1986). *Understanding Computers: Input/Output.* Alexandria, VA: Time-Life Books.

Editors of Time-Life Books. (1987). *Understanding Computers: Memory and Storage.* Alexandria, VA: Time-Life Books.

Encyclopedia Britannica Educational Corporation. (1982). *Understanding Computers.* Skokie, IL.

Falk, B. (1994). *The Internet Roadmap.* Alameda, CA: SYBEX.

Finkelstein, C. B. (1983). IBM Card. In A. Ralston and E. D. Reilly, Jr. (Eds.), *Encyclopedia of Computer Science and Engineering* (2d ed.) (pp. 706–709). New York: Van Nostrand Reinhold.

Fisher, S. (1993). *Riding the Internet Highway.* Carmen, IN: New Riders.

Frankenhaus, J. P. (1982, May–June). How to get a good mini. *Harvard Business Review,* 139–149.

Freeman, D. N. (1983). Memory: Auxiliary. In A. Ralston and E. D. Reilly, Jr. (Eds.), *Encyclopedia of Computer Science and Engineering* (2d ed.) (pp. 955–956). New York: Van Nostrand Reinhold.

Garfield, J. (1984, Aug.). Buying your first modem. *Cider,* 58–60.

Gookin, D., and Rathbone, A. (1992). *PCs for Dummies.* San Mateo, CA: IDG Books.

Graham, N. (1986). *The Mind Tool: Computers and Their Impact on Society* (4th ed.). New York: West.

Hedberg, A. (1982, Nov.). Choosing the best computer for now. *Money,* 68–117.

Heller, R. S., and Martin, D. C. (1982). *Bits'n Bytes about Computing: A Computer Literacy Primer.* Rockville, MD: Computer Science Press.

Hopper, G. M., and Mandell, S. L. (1987). *Understanding Computers* (2d ed.). New York: West.

Hutchison, S. E., and Sawyer, S. C. (1988). *Computers: The User Perspective* (2d ed.). Boston: Irwin.

IBM Corporation. (1974). *More about Computers.* Armonk, NY.

IBM Corporation. (1981). *Introduction to IBM Data Processing Systems.* Poughkeepsie, NY.

Korfhage, R. R. (1983). Boolean algebra. In A. Ralston and E. D. Reilly, Jr. (Eds.), *Encyclopedia of Computer Science and Engineering* (2d ed.) (pp. 179–184). New York: Van Nostrand Reinhold.

Libes, S. (1983). Editor's page. *Microsystems, 4*(5), 8–9.

Lindberg, K. P. (1993). *Novell's Guide to Managing Small Netware Networks.* San Jose, CA: Novell Press.

Logitech. (1990–1992). *Microsoft Windows Operating System: Version 3.1: User's Guide.* Freemont, CA: Logitech.

Logitech Inc. (1991). *MouseWare User's Guide: Getting the Most from Your Mouse.* Fremont, CA: Logitech.

Mandell, S. L. (1985). *Introduction to Computers Using the IBM PC.* New York: West.

Mandell, S. L. (1986). *Computers and Data Processing Today: With Basic* (2d ed.). New York: West.

McGlynn, D. R. (1982). *Personal Computing: Home, Professional and Small Business Applications* (2d ed.). New York: John Wiley.

McKeown, P. G. (1986). *Living with Computers.* New York: Harcourt Brace Jovanovich.

McLeod, R., Jr., and Forkner, I. (1982). *Computerized Business Information Systems: An Introduction to Data Processing.* New York: John Wiley.

Morris, G. J. (1983). Digital computers: General principles. In A. Ralston and E. D. Reilly, Jr. (Eds.), *Encyclopedia of Computer Science and Engineering* (2d ed.) (pp. 524–533). New York: Van Nostrand Reinhold.

Necas, J. (1983). Input-output devices. In A. Ralston and E. D. Reilly, Jr. (Eds.), *Encyclopedia of Computer Science and Engineering* (2d ed.) (pp. 735–766). New York: Van Nostrand Reinhold.

Nimersheim, J. (1990). *The First Book of Microsoft Windows 3.0.* Carmel, IN: SAMS.

Owen, B. (1991). *Personal Computers for the Computer Literate: The What, When, Why, Where, and How Guide.* New York: Harper Perennial.

Person, R., and Rose, K. (1990). *Using Microsoft Windows 3: 2d Edition.* Indianapolis, IN: Que Corp.

Pfaffenberger, B. (1991). *Que's Computer User's Dictionary.* Carmel, IN: Que Corp.

Popyk, M. K. (1988). *Up and Running! Microcomputer Applications.* New York: Addison-Wesley.

Prichard, K. (1982). Computers: I. An introduction. *Nursing Times, 78*(5), 355–357.

Ralston, A., and Reilly, E. D., Jr. (Eds.). (1983). *Encyclopedia of Computer Science and Engineering* (2d ed.). New York: Van Nostrand Reinhold.

Rinder, R. M. (1981). *A Practical Guide to Small Computers for Business and Professional Use.* New York: Monarch Press.

Rosen, S. (1983). Digital computers: History: Contemporary and future. In A. Ralston and E. D. Reilly, Jr. (Eds.), *Encyclopedia of Computer Science and Engineering* (2d ed.) (pp. 540–554). New York: Van Nostrand Reinhold.

Sanders, D. H. (1968). *Computers in Business: An Introduction* (4th ed.). New York: McGraw-Hill.

Schnaidt, P. (1990). *LAN Tutorial with Glossary of Terms.* New York: Miller Freeman.

Shea, T. (1983). Personal computer graphics: Pushing technology to the limit. *InfoWorld, 5*(51), 34–36.

Shelly, G. B., and Cashman, T. J. (1980). *Introduction to Computers and Data Processing.* Brea, CA: Anaheim.

Shore, J. (1989). *Using Computers in Business.* Carmel, IN: Que Corp.

Stern, R. A., and Stern, N. (1982). *An Introduction to Computers and Information Processing.* New York: John Wiley.

Sullivan, D. R., Lewis, T. G., and Cook, C. R. (1985). *Computing Today: Microcomputer Concepts and Applications.* Boston: Houghton Mifflin.

Vacroux, A. G. (1975). Microcomputers. *Science America, 232*(5), 32–40.

Walsh, M. E. (1982). *Understanding Computers: What Managers and Users Need to Know.* New York: John Wiley.

Wang, W. E., and Kraynak, J. (1990). *The First Book of Personal Computing.* Carmel, IN: Sams.

Yau, S. S., and Brasch, F. M. (1983). Computer circuiting. In A. Ralston and E. D. Reilly, Jr. (Eds.), *Encyclopedia of Computer Science and Engineering* (2d ed.) (pp. 306–317). New York: Van Nostrand Reinhold.

*4*

• • • • • • • • • • • • • • • • • • • • • • • •

# COMPUTER SOFTWARE

## OBJECTIVES

- Discuss computer software.
- Discuss computer programs.
- Identify software packages.
- Describe programming languages.
- Understand computer programming.

Computer software makes a computer run and controls a computer's resources. It tells the computer "what to do." Computer software includes all the intangible components that are not considered hardware and are not visible. Software refers to the various types of computer programs, including systems programs, applications programs, programming languages, and the programming process.

This chapter describes several aspects of computer software. It discusses the different uses and types of computer programs and highlights software packages, including the major applications for microcomputers. The traditional programming languages are described. Finally, this chapter describes programming, the process of writing of a program. The major areas of software include the following:

- Computer programs
- Software packages
- Programming languages
- Computer programming

# COMPUTER PROGRAMS

The stored computer program was first described by Ada, Countess of Lovelace, in reference to Charles Babbage's analytical engine. She theorized about the automatic repetitious arithmetic steps the analytical engine would follow to solve a problem: the loop concept. This concept gave her the title of the "first programmer" in computer history. However, it was Von Newmann who proposed that both data and instructions could be stored in the computer and that the instructions could be carried out automatically. The stored program concept was subsequently implemented as a major advance in the evolution of the computer.

## Definition

A computer program is a set of stored instructions that tells the computer what to do. It enables the computer to automatically perform a desired action, function, or procedure and solve a problem. It is an algorithm, logically organized in a proper sequence of steps, that directs the execution of a task.

Different types of computer programs are described according to how they function. Some computer programs are prepared by the manufacturer for the internal management of the hardware resources; others are prepared by programmers to carry out specific applications or are developed as software packages for multipurpose users; still others are prepared by microcomputer users for their own applications. Two major categories of computer programs exist:

- System programs
- Applications programs

## System Programs

System programs are all the software used to operate and maintain a computer. A system program enables a computer to manage its own operations. System programs include the operating system, translation programs, utility programs, and other programs that manage the resources of a computer. System programs are designed to carry out, maintain, supervise, and control all the automatic functions of the computer. These programs are stored in read-only memory (ROM). They are generally not visible and not accessible to users and are designed to ensure the smooth functioning of the computer system. System programs are prepared by the manufacturer and are essential for running computer hardware.

All computers require system programs. Mainframes and minicomputers require system programs to carry out their many functions, which are different from those of microcomputers because they are larger and more complex. In a mainframe, system programs supervise and schedule the concurrent processing of multiple programs for many users. They function as interpreters, compilers, assemblers, editors, and debuggers. Microcomputers, by contrast, need fewer programs because they were originally designed to process only one computer program at a time. However, later high-end microcomputers, especially with Windows, began to run more than one program at a time. System programs can be further described by the different functions they perform:

- Operating systems
- Translation programs
- Utility programs

### Operating Systems

The operating system is a set of programs that direct "traffic." It acts as the "traffic cop" and supervises, coordinates, and controls computer resources to manage data and run computer programs. The operating system is a collection of computer programs that control the computer's resources and are responsible for its housekeeping tasks. It runs the software, translates the programming languages, and manages the data. It is used to direct, schedule, and control all input/output devices (monitor, keyboard, printer) and functions, manage the flow of data into and out of memory, and assign data to memory and storage locations. This system also is used to automatically control computer programs (software) that run concurrently (multiprogramming), share resources, and manage timesharing and other special automatic features in large computer systems. The operating system has many commands and functions; some are used for internal control of the computer, and others are used for external control and are executed by the user.

The operating system, a major program in the control system in early mainframe computers, is developed for a specific brand of computer hardware. The operating system is specifically tailored to fit a certain type of computer hardware to ensure its efficient operation. It is used to "boot" a computer, which means that it is loaded into the main memory that turns the computer on. All computers, regardless of type or size, require an operating system to function efficiently.

The operating system is designed not only for internal but also for external control of a computer. An example of an internal control program is the BACKUP program designed to automatically save files being created or edited. An external control program uses commands to activate a computer program such as the FORMAT A DISK program. Such a program allows the user to format a disk for that specific computer to store data. The common commands used to manage microcomputer files are listed in Table 4.1.

Operating systems differ in the various brands of computers. For example, AppleWorks is used exclusively by Apple Macintosh, and MS-DOS (Microsoft Disk Operating System) by IBM and IBM-compatible (clones) microcomputers. Each was developed specifically for one type of equipment and cannot be used for the other. In 1981, Bill Gates developed MS-DOS as the operating system for the first personal computer introduced by IBM. MS-DOS was a separate operating system that was loaded to run the computer; it became the most widely used operating system.

The IBM PC was different from the Apple PC in that the AppleWorks operations system was designed as an integral part of the microcomputer. As a result, Apples could not be cloned, whereas IBM PCs could. This led to the introduction of several compatible clones of the IBM PC that were developed by numerous companies using minor adaptations of MS-DOS. In the late 1980s Microsoft Corporation introduced MS-Windows with several innovative concepts. It was a newer operating system developed as technological capabilities advanced and microcomputers became less expensive. It was designed to reach additional users by providing a more user-friendly graphical interface, making the microcomputer easier to use.

MS-Windows is a computer application that runs on microcomputers that use only the MS-DOS operating system, primarily IBM and IBM-compatible microcomputers. It acts as a "shell" that enables microcomputers to run more than one application at a time and allows for the transfer of information between applications. It also has a "graphical user interface"

**TABLE 4.1**    COMMON MICROSOFT DISK OPERATING SYSTEM
                (MS-DOS) COMMANDS

| Command | Purpose | Syntax |
|---------|---------|--------|
| FORMAT | To prepare a disk for storage | Format <drive name> |
| DIR | Directory: to list stored files by name | Dir <drive name> |
| COPY | To copy a file | Copy <drive name> <file name> to <drive name> |
| DEL | To delete a file from storage | Del <drive name> <file name> |
| CHKDSK | Check disk: to check the status of files and the amount of memory used | Chkdsk <drive name> |
| NAME | To name a file | Name <drive name> <file name> |
| RENAME | To change the name of a file | Rename <drive name> <file name> <new file name> |

that uses prompts, pull-down menus, icons (pictures or symbols), buttons, and dialog boxes that allow the user to perform tasks and/or carry out commands. Thus, the graphical interfaces represent different computer entities. MS-Windows also uses a mouse pointer or cursor as an input device. MS-Windows also offers other applications and utility programs. It enables users to quickly change or update hardware devices without altering or reprogramming each application. Device drivers such as printer drivers can be installed during the system setup, independent of applications. Users do not have to install drivers with each application, as they do with other operating systems.

Computer packages developed for Windows have a common look and feel, lessening the time spent in the initial learning process. MS-Windows eliminates the need to memorize different commands for different software packages and makes computer programs more user-friendly.

MS-Windows/NT is the newest version of the operating system and offers several advanced features. It allows the microcomputer to perform multiuser and multitasking processing. Further, it can run applications developed for different operating systems, such as those used to run the Apple Macintosh. It also has a built-in networking capability, making it possible to share processing resources and facilitating communication within and between local area networks (LANs). A preview version of MS-Windows 95 "Chicago" reveals that it is a true operating system that will enhance prior versions and make Windows easier to use. Similar advances are also offered in Version 2 of the IBM OS/2 system, the Solaris Unix workstations offered by Sun Microsystems, Power PC for both the Apple Macintosh and the IBM PC, and several other emerging microcomputer systems.

### Translation Programs

The major function of a translation program is to translate programming languages into machine language. Translation programs, which are called compilers, interpreters, or assemblers, are machine-dependent; that is, a computer has a specific compiler, interpreter, or assembler to translate the general programming language of the computer program into the language specific to the brand of computer. For example, if a program is written in FORTRAN, the computer needs to have a translation program to translate FORTRAN into machine language or the computer will not be able to run the program.

### Utility Programs

A utility program is designed primarily to handle a computer's housekeeping procedures. Utility programs take care of repetitive tasks and are used to manage and streamline computer resources and operations. They improve and maintain the efficiency of the operating system. A utility program can, for example, update files, convert one type of output medium to another (e.g., paper copy to microfilm), and improve the storage process. Utility programs are used in all computers. In mainframes and minicomputers they may be separate and/or different programs (optional programs), whereas in microcomputers they are generally internal programs that are included in the operating system.

## Applications Programs

Applications programs process data to perform a desired action. Unlike system programs, they are written by or for system users and are stored in random access memory (RAM). They were traditionally written by computer programmers in a programming language to solve a problem, perform a task, or produce a result. They were prepared for a specific manufacturer's computer and could run on a computer only if it also had a translation program. However, with the advancing language generations, user-friendly applications programs started to be provided as off-the-shelf software packages.

## SOFTWARE PACKAGES

Software packages are application programs that are developed for a specific function for many different microcomputer users. They are ready-to-run programs that include utility programs and documentation. For example, a word-processing software package can be used by any user preparing a document. Generally written in an English-like computer language, they require little or no programming knowledge and are ready to use.

Software packages are being developed and marketed by an increasing number of vendors. They are standardized and sometimes are called generic computer programs. They are designed to process a specific type of application, such as word processing, spreadsheets, and database management, and they are available for all brands of microcomputers. The packages are available on disks that have to be loaded into the microcomputer for the application to be activated.

## Software Package Types

There are many types of software packages. Early packages were keyboard-driven, using commands and/or menus, whereas newer Windows packages are "mouse-driven," using pull-down menus, pop-up menus, buttons, icons, and dialog boxes.

### Keyboard-Driven Packages

Keyboard-driven software packages use menus to activate commands. The command labels (names) are typed with the keyboard, selected from a coded menu displayed on the screen, or selected from one function key or a combination of function keys to activate the different functions. Typing in the command labels to activate a function requires the user to know the labels used by the software package. The commands listed on a menu are selected by keying a number or letter to activate a function. Generally, the menus consist of a standard list of command labels that are logical and easy to understand and lead the user through a sequence of steps to carry out a function. For example, in one word-processing package a menu consists of labels such as: TYPE, PRINT, GET, SAVE, REMOVE, and EXIT. The commands selected using one function key or a combination of keys perform similarly to menus but are activated by the **magic** keys. For example, the F10 function key is used to activate the function GET, the F7 key to execute the EXIT function, and the Shift and F7 keys to display the Print Menu options.

### Mouse-Driven Packages

Newer software packages are using a mouse to activate a command or select an icon that represents an application. A mouse is a hand-held device that is used as a pointer or cursor to point and move things around the screen. A mouse is designed to activate a command, operation, or function by "pointing" and then "clicking" at a prompt or "dragging" to cover a block of text. A user points and clicks the mouse to make specific selections, initiate operations, and run the program functions.

Mouse-driven software packages are becoming the most popular packages. They offer a series of icons (graphic symbols or pictures) designed to represent computer entities. For example, a piece of paper is used to depict a sheet of paper and a trash can is used to depict the deletion of a file. Icons and/or buttons also depict data files, program files, and other commands and functions.

Mouse-driven software packages also use menus, pull-down menus, buttons, and dialog boxes. The main menu consists of main commands listed in a menu bar at the top of the screen. When activated, each main menu command displays a "pull-down menu" that lists several functions. Pull-down menus are designed to manage the standard commands, such as opening and closing files. Pull-down menu options can activate a function, bring up another pull-down menu with other options, and bring up a dialog box that contains multiple options for other functions. If the dialog box appears as a template with options, each option has to be addressed. Still other functions can be activated by selecting the options on a button bar. The button bar consists of graphic or labeled "buttons" on a list placed on the top or on the side of the screen (Fig. 4.1).

## Software Package Commands

Generic software packages are ready-to-use packages that offer a specific type of application. They are generally produced by commercial vendors,

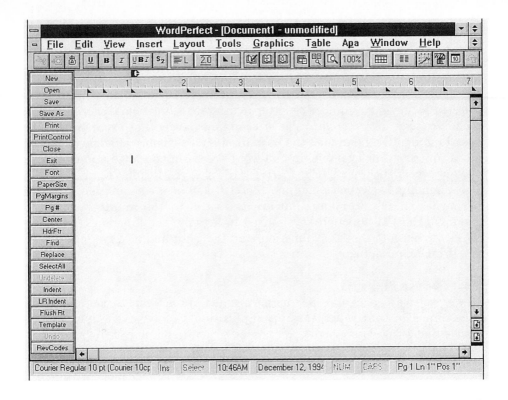

## Parts of a Window

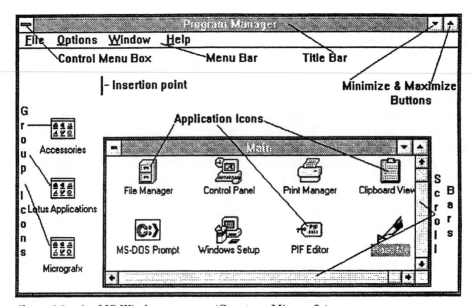

**Figure 4.1** An MS-Windows screen. (Courtesy Microsoft.)

which usually retain ownership rights, limiting the manufacture of copies for resale. Many of the newer packages are available using both MS-DOS and MS-Windows commands. A comparison for one package is shown in Fig. 4.1.

## MS-DOS Commands

Software packages that use MS-DOS commands are activated by pressing different keys on the keyboard. That is, the function keys are used separately or in combination with other keys to carry out a command.

- **Save a document:** F10 (a function key) is pressed to activate the statement "Document to be saved," which appears at the bottom of the screen. The user has to (1) enter the label for a disk drive (A:, B:, or C:) to indicate where the document is to be stored, (2) name the file, and (3) activate the command with the Enter key, which sends the file to the disk in the named drive. The file name cannot exceed eight characters, plus a decimal point and three more characters (B: Sabatble.New).
- **Print a document:** Shift and F7 are pressed together. They activate the "Print Menu," which appears on a separate screen. The print menu offers the user several printing commands for different options.

## MS-Windows Commands

Software packages that use MS-Windows do not use the function keys but are activated by pointing and clicking the mouse at menu labels on the menu bar, pull-down menus, buttons (icons or labels) on the button bar, or icons on the screen to activate similar commands.

- **Save a document:** Click the mouse on "File" on the control menu bar at the top of the screen. This activates a pull-down menu with several labels, including "Save" and "Save As." To save a new file, "Save As" is chosen. Next, the "Save Dialog Box" appears on the screen, requesting the disk drive and file name. Once the file name has been entered (the same as the file name used for MS-DOS above), the "Save" command is clicked and the document is sent to storage.
- **Print a document:** Click the mouse on "File" on the control menu bar at the top of the screen to activate a pull-down menu with several labels. Choose "Print" to print a document. Next, the "Print Dialog Box" appears on the next screen, and the user selects and/or enters the desired print options. Once the options have been selected, click the "Print" command to print the document.

Software packages are being used by health professionals to process all types of data. They are being employed to document daily administrative activities regardless of the setting. Generic software packages make microcomputers an integral part of every health professional's daily functions. They include

- Word-processing packages
- Desktop publishing packages
- Spreadsheet packages
- Database management packages
- Graphic packages
- Communication packages
- Statistical packages

## Word-Processing Packages

A word-processing software package is the most common package used on microcomputers. These packages are designed to process words and prepare documents. They have streamlined the preparation of documents that traditionally were prepared on a typewriter. The tedious steps involved in the physical composition, revision, and correction of text have been removed. With word-processing packages, the written language is easy and flexible and corrections can be made quickly. The transition of a document from its conception to the final copy has been made easy, efficient, and error-free.

### Document Cycle

A word-processing package provides commands and functions that enhance the preparation of a document. The major ones include (1) entering and creating text, (2) editing and manipulating text, (3) naming, saving, storing, and retrieving text, and (4) printing text. Each step in the document cycle uses a number of different features of the word-processing package. The commands used to carry out a function generally vary with different packages.

### Enter Text

The major way to enter text is by keying it in, using the keyboard. The version of the text that appears on the video screen uses several major features of word processing, including word wrap and scroll. Word wrap allows for the automatic carrying of words to the next line. Scrolling allows the automatic movement of lines of text up and down on the screen. The scroll feature is also used to carry lines over from one page to the next without stopping or being concerned with the bottom of the page.

Other features used for entering text include the preparation of the physical appearance of the document: margins, spacing, tab, page numbers, headers, and footers. These features are generally determined by using menus with several options. A page is formatted by setting the margins either in inches or by the number of spaces on the line, which consists of 120 spaces. Spacing (single, double, or triple) between lines can be set, and **tabs** can be set by the number of spaces. Pages can be formatted by setting the location and sequence of the page numbers and can be labeled by inserting headers and footers.

## Edit Text

Editing text involves several features for the efficient preparation of a document. The major ones include insert, delete, copy and move, and merge. To insert and delete text, the user employs the insert and delete keys and/or the space bar. To copy and move refers to copying and moving blocks of text to any place on the document. Merging refers to moving text from other documents into a document. Several of these functions are accomplished with the block feature. In addition, functions are used to center, boldface, and underline text. Search and replace can be used to search for and replace a specific word or phrase. Other editing options include the spell check, a review of synonyms that uses the thesaurus, and a grammar check. The preparation of footnotes and references can also be done by the word-processing package.

## Save and Retrieve Text

Saving and retrieving text makes it possible to save a document in storage, on a floppy disk or on the hard disk. The major feature for carrying out this function requires naming the file. In most software packages an eight-character name is used to label the document. Once named, the file can be saved and retrieved by using the saving and retrieving commands. In most packages the name of the file is listed on a directory, making it possible to find and select a file, even if the name has been forgotten.

## Print Text

Printing text refers to the final production of a document. It includes selecting the font type and size and reviewing the margin options to determine whether the text margins will be evenly aligned or ragged and whether words will be hyphenated. Finally, it includes activating the printer by using the print command for the specific printer to print a paper copy of the document. Some word-processing packages offer other features that provide simple statistical calculations and generate statistical tables and graphics.

# Desktop Publishing Packages

As part of the preparation of final reports and manuscripts, text editing and desktop publishing packages are available. They are packages that make project documentation easier and information dissemination more timely. Generally, they are available as a single package or can be part of a word-processing package. These packages can create pages similar to those that appear in newspapers, magazines, and newsletters. They can manipulate words, add headlines, include pictures, and arrange words into columns so that the paper looks professionally prepared. Desktop publishing software also allows for the direct publication of articles via electronic dissemination to research journals. Manuscripts can be transmitted by a communication network system with a computer modem to a publisher, library, or vendor.

## Spreadsheet Packages

Spreadsheet packages, also called electronic spreadsheets, are used to manage numbers and are called "number crunchers." They are designed to calculate, store, and manipulate numbers, formulas, and accounts. They do for numbers what word processing does for writing. The first software package was a spreadsheet package called VisiCalc, which made numeric processing available to a user without programming knowledge.

Electronic spreadsheet packages are widely used for the preparation of financial statements, budgets, and cash projections. They can perform mathematical calculations, including addition, subtraction, multiplication, and division. Calculations are prepared by formulas, allowing for automatic immediate recalculation of the numbers when a spreadsheet number is altered. Spreadsheet packages are similar to word-processing packages in that commands are used to carry out functions for manipulating numbers. Spreadsheets can be created, edited, named, saved, stored, and retrieved. A spreadsheet that requires labeling of the rows and column should be manually designed before it is programmed. A spreadsheet requires a plan, the variables must be identified, and the spreadsheet needs to be tested before it is used (see Fig. 4.2, p. 136).

### Spreadsheet Size

An electronic spreadsheet resembles a ledger pad consisting of intersecting rows and columns, ranging in size from 128 to 256 columns and 2,048 to 9,999 rows, for a total of more than 2 million cells. A cell is the rectangular area identified by the intersection between a row identified by a number and a column identified by a letter. For example, C1 is the address that refers to the cell formed by the intersection of row 1 and column C. Using an electronic spreadsheet involves three major operations: (1) enter and manipulate data, (2) edit data, which includes naming, storing, and retrieving data, and (3) print a spreadsheet, also called a document or file.

### Enter and Manipulate Data

Data are entered into cells as numbers, labels, or formulas. They are entered by positioning the cursor in the cell to enter labels, numeric values, or formulas that are activated by pressing the enter key. A label provides descriptive text (nonnumeric) about the data in the cell. Labels are used to name the columns and rows in the table. A label can also include a number that is used not mathematically but as a fact, such as a street address. A numeric value is a number to be calculated. It can represent a whole or decimal number, currency, percent, or any other numeric value.

A formula is used to calculate a total, percent, ratio, or financial payment. It is designed to perform mathematical, scientific, or financial operations easily. A mathematical formula refers to computation or addition, such as a sum of numbers in several cells that signify subtotals and totals. A statistical function refers to the computation, such as an average, mean, or ratio, of the numbers in a range of cells. A financial formula refers to the computation of financial functions, such as computing the amount in dollars needed to pay off the principal of a loan.

### Edit Data
Editing data refers to operations that are activated primarily through the use of menus. The menu system is hierarchically arranged and generally is composed of two lines displayed along the top of the screen. The first line lists the major commands, and the second line lists a different set of commands. The major functions include commands such as worksheet, copy, move, file, print, graph, and quit. For each of these commands other commands appear, such as global, column, erase, status, and page; when one is selected, other commands appear sequentially and lead the user through a series of options to complete the function.

To format the size of cells, for example, the following commands might be used. First, the menu feature is turned on, activating the two menu lines, which appear on the screen. If the worksheet command is selected from the first line, a second line of commands appears. If global is selected from the second line, a query appears, asking the user to indicate the width by entering the number of spaces for the spreadsheet columns. Global commands allow the user to set the width of one column or all the columns on the spreadsheet. Menu commands are used to edit the spreadsheet. They include commands to (1) save, store, and retrieve a spreadsheet, (2) copy, move, and delete cells, rows, and columns, (3) calculate totals, percents, or ratios with formulas, (4) transfer data between spreadsheets and storage, and (5) print a spreadsheet as a table or graph. Spreadsheets use menu commands that are similar to those used for word-processing packages. They are activated by following the menu sequences.

### Print Spreadsheet File
Spreadsheets can be printed as tables or graphs. Tables require the user to identify the range of the rows and columns and the labels for them. Graphs require a similar set of commands. Graphs can be line, bar, or pie charts. A line graph is designed to map trends over time and is used to compare two variables on the same graph. A bar graph is used to compare different sets of data, with each bar on the chart used to present one data element. A pie chart plots one variable at a time. It is generally a circle with wedges that look like slices of pie. It can show relationships in a single set of data items, with each data item represented by a slice of the pie.

Spreadsheet packages are used to prepare two- and three-dimensional spreadsheets to perform complex financial analyses. The formula options are used to answer "what if–then" questions for any mathematical calculation required for the research. For example, "what if" the number of bed census increases? "Then" how many more nursing staff hours will be needed to provide care? Electronic spreadsheets are used primarily for financial applications such as budget projections and mortgage amortization. They are used for preparing a budget; presenting tables and graphs; preparing forecast projections of time, cost, and personnel; and outlining milestone tasks and charts (Fig. 4.2).

## Database Management Packages

Database management packages are designed to process data. They do this similarly to the way words are processed by word-processing packages and numbers are processed by spreadsheet packages. Database management packages process data, which can be a name, number, or concept. Database management programs are described in Chap. 5.

```
A:A1: [W14] 'PERSONNEL DATA: Sloane Camera and Video
Worksheet  Range  Copy  Move  File  Print  Graph  Data  System  Quit
Global  Insert  Delete  Column  Erase  Titles  Window  Status  Page  Hide
```

| | A | B | C | D | E |
|---|---|---|---|---|---|
| 1 | PERSONNEL DATA: Sloane Camera and Video | | | | |
| 2 | | | | | |
| 3 | EMPLOYEE# | LASTNAME | FIRSTNAME | LOCATION | DATE_HIRED |
| 4 | 000220 | Edwards | Jack | Atlanta | 14-Feb-87 |
| 5 | 000297 | Percival | James | Atlanta | 18-Dec-87 |
| 6 | 000348 | Reese | Carl | Atlanta | 13-Sep-88 |
| 7 | 000190 | Santos | Elizabeth | Atlanta | 17-Jul-86 |
| 8 | 000247 | Savage | Elaine | Atlanta | 27-May-87 |
| 9 | 000281 | Adamson | Joy | Boston | 21-Oct-87 |
| 10 | 000262 | Bird | Lance | Boston | 13-Aug-87 |
| 11 | 000159 | Caulfield | Sherry | Boston | 19-Mar-84 |
| 12 | 000139 | Cobb | William | Boston | 28-May-82 |
| 13 | 000367 | Fletcher | Amanda | Boston | 03-Jan-89 |
| 14 | 000185 | Johnson | Rebecca | Boston | 04-Feb-86 |
| 15 | 000118 | Kaplan | Janet | Boston | 22-Jun-81 |
| 16 | 000307 | Bjorkman | Robert | Chicago | 24-Feb-88 |
| 17 | 000146 | Krauss | Edward | Chicago | 13-Jul-83 |
| 18 | 000162 | Lerner | Kimberly | Chicago | 28-Jun-84 |
| 19 | 000284 | Morse | Miriam | Chicago | 02-Nov-87 |
| 20 | 000324 | Tallan | George | Chicago | 20-May-88 |

```
DBT13S.WK3                                          NUM
```

**Figure 4.2**  A spreadsheet.

# Graphic Packages

Graphic packages communicate ideas via pictures. They are used to display visual representation of data. There are several different types of graphs, including (1) analysis graphs, (2) presentation graphs, (3) computer-aided design, and (4) paint packages.

### Analysis Graphs

Analysis graphs are primarily charts for the presentation of data, such as line and bar graphs, pie charts, and cluster graphs and scattergrams. A graphic display is a useful way to describe data and reveal trends, unusual values, and relationships between variables. These displays are primarily produced from spreadsheet and/or statistical packages.

### Presentation Graphs

Presentation graphs are used for illustrations that are multidimensional. They generally use full color and are designed to enhance the presentation of data. Some packages offer the ability to enlarge and change the composition of an illustration while viewing the screen. They are used to illustrate survey data.

### Computer-Aided Design

Computer-aided design (CAD) packages are employed for electronic and structural design activities. They are used primarily by architects, engineers, and other specialists who require design and mapping features.

### Paint Packages

Paint packages are used to replicate pictures. Such packages can draw pictures and/or select a picture from a dictionary of illustrations. Graphics can be also produced from statistical packages that run on a mainframe, a minicomputer, or a microcomputer connected to a plotter printer with graphic capabilities.

### Virtual Reality

Virtual reality refers to the use of advanced computer graphics that enable a user to graphically view the environment being depicted. It simulates real-life situations and/or environments. It requires virtual reality technology (advanced hardware), a headset to view the actual images by using some form of video display, and the appropriate software. Virtual reality is being used in health care to view surgical operations and medical procedures. Such graphic techniques also can be used to educate not only professionals but also laypersons about new specialized techniques and treatments.

## Communication Packages

Communication packages are applications programs that enable the user to connect to and transmit data to and from other distant computers via a modem for the purpose of sharing and exchanging information. Several communication software programs can be used on a microcomputer, but they will not work unless the computer has a modem or another communication device. Communication software packages allow the user to communicate with, transmit to, or access common resources and/or services from a remote location.

## Statistical Packages

Statistical packages are designed to analyze data. They perform statistical operations and use analytic techniques to process data. Researchers and administrators are the health professionals who most often use statistical packages. These packages are defined and described in Chap. 15.

## PROGRAMMING LANGUAGES

A programming language, a language used to communicate with a computer, is defined by the American National Standards Institute (ANSI) as "a language used to prepare computer programs" (Sammet, 1969). It contains a defined set of characters (symbols) and rules (semantics); the rules clearly define how the symbols are used.

Computer programming languages, also called software, have their own history and have gone through several generations. With the invention of the computer in 1946, machine languages emerged, followed by assembly languages. High-level programming languages followed in the 1950s. Instrumental in this development was Commodore Grace Hopper, U.S. Navy, who with associates developed one of the first automatic coding systems or high-level languages: COBOL (**Co**mmon **B**usiness **O**riented **L**anguage). COBOL is used primarily for business applications.

The five levels of computer programming languages are as follows:

- Machine language
- Assembly language
- High-level languages
- Natural languages
- Object-oriented languages

## Machine Language

Machine language, a low-level language, is the true language of the computer. Every program must be translated into machine language before the computer can execute it. The machine language consists only of the binary numbers 1 and 0, representing **on** and **off** electrical impulses.

All data—numbers, letters, and symbols—are represented by combinations of binary digits. For example, the number 3 is represented by eight binary numbers (0000 0011), and 6 is represented by 0000 0110. Traditionally, machine languages are machine-dependent and dissimilar; thus, each machine has its own unique language (Fig. 4.3).

## Assembly Language

Assembly language, another low-level language, was developed to make writing computer programs less burdensome. Assembly languages use abbreviations or mnemonic codes instead of binary codes; symbols are used for programming instructions. For example, "A" might be used for "ADD" and "S" might be used for "subtract." Assembly language is written on a one-to-one basis, as is machine language. For each line of assembly language code there is an equivalent line of machine language code. To code the instruction "ADD 6 and 3," the assembly language might read "A 6,3." One line of code is used for the instruction. An assembly program needs an assembler to translate assembly language into machine language. Like machine language, assembly language is machine-dependent.

## High-Level Languages

Like assembly language, high-level languages were the next generation developed to make writing programs easier. They approximated the language used to state or solve a problem, and they resembled English

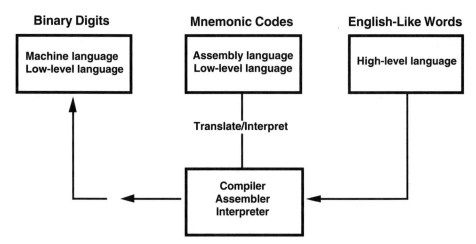

**Figure 4.3**   Computer programming language levels.

and used English-like words to code programs. Scientific problems were more readily understood because mathematical formulas could be expressed clearly in the coding; by the same token, business terms were more readily understood because their common terms were used for naming variables. Over 200 programming languages are considered high-level languages.

Software command languages have also been developed. They are high-level programming languages designed to work on a generic software package such as a spreadsheet or a database management program. Software command languages vary, but they all enable users to create custom applications, perform logical branching, and execute operations with ease.

High-level languages have many advantages over machine and assembly languages. They are written not for a specific machine but for programmers, thus requiring little or no knowledge of a specific computer; however, they do require learning the rules of the language. A programmer can write a program with little or no knowledge of the specific computer the program will be run on. Program instructions are relatively easy to write because they are written in terms similar to those used in solving a problem. Each instruction is translated into several lines of machine language code. For example, the instruction to read two variables, "READ A, B," will be translated into several separate instructions in machine language code.

All high-level languages are machine-independent. The instructions cannot be executed unless the computer translates them into machine language, and so they require the use of a compiler program or interpreter program. The major programming languages developed for a specific purpose are FORTRAN, COBOL, and BASIC; the general-purpose ones are ADA, PASCAL, and C/C++. Other languages developed for the new generation of microcomputers include LISP and PROLOG.

### FORTRAN

FORTRAN (**For**mula **Tran**slator), a programming language used primarily for scientific and mathematical applications, was introduced by IBM in 1954. It was the first and is the oldest high-level language. Originally developed for scientists, engineers, and business statisticians, it has proved to be an excellent language for all scientific fields. A major advantage of FORTRAN is its application for complex mathematical calculations and problems.

### COBOL

COBOL, one of the earliest high-level languages, was the most widely used programming language for business applications. It was developed in 1959 by Grace Hopper and her associates, who pioneered the development of the COBOL compiler. COBOL is machine-independent, has an English-like feature, and is still used in many different types of computer systems.

## BASIC

BASIC (**B**eginners **A**ll-Purpose **S**ymbolic **I**nstruction **C**ode), which was introduced in 1965 at Dartmouth College under the direction of Professor John Kemeny, is an interactive English-like language that is easy to learn and use. Developed for use on a timesharing computer system by students, it is mathematical but also allows for free-form text. It is simpler than most other languages and has become one of the major languages in the microcomputer field.

## ADA

Named for Ada, Countess of Lovelace, ADA was developed for the Department of Defense. Completed in 1984, it is designed to meet the department's technical, management, and cost criteria requirements. Designed to provide greater reliability and efficient maintenance of computer programs, ADA is structured to be used for scientific, business, and command and control applications.

## PASCAL

Named after Blaise Pascal, PASCAL was developed in 1972 by the Swiss professor Nicklaus Wirth. It was developed for all types of applications and for applying structured programming. PASCAL is notable for its efficiency, portability, and all-around usability. A popular language for teaching, it is widely used on many microcomputers.

## C/C++

C/C++ is an upgraded version of C and is similar to PASCAL in many ways. This language was developed by Bell Laboratories in 1972. It is an economical language that allows an experienced programmer to write programs that make more efficient use of computer hardware. It is machine-independent and is considered a portable program. Programs are currently being developed in this language that may enable users to emulate knowledge-based systems.

## LISP

LISP (**Lis**t **P**rocessor) was designed at about the same time as ALGOL. It aided scientists in working on problems of artificial intelligence in an attempt to make computers translate human languages.

## PROLOG

Researchers recently have chosen PROLOG (**Pro**gramming **Log**ic) for a new generation of computers. PROLOG is convenient for programming logical processes and making deductions automatically. It is the language that will be used in artificial intelligence systems of the future.

### MUMPS

MUMPS (**M**assachusetts General Hospital **U**tility **M**ulti **P**rogramming **S**ystem), in use since 1965, was developed for clinical health care applications. It uses a hierarchical structure that permits large volumes of data to be handled easily. MUMPS is available primarily on minicomputers. Because many computers do not have compilers or interpreters that can translate this language, it has had limited use.

Other significant high-level programming languages include the following:

### PL/1

PL/I (**P**rogramming **L**anguage **1**) is a symbolic general-purpose language that was developed by IBM in 1964 for a variety of business, engineering, and scientific applications. A powerful and flexible language, it incorporates the major advantages of COBOL and FORTRAN.

### RPG

RPG (**R**eport **P**rogram **G**enerator) appeared in 1964. Developed for IBM computers and relatively easy to use, it was designed to allow for rapid generation of business reports.

### ALGOL

ALGOL (**Algo**rithmic **L**anguage) is an international algebraic language. Introduced in 1960 by European and American scientists, it was developed primarily for scientific applications and is similar to FORTRAN and PASCAL. It has been replaced by PASCAL as the language used by computer scientists for the formal descriptions of algorithms.

## Natural Languages

Natural language, also called fifth-generation language, translates all terminology to a binary code that the computer understands. A true natural language resembles "natural" spoken English, in that it is humanlike and is based on rules or syntax. Most natural language programs are relatively crude and are based primarily on pattern-matching techniques. That is, they are translation programs with rules designed to recognize the syntax of sentences. However, translating a natural language in depth also requires an understanding of the sentence before a correct translation can be made.

Preparing a translation program for a natural language requires several levels of analysis. First, the sentence needs to be parsed to identify the parts of speech, for example, the subject. The next level is called semantic analysis, by which the grammar of each word in the sentence is analyzed. This level attempts to recognize the action described and the object of the action. There are several computer programs that translate natural languages on the basis of the rules of English. They generally are specially written programs designed to interact with databases on a specific topic. When the program is limited to querying the database, it is possible to process the natural language terms.

Another level of analysis is contextual analysis, which determines the meaning of the sentence. Since this level overlaps, it is a difficult task to program. However, advanced natural language processing, also referred to as a knowledge-based language, interacts with a base of knowledge on a particular subject. Thus, the use of a natural language is critical to accessing a knowledge base and is the basis for artificial intelligence. Therefore, advanced natural languages are associated with artificial intelligence. In fact, the Japanese have selected natural language as the official language for the next generation of computers.

The advanced natural languages have emerged with advances in computer technology and algorithms. They are algorithms that can be developed with instructions that can be executed simultaneously instead of one set of instructions at a time. That is, they represent parallel processing. These newer languages are used to develop decision support systems, expert systems, and artificial intelligence. They are making it possible to progress to the next programming generation.

## Object-Oriented Languages

An object-oriented language is a nonprocedural programming language that conceptualizes program elements as objects, each of which has its own data and programming code. Each object is a modular program, which makes it possible to add, copy, and move to other programs without having to reconstruct the object elements.

## COMPUTER PROGRAMMING

Computer programming refers to the process of writing a computer program, which is a series of instructions written in the proper sequence to solve a specific problem or accomplish a stated goal. A program primarily encompasses the program instructions and is generally written by a computer programmer. The five major steps in writing a computer program are as follows:

1. Problem definition
2. Program design
3. Program preparation

4. Program testing
5. Program implementation/documentation

## Problem Definition

Problem definition is the most critical step in programming, as it requires a thorough understanding of the problem at hand. The definition must state the problem that requires a solution, including the relevant data and where to find them. In essence, the problem and/or stated goal must be analyzed and outlined in detail to determine its scope and all the data elements needed. For example, a very simple problem definition for the cost of a nursing visit might read as follows: "Calculate cost of nursing visit C by totaling cost of nurse A and cost of supplies B."

## Program Design

The program design is the plan designed to solve the problem and/or achieve the stated goal preliminary to the actual preparation and coding. The plan must be detailed enough to outline the way to produce the desired output. It must be analyzed and broken down into a set of logical sequential steps called an algorithm. An algorithm is actually the procedure or "recipe" that solves a problem and/or accomplishes a stated goal. The steps of the algorithm are generally listed and illustrated with a flowchart.

### Flowchart

A flowchart employs a series of symbols to illustrate graphically or a set of instructions to identify the logical solution to a problem and/or the way to accomplish a stated goal. It specifies the sequence of instructions or groups of instructions in a computer program. A flowchart can be an illustration that clarifies essential details and their relationships in the computer program. Various operations, data, tasks, and the flow process are presented graphically or in a sequence of instructions.

### Loops

Loops represent graphically the repetitive operations or instructions in a computer program. A unique feature of programming and the major characteristic of a computer program, loops require both lines and symbols. Figure 4.4 illustrates a flowchart with a loop.

## Program Preparation

Program preparation—the actual writing of a program—entails coding the program in a programming language. The program instructions (algorithms) must be coded in detail and in logical sequence so that the program can be processed correctly. The programming language selected not

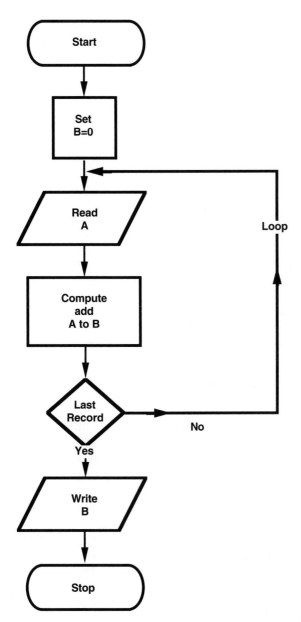

**Figure 4.4**
A flowchart with a loop.

only must be appropriate for processing the problem but also must be translatable by the computer for which it is written. The language rules must be followed precisely because a single coding error can stop the program from running or cause a program malfunction.

A mathematical problem might be coded with a high-level language as follows:

```
START
READ A
READ B
COMPUTE C = A + B
PRINT C
```

# Program Testing

Program testing occurs after coding. Actual data should be used to test the program to ensure correct output and program writing and coding. The program also is tested to determine whether the programming language is correct, the processing logic is sound, and the program runs correctly. The program can be implemented after it has been judged correct.

A major activity in testing is debugging, which entails checking the program to ensure that it is free of error. The term "debugging" was coined by Grace Hopper. In 1945, when working at Harvard on MARK II, she removed from the computer a moth that had caused it to stop. As a result, the term was used to refer to any correction of a computer problem.

# Program Implementation/Documentation

Program implementation/documentation is the final step in programming. Once a program has been tested and debugged, it is ready to produce the defined output; however, detailed documentation (according to accepted standards) of each programming step is required. Documentation generally should be prepared to aid the program users and programmers who will perform program maintenance (changes, revisions, updates). The program must be documented sufficiently to satisfy the reference needs of both groups.

The popularity and ease of use of software packages have enabled nonprogrammers to select a preprogrammed set of instructions that most clearly matches an application. Users design forms or screens for data input and report formats for data output. Although such packages free the user from writing the actual program code in a selected language, the user must still consider the five steps of computer programming defined above.

The problem definition and/or stated goal is still the most critical step. Users must clearly understand the task of selecting the proper software package. Program design becomes form or report design. The user must consider how the data are to be input into the system and select a clear and understandable format for reporting the output. Program preparation can be compared to screen design. The user "places" fields of data on the screen and with special function keys "moves" the fields about to get a more logical arrangement. All programs, whether created by direct code or by a software package, must be tested before they can be implemented. Completed screens can be tested or debugged with a small sample subset of the data to ensure that the program produces the correct output.

A final caution for users of software packages: Users may design screens and report formats, but they must be aware that all copyrights remain with the software package creators. Any plans to distribute designed screens or report formats must be cleared with the package creator.

## SUMMARY

This chapter highlighted computer software, which includes computer programs and the programming languages that run a computer. Computer programs are sets of instructions stored in computer memory that are used to make the computer run. The newer computer programs called software packages are sets of computer programs designed for many users and different computers. They are generally written in a language that uses English-like words and require little or no programming expertise. Several of the most common generic software packages were also described.

Software also refers to the programming languages that are needed to communicate with the computer. Several levels of programming languages—machine, assembly, high-level, natural, and object-oriented—were presented, along with the different programming languages. The five major programming steps are problem definition, program design, program preparation, program testing, and program implementation and documentation.

## REFERENCES

Sammet, J. E. (1969). *Programming Languages: History and Fundamentals* (p. 8). Englewood Cliffs, NJ: Prentice-Hall.

## BIBLIOGRAPHY

Bentley, M. B. (1988). *The Viewpoint Technician: A Guide to Portable Software Design.* Glenview, IL: Scott, Foresman.

Brookshear, J. G. (1991). *Computer Science: An Overview* (3d ed.). New York: Benjamin/Cummings.

Cain, N. W., and Cain, T. (1987). *Hard Disk Manager.* New York: Prentice-Hall.

Capron, H. L. (1990). *Computers: Tools for the Information Age* (2d ed.). Menlo Park, CA: Benjamin/Cummings.

Capron, H. L., and Williams, B. K. (1984). *Computer and Data Processing* (2d ed.). Menlo Park, CA: Benjamin/Cummings.

DATAPRO Research Corporation. (1981). *An Evaluation of the MUMPS Language*. Delron, NJ.

Davis, R. M. (1977). Evolution of computers and computing. *Science, 195*(4283), 1096–1102.

Denning, P. J. (1971). Third generation computer systems. *Computer Survey, 3*(4), 175–213.

Denning, P. J. (1983). Operating systems. In A. Ralston and E. D. Reilly, Jr. (Eds.), *Encyclopedia of Computer Science and Engineering* (2d ed.) (pp. 1053–1075). New York: Van Nostrand Reinhold.

Desposito, J., Marcim, J., and White, D. (1992). *Que's Computer Buyer's Guide: 1992 Edition*. Carmel, NY: Que Corp.

DeVoney, C. (1987). *Using PC DOS*. Indianapolis, IN: Que Corp.

Editors of Time-Life Books. (1985). *Understanding Computers: Software*. Alexandria, VA: Time-Life Books.

Editors of Time-Life Books. (1986). *Understanding Computers: Computer Languages*. Alexandria, VA: Time-Life Books.

Editors of Time-Life Books. (1988). *Understanding Computers: The Software Challenge*. Alexandria, VA: Time-Life Books.

Encyclopedia Britannica Educational Corporation. (1982). *Understanding Computers*. Skokie, IL.

Enlander, D. (1980). *Computers in Medicine: An Introduction*. St. Louis: Mosby.

Falk, B. (1994). *The Internet Roadmap*. Alameda, CA: SYBEX.

The first lady of computers. (1982, Nov. 14). *Washington Post Parade Magazine*, 21.

Frenzel, L. E. (1979, Winter). Understanding personal computer software. *On Computing*, 17–25, 77–99.

Gookin, D., and Rathbone, A. (1992). *PCs for Dummies*. San Mateo, CA: IDG Books.

Grace M. Hopper: Programmer's programmer. (1982, Nov. 28). *Washington Post Magazine*, 113–114.

Harm, L. W. (1983). Software packages. In A. Ralston and E. D. Reilly, Jr. (Eds.), *Encyclopedia of Computer Science and Engineering* (2d ed.) (pp. 1364–1370). New York: Van Nostrand Reinhold.

Hart, A. (1992). *Knowledge Acquisition for Expert Systems*. (2d ed.). New York: McGraw-Hill.

Heller, R. S., and Martin, D. C. (1982). *Bits 'n Bytes about Computing: A Computer Literacy Primer*. Rockville, MD: Computer Science Press.

Hopper, G. M., and Mandell, S. L. (1987). *Understanding Computers* (2d ed.). New York: West.

Hutchison, S. E., and Sawyer, S. C. (1988). *Computers: The User Perspective* (2d ed.). Boston, MA: Irwin.

IBM Corporation. (1981). *Introduction to IBM Data Processing Systems* (5th ed.). White Plains, NY.

ICP Interview with Grace M. Hopper. (1980, Spring). *ICP INTERFACE Administrative and Accounting*, 18–23.

Joos, I., Whitman, N. I., Smith, M. J., and Nelson, R. (1992). *Computers in Small Bytes: The Computer Workbook*. New York: National League for Nursing Press.

Johnson, S. (1982, Sept.). Grace Hopper—a living legend. *All Hands*, 3–6.

Kemeny, J. G. (1972). *Man and the Computer*. New York: Scribner.

Logitech. (1990–1992). *Microsoft Windows Operating System: Version 3.1: User's Guide*. Freemont, CA: Logitech.

Logitech. (1991). *MouseWare User's Guide: Getting the Most from Your Mouse*. Fremont, CA: Logitech.

Mace, S. (1982). Mother of COBOL—still thinkin', still workin'. *InfoWorld*, 5(18), 29–31.

Mandell, S. L. (1985). *Introduction to Computers Using the IBM PC*. New York: West.

McKeown, P. G. (1987). A *Personal Computer Toolbox: Software Applications for the IBM PC*. Washington, DC: Harcourt Brace Jovanovich.

Morris, R. A. (1980). Comparison of some high-level languages. *BYTE, 5*(2), 128–139.

Nimersheim, J. (1990). *The First Book of Microsoft Windows 3.0*. Carmel, IN: SAMS & Co.

Owen, B. (1991). *Personal Computers for the Computer Illiterate: The What, When, Why, Where, and How Guide*. New York: Harper Perennial.

Person, R., and Rose, K. (1990). *Using Microsoft Windows 3: 2d Edition*. Indianapolis, IN: Que Corp.

Pfaffenberger, B. (1991). *Que's Computer User's Dictionary*. Carmel, IN: Que Corp.

Pogue, R. E. (1980). The authoring system: Interface between author and computer. *Journal of Research and Developmental Education, 14*(1), 57–68.

Popyk, M. K. (1988). *Up and Running! Microcomputer Applications*. New York: Addison-Wesley.

Price, D. (1980, June). Questions and answers on programming languages. *Microcomputing*, 82–85.

Pritchard, K. (1982). Computers: I. An introduction. *Nursing Times, 78*(5), 355–357.

Product Line Brief. (1993). *Apple Newton MessagePad*. Cupertino, CA: Apple Corp.

Ralston, A., and Reilly, E. D., Jr. (Eds.). (1983). *Encyclopedia of Computer Science and Engineering* (2d ed.). New York: Van Nostrand Reinhold.

Rosen, S. (1983). Software. In A. Ralston and E. D. Reilly, Jr. (Eds.), *Encyclopedia of Computer Science and Engineering* (2d ed.) (pp. 1346–1348). New York: Van Nostrand Reinhold.

Ross, S. C., Lund, P. H., Hayden, B. A., and Smith, M. T. (1987). *Understanding and Using Application Software: Vol. 2*. New York: West.

Sagman, S. W., and Sandler, J. G. (1990). *Using Harvard Graphics* (2d ed.). Carmel, IN: Que Corp.

Sammet, J. E. (1983). Programming languages. In A. Ralston and E. D. Reilly, Jr. (Eds.), *Encyclopedia of Computer Science and Engineering* (2d ed.) (pp. 1228–1232). New York: Van Nostrand Reinhold.

Schnaidt, P. (1990). *LAN Tutorial with Glossary of Terms*. New York: Miller Freeman.

Shelly, G. B., and Cashman, T. J. (1980). *Introduction to Computers and Data Processing*. Brea, CA: Anaheim.

Shore, J. (1989). *Using Computers in Business*. Carmel, IN: Que Corp.

Smith, B. (1990). *UNIX: Step-by-Step*. Carmel, IN: Sams & Co.

Stern, R. A., and Stern, N. (1982). *An Introduction to Computers and Information Processing* (2d ed.). New York: John Wiley.

Sullivan, D. R., Lewis, T. G., and Cook, C. R. (1985). *Computing Today: Microcomputer Concepts and Applications*. Boston: Houghton Mifflin.

Tropp, H. S. (1983). Hopper, Grace Murray. In A. Ralston and E. D. Reilly, Jr. (Eds.), *Encyclopedia of Computer Science and Engineering* (2d ed.) (pp. 685–686). New York: Van Nostrand Reinhold.

Wang, W. E., and Kraynak, J. (1990). *The First Book of Personal Computing.* Carmel, IN: Sams.

Wilkes, M. V. (1983). Charles Babbage. In A. Ralston and E. D. Reilly, Jr. (Eds.), *Encyclopedia of Computer Science and Engineering* (2d ed.) (pp. 157–158). New York: Van Nostrand Reinhold.

WordPerfect Corp. (1991). *WordPerfect for Windows: Workbook.* Orem, UT.

Zin, K. L. (1983). Authoring languages and systems. In A. Ralston and E. D. Reilly, Jr. (Eds.), *Encyclopedia of Computer Science and Engineering* (2d ed.) (pp. 144–146). New York: Van Nostrand Reinhold.

# 5

. . . . . . . . . . . . . . . . . . . . . . . . .

# DATA PROCESSING

## OBJECTIVES

- Understand what data are.
- Identify data structure and storage.
- Describe database management systems.
- Interpret data processing.
- Discuss data security, privacy, and confidentiality.

Computers process data: facts, figures, names, and a variety of patient characteristics. Once processed, data become the information needed to solve a problem or carry out an application. Computer hardware—the machine—processes data as instructed by computer software, making data processing the interaction between hardware and software that changes data into information. Previous chapters described computer hardware and software. This chapter discusses data storage, organization, and structure; database management systems; data processing; and data security, privacy, and confidentiality. Specifically, it includes the following:

- Data
- Data structure and storage
- Database management systems

- Data processing
- Computer security
- Privacy and confidentiality

## DATA

Data are raw facts that represent single pieces of information. A fact, also called a data element, is a word or a numeric value representing a piece of information. Data are the smallest units of information that can be stored, retrieved, and/or edited. Data are stored in computer memory and secondary storage. All data are organized in a logical structure so that they can be labeled, indexed, and easily located and retrieved.

## DATA STRUCTURE AND STORAGE

Data are organized and stored in logical entities. These entities are arranged in a hierarchy consisting of the following:

- Bytes/characters
- Fields/data elements
- Records
- Files
- Databases

## Bytes/Characters

A byte, also called a character, is the smallest logical entity stored in the computer. A byte consists of a combination of 8 bits (**bi**nary dig**its**), which are either 0s or 1s. A byte represents a character—a letter, number, or symbol—that is entered into the computer, coded, and stored as machine language. There are a maximum of 256 different bytes to represent all uppercase and lowercase letters of the alphabet, numbers from zero to nine (0–9), and special symbols such as percent, dollar sign, and semicolon. For example, the letter "A" is coded as 0100 0001 (8 bits) and the number 1 is coded as 0011 0001 (8 bits) in ASCII code.

Computer processing is based on arithmetic calculations and logical comparisons of bytes. These functions are conducted in the arithmetic logic unit (ALU) in the central processing unit (CPU) of the computer. The arithmetic operations—addition, subtraction, multiplication, and division—are performed using binary numbers. Logical operations are performed by comparing one byte with another to determine whether the data are "true" or "false," using Boolean logic.

## Coding Schemes

Two coding schemes have emerged as the standards for coding binary characters: ASCII (**A**merican **S**tandard **C**ode for **I**nformation **I**nterchange) and EBCDIC (**E**xtended **B**inary **C**oded **D**ecimal **I**nterchange **C**ode). ASCII has been adopted by the U.S. government as the standard code for the computer industry (see Chap. 3). It uses 8 bits to form a byte. EBCDIC is an 8-digit bit coding scheme that was developed by IBM primarily to represent graphic and special characters. EBCDIC may still be found as machine language in early mainframes and minicomputers.

## Storage Structure

Computer memory is characterized by its capacity in terms of the number of bytes it can hold. Bytes are stored in locations, each of which has its own unique electronic address. The locations identify the address of the characters, as is done with post office boxes. The address changes as the data move in and out of the locations, as when people move from address to address. Bytes (bit words) move around the computer components via a "data bus," a bootstraplike data path (see Chap. 3).

The bus accommodates the (bit) word size, which varies based on the number of bits in a word. Each doubling of the number of (bit) words on the bus increases the speed of the computer twofold. Thus, the 8-bit (one-word) machine is half as fast as the 16-bit (two-word) machine, which is half as fast as the 32-bit (four-word) machine. The larger (bit) word size makes the computer faster and increases its processing power.

# Fields/Data Elements

A field or data element is a group of characters that represents a single fact, value, or item. It is a piece of information composed of combinations of bytes that represent a word or a numeric value, for example, a patient's name, identification number, address, city, state, or zip code. Each of these six separate pieces of information represents a different data field (Table 5.1).

# Records

A record is a group of separate related data fields/elements that form a single unit of information. For example, the identification data for John Smith is a record composed of six data fields that form one record (unit) (Fig. 5.1). A record may be of fixed length or variable length, depending on the computer and the method and type of storage media. A fixed-length record allows a fixed number of spaces for a field or data element; a variable-length record takes only the spaces it actually needs. For example, John Smith's name, identification number, and address require 43 spaces.

**TABLE 5.1**    EXAMPLE OF A PATIENT IDENTIFICATION DATA RECORD

| | |
|---|---|
| Name: | John Smith |
| Identification Number: | 03662 |
| Street Address: | 120 N. Wayne St. |
| City: | Washington |
| State: | DC |
| Zip Code: | 30007 |

If the record were stored as a fixed-length record, 60 spaces might be set aside to accommodate different records, leaving 17 spaces empty. However, as a variable-length record, it would use only 43 spaces.

These two different record structures affect computer processing capability, since fixed-length records are not very flexible even though the programs written to process them are easier to prepare. It is easier to process variable-length records but more difficult to prepare computer programs using them. Also, even though variable-length records store data more efficiently, they cost more to process.

## Files

A file is the next level of data storage. A file is a group of related records that have the same data fields. Files are critical in organizing data in a database. For example, the patient identification file that contains John

**Figure 5.1**   Illustration of data organization by category.

| Category | | Data | |
|---|---|---|---|
| Field | Patient ID Number | 0 3 6 6 2* | Record (Name & Address of Patient) |
| Field | Patient Name | John Smith* | |
| Field | Patient Address | 120 N. Wayne St. | |
| Field | City | Arlington* | |
| Field | State | MA* | |
| Field | Zip Code | 10638* | |
| Record | Name and Address of John Smith | | File (Names and Addresses of All Patients) |
| Record | Name and Address of Nancy Doe | | |
| Record | Name and Address of Virginia Green | | |
| Record | Name and Address of Dick Jones | | |
| File | Names and Addresses of Patients | | Databases (Patients' Accounts) |
| File | Patients' Accounts | | |
| File | Patient Drug Accounts | | |
| File | Other Accounts | | |

* Each number, letter, or symbol is a character (byte).

Smith's identification record could also contain the identification records of all the other patients on the same nursing unit or in the entire hospital (Fig. 5.1).

Computer files are the key to efficient data processing. They resemble office files organized in file cabinets. A file is named and listed in a directory like the names in a telephone book. File names are used to keep track of all files, including their locations and addresses (where they are stored for a specific application). Different file types, storage sizes, and processing methods also influence efficient data processing, including their organization, a crucial element. Many computers use a hierarchical directory, a treelike structure that can also arrange records in different subdirectories used for different purposes.

There are many different types of files for various aspects of data processing, including the following:

- Master files
- Transaction/update files
- Report/sort files

### Master Files

A master file contains all the permanent raw data elements for a specific application. An example is the identification file for all patient identification records in a hospital.

### Transaction/Update Files

A transaction/update file contains all the corrections and additions needed to update records in the master file, such as corrections or changes in a patient's name, insurance number, or address and new hospital admissions.

### Report/Sort Files

The report/sort file (also called the report generator) contains records needed for processing special data, such as the records of all patients with a particular diagnosis. These files are primarily organized according to how the records are structured and stored. The structure will influence the method by which data are accessed, processed, and retrieved. Three common file structures are used:

- Sequential access files
- Direct random access files
- Indexed access files

### Sequential Access Files

The sequential file, the simplest method of structuring files, organizes records sequentially. That is, the records are accessed in the same order in which they are physically stored. They can be organized alphabetically or serially or by some type of special arrangement (e.g., name or diagnosis). Sequential file organization was the earliest type of file organization because magnetic tape could store files only sequentially. In this method, records are accessed one after the other, which means that access is slow and accessibility of data is limited. For example, if records were in alphabetical order, all records from A to S would have to be read before John Smith's record could be accessed.

### Direct Random Access Files

The direct access file allows records to be organized randomly and allows direct access without having to review all the intervening records. The record files are arranged and stored in any order and identified with labels or keys to allow easy direct random access. The random access method makes it possible to access data quickly and instantly. For example, John Smith's record, if organized randomly, could be instantly accessed with one key, such as his identification number. This method is used to process data stored on any of the common on-line magnetic storage devices used today. With this type of storage, data are accessed on-line and processed instantly or in real time.

### Indexed Access Files

The indexed access file, also called the indexed sequential access file, combines features of the sequential and the direct random access files. Generally, records with like key field values are arranged sequentially, but also are indexed so that they can be found either sequentially or directly. In this type of file the records are indexed in a directory that contains a key or pointer to each record stored in the file.

## Databases

A database is the highest level of data storage. It consists of groups of interrelated files that are stored together. It is an organized collection of data. A database organizes and stores all related files with like records and fields. A database can be processed and shared for one or more applications and/or connected to other databases. For example, the patient database contains John Smith's record in the patient identification file, the drug file, the radiology file, and any other files in the database of the hospital information system.

Building a database is as critical for accessing data as is organizing files and records. Data stored in databases are generally managed by a software package called a database management system (DBMS). There are several types of database structures; the major database structures are:

- Hierarchical databases
- Network databases
- Relational databases
- Object-oriented databases

## Hierarchical Databases

A hierarchical database, also called a tree structure database, arranges data in order of rank, with all data records connected to the same base or root. The hierarchical structure is characteristic of mainframes and mini-computer systems. Beginning at the base, an index record points to successive layers of branches. Although in this structure all records are based on one particular root, levels do occasionally exist. In the patients' accounts database, for example, John Smith's name or identification number could be the root for his identification information records in other accounting files. His nursing diagnosis might be the root for a database containing nursing information.

## Network Databases

In a network database records are structured by linking them together by **pointers** using some type of relationship (key), such as patient name, physician name, or diagnosis. Thus, John Smith's records in the different files can be linked on the basis of his medical diagnosis, his name, his physician's name, or any other variable. The selection of variables to be linked together influences the structure of the database and the way the database is accessed.

## Relational Databases

In a relational database two or more interrelated records are connected by the attributes of field (data element) types. This type of structure allows files from one database to be linked with files from another, a process that allows for easy access to and manipulation of records. Generally, in this structure a table is designed with rows and columns. The rows correspond to the records in the files, and the columns to the fields in the database. In this structure the relationships are linear and only relate one data element to another.

## Object-Oriented Databases

The most recent database structure is the object-oriented database, which is based on the concept that databases reflect the meaning of the data, not just the relationships between the data elements. This structure consists of a collection of data objects that belong to a class and have their own characteristics. Each object has its own list of data elements and a programming code, making it possible to pass messages between objects. Each object represents a highly cohesive module containing the activities required to simulate the actions of the object. In this structure, objects can be linked and the relationships between objects can be linked.

Object-oriented databases have grown out of object-oriented programming languages, so that these databases have added characteristics which make it possible to control, manage, and query the databases. The object-oriented programming language processes the program elements conceptualized as independent objects. The processing of objects instead of data elements not only reduces the number of possible combinations of attributes and values to solve the problem but also makes programming easier. Object-oriented structures and programming are being used with the newer hardware and software technology, reducing the data-processing time while increasing processing capabilities.

This type of database may evolve to a combination of object and constraint database models by the turn of the century. New products are being described with virtual multidimensional object-oriented databases.

## DATABASE MANAGEMENT SYSTEMS

A DBMS is a set of computer programs with a unique query (high-level programming) language for manipulating the data in a database. A DBMS is designed to create, access, manage, and monitor a database. The query language allows users to communicate easily with the database without having extensive programming skills.

A DBMS is designed to store and retrieve data, manipulate and rearrange data, and create reports. It is similar to a file cabinet with different drawers, each with hanging file folders containing separate files, all of which are differently and uniquely labeled. DBMSs reduce the amount of programming needed to manipulate large amounts of data. These packages usually have their own software programming language, and different packages have different capabilities. For example, some packages allow for tracking of the data using sequence of dates and others for listing of events. A DBMS may also be designed to organize and structure data in a relational database. In this type of system the data elements are related to one another, providing relationships not previously possible. The relationships do not necessarily have to be predetermined, but can be determined during the analysis. This capability allows the user to obtain inferences from processing the data without being limited by the programming language or by a computer program that was specifically written to process the study data that were required in the past.

A DBMS also is used to manipulate a large database because it allows a computer user to work with the database without having to write a program. Sometimes it can help a user design an efficient database more quickly and more easily. It can also edit data being entered into the computer and provide computer security by controlling access to data. A DBMS is the key to an integrated computer system, as it can manipulate data using a relational structure.

Usually developed by computer manufacturers and software vendors, DBMSs are available for all sizes of computers. Many of the large computerized information systems that contain patient data and generate patient care reports use a DBMS. They are also used in microcomputer systems to manage databases such as personnel, patient classification, or nurse staffing and scheduling. As the processing capability of microcomputers approaches that of the larger computers, they are being used more frequently to manage large databases. There are several DBMS software packages available for microcomputers that are menu-driven and user-friendly.

## Database Tasks

The major commands in a DBMS software package generally include Create, Use, Append, Edit, Modify, List, Browse, Go To, Next, and Delete. Using a DBMS package generally involves four basic steps: (1) set up data, (2) maintain data, (3) manipulate data, and (4) output data.

The first step, set up data, involves creating the structure that will hold the data. The user must name the database file and define the fields (field name, type, and size). Once defined, the data structure is ready to store the records, including their names and sizes. Maintaining data involves periodically revising and updating records, adding new records, and deleting obsolete ones. Data records can be manipulated and searched in a variety of ways. A user can browse through the records, list the data from records, and search for a specific record or type of data. For example, records can be ordered alphabetically or numerically, or they can be filtered so that only records matching a user-specified criterion are selected. The data, once selected, can be prepared as output data. This last step generates formatted reports or graphs to depict the information.

Although a database technically includes only one body of information, it is often made up of two or more structures related or linked by a common field (data element). Programs capable of relating data in this fashion are known as relational DBMS software programs.

## Relational DBMS

There are several relational DBMS software packages for microcomputers. They all provide a menu-driven interface for user-friendly operation by nonprogrammers, and a query (programming) language that includes instructions for manipulating the data using a relational structure. A relational DBMS uses a table with a unique format consisting of related rows and columns rather than a directory or list. The table corresponds to a file, the rows correspond to records, and columns correspond to the fields

**TABLE 5.2**     EXAMPLE OF A RELATIONAL DATABASE: NURSES DATABASE

| NURSLIST | NURSADDS | NURSINFO |
|----------|----------|----------|
| Nursid | Nursid | Nursid |
| Ntitle | City | CEU |
| Salary | County | Eval |
| Dept | State | Vac |
| DOH | Zip | Sick |

in the records. The table structure is simple, and a set of rules is used to carry out the processing operations.

A relational database can be illustrated by the structure in Table 5.2. Collectively, it consists of the following three tables (files) and is known as the NURSES DATABASE.

- **NURSLIST** contains a list of nurses with their titles, salaries, departments, and dates of hire (Table 5.3).
- **NURSADDS** contains a list of nurses with their addresses.
- **NURSINFO** contains a list of nurses with their continuing education credits, evaluation review, and vacation and sick leave taken.

Data for each nurse are entered into the database composed of these three tables or files. *Note:* Only one field is common to all the files— "NURSID." It provides the relational "link" between the three tables. As a result, in processing this database, the data fields from each file can be mapped to the others via this identifier.

Each database in the relational database structure represents a data file and consists of records with identical data fields. There are several advantages of relational databases. They include:

- Reduced repetitious information. If a field (data element) changes, it only has to be changed in one table; it will automatically be changed in the others.

**TABLE 5.3**     EXAMPLE OF A TABLE OF DATABASE RECORDS: NURSELIST TABLE/FILE

| Nursid | Ntitle | Salary | Dept | DOH |
|--------|--------|--------|------|-----|
| 4352 | Sup | $40,000 | 3E | 1/1/80 |
| 6684 | HN | $35,000 | 3E | 6/6/85 |
| 3289 | Staff | $32,000 | 3E | 8/5/89 |
| 1111 | Staff | $30,000 | 3E | 9/9/90 |
| 9864 | LPN | $25,000 | 3E | 6/6/80 |

- Manageable data files. Computer programs written for specific tables do not have to read unnecessary fields of information.
- Efficient access to data. Individual users have access only to the data they require. Data which they need access to on an infrequent or scheduled basis may be accessed by linking the tables.
- Secure data. Data can be kept in tables with limited access.

## DATA PROCESSING

Data processing is the changing of raw data into information as instructed by computer programs. Raw facts are data elements that represent pieces of data. The computer can process data that are used to describe a patient, such as age, identification number, race, and sex. Other data such as temperature, pulse, respiration, and blood pressure can be used to analyze a patient's vital signs. In this example, the instructions (software programs) used to analyze (process) the raw data—patient's vital signs— would use logical comparisons to compare the patients' vital signs with normal measurements to determine if they were within acceptable ranges.

   Data are always processed in the same manner; that is, they are processed as directed by the instructions in the software programs. Both the raw data and the computer program that is to process them must be entered as input into computer memory, where they remain until processing begins. When ordered, the program instructions and data are transmitted on a data bus to the arithmetic logic unit (ALU) for processing. The ALU is the only location in the CPU where data are processed according to the instructions in the software programs. In this unit only one instruction is processed at a time, but the speed of processing is so fast that it appears to the user that multiple instructions are being processed. Once processing is completed, the processed data are sent back by "data bus" to be stored in memory. The processed data, now information, remain stored in memory until instructed to be produced as printed output.

## Data Processing Operations

A computer performs a number of different data processing operations. The common operations include the following:

- Input
- Store
- Inquire
- Update
- Retrieve
- Sort
- Transform
- Classify
- Compare
- Compute
- Summarize
- Report
- Output

These processing operations are performed at different times in the data processing cycle. They are based on the instructions in the computer programs. Some are used to manipulate data, such as input, store, and update. Other operations are used to compare, compute, and classify data, and then summarize data and produce output.

The processing operations can be illustrated in a hospital information system as follows. On admission to a hospital, patient data are input and stored in memory. Once they are entered, the patient database can be queried, "inquire," to determine the location of the patient, and updated if errors are found. Patient data can be retrieved by the nurse to review physician orders. The patient data can be sorted in a particular sequence (e.g., alphabetically or diagnostically); classified according to a particular characteristic, such as sex, age, or ethnic origin; and summarized, as in the census report for each nursing shift. Data such as the patient's vital signs can be compared to normal values. Drug dosage can be computed when calculations are needed (if, for example, the drug dosage is based on patient weight). And finally, a shift report listing the status of the patients can be produced as printed output. Data can be also transformed for a specific application, such as converting a drug order to a patient order and/or billing voucher. The data elements are then returned to their original format for other data processing and storage operations.

## Data Processing Types

Data processing types, the different ways of processing data, include the following:

- On-line processing
- Interactive/real-time processing
- Batch processing
- Transaction processing

### On-line Processing

On-line processing directly connects a computer terminal to a computer. In such systems data are entered from a VDT or CRT terminal or other data input terminal. The data are transmitted directly to the CPU of the computer and stored, to remain until needed. In this method, the terminal is used to transmit or receive data. An example of an on-line computer system may be found in patient care units where an on-line terminal is used to process patients' bills. Patient care services are recorded on a terminal, and data are transmitted directly to the accounting office. Similarly, in some public health and community health agencies, data on patient care services are transmitted on-line to an offsite service bureau computer for processing.

## Interactive/Real-Time Processing

Interactive/real-time processing, the most common type of processing used for random access, generally refers to mainframes and minicomputers that process data immediately upon instruction. Data are entered through on-line terminals directly connected or linked via a communication network to the computer's CPU. The data are processed, and results are transmitted directly back to system users. Such computer systems allow the user at the terminal to interact with the computer database. This type of processing is also available via a microcomputer with hard disk storage which is on-line to the CPU. Using the terminal, a user can prepare, edit, and correct data as they are entered into the terminal. This interactive processing can be used to update files, revise computer programs, and design and generate outputs.

Different levels of interactive/real-time processing are available. They include the processing of a sequential transaction, processing of a problem, and continuous processing. In the first instance, each transaction is completed before another one is initiated. In the second instance, the problem is formulated and executed and the results are retrieved on-line. In continuous processing, computer applications are ongoing, such as those found in the processing of a hospital information system.

Interactive/real-time processing has been made possible by magnetic disk storage. Magnetic disk packs and hard disks are used to expand computer storage and make the size of databases to be processed almost unlimited. Any of these levels of processing can be used in the newer patient information systems being introduced in hospitals. In such systems, nursing personnel enter information on a patient through on-line terminals located at the bedside or in different hospital units. Simultaneously, the user interacts directly with the computer's CPU to maintain complete, up-to-date computer-based patient records. Microcomputers and/or workstations are being introduced on patient care units in hospitals to function as stand-alone systems or as an integral component of local area networks (LANs) that function similarly to mainframe and minicomputer systems.

## Batch Processing

In batch processing data are assembled and processed at once or at specially designated times without further instruction from the user. Generally, data are not processed as they enter the computer but are stored for processing later. Batch processing is used in any system where data are processed at fixed intervals, such as a hospital payroll. The computer program and data to be processed are generally stored off-line on magnetic tapes or magnetic disk packs that are mounted onto the computer when the computer programs are run.

## Transaction Processing

In transaction processing, transactions are processed in the order in which they occur. Whenever a transaction is processed in real time, that means it is processed fast enough to be acted upon instantly. An example is a bank teller being able to retrieve your balance or account transactions.

## COMPUTER SECURITY

A major consideration for any computer system is computer security, which involves protecting the computer system and data against deliberate destruction, accidental access, or loss by unauthorized persons. Computer security involves protecting the hardware and software functions, features, and/or characteristics against illegal access and illicit use. It refers to the methods by which access to confidential information is limited and includes the physical security of the computer system equipment (input/output devices, storage units, and CPU) and protecting the data themselves. Computer security includes physical, communication, data, and system security. These are described below.

### Physical Security

Physical security encompasses protecting the computer system against physical threats, such as theft and deliberate destructive acts, environmental hazards, and/or disasters such as fire and floods. It includes a variety of controls to prevent damaging equipment through simple carelessness, such as dropping it. It also includes physical control of access to where the hardware is located and personnel security, which refers to authorized access to the hardware. Controls can be maintained by installing door locks, closed-circuit television, and other alarm systems. A special unique identifier can be used to limit access to the computer facility or mainframe or minicomputer equipment to authorized personnel. A duplicate computer system installed in a second location can provide a backup for any loss of physical equipment.

### Communication Security

Communication security refers to the authenticity of data communicated via telecommunication devices. Protection of data during transmission to and from the computer system is also part of data security. Wiretapping and eavesdropping are security threats that computer users can take measures to prevent. If telephone lines are tapped, data can be copied. Data being transmitted over telecommunication lines can be protected by scrambling; that is, the data are encrypted (encoded) by the sender, sent, and decrypted (decoded) by the authorized receiver.

Communication security includes communication line security, which means protecting the connections between one location and another, such as communication cables, telephone lines, and junction boxes. Transmission security includes security of the transmission of data from one or more locations. It includes securing test messages, operator procedures, message formats, and speech privacy. Crytographic security provides security to cryptographic equipment and materials such as overview ciphers, message lengths, signature analysis, and other operations involved in the cryptographic operations and maintenance. Emission security includes review of device fingerprints and acoustical materials, and technical security includes verification checking, voice recognition checking, and checking for viruses.

## Data Security

Data security refers to the secure access of the computer system data by a user. Terminals can be secured by limiting access through the use of random passwords, identification numbers, card-keys, or other forms of security codes. Database design can limit access to identified authorized users by giving different groups of hospital personnel different security codes. For example, a nurse's aide's security code might allow access to certain items in the database, such as vital signs, but deny access to other information, such as medication orders or laboratory results. New identification methods are being considered, such as handwriting recognition, voice recognition, eye patterns, handprint patterns, and fingerprint mapping. Data security also includes protecting the data against being destroyed with computer viruses.

### Computer Viruses

Computer viruses are often destructive programs that travel concealed in other programs that they have infected. They are pieces of self-replicating computer code hidden in the program code that attach themselves to other programs and files, causing them to function improperly. Sometimes viruses are programmed not to appear for specific periods of time. That way they can spread from disk to disk and system to system. Generally viruses are transmitted by downloading through modems and through shared disks, illegally copied programs, or free computer programs. To combat viruses, computer programs are available that check for and wipe out known viruses. Viruses can be prevented by being cautious about sharing software programs and by backing up data files on a regular basis.

## System Security

System security involves methods to ensure that the data input, processing, and output for the entire system are accurate and reliable. Assorted checks and audits enable users to ensure that data are not lost, altered, or used incorrectly. Data integrity is critical to the life cycle of a system. One type of check is the automatic recording of all uses and transactions performed by the computer system; such a method can detect any unlawful user or unauthorized transaction. Another is the use of audit trails to ensure that computer programs process data correctly and that they have not been tampered with. System security can be costly, but every computer system requires some level of security.

System surveillance includes monitoring data acquisition, and using analysis and reports in order to ensure system reliability and security. Site licenses are required if copyrighted software packages are to be used throughout the system. The Computer Software Copyright Act of 1980 protects computer programs and treats them similarly to literary works, allowing them to be copyrighted.

## PRIVACY AND CONFIDENTIALITY

### Privacy

Privacy is the ability to control the use of information about individual patients. Individuals have the right to control disclosure of their personal information. Privacy of a computer system assures people that personal data are protected against improper access. Such protection is critical to the integrity of any computer system. As computer systems multiply in number and increase in size and scope, data on individuals are becoming increasingly available. Several legislative acts have been passed in an effort to protect people's privacy:

- Freedom of Information Act of 1966: This law gives people access to their personal data collected by federal agencies.
- Fair Credit Act of 1970: This law gives people access to their credit records.
- Privacy Act of 1974: This is one of the most significant acts. It established safeguards for protecting records that the government collects and keeps on citizens. It stipulates that federal agencies cannot maintain any secret files on citizens and that citizens have the right to know what government files say about them. A Privacy Commission set up as a result of this act formulated and published a basic document on protecting the privacy of citizens that recommended six basic principles for the private sector:

1. All personal records should be made public.
2. Individuals must be allowed to find out when information is stored about them and how it is used.
3. Personal information should be used only for its intended purpose.
4. Individuals must be able to amend records about themselves.

5. Personal information must be obtained in such a way as to ensure that it is complete, accurate, relevant, timely, and secure.
6. All uses of personal information should be accounted for by a responsible manager (Capron and Williams, 1984, p. 387).

This act also recommended that social security numbers be used only in connection with official government business and that any new private-sector computer systems not use them for identification purposes. As a result of this commission, several state and local governments passed similar legislation protecting the privacy of data on their residents. A new privacy act is being proposed to accommodate the National Information Infrastructure (NII) and use of health information on the nation's information superhighway.

Other laws that affect data on individuals that can be stored in computer systems include:

- Privacy Protection Act of 1980 (Title 11): This law allows the attorney general to access documents that are confidential, such as medical records.
- Electronic Communications Privacy Act of 1986: This law makes it a crime to own any electronic, mechanical, or other device primarily for the purpose of the surreptitious interception of wire, oral, or electronic communication.
- Computer Fraud and Abuse Act of 1984, amended in 1986: This law specifies that it is a crime to access a federal computer without authorization in order to alter, destroy, or damage information.
- Copyright Act: This law protects the textual, pictorial, or musical expression embodied in a work. It stipulates that it is a federal offense to reproduce computer software without authorization.

## Confidentiality

Confidentiality is the expectation that information provided to an authorized user will not be redisclosed. Confidentiality is an ethical obligation health professionals are expected to honor. However, if abused, confidentiality may not be enforced through the courts. Confidentiality of health information has historically been addressed at the state level. Thus there is a morass of laws defining the confidentiality obligation of health care providers. The *Code for Nurses* clearly states, "The nurse safeguards the clients' right to privacy by judiciously protecting information of a confidential nature" (American Nurses Association, 1975). However, the providers' ability to carry out their obligation to ensure confidentiality can be greatly affected by use of electronic media to store and transmit health information.

Historically, providers have stored health information on paper records. Even though the paper medium is cumbersome and expensive, it minimizes confidentiality problems because of the sheer difficulty of obtaining and reviewing large volumes of health care data, records, and claim forms. The major concern about using electronic media to transmit claims information with health information is that they provide ample opportunity for access and breaching confidentiality.

## Current Initiatives

Beginning in the early 1990s, several organizations began to focus on the privacy, security, and confidentiality of electronic and/or computer-based patient records (CPR). The Work Group for Electronic Data Interchange (WEDI), initiated by the secretary of the Department of Health and Human Services, made recommendations, including possible legislation on data security for health information. WEDI explored many issues related to filing patients' health insurance claims, including electronic claims processing, that will affect providers who participate in those functions. The WEDI work group recommended that uniform national standards be developed for documenting and sharing patient information and for protecting the privacy and confidentiality of patient information (Work Group for Electronic Data Interchange Technical Advisory Group, 1992).

The Computer-Based Patient Record Institute (CPRI) also recommended that appropriate mechanisms, including data protection standards, be established that would give patients and their providers the ability to control access to electronic transmission of CPR data. The CPRI Work Group on Confidentiality, Privacy, and Legislation focuses on the protection of the CPR. It indicated that the national information infrastructure (NII), the nation's information superhighway being developed to connect computer systems, made sharing of massive amounts of information fast, simple, and easy (Dick and Steen, 1991). It indicated that the NII will be used to transmit the CPR and carry information between nurses, doctors, payers, and health care facilities. It stated that the need to protect these highways from misuse and provide security for them is critical and will be of concern for many years (Work Group on Computerization of Patient Records, 1993).

## SUMMARY

This chapter described data processing, which is essentially what computers do. It highlighted the various operations possible with data processing and described the organization and structure of data, including the logical entities organized in a hierarchy—byte (a byte is a character), field, record, file, and database. Data structure and organization and how data are accessed and processed were described. The differences between on-line, interactive real-time, and batch processing were reviewed. Finally, the various types of data security methods were outlined. The differences between the physical security of the system and the security of the data were stressed, and how data on individuals are protected was discussed. A brief overview of privacy and confidentiality, highlighting the most recent initiatives, concluded the chapter.

## REFERENCES

American Nurses Association. (1975). *Code for Nurses with Interpretative Statements* (p. 6). Kansas City, MO.

Capron, H. L., and Williams, B. K. (1984). *Computer and Data Processing.* Menlo Park, CA: Benjamin/Cummings.

Dick, R. S., and Steen, E. B. (Eds.). (1991). *The Computer-Based Patient Record: An Essential Technology for Health Care.* Washington, DC: National Academy Press.

WEDI Technical Advisory Group. (1992). *WEDI Technical Advisory Group White Paper: Appendix 4: Confidentiality and Antitrust Issues.* Report to Secretary of U.S. DHHS. Washington, DC.

Work Group on Computerization of Patient Records. (1993). *Toward a National Health Information Infrastructure.* Report to Secretary of U.S. DHHS. Washington, DC.

## BIBLIOGRAPHY

Blasgen, M. W. (1982). Database systems. *Science, 215*(4534), 869–872.

Boraiko, A. A. (1982). The chip: Electronic minimarvel that is changing your life. *National Geographic, 162*(4), 421–458.

Brewer, S. C. (1983). Data security. In A. Ralston and E. D. Reilly, Jr. (Eds.), *Encyclopedia of Computer Science and Engineering* (2d ed.) (pp. 493–497). New York: Van Nostrand Reinhold.

Bronzino, J. D. (1982). *Computer Applications for Patient Care.* Reading, MA: Addison-Wesley.

Brookshear, J. G. (1991). *Computer Science: An Overview* (3d ed.). New York: Benjamin/Cummings.

Brown, W. F., and Jacobsen, R. V. (1983). Security of computer installations, physical. In A. Ralston and E. D. Reilly, Jr. (Eds.), *Encyclopedia of Computer Science and Engineering* (2d ed.) (pp. 1308–1310). New York: Van Nostrand Reinhold.

Capron, H. L. (1990). *Computer: Tools for the Information Age* (2d ed.). Menlo Park, CA: Benjamin/Cummings.

Carroll, J. M. (1979). *Computer Security.* Boston: Butterworth Publishing.

Chorafas, D. N. (1983). *DBMS for Distributed Computers and Networks.* New York: Petrocelli Books.

Covvey, H. D., and McAlister, N. H. (1980). *Computers in the Practice of Medicine:* Vol. 1. *Introduction to Computing Concepts.* Reading, MA: Addison-Wesley.

Cox, H. C., Harasanyi, B., and Dean, L. C. (1987). *Computers and Nursing: Applications to Practice, Education and Research.* Norwalk, CO: Appleton and Lange.

Desposito, J., Marcim, J., and White, D. (1992). *Que's Computer Buyer's Guide: 1992 Edition.* Carmel, NY: Que Corp.

DeVoney, C. (1987). *Using PC DOS.* Indianapolis, IN: Que Corp.

Editors of Time-Life Books. (1986). *Understanding Computers: Artificial Intelligence.* Chicago: Time-Life Books.

Editors of Time-Life Books. (1986). *Understanding Computers: Computer Security.* Chicago: Time-Life Books.

Encyclopedia Britannica Educational Corporation. (1982). *Understanding Computers.* Skokie, IL.

Enlander, D. (1980). *Computers in Medicine: An Introduction.* St. Louis: Mosby.

Frankenhais, J. P. (1982, May–June). How to get a good mini. *Harvard Business Review*, 139–149.

Freeman, D. N. (1983). Processing modes. In A. Ralston and E. D. Reilly, Jr. (Eds.), *Encyclopedia of Computer Science and Engineering* (2d ed.) (pp. 1217–1218). New York: Van Nostrand Reinhold.

Fry, J. P., and Sibley, E. H. (1976). Evolution of data-base management systems. *Computer Survey, 8*(1), 7–42.

Gookin, D., and Rathbone, A. (1992). *PCs for Dummies.* San Mateo, CA: IDG Books.

Hart, A. (1992). *Knowledge Acquisition for Expert Systems* (2d ed.). New York: McGraw-Hill.

Head, R. V. (1983). Real-time applications. In A. Ralston and E. D. Reilly, Jr. (Eds.), *Encyclopedia of Computer Science and Engineering* (2d ed.) (pp. 1265–1272). New York: Van Nostrand Reinhold.

Heller, R. S., and Martin, D. C. (1982). *Bits 'n Bytes about Computers: A Computer Literacy Primer.* Rockville, MD: Computer Science Press.

Hopper, G. M., and Mandell, S. L. (1984). *Understanding Computers.* New York: West.

Hopper, G. M., and Mandell, S. L. (1987). *Understanding Computers* (2d ed.). New York: West.

Hume, J. P. (1983). Data security. In A. Ralston and E. D. Reilly, Jr. (Eds.), *Encyclopedia of Computer Science and Engineering* (2d ed.) (pp. 493–497). New York: Van Nostrand Reinhold.

Hutchison, S. E., and Sawyer, S. C. (1988). *Computers: The User Perspective* (2d ed.). Boston: Irwin.

IBM Corporation. (1981). *Introduction to IBM Data Processing Systems.* Poughkeepsie, NY.

Johnson, D. G. (1985). *Computer Ethics.* Englewood Cliffs, NJ: Prentice-Hall.

Joos, I., Whitman, N. I., Smith, M. J., and Nelson, R. (1992). *Computers in Small Bytes: The Computer Workbook.* New York: National League for Nursing Press.

London, K. R. (1973). *Techniques for Direct Access.* Philadelphia: Auerbach.

MacLeod, R. J., and Forkner, I. (1982). *Computerized Business Information Systems: An Introduction to Data Processing.* New York: John Wiley.

Martin, J. (1982). *Introduction to Teleprocessing.* Englewood Cliffs, NJ: Prentice-Hall.

Murphy, G. (1992). System and data protection. In M. J. Ball and M. F. Collen (Eds.), *Aspects of the Computer-Based Patient Record* (pp. 201–211). New York: Springer-Verlag.

National Bureau of Standards. (1980). *Guidelines for Security of Computer Applications* (Fips Publication No. 73). Washington, DC.

Olle, T. W. (1983). Database management. In A. Ralston and E. D. Reilly, Jr. (Eds.), *Encyclopedia of Computer Science and Engineering* (2d ed.) (pp. 441–447). New York: Van Nostrand Reinhold.

Owen, B. (1991). *Personal Computers for the Computer Illiterate: The What, When, Why, Where, and How Guide.* New York: Harper Perennial.

Pfaffenberger, B. (1991). *Que's Computer User's Dictionary.* Carmel, IN: Que Corp.

Popyk, M. K. (1988). *Up and Running! Microcomputer Applications.* New York: Addison-Wesley.

Ralston, A., and Reilly, E. D., Jr. (Eds.). (1983). *Encyclopedia of Computer Science and Engineering* (2d ed.). New York: Van Nostrand Reinhold.

Report of the Secretary's Advisory Committee on Automated Personal Data Systems. (1973). *Records Computers and the Rights of Citizens* (DHEW Publication No. OS 73–94). Washington, DC: U.S. Government Printing Office.

Romano, C. A. (1987). Privacy, confidentiality, and security of computerized systems. *Computers in Nursing, 5*(3), 99–104.

Sanders, D. H. (1979). *Computers in Business: An Introduction.* New York: McGraw-Hill.

Schnaidt, P. (1990). *LAN Tutorial with Glossary of Terms.* New York: Miller Freeman Pubs.

Shelly, G. B., and Cashman, T. J. (1980). *Introduction to Computers and Data Processing.* Brea, CA: Anaheim.

Shore, J. (1989). *Using Computers in Business.* Carmel, IN: Que Corp.

Sibley, E. H. (1976). The development of data-base technology. *Computer Survey, 8*(1), 1–5.

Stern, R. A., and Stern, N. (1982). *An Introduction to Computers and Information Processing.* New York: John Wiley.

Sullivan, D. R., Lewis, T. G., and Cook, C. R. (1985). *Computing Today: Microcomputer Concepts and Applications.* Boston: Houghton Mifflin.

Walsh, M. E. (1982). *Understanding Computers: What Managers and Users Need to Know.* New York: John Wiley.

Wang, W. E., and Kraynak, J. (1990). *The First Book of Personal Computing.* Carmel, IN: Sams.

Work Group on Computerization of Patient Records. (1993, April). Appendix D: Computer-based patient records: Confidentiality, privacy and security concerns. In *Toward a National Health Information Infrastructure.* Washington, DC: U.S. DHHS.

Yovits, M. C. (1983). Information and data. In A. Ralston and E. D. Reilly, Jr. (Eds.), *Encyclopedia of Computer Science and Engineering* (2d ed.) (pp. 714–717). New York: Van Nostrand Reinhold.

# COMPUTER SYSTEMS

# 6

• • • • • • • • • • • • • • • • • • • • • • • •

# COMPUTER SYSTEMS

## OBJECTIVES

- Discuss systems.
- Describe computer systems.
- Identify types of information systems.
- Describe management information systems.
- Discuss hospital information systems.
- Describe patient record systems.
- Identify data standards.
- Describe CPR standards initiatives.

The use of systems in computer technology is based on systems theory. Previous chapters described computer hardware, computer software, and data processing; added together, these explain a computer system. Systems theory provides the basis for viewing a computer system, and the systems concepts provide a framework for understanding the relationships of all parts of the computer system; together, these concepts also explain a computer system.

This chapter provides an overview of systems, including their different types, elements, and characteristics. It focuses on computer systems, information systems, management information systems (MISs), and hospital information systems (HISs). It also focuses on computer-based patient record systems, data standards for systems, and communication networks, and provides an overview of the national information infrastructure. Specifically, this chapter describes the following:

- Systems
- Computer systems
- Information systems
- Management information systems
- Hospital information systems
- Patient record systems
- Data standards
- Standards initiatives

## SYSTEMS

Systems theory provides the conceptual basis for a system and is defined as several interrelated parts all working together to achieve a desired result. It also provides the basis for a computer system, which consists of computer parts, all of which are interrelated and needed to make the computer run; without them, the computer cannot run and is useless.

General systems theory was introduced in the 1930s and developed in 1950 by the biologist Ludwig von Bertalanffy (1968). He formulated systems theory as a framework for integrating and interpreting scientific knowledge. He indicated that to understand all living organisms, it is necessary to view them as parts of a whole. He also advocated that his theory be used to view the empirical world as one whole made up of varying interrelated parts. He argued that all living organisms interact with their environment and, as such, are open systems.

In 1956 Kenneth Boulding, a biologist, developed the Classification of General Systems Theory, which identified nine levels in a complex progressive hierarchy. The levels ranged from a static closed level to classify the lowest structure of basic elements to the most complex transcendental level to describe the highest structure and relationships among its changing elements. This classification was proposed as a means of bridging the gap between theoretical models and empirical knowledge (Boulding, 1956).

During World War II, systems theory, also called systems analysis, emerged as a holistic approach for solving problems. It was first applied by British scientists in the area of radar technology. They pioneered in combining the skills of many experts to deal with unresolved mathematical problems. They also used this technique of integrating different groups of people and pooling all types of resources to solve a critical problem at that time, saving their cities. During World War II, systems theory was also applied for the first time in the United States. The military used it to facilitate the development of improved weapons. Systems theory was also used to research other military projects and develop military equipment, such as the supersonic bomber.

After World War II, systems theory concepts influenced the development of computer hardware and software. They influenced the design of computers and computer systems for solving military and other scientific problems. During this time, systems theory applications expanded into other areas of computer science and into social sciences, medicine, and nursing. During the 1960s, systems theory influenced the development of nursing theory (Donnelly et al., 1980). Nurse theorists began to view a nursing model of practice as unique and distinct, and began to separate it from nursing practice in a traditional medical model. They began to use systems theory concepts found in other disciplines to analyze nursing practice in terms of a holistic approach and create several nursing theories.

## System Concepts

A system is a concept that describes a single unit composed of a set of interrelated subunits or parts. Each part works independently but is essential to the whole system. The unit is greater than any of its parts, but if any one part changes, all other parts are affected. Systems are described as follows:

- System types
- System elements
- System characteristics

### System Types

The type of system refers to its structure. Different types of systems describe different types of structures, such as mechanical, organizational, or human structures or a combination of structures. For example, a computer, a hospital, and even the nursing profession are different types of systems.

An automobile can be described as a mechanical system. Its parts work together to make it run. A community health care delivery system is an organizational system. Different health care facilities (parts) such as a hospital, nursing home, community health agency, home health agency, and health maintenance organization (HMO) work together to provide health care services in a community. Even though each facility has its own goals and its own system, each facility is also a part of the community health care system (Fig. 6.1). A nursing department in a hospital is a human system. It is composed of nursing personnel in different nursing units (parts)—patient care units, a research unit, and an educational unit (Fig. 6.2). All nursing personnel work together to achieve the overall goal of the hospital, and the nurses in each unit work to achieve the goals of their respective units.

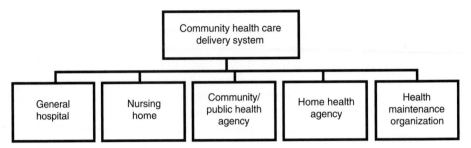

**Figure 6.1**  An example of an organizational system.

## System Elements

A system is described by the following five major elements: input, process, output, feedback, and control (Optner, 1975).

***Input***  Input is the start-up force that puts a system into operation; it consists of the raw facts and the other requirements the system needs in order to operate.

***Process***  Process is the activity that transforms input into output, and is the mode of operation. It can be modified in response to feedback and control.

**Figure 6.2**  An example of a human system.

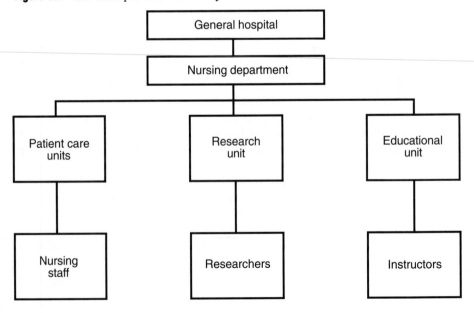

***Output***   Output is the result of the process and is the final product of the operation.

***Feedback and Control***   Feedback and control are two interrelated elements that control the system. Feedback is a function which allows adjustments to be made to control—monitor, evaluate, and direct—the system. Control regulates the functions of input, process, and output and provides the rules and procedures for their operations. Control regulates (1) input by checking, validating, and verifying data, (2) process by completing the operations and detecting errors, and (3) output by ensuring conformity, checking validity of content, and correcting errors. The constraints of a system are an additional control and impose the boundaries for a specific processing problem.

The five elements of a system make up the framework of a computer system, which is primarily an open system that allows all types of constraints based on feedback and control regulations (Fig. 6.3). An episode of care or a hospitalization can also be compared to the various elements of a computer system (Fig. 6.4).

The elements of a hospitalization of a burn patient can be described as follows. The admission of the burn patient is the input into an acute care hospital, the actual patient care is the process, and once care has been com-

**Figure 6.3**   Five elements of a system.

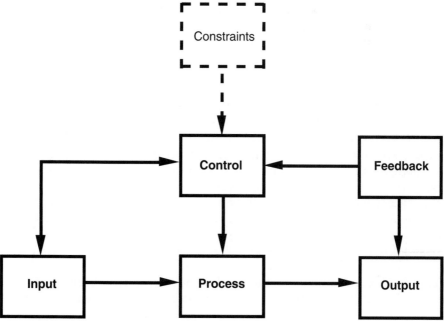

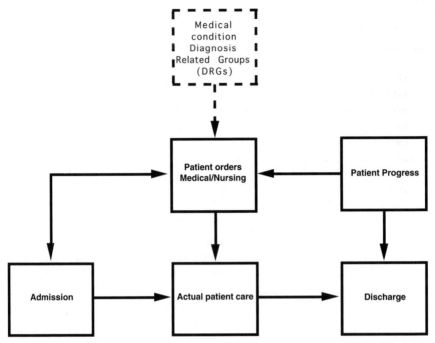

**Figure 6.4**   An example of the five elements of a system.

pleted, the patient is discharged, or output. The feedback consists of information on the patient's progress, and control refers to medical and nursing orders; the actions resulting from the orders provide feedback information. Feedback and control affect the care process. A constraint for the patient care process is a DRG regulation which limits the number of days the patient can stay in the hospital for the patient's specific medical condition.

## System Characteristics
Systems are also characterized as closed systems or open systems.

*Closed Systems* A closed system is generally one with complete, fixed, and unchanging elements. It does not interact with its environment and does not change. It is self-contained, automatically controls its own operation, and is self-regulating. This type of system has been defined as a "black box" which is characterized by a given set of inputs and outputs. An example of a closed system is a physiological monitoring unit, which contains an alarm that is set off automatically when a patient's heart rate deviates from normal.

*Open Systems* An open system is dynamic. Because its elements are affected by and respond to external forces, it allows for change and adjustments. An example of an open system is a hospital census system; the number of discharges influences the number of admissions.

## COMPUTER SYSTEMS

A computer system is the application of systems theory to the computer. It refers to the hardware and software that interact to process data into information. This interaction is essential to make the computer function, since without it computer hardware is useless. A computer system consists of a configuration of components. It is a machine that can be programmed to accept data (input) and manipulate (process) those data into usable information (output). A computer system is based on computer science, the discipline that provides the scientific foundation for it (Perreault and Wiederhold, 1990b).

Computer science encompasses a wide array of topics that address the advancing technology. It encompasses the design and construction of computer hardware and software. The previous chapters described computer hardware (architecture), computer software (programs), and data processing, which together provide the basis for a computer system.

### Hardware Architecture

Hardware refers to an electronic computer and all the peripheral equipment (terminals, central processing unit, memory, storage devices, communication devices). It refers to any size of computer (supercomputer, mainframe, minicomputer, microcomputer) and any type of computer (analog, digital, hybrid). Hardware architecture refers to the computer hardware standards for specific computers, such as IBM or Apple. It also refers to the type and size of the microprocessor which determines the internal capabilities of the central processing unit—operating system, arithmetic logic unit, and main memory (see Chap. 3).

### Software Programs

Software programs refer to the computer programs that make the computer run. The term "software" has several meanings. It refers to (1) the language of the computer programs, (2) system programs written to control the computer (the operating system, utilities, etc.), and (3) application programs written to process computer data.

A fundamental concept of a computer program is an algorithm, which is a sequence of steps designed to direct the execution of a task. An algorithm is a computer program stored in a computer system which is executed automatically to solve a problem or accomplish a stated goal. An algorithm also refers to how the data are processed by the computer system—how the problem is solved and/or the goal accomplished (see Chap. 4).

## Computer System Characteristics

A computer system is characterized by its high speed and reliability in processing data. It can

- Document, organize, store, and process large volumes of data.
- Communicate and retrieve information for timely decision making.
- Generate aggregate information for quality control, cost control, evaluation, and research.
- Educate and instruct students.
- Support the research process.

## INFORMATION SYSTEMS

An information system, sometimes called an information processing system or data processing system, uses a computer system (hardware and software) to process data into information. Designed for human-machine interaction, an information system consists of computer programs written for a specific purpose and a database containing raw facts or data elements. A computer system is designed to solve a problem or accomplish a stated goal by accepting data into a database, processing the data, and producing the results (information) as output.

## Information System Types

Information systems are found in hospitals, community health agencies, research facilities, and educational institutions. They vary widely depending on how they are used and/or described. Systems can be described (1) by the purpose or focus of the application, (2) by the type of use or service they provide, or (3) as tools used for developing other information systems. They also can be described by (1) how they process information (on-line, interactive real-time, and/or batch processing), (2) how they are configured (modular, network, stand-alone systems), and (3) their other characteristics—memory size, storage capacity, and processing power (Blum, 1986; Perreault and Wiederhold, 1990a; Wiederhold and Perreault, 1990).

There is a wide range of information systems in health care facilities that perform different functions. They have different titles/names which overlap depending on the context in which they are used. The major ones to be described include:

- Information storage and retrieval systems
- Bibliographic retrieval systems
- Dedicated systems
- Transaction systems
- Monitoring systems
- Decision support systems
- Expert systems
- Natural language systems

### Information Storage and Retrieval Systems

An information storage and retrieval system is a general term for a large mainframe computer system that stores, processes, and retrieves vast amounts of information. It is a system with a collection of data available to the user. The data are stored in a database from which desired elements can be retrieved. Essentially this type of system is the basic computer system used to manage and communicate information in a large health care facility. It is generally an interactive real-time computer system.

The large storage and retrieval systems are divided into subsystems on the basis of the different types of data collected and stored in the database. For example, the patient drug data in a patient information storage and retrieval system database is "downloaded" to the pharmacy department for a drug subsystem. The pharmacy system uses the patient drug subsystem to manage different uses of the drug data, such as processing drug orders for patients, ordering drugs, or dispensing patient educational material. Another example can be downloading patient care data to a patient acuity/classification subsystem in the nursing department, where the data are used to determine staffing requirements.

### Bibliographic Retrieval Systems

A bibliographic retrieval system is a retrieval system that generally provides bibliographic data, document information, or literature. Such a system is primarily used to store and retrieve data and does not conduct any computations per se. The textual data are input, stored, and available for retrieval in a user-friendly format which is easy to read and understand. The system is designed to provide bibliographic data on journal articles, books, monographs, and textual reports. It generally contains not only the actual citations, but also keywords, abstracts, and other pertinent facts on the documents in the database.

### Dedicated Systems

A dedicated system, or a special-purpose system, is an information system developed for a single application or function. Most dedicated systems are described by their purpose, such as the specialty information systems found in the pharmacy, laboratory, and/or radiology departments in a hospital. Patient classification/acuity systems for nurse staffing, can also be special-purpose or dedicated systems. Generally, special-purpose systems are stand-alone systems that run on a microcomputer.

Another type of special-purpose system is one that processes a single application, such as a survey or a study conducted to solve a problem. Generally, for this type of application, a software package is selected and modified or a computer program is written to input, store, and process the survey data in a database. Once the survey results are processed and reports generated as output, the computer program has fulfilled its purpose, and the computer system per se is no longer needed.

### Transaction Systems

A transaction system is used to process predefined transactions and produce predefined reports. It is designed for repeated operations using a fixed list. From this list, displayed on a computer terminal, a user selects the names of transactions to be processed. A computer program is written so that it can be used repeatedly to process the same type of transactions and generate the same type of reports or products. The computer program and the list of transactions are retained in storage and retrieved as needed.

An inventory system is an example of a transaction system. It is used to monitor the distribution of supplies, update the quantity on hand, and reorder; these actions are repetitious and always processed in the same manner. A standard list of items is initially developed; depending on the system, quantities on hand can be automatically updated and supplies reordered as they are needed. The transactions can also be summarized and reports developed to produce monthly bills, prepare order vouchers, and summarize the inventory status for any given time period. In this type of system, the computer program is specifically written to process the transactions (raw data).

A transaction system can also process routine medical or nursing orders, which can be updated in real time. This is done to ensure that the orders, once entered, are current in the system. The updated medical and nursing orders can also be used for documenting care plans, change of shift reports, discharge summaries, quality reviews, research studies, etc.

### Monitoring Systems

A monitoring system, a physiological control system, is primarily used to assist in monitoring specific patient physiological equipment. The electronic system provides alarm signals from sensors for predefined emergency conditions. Monitoring systems are found primarily in intensive care, critical care, emergency room, and operating room units of hospitals.

Physiological monitoring systems are being used more frequently to measure and monitor continuous automatic physiological findings such as heart rate, blood pressure, and other vital signs. Monitoring systems provide alarms to detect significant abnormal findings when personnel are needed to provide patient care and save lives. The early monitoring systems were analog and displayed physiological signals on the terminal video screens. Computer-based monitoring systems can also provide a logic module that processes the data (see Chap. 11).

## Decision Support Systems

A decision support system is a computer system that supports decision making. It uses a model or a simulation of a real-life situation, which is a mathematical representation using "what if" options. A decision support system does not replace the information system but enhances it. Modeling of the computer constructs is used to simulate live situations in order to make a decision using the same information that experts in the field would use. These systems are also called expert systems (Hart, 1992; Shortliffe, 1990).

## Expert Systems

An expert system is a computer system containing the information supplied by an expert to assist nonexperts in decision making. An expert system is designed to enable users to simulate the cause-and-effect reasoning that an expert would use if confronted with the same situation in a real environment.

The heart of an expert system has two parts: (1) a knowledge base incorporating the experience and expertise of expert clinicians, and (2) an inference mechanism, on which the operation of the system is based. The rules for analyzing the data are "what if–then" rules. They are used to draw inferences from the knowledge base to solve a problem or provide possible solutions in a given situation. The inference system is based on a method of reasoning which can be either inductive or deductive. Expert systems can be used to help practitioners implement clinical practice guidelines.

*Artificial Intelligence*   An artificial intelligence (AI) system is also an expert system. This field of computer science field is attempting to improve computer systems by giving them characteristics of human intelligence, such as the capability to understand natural language and to reason under conditions of uncertainty. Artificial intelligence uses rules that are referred to as "heuristic" to represent a knowledge base. The knowledge is specific to the focus of the system. The rules are searched to produce "smart results." An AI system goes beyond an expert system, which is based on a set of rules and an algorithm to process data; it is expanded to include heuristic reasoning. The term "artificial intelligence" is also applied to using natural languages and object-oriented programming to manipulate the object-oriented structure of a knowledge database (Brookshear, 1991; Graham, 1986).

### Natural Language Systems

A natural language system is a system which requires teaching the computer to understand a wide range of words and sentence structures' syntax. It does not require a special vocabulary and rules for the computer instructions, nor does it require a user to learn a special computer language. A natural language command is shorter and more precise than a higher-level language command and requires less memory. Some computer programs that accept and process natural language input are being marketed. They use relatively crude matching techniques to process the input. The newer natural language systems are those that can recognize and process human speech and/or handwriting.

## MANAGEMENT INFORMATION SYSTEMS

An MIS is another type of information system that supports management information activities and functions. An MIS is defined as an organized standardized system for managing the flow of information in an organization in a timely manner; it therefore assists in the decision-making processes.

   When properly designed and implemented, an MIS helps an organization analyze and manage its information logically. It can effectively meet organizational objectives, be responsive to decision-making functions, and provide relevant feedback for short-range and long-range planning. It can be separate or an integral module of a hospitalwide information system, or it can be designed as a special dedicated system to be used by, for example, the nursing department in a hospital, community health agency, educational institution, or research facility (Saba, 1974).

### Levels of Management

An MIS is based on the structure and functions of any organization and provides the information needed to satisfy these components. The structure of an agency generally refers to the three levels of management (top, middle, and lower) and to their three functional areas of control (strategic planning, management control, and operational control) (Fig. 6.5).

#### Strategic Planning

Strategic planning in a nursing department refers to the policy decisions made by the top-level nursing administrator. An administrator requires summary information to administer the department, plan the agency program, and forecast future needs to meet agency goals.

#### Management Control

The management control function refers to the program and personnel decisions made by middle-level managers, supervisors, and head nurses.

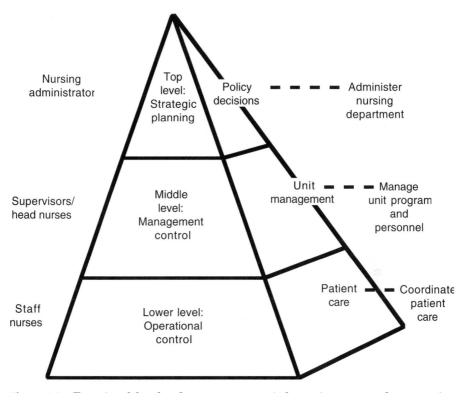

**Figure 6.5**   Functional levels of a management information system for a nursing department in a health care facility.

They need information to measure performance standards and to control, plan, and allocate resources.

### Operational Control

The operational control functions are needed by the lower-level nursing staff to manage, coordinate, and provide patient care. They need information so that they can effectively and efficiently carry out patient care.

An MIS can provide information to personnel at the three functional levels to enable them to perform activities and to make decisions. A carefully structured MIS provides the essential management information needed so that data can flow vertically and horizontally. The vertical flow of information upward starts with the data collected at the operations level; these are used by the nursing staff to coordinate patient care. From this data set, selected information is generated for the head nurses and supervisors so that they can manage their respective units, and finally summary information is identified for the nursing administrator. Information also flows horizontally across and between patient care units and across departments such as the operating room and specialty units. Such information is shared so that the operating units function consistently (Fig. 6.6).

Most MISs in health care facilities are separate from the HISs or other systems in the agency. According to Dr. Morris Collen (1983), an authority on HISs, an MIS subsystem should be integrated into a hospital information system to support management. He indicated that the HIS could provide management information for such things as patient registration and tracking, quality assurance, utilization review, and educational and research needs. A great deal of information can be shared between the HIS's extensive database and the MIS.

**Figure 6.6** Vertical and horizontal flow of information for a management information system in a nursing department of a health care facility.

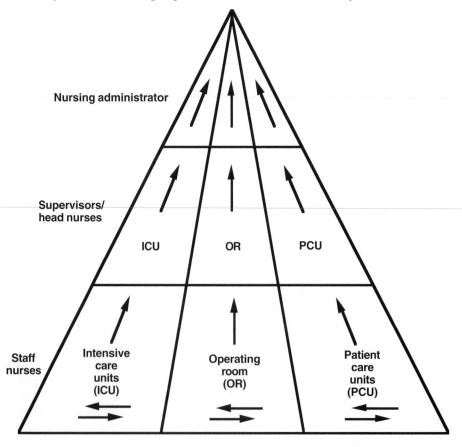

# HOSPITAL INFORMATION SYSTEMS

An HIS, sometimes called a patient care system (PCS), focuses on hospital functions. The purpose of an HIS is to manage the information needed to facilitate daily hospital operations by all health care personnel. Administrators manage financial budgets and establish charges for services; physicians diagnose, treat, and evaluate patient conditions; nurses assess, plan, and provide patient care; and a variety of other personnel provide ancillary services, and support the delivery of patient care services.

The term "HIS" generally refers to the large information systems used in the delivery of patient care services and designed to manage the integration and communication of client data in a hospital. An HIS can be either one big central integrated system or a modular system in which individual modules are linked together in order to share patient data. Hospitals may also have other separate dedicated information systems for special purposes, such as a nurse staffing, pharmacy, or laboratory system (Blum, 1984; Collen, 1983, 1994; Shortliffe and Perreault, 1990; Wiederhold and Perreault, 1990).

A discussion of HISs includes the following:

- HIS definitions
- HIS trends
- HIS types
- HIS configurations

## Hospital Information System Definitions

An HIS is "the dedicated use of a computer with associated hardware, software, and terminals to collect, store, process, retrieve and communicate relevant patient care and administrative information to support primarily the professional specialty group providing direct patient care within a hospital, its associated clinical departmental subsystems, and its outpatient services" (Collen, 1983). The major functions of an HIS are to communicate and integrate the subsystems or components and to provide management support.

Another authority on HISs restates Collen's points and stresses the need for data files in the system to be integrated (Austin, 1983). Both authors concur that the major purpose of any HIS is to facilitate the communication and integration of data necessary to deliver patient care and associated services.

However, Blum (1986), another authority, believes that an HIS performs two major functions: (1) it supports communications, and (2) it organizes data to facilitate decision making in a hospital. He indicated that the HIS provides the tools to enable each operational unit in a hospital to communicate with other units as well as support its internal operations. Such an approach uses the integrated model, which is becoming the system of choice (Fig. 6.7).

## Hospital Information System Trends

Hospitals have been slow in buying HISs or PCSs. According to Dorenfest (1987), they were slow because the systems being offered did not meet their needs. The hospital executives wanted integrated systems that could be updated simultaneously as the services were provided. He maintained that at that time, none of the PCSs implemented were truly integrated. He indicated that the typical computer-based HIS allowed for entry of only 50 to 75 percent of the physician orders, and that the nursing and ancillary orders were still being transcribed manually.

In the fifth and sixth surveys of 3,000+ community hospitals with patient care systems, Dorenfest found that of the approximately 5,500 community health hospitals in the country, only 2,241 (41.1 percent) had patient care systems in 1991, and only 2,348 (43.6 percent) had systems in 1992. This was lower than he had estimated in his study of 1987, when he predicted that 3,200 (58.1 percent) would have systems by 1990. The slow progress reflected the reduced budgets and changes in hospital services from inpatient to outpatient. Each of these patient care community hos-

**Figure 6.7** Hospital information system (HIS) showing subsystem and functional components. (Edward H. Shortliffe and Leslie A. Perrault, *Medical Informatics: Computer Applications in Health Care* (p. 166), © 1990 by Addison-Wesley Publishing Company, Inc. Reprinted by permission of the publisher.)

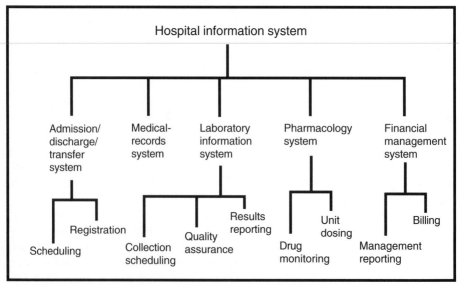

**TABLE 6.1**    TRENDS IN HOSPITALS WITH AUTOMATED PATIENT CARE
SYSTEMS

| Year | Hospitals with Systems | Percent of all Hospitals (n-5759) |
|------|------------------------|-----------------------------------|
| 1980 | 625 | 10.7% |
| 1982 | 940 | 16.1% |
| 1984 | 1,475 | 25.4% |
| 1986 | 1,800 | 31.3% |
| 1990 | 2,241 | 41.1% |
| 1992 | 2,348 | 43.6% |

Source: The Dorenfest 3000 + Database and The Dorenfest Guide to the Hospital Information Systems Market
(Dorenfest, 1987, 1992).

pitals had a computer-based patient care system with automated order
entry capability at the nurses' station. However, the 1990 increase did represent a 400 percent increase in one decade, from 1980 to 1990 (Table 6.1)
(Dorenfest, 1987, 1992).

## Hospital Information System Types

HISs vary widely, but most consist of various applications centering around
services, including nursing, provided to and received by patients. They are
designed to incorporate administrative, clinical, and special-purpose applications to satisfy medical, nursing, and other departments in a hospital.

### Administrative Applications

Administrative applications are those that support the administrative
functions of patient care. They generally include budgeting and payroll,
cost accounting, patient billing, inventory control, bed census, and medical
records. They also include the admission, discharge, and transfer (ADT)
systems which control the flow of patients in a hospital from admission to
discharge. They are used to prepare the midnight census and activity
reports. ADT changes and generation of bed charges provide the census,
which is a key factor in planning hospital resources (see Chap. 9).

### Clinical Applications

Clinical applications generally include applications that focus on patient
care services during a hospitalization or an episode of care. They are
essentially short-term databases. They include order entry/results reporting, vital signs, shift report, nursing care plans, nurses' notes, and other
nursing documentation activities. The order entry application generally
includes all physician and nursing orders, requested tests (laboratory,
radiological, etc.), procedures, drugs, and other services provided in the
hospital. The results reporting applications produce reports of the test

results, evaluations and/or outcomes of the procedures, outcomes of medications administered including medication profiles for the patients, and results of the other identified services (see Chap. 10).

## Special-Purpose Applications

Special-purpose applications generally refer to the services other than medical and nursing services that are provided for patient care. They are generally ancillary services such as laboratory, pharmacy, and radiology. These applications are used not only to track requests but also to provide the needed results and reports to personnel who manage them.

A typical laboratory system, for example, receives a laboratory test request, generates the specimen labels, tracks the specimen through the various laboratory stages, generates the results, and communicates the findings to the patient's medical record. Such a system generally includes a database that contains the Physician Drug Reference (PDR) Manual to provide a knowledge base for the system users.

Other special-purpose systems include patient monitoring systems using physiological monitoring equipment connected to a patient database management system; patient classification for nurse staffing systems and nurse scheduling and personnel systems; and quality care and outcomes applications that are not a part of the large integrated patient care system.

Newer systems include graphic and imaging capabilities that provide visual displays of diagnostic conditions. These enhancements have added new dimensions to systems. They are also forming the basis for diagnosing visual conditions and will improve the decision-making applications.

## Hospital Information System Configurations

HISs can use several different computer system configurations, the most common being stand-alone large mainframe systems, which are on-line interactive systems with real-time processing. Other HISs run on minicomputer and microcomputer systems that combine the various computer configurations, and many of the newer systems are described as modular, local area network, point of service, and/or workstation systems. These different descriptions overlap depending on the context in which they are used (Blum, 1986; Shortliffe, 1990).

### Mainframe Systems

A mainframe computer system is traditionally a distributive system with hundreds of remote terminals located in and outside a large health care facility. The computer terminals are used to communicate with and access the mainframe computer, which is generally centrally located in one facility or shared with another facility. This type of system is on-line interactive with real-time processing and is used to manage the information on patient services. The system is designed to transmit and communicate patient service data (orders) to the accounting, pharmacy, and pathology departments, and acts as a messenger service. This type of system processes data in a real-time mode, producing information needed to document the care process and deliver care. It allows for both real-time and batch processing and generally has a large secondary storage capability (Fig. 6.8).

## Minicomputer Systems

In smaller health care facilities, minicomputer systems are still being implemented. Generally, they are configured identically to a mainframe system but on a smaller scale. The concept is the same, but the computer terminals or video display monitors used to communicate with and access the computer are fewer in number, and the size of the computer is smaller.

Minicomputers also are generally networked and function like mainframes. This type of configuration allows for distributed processing of dif-

**Figure 6.8**   An integrated on-line real-time hospital information system.

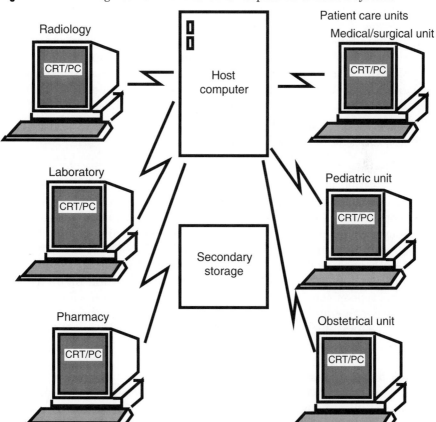

ferent applications by different minicomputers; however, because they are in a network, they appear to be one computer system. Both mainframe and minicomputer systems are also being configured with microcomputers or personal computers (PCs) as remote terminals. In this configuration the PCs not only perform as terminals to support a mainframe computer but also are used to run separate generic software packages. This configuration allows for different users and different levels of data processing, and at the same time allows a variety of computer applications to be conducted.

### Microcomputer Systems

Microcomputer, or PC, systems have emerged in all work environments. Generally, microcomputers have two functions: (1) to communicate on-line and interact in a real-time mode with the central computer, and (2) to run specific applications that are not integral components of the central HIS. With this combination, the microcomputer is used to download and upload data to and from the HIS mainframe for specific purposes. For example, a microcomputer can capture nursing service variables from the documentation system, download them for the patient classification staffing system, and then upload the actual staffing for the patient units to the HIS for the payroll system.

Microcomputers can be used to run software packages which do not require processing by the mainframe computer. A microcomputer can run a word-processing package for producing unit documents, a spreadsheet for preparing a budget, or a database management package for personnel evaluations. Other software packages can be used to teach a new procedure by reviewing computer-assisted instruction (CAI) or to apply statistical techniques for conducting research.

### Modular Systems

A modular system is a system which links several computers together to support a mainframe computer. In this configuration, an HIS consists of several departmental computers which are connected to the central computer to form a customized modular system. In this arrangement, which is essentially a distributed system, each computer integrates only selected common data, such as patient identification, and processes its departmental applications, such as patient acuity for nurse staffing or pharmacy orders. This type of configuration allows the HISs to remain small and relatively inexpensive and yet perform functions similar to those of a large integrated system. Such a topology is primarily found in many medium-sized hospitals that cannot afford a mainframe system (Fig. 6.9).

### Local Area Network Systems

A local area network (LAN) system functions the same as a modular system, but differs in size, scope, and configuration. A LAN consists of several

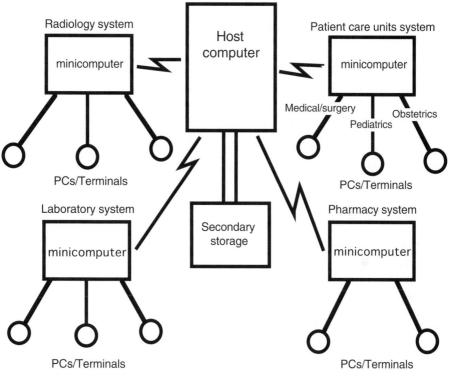

**Figure 6.9** An integrated hospital information system using a network of computers.

microcomputers linked together to share and process patient data for a specific hospital unit or specific environment, such as a specific patient care unit, computer classroom, or research environment. There are several different configurations for LANs, which are described in Chap. 3.

### Point-of-Service Systems

A point-of-service or point-of-care system uses a "bedside terminal" to minimize the manual charting which occurs at the nurses' station. The system uses a dumb terminal, microcomputer, or some other type of device such as a notebook or hand-held computer for data collection. Each of these devices offers different degrees of processing and distributing information throughout a health care facility. This new concept is believed to improve the efficiency of the HIS in processing patient data and communicating timely information to the users.

A point-of-service system is designed to save time by recording critical clinical data such as patient assessment, drug administration, vital signs, etc., at the time by the provider of the service. It also gives all care providers involved with the patient immediate access to key patient information. It can retrieve the patient's care plan, latest vital signs, or medication administered. Point-of-service systems are generally installed in direct patient care units such as intensive or critical care units, but can be also found in patient care units in a facility where an HIS is installed (Massengill, 1993; Wiederhold and Perreault, 1990).

## Workstation Systems

A workstation system is another new approach being introduced in several hospitals. A workstation system combines the central, modular, and local area network system configurations. This new approach is possible because of the advances in hardware technology whereby computers are getting smaller and faster and have the ability to store and process increasing volumes of data.

In a workstation system, a workstation computer is located on each hospital patient unit instead of a central mainframe. This computer is essentially a large microcomputer which is designed to integrate all patient data at the unit level. A workstation system is also modular, in that it communicates with other dedicated systems in the hospital, such as the laboratory system, and receives data for the unit. It can also function as a "server" for a LAN with terminals located on a nursing unit.

A workstation system is generally configured with open architecture that allows expansion of storage capacity and a software platform that allows enhancements and/or changes in the computer programs to meet the needs of a variety of users. This type of system can also include a communication network outside the hospital linking other health care facilities, referrals to home health agencies, libraries, national databanks, physician offices, and other authorized users of the information. It also offers several other applications such as Internet services and resources, including E-mail. It can be used to display digitized images and photographs and present graphic displays of data, and in time it will accept voice input. A workstation system includes all the tools and data needed to document and provide patient care services on the unit, including the standard data for the computer-based patient record.

## Stand-Alone Systems

A stand-alone system is a microcomputer designed for a single user that generally runs one application at a time. It is used as a PC for personal, home, or private use. These systems generally employ user-friendly software packages to develop specific applications. They do not rely on a central database, nor do they share computing resources. However, with the introduction of the Internet, communication with other services, resources, and databases is possible.

## PATIENT RECORD SYSTEMS

### Paper-Based Patient Record

The patient record is the major document that contains data about the patient's health care. It has been in use since 1918. The patient record is used by all providers of health care services to record, store, and review information. Paper-based patient records differ from hospital to hospital, and in some hospitals from patient unit to patient unit, as well as varying for the different types of health care facilities providing patient care.

As the computer industry grew, the use of computers, including HISs, in the health care industry also grew. The paper-based patient record began to change to an automated patient record. In 1991, it was determined by the U.S. General Accounting Office in a Report to the Chairman, Committee on Governmental Affairs, that a fully automated patient record offered a means to improve patient care, increase efficiency, and reduce cost. The report further indicated that as of 1991 such a record had not yet been developed and that the technological advances had not led to a standardized computer-based patient record (General Accounting Office, 1991).

### Computer-Based Patient Record

The automated patient record, also referred to as the computer-based patient record (CPR), was determined to have many advantages over a paper-based record and has emerged as a new structure for the traditional paper patient record. Such a record can (1) improve health care personnel's ability to deliver health care, (2) enhance outcomes research programs, and (3) increase hospital efficiency. Automation provides a solution to many information gathering and dissemination problems and can be used to more effectively and efficiently provide data for outcomes research (Fig. 6.10) (Dick and Steen, 1991).

Despite the technological advances, including the development of HISs, there is no consensus on the composition of the CPR—that is, what data the CPR should include; how the data should be structured, organized, or stored; and how the data should be communicated within and outside the health care facility. However, the need for a standardized CPR has been identified by all members of the health care community (Ball and Collen, 1992; Milholland and Heller, 1992).

To address this concern, the Institute of Medicine (IOM) initiated a study of the patient record in June 1986 and completed it in 1990. The IOM established a Patient Record Study Committee with a mandate to examine the problems of the existing medical and patient record systems in order to recommend actions and research for their improvement using

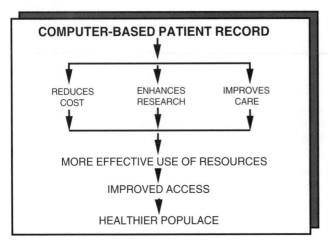

**Figure 6.10**   Computer-based patient record model. (Courtesy Computer-Based Patient Record Institute [CPRI].)

new computer technologies. The committee, which consisted of representatives from patient groups, software and hardware vendors, third-party payers, government agencies, and professional organizations, was divided into five subcommittees, each with a different focus. The committee agreed that the CPR be defined as follows:

> A computer-based patient record (CPR) is an electronic patient record that resides in a system specifically designed to support users by providing accessibility to complete and accurate data, alerts, reminders, clinical decision support systems, links to medical knowledge and other aids (Dick and Steen, 1991).

The IOM CPR committee concluded that automation could improve patient records, which in turn could improve the management of health care data, an essential element of our nation's health care system. They made several recommendations, which are listed in Table 6.2. The major recommendation was for health care professionals and organizations to adopt the CPR as the standard for all records related to patient care. They also urged that a private nonprofit organization be formed to implement the CPR. As a result, the Computer-Based Patient Record Institute (CPRI) was formed and officially incorporated in January 1992.

## Computer-Based Patient Record Institute

The CPRI, once formed, was instrumental in promoting the CPR. The initial structure consisted of an executive board with five founding members, one of which was the American Nurses Association. The CPRI believes that the CPR is critical to implementing the proposed Agenda for Health

**TABLE 6.2**   RECOMMENDATIONS OF THE INSTITUTE OF MEDICINE
COMMITTEE ON IMPROVING THE PATIENT RECORD

The Committee recommends the following:

1. Health care professionals and organizations should adopt the computer-based patient record (CPR) as the standard for medical and all other records related to patient care.

2. To accomplish Recommendation No. 1, the public and private sectors should join in establishing a Computer-Based Patient Record Institute (CPRI) to promote and facilitate development, implementation, and dissemination of the CPR.

3. Both the public and private sectors should expand support for the CPR and CPR system implementation through research, development, and demonstration projects. Specifically, the committee recommends that Congress authorize and appropriate funds to implement the research and development agenda outlined herein. The committee further recommends that private foundations and vendors fund programs that support and facilitate this research and development agenda.

4. The CPRI should promulgate uniform national standards for data and security to facilitate implementation of the CPR and its secondary data bases.

5. The CPRI should review federal and state laws and regulations for the purpose of proposing and promulgating modes legislation and regulations to facilitate the implementation and dissemination of the CPR and its secondary data bases and to streamline the CPR and CPR systems.

6. The costs of CPR systems should be shared by those who benefit from the value of the CPR. Specifically, the full costs of implementing and operating CPRs and CPR systems should be factored into reimbursement levels or payment schedules of both public and private sector third-party payers. In addition, users of secondary data bases should support the costs of creating such data bases.

7. Health care professional schools and organizations should enhance educational programs for students and practitioners in the use of computers, CPRs, and CPR systems for patient care, education, and research.

*Source:* Reprinted with permission from *The Computer-Based Patient Record.* Copyright 1991 by the National Academy of Sciences. Courtesy of the National Academy Press, Washington, DC.

Care Reform. The mission of the CPRI is to initiate and coordinate activities which will facilitate and promote the routine use of the CPR in health care. The goals of the CPRI that were identified were to

- Promote the development and use of standards for CPR messages, codes, and identifiers.
- Demonstrate how CPR systems can lead to improvements in effective and efficient patient care.
- Encourage the creation of policies and mechanisms to protect provider confidentiality and ensure data security.
- Educate health professionals and the public about CPRs.
- Coordinate the building of technical and legal infrastructures that enable the use of CPRs.
- Promote CPR research activities (Computer-Based Patient Record Institute, 1993).

CPRI initiated several work groups, each of which is involved in different activities that will ultimately provide recommendations for not only a comprehensive CPR, but also a CPR system and ultimately a longitudinal CPR system that would provide clinical, financial, and research data. The work groups that were created have changed over time but continue to focus on (1) data codes and structure, (2) confidentiality, privacy, and legislation, (3) professional and public education, and (4) CPR systems evaluation.

The mission of the Codes and Structure Work Group focuses on the development and use of standards for CPR structure and associated messages, communications, codes, and identifiers. This work group is involved in several activities, including (1) the promotion of a universal identification for the patient and provider, (2) evaluating disease and procedure coding systems, and (3) providing input into data and message communication standards.

## DATA STANDARDS

A standard is defined by the National Standards Policy Advisory Committee as: "A prescribed set of rules, conditions, or requirements concerning definitions of terms; classification of components; specification of materials, performance, or operations; delineation of procedures; or measurement of quantity and quality in describing materials, products, systems, services, or practices" (National Standards Policy Advisory Committee, 1978, p. 6).

The evolution of a standard goes through several stages: conceptualization, discussion, development, implementation, and promulgation. The conceptualization of health care standards for data interchange emerged in the 1980s as health care information systems expanded in the health care industry. Several standards have emerged for different types of computer data. They include clinical data standards and communication standards for the interchange of data inside and outside health care facilities. They also include disease and procedure classification systems which have been considered to be standards for reporting mortality and morbidity and for reimbursement systems. Nursing care standards and classification schemes are described in Chap. 7.

The major areas that need to be addressed in relation to data standards for health care information systems including CPR systems comprise the following:

- Clinical data standards
- Clinical data standards organizations
- Clinical data communication standards
- Clinical data communication standards organizations
- Disease and procedure classification systems

# Clinical Data Standards

National clinical data standards are being developed to provide a guide for policy, law, and systems development. Standards are also being developed to establish formats for electronic communication and data interchange. Without nationally accepted computer formats, data compatibility, which is needed to achieve electronic communication of the CPR, will not be achieved.

There are many kinds of clinical patient data incorporated in the CPR. They include narrative progress notes, laboratory and radiology reports, history and physical examination reports, medication administrations, treatments and procedures, nursing care reports, discharge summaries, etc. Data come from many sites, including hospitals, physicians' offices, skilled nursing facilities, home health agencies, community health departments, etc. However, for each kind of data and each site of care, hundreds of providers exist, and standards for terminology span more than one provider's domain. It is nevertheless agreed that a common language combining data structures and grammar should be developed so that meaningful "coded" messages could be sent between CPR systems.

Clinical data standards which act as guides are by consensus the best way to develop appropriate practices in the rapidly developing field of computers. They allow options and can be less specific than other forms of standards; however, standards specifications are being developed which require strict adherence. One of the major standards efforts is the determination of universal identification codes for CPR systems.

## Universal Identification Codes

One of the primary obstacles to fully utilizing computers in health care and the patient record is the absence of a unified set of clinical data standards. Universal identifiers for people and places are a prerequisite for sharing and integrating patient data. They must be designed to prevent unauthorized access to confidential patient data. In addition, they must also include universal provider and place identifiers for use by the new technology.

The properties of a Universal Health Care Identifier (UHID) proposed in 1993 is limited to the U.S. population (Medical Records Institute, 1993). Its purpose is to encompass four functions: (1) provide positive identification of patients when health care services are provided, (2) enable automated linkages of other CPRs on the same patient, (3) provide adequate data security, and (4) use new technology to minimize cost (Gabrieli and Hieb, 1994).

## Patient Identifiers

The CPRI and several of the other professional organizations have recommended that the social security number (SSN) be used as the patient identifier. It was recommended that a self-check digit be added to the SSN to reduce errors in identification, and that temporary numbers be assigned to accommodate infants and others who would not ordinarily have assigned SSNs. The patient identification should encompass multiprovider records in all health care settings and at all levels (regional, national, and international settings). Another standard for a UHID that consists of 19 digits has been proposed by Gabrieli and Hieb as members of the ASTM E-31.12-5 standards committee. This proposal not only provides a unique identifier but also ensures data security.

### Provider Identifiers

There are several existing alternatives for the provider identifiers. Provider identifiers are essential so that physicians, nurses, and other health care professionals can access patient information in order to provide continuity of care. The Health Care Financing Administration (HCFA) supports the use of a universal physician identifier number (UPIN) system which it has already developed and absorbed the cost of implementing. It is a coding scheme used to identify physicians and other providers (e.g., nurse practitioners) of patient services reimbursed by Medicare and/or Medicaid. However, it does not include physicians who do not care for Medicare or Medicaid patients, nor does it include other care givers who do not receive reimbursement for services, such as hospital staff nurses. A proposed solution is to have health care providers without a UPIN use their SSN until a UPIN could be issued.

### Site of Care Identifiers

A single universal identifier is also proposed for all sites where health care is provided, regardless of whether the site is a hospital, home, agency, clinic, or physician's office. HCFA has a provider identification scheme already in place for all health care organizations certified to provide Medicare and/or Medicaid services.

## Clinical Data Standards Organizations

Data standards are also being developed by private groups and government agencies. There are different standards for different kinds of messages depending upon the subject matter and method of communication. Within institutions there are different message communications data standards for the institution and for the clinical areas, and these differ from clinical data standards. Institutions include hospitals, nursing homes, clinics, physician offices, community health departments, and other care-providing institutions. Clinical data refer to results of diagnostic studies, history and physical examination records, visit notes, nursing notes, progress notes, vital signs, discharge summaries, and other clinically relevant information about the patient.

Several national and international organizations are involved in the development and coordination of data standards, the structure and organization of each data element in the CPR, and the communication of data between units in a hospital and to outside facilities (McDonald and Hirpcsak, 1992; Office of Science and Data Development, 1994). Federal agencies also develop health related data standards. Several professional organizations additionally have become involved in setting standards. The major ones are described below.

### American National Standards Institute

The American National Standards Institute (ANSI) serves as the coordinator of voluntary standards activities in the United States and is the agency that approves standards as American National Standards. ANSI has developed the consensus methodology for approving these national standards.

ANSI is another organization establishing standards. ANSI Z39.50 is a standard for transmitting requests for bibliographic information to bibliographic retrieval systems.

### American Society for Testing and Materials

ASTM was organized in 1898 and has grown into one of the largest voluntary standards development systems in the country. ASTM has been active in medical computing and has initiated several committees to develop standards for different aspects of the CPR. The ASTM Committee E31 on Computerized Systems was organized in 1970. It was established to develop standards for computer systems in medical applications. The early standards were guides for the best ways to do things. However, as computers advanced, subcommittees were formed to help computer developers in their profession (American Society for Testing and Materials, 1992). Several of the subcommittees are described below.

The ASTM E31.12 Computer-Based Patient Records Subcommittee is responsible for content and structure of the CPR and CPR systems. This committee has been involved for several years in developing standards for electronic patient records. Included are classifications, guides, and terminology needed to define patient records in sufficient detail that information gathered in one setting is consistent with information gathered in another setting and usable at another institution (Murphy, 1993).

The standard developed by this subcommittee in 1992 defines the organization of the information, the meaning of terms, and a logical structure for the CPR. The guide sets forth the fundamental principles for the CPR, including its major attributes. The standards being developed have application to use of the CPR in health care delivery, health education, and biomedical research.

ASTM is also concerned with the minimal essential content and logical structure for the electronic longitudinal patient health record. In the early 1990s ASTM formed several other subcommittees related to the automated patient record. The major ones include ASTM E31.17 on Access, Privacy, and Confidentiality of Medical Records, E31.18 on Health Data

Cards, E31.19 on CBPR Content and Structure, and a subcommittee concerned with the extension of the CPR called the automated longitudinal health record (ALHR). The ALHR is considered to be a component of the CPR and is applicable to all types of health care services in all settings, e.g., acute hospital care, long-term care, home health care, ambulatory care, etc.

ASTM E31.12 Standard 1384: Automated Primary Record of Care, proposed in 1993, focuses on the primary legal record documenting health care services provided to a person in any aspect of health care delivery. It outlines a draft of the standards with the data presentations and coded values.

Several other ASTM subcommittees focus on different aspects of standards for computer systems in medical applications and on standards for data transmission and communication across settings and outside a hospital and/or health care facility.

ASTM E31.11: Data Exchange for Clinical Observations develops standards for the two-way transmission of clinical observations between independent computer systems. The purpose of the standards is to facilitate the use of computerized medical records and increase the availability, accuracy, and completeness of clinical data for medical practice and research.

### Healthlevel 7
HL7 focuses on standards for transmitting and communicating clinical data within an institution. It has instituted several technical committees and special-interest groups which meet periodically to develop data standards. The focus is primarily on the internal transfer of medical orders; clinical observations; clinical data (including test results); admission, transfer, and discharge records (ADT); and charge and billing information. HL7 standards are used in many hospitals and other health care institutions, and are supported by several vendors and developers of patient care systems.

### Institute of Electrical and Electronic Engineers
The IEEE standard IEEE P1073 Medical Information Bus (MIB) is another standard used to control and link medical instrumentation such as that used in critical care equipment. Several standards for medical device communications have also been developed.

### European Technical Committee for Standardization
The European Technical Committee for Standardization (CEN) established Technical Committee 251 (Medical Informatics) in early 1990. This committee CEN-TC PT 251 was formed to develop standards for the interchange of clinical and management data among independent medical information systems. CEN recognized that such an effort required international cooper-

ation. Liaison activities with the United States will involve ANSI, which will play a coordinating role for different U.S. standards efforts.

## International Standards Organization

The International Standards Organization (ISO) oversees the development of standards internationally. The United States standards are brought to ISO through the American National Standards Institute (ANSI) via the Technical Advisor Groups (TAGS).

## Healthcare Informatics Standards Planning Panel

One of the organizations that have been working on establishing data standards is the American National Standards Institute (ANSI), which has made efforts to coordinate U.S. and international standards development through the Healthcare Informatics Standards Planning Panel (HISPP). The ANSI HISPP was convened in 1991 to coordinate the standards groups for health care data interchange and health care informatics and other relevant standards groups. This group works toward achieving a unified set of nonredundant nonconflicting standards that are compatible with communication environments. This group is working directly with the CPRI Work Group on Codes and Structures. Like CPRI, ANSI HISPP will not write standards but will serve as a coordinator, identifying needs and coordinating committees related to health care standardization.

## Workgroup for Electronic Data Interchange

The Workgroup for Electronic Data Interchange (WEDI) is an industry-led task force created to streamline health care administration through standardized electronic communications. WEDI was formed to develop an action plan following a national summit on health care paperwork convened in November 1991 by Secretary Sullivan of HHS. In 1992 WEDI convened national leaders to outline the steps to make electronic data interchange for the health care industry a reality by 1994. WEDI envisioned a public-private partnership to achieve one national standard format and interconnecting networks for users conducting business via computer (Workgroup for Electronic Data Interchange, 1992).

WEDI reconvened in 1993 to resolve other obstacles regarding electronic communication. The major goal was to monitor the health care industry's progress toward EDI and the use of standardized data. It expanded its financial analysis and formed eleven technical advisory groups. They prepared recommendations which included the financial impact on the health care industry. The financial analysis included the cost of implementation, estimated cost savings for employers and payers, and net savings to reallocate activities to enhance patient care, quality care, and client services (Workshop for Electronic Data Interchange, 1993).

# Disease and Procedure Classification Systems

Several disease, diagnostic, and procedure classification systems that affect the CPR are being used to code, classify, and label clinical patient care. Each has a different focus and purpose, and is used to code and document different aspects of clinical patient care, such as diagnostic conditions, reason for encounters, or procedures provided to patients inside and outside of a hospital. The major ones include classification schemes that are used to code and classify (1) diagnostic conditions, (2) procedures, or (3) combinations of diagnostic conditions and procedures.

## Disease Classifications

***International Statistical Classification of Diseases and Related Health Problems: Tenth Revision*** The *International Statistical Classification of Diseases and Related Health Problems: Tenth Revision* (ICD-10) (World Health Organization, 1992) is a system of categories to which mortality and morbidity entities are assigned according to established criteria. It encompasses not only diagnostic labels but also nomenclature structures. This revision is the latest in a series that was formalized in 1893 as the Bertillon Classification or International List of Causes of Death. It is anticipated that ICD-10 will not be fully implemented and used to collect both mortality and morbidity statistics until the turn of the century.

***International Classification of Diseases: Ninth Revision: Clinical Modifications*** The *International Classification of Diseases: Ninth Revision: Clinical Modifications* (ICD-9CM) (World Health Organization, 1980a) codes are traditionally used for morbidity and mortality conditions. ICD-9 is used to classify and code mortality statistics internationally. It is also being used to classify and code morbidity data for medical records, research, health care services, etc. ICD-9 also provides the basis for the diagnosis related groups (DRGs) which are used for payment and reimbursement for treatment of medical conditions in hospitals.

This classification is published by the World Health Organization (WHO); however, the ICD-9 CM (Clinical Modification) is a special edition published for use in the United States. It is updated periodically with additions, deletions, and corrections.

***International Classification of Impairments, Disabilities, and Handicaps*** The *International Classification of Impairments, Disabilities, and Handicaps* (ICIDH) (World Health Organization, 1980c) is a supplementary classification published by WHO beginning in 1980. This classification is endorsed by WHO since it conforms to the coding structure of the ICD classifications. The ICIDH does not focus on disease processes as

ICD-10 does, but rather follows three levels of experiences consequent upon disease: (1) impairments, or abnormalities of body structure, (2) disabilities, defined as a restriction or lack of ability in functional performance and activity by an individual; and (3) handicaps, or disadvantages experienced by an individual as a result of impairments and disabilities.

***International Classification of Primary Care***   The *International Classification of Primary Care* (ICPC) (World Organization of National Colleges, 1987) is a classification prepared for the World Organization of National Colleges, Academies and Academic Associations of General Practitioners/Family Physicians. It was developed by the ICPC Working Party and is designed to classify three elements of health care encounters: (1) reasons for the encounter, (2) diagnosis or problems, and (3) the process of care. This classification is unique in that it uses patients' own words for the reasons they are seeking health services. It is structured as a multi-axis classification that links diagnoses/problems with interventions. The reason for seeking health services is coded according to body system. Two chapters depict "general" and "social" reasons. This classification could be used by primary health care nurse specialists for coding and classifying some aspects of their protocols of care (Lamberts and Wood, 1987).

***Diagnostic and Statistical Manual Mental Disorders***   *Diagnostic and Statistical Manual Mental Disorders* (DSM-III-R) (American Psychiatric Association, 1987) is developed by the American Psychiatric Association. It originated in 1952 and was the first official manual of mental disorders to contain a glossary of diagnostic conditions. DSM was revised in 1987. It provides a classification of mental disorders, which are clinically significant behaviors or psychological syndromes or patterns that occur in a person and are associated with stressful conditions.

DSM-III-R is accepted in the United States as the common language of mental health clinicians and researchers for documenting disorders for which they have professional responsibility. It also conforms with the ICD-9 R codes. Examples of DSM classifications are 317.00, Mild mental retardation, and 303.00, Alcohol intoxication.

## Procedure Classifications

***Current Procedural Terminology***   The *Physicians' Current Procedural Terminology, Fourth Revision* (CPT-4) (American Medical Association, 1992) is a comprehensive listing of medical terms and codes for uniform coding of medical procedures and services provided by physicians. The list was first developed by the American Medical Association in 1966 primarily for reimbursement of medical services and procedures performed by physicians and other authorized health care providers, such as nurse practitioners and clinical nurse specialists. CPT lists and codes procedures and services performed in outpatient clinics, ambulatory surgery, ambulatory care centers, physician offices and clinics, and other settings outside the hospital where medical services are provided.

The CPT codes are listed in five sections, and within each section are subsections with anatomic, procedural, condition, or descriptor subheadings, all presented in numeric order. These codes are used for reimbursement and payment for services performed in outpatient clinics, physicians' offices, and other settings outside a hospital.

Many of the CPT codes are routinely used by nurses. Seven nursing specialty groups indicated in a recent study that they use approximately 493 CPT codes to document as well as to be reimbursed for the services they provide. The major nursing groups include family nurse practitioners, midwives, and specialty nurses such as school, orthopedic, oncology, rehabilitation, and critical care nurses (Griffith and Robinson, 1993).

***HCFA Common Procedure Coding System*** *HCFA Common Procedure Coding System* (HCPCS) was developed in 1983 by the HCFA for the purpose of standardizing the coding system used to process Medicare and some Medicaid claims on a national basis. HCPCS is used to bill Medicare primarily for supplies, materials, and injections. It is also used for noninstitutional providers of health care services and procedures which are not defined by CPT. The major portion of the HCPCS coding system is CPT, which is used for most of the procedures and services performed. HCPCS also has two other levels: level 2, used to describe services covered by Medicare intermediaries; and level 3, used to describe new procedures, services, and supplies (HCFA, 1983).

***International Classification of Diseases: Volume 3: Procedures*** *International Classification of Diseases: Volume 3: Procedures* (ICD 9CM Procedures) (World Health Organization, 1980b) is used for morbidity coding of surgical procedures for hospitalized patients. It is published by the U.S. government using a classification similar to ICD-9, which is used to code the cause of death (mortality). It is based on anatomy and in some cases surgical specialty. This scheme is not as precise as CPT. This coding scheme is also used by nurse practitioners. However, because nurses do not generally get reimbursed for specific services in hospitals, the coding scheme is not widely used.

### Combined Diagnostic and Procedural Classification

***Systematized Nomenclature of Medicine*** *SNOMED International: The Systematized Nomenclature of Human and Veterinary Medicine* (College of American Pathologists, 1993) is a structured nomenclature and classification of terminology used in human and veterinary medicine. SNOMED International is intended to be a comprehensive coding system capable of recording all events described in the medical record, including the diagnostic conditions and procedures. SNOMED is being used by an increasing number of health professional specialty groups. Terms can be linked to one another using the General Linkage Modified Module, making it possible to code complex entities.

SNOMED International contains eleven independent modules, each an independent taxonomy, representing the semantic categories necessary for describing and indexing events in the medical record. They include (1) Topography, (2) Morphology, (3) Function, (4) Living Organisms, (5) Chemicals, Drugs and Biological Products, (6) Physical Agents, Forces, and Activities, (7) Occupations, (8) Social Context, (9) Disease/Diagnosis, (10) Procedures, and (11) Procedures, General Linkage/Modifiers (Cote et al., 1993; Henry et al., 1994).

## STANDARDS INITIATIVES

Several initiatives have been started that affect the clinical and data standards for CPRs. The unified medical language system (UMLS) project will ultimately produce a unified medical language that may become the standard nomenclature for the CPR. Other initiatives that are influencing the standardized CPR are the proposed Agenda for Health Care Reform, the High Performance Computing and Communication (HPCC) Program, and the National Information Infrastructure (NII).

## Unified Medical Language System

The UMLS was initiated in September 1986 by the National Library of Medicine (NLM) as a long-term research and development effort. The goal of the UMLS project is to link the vocabularies of several knowledge sources so that health professionals could locate, retrieve, and integrate relevant machine-readable information. The vocabularies include the scientific literature, patient records, knowledge-based expert systems, factual databanks, and directories of institutions and individuals. The resulting system is a biomedical information system which supports three new knowledge sources: (1) a Metathesaurus of terms and concepts from the various vocabularies of the different databases, (2) a Semantic Network of the relationships among the broad categories to which the concepts of the Metathesaurus are assigned, and (3) an Information Sources Map of the machine-readable biomedical databases.

In 1990 the NLM released Meta-1, which matches appropriate terms and link them together. By 1991 the Metathesaurus contained 67,242 concepts and 220,792 terms, including synonyms. The initial vocabularies included the NLM's Medical Subject Headings (MeSH), ICD-9CM, CPT, and several other specialized medical vocabularies. The UMLS is creating new data structures and computer-based tools to link core concepts of biomedical terminologies (Humphreys and Lindberg, 1992; Masys and Humphreys, 1992). In 1993 and 1994, the UMLS added the four nursing classification schemes recommended by the American Nurses Association (ANA) Database Steering Committee.

## Agenda for Health Care Reform

The Agenda for Health Care Reform was introduced by President Clinton in September 1993 and proposed as the Health Security Act of 1993, which Congress did not pass. As it was conceived, it would have created major changes in the way Americans pay for and receive medical services. The goals of health care reform were to (1) increase access (universal coverage), (2) improve quality, and (3) reduce costs. The capabilities of computers and information technology were viewed as essential to achieving these goals (White House Council on Domestic Policy, 1993). Health care reform has started in the private sector and will be ongoing for the next decade.

## High Performance Computing and Communications Program

The High Performance Computing and Communications (HPCC) program is a multiagency effort designed to apply high-speed and high-performance computers to help solve the nation's problems, including health. The program was initiated to implement the High Performance Computer Act of 1991, which authorized the construction of a new high-speed computer communication network to connect government agencies, educational institutions, and scientific organizations. A total of ten federal departments and agencies are participating in this initiative.

The first phase of the program identified a group of problems; the second phase proposed information technology applications as well as the creation of a national information infrastructure. Six types of applications were identified: (1) test beds for linking hospitals and settings where health care professionals need to share medical data and images, (2) software for imaging technology, (3) virtual reality technology, (4) collaborative technology in remote locations whereby health care providers treat patients using real-time computer processing, (5) database technology for accessing relevant medical information and literature, and (6) database technologies for accessing, transmitting, and storing patient record information while protecting the accuracy and privacy of the CPRs (Elmer-Dewitt, 1993; Little, 1992; Office of Science and Technology Policy, 1993; Work Group on Computerization of Patient Records, 1993).

The HPCC, by streamlining health care processing, is being viewed as a viable cost containment component of the Agenda for Health Care Reform.

The "information highway" will be used for the automatic transmission of a single standardized claims form which can be completed on the computer. The information highway is an interconnected seamless broad-based web of communication networks, computers, databases, and consumer electronics that will put vast amounts of information at users' fingertips and that connects everyone—providers, patients, and administrators.

The HCPP includes a wide range of devices used to transmit, store, process, and display voice, data, and images. It integrates and interconnects the physical components in a technological network. HCPP allows researchers and health care policy makers to access information from libraries, databases, and supercomputers. It links health care facilities, health care providers, and health resources together, creating a national health information infrastructure system. The development of the NII will help unleash an information revolution that will change forever the way people live, work, and interact with one another. This is illustrated by the NSFNET as shown in Fig. 6.11.

## National Information Infrastructure

The vision that an NII be developed to support health and health care service in the United States emerged from a forum convened in 1991 by the

**Figure 6.11**   NSFNET: Bringing the World of Ideas Together. (Courtesy Donna Cox and Robert Patterson, NCSA/University of Illinois at Urbana–Champaign.)

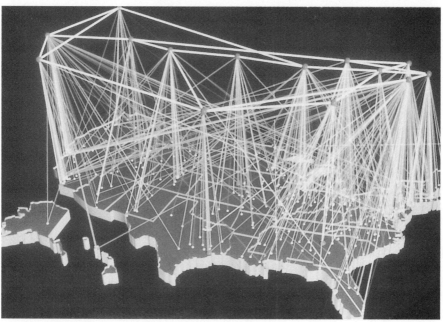

secretary of the Department of Health and Human Services (DHHS). The primary purpose of the NII was to transmit electronic claims data and payment transfers for federal payment as a means of reducing the cost of processing paper claims forms. It was also considered as a means of linking all participants in the U.S. health care system to one another. Each health care facility and practitioner would connect to the network via its own CPR system.

In this context, the CPR would have the ability to create, store, retrieve, transmit, and manipulate patients' health data. It will be designed to support decision making, analyze the outcomes, and provide aggregated data to use in knowledge-based systems. This strategy could improve logic and practice guidelines for health care providers making decisions about diagnoses and treatment options. The CPR would also be a lifelong longitudinal health record (Fitzmaurice, 1994; Report of the Work Group on Computerization of Current Records, 1993).

The NII is needed to obtain timely and reliable information for: (1) supporting the administration and operation of the health care system at all levels, (2) supporting public health objectives and programs, and (3) monitoring the implementation of health care reform and assessing its impact. The NII components will require at least an administrative data system which consists of an enrollment and encounter data system and provider and plan characteristics, as well as a survey program. The administrative data systems should address the following:

- Universal health security cards
- Uniform health data sets for enrollment and claims/encounters
- Electronic data transmission formats and standards
- Electronic data networks
- Regional data centers linking plans, alliances, states, and the federal government
- Standards and unique identification numbers for providers, plans, employers, and enrollees
- Privacy protection safeguards through national legislation
- Support for point-of-service systems

The electronic data network is viewed as a public-private partnership which will include enrollment data, claims/encounter data, and provider and health plan characteristics. To implement the electronic network will require determining data needs and uses in the areas of budgeting, premiums, risk factors, rate negotiations with providers, monitoring performance on quality (access, under/over service, and outcomes), providing clear and useful information to consumers, and detecting fraud and abuse. It will require information on public health (PH) obtained by monitoring progress toward PH objectives and supporting PH surveillance and assessment. In the area of research for planning and policy development, information is needed on effectiveness, outcomes, and program evaluation. The surveys to be conducted will focus on consumers by health plan and on employers, providers, health insurers, plans, and households on the national and state level.

Technology is central to the implementation of a national health information infrastructure vision. The NII will provide the framework for the standards that facilitate data exchange and interpretation between different health care applications. The CPR is viewed as a critical source of data and information required for the Agenda for Health Care Reform.

## Internet

The Internet was started by the Pentagon in 1969 to support U.S. Department of Defense military research by linking phone lines and computer databases. The initial electronic network was called the Advanced Research Projects Agency Network (ARPANET). This was replaced by the National Science Foundation Network (NSFNET), which consisted of a small number of links connecting six nationally funded supercomputer centers so that they could share their resources for scholarly research. This led to the need for more advanced networking technology to support the increased growth in traffic on this network. As a result, in 1987 the NSF issued a competitive solicitation for a new and still faster network service. NSFNET was upgraded and expanded and became a new network resource that universities could use to access supercomputer resources.

This network led to the concept of a network of networks called the Internet. The Internet is the world's largest collection of computer networks. It is not a network but a collection of individual telecommunication networks which communicate with one another. The NSFNET is the backbone and the largest service of the Internet, which has grown to over 11,252 interconnected networks in over 40 countries. The Internet is a high-speed telecommunication network which allows the exchange of data, mail, and even video. A user can transfer large data files from one computer to another, send electronic mail (E-mail) to other users on the network or use a bulletin board to communicate with them, and access other computer resources such as a supercomputer or large computer system via a remote terminal (Falk, 1994; Krol, 1993; Schneider, 1993).

To use the Internet, a user must have a dial-up connection that has been hooked to one of the many independent networks. Each network in the collection uses routers which connect networks together to transfer data from one computer to another. Networks can also access other networks using gateways which translate between them.

The Internet is also an international network. The protocols for access use standards established by the Organization for International Standardization (OSI). The major drawback at this time is the lack of a national health information infrastructure needed to make the system standardized and efficient.

## SUMMARY

This chapter discussed systems theory, when and how it was introduced, and how it influenced the development of computers and computer systems. The concept of systems, including types, elements, and major characteristics, was discussed. Computer systems were also defined, followed by a discussion of major types of information systems—namely, dedicated, transaction, retrieval, monitoring, decision support, and expert systems and artificial intelligence.

A review of MISs was provided, including how the three levels of management in any organization benefit from MISs. HISs were defined and various types described, including the basic hardware configurations of several major models. Another section focused on classification systems used to code, classify, and document CPR clinical care services, and provided an overview of the clinical data standards and data communication standards and the organizations involved in their development.

The final section focused on computer-based standards initiatives. The HPCC program, which is being implemented as part of a new initiative in the health care industry and is recognized as a key technology for the future biomedical sciences, was discussed. Also an overview of the National Information Infrastructure, the Internet, and Telenet is provided.

## REFERENCES

American Medical Association. (1992). *Physicians' Current Procedural Terminology. CPT-4.* Chicago.

American Psychiatric Association. (1987). *Diagnostic and Statistical Manual of Mental Disorders* (DSM-III-R) (3d ed. revised). Washington, DC.

ASTM Committee E31. (1992). *Medical Computing Standards: A Review of Published Standards and Current Projects.* Philadelphia: American Society for Testing and Materials.

Austin, C. J. (1978, 1983). *Information Systems for Hospital Administration* (2d ed.). Ann Arbor, MI: Health Administration Press.

Ball, M. J., and Collen, M. F. (Eds.). (1992). *Aspects of the Computer-Based Patient Record.* New York: Springer-Verlag.

Bertalanffy, L. von. (1968). *General Systems Theory.* New York: George Braziller.

Blum, B. I. (Ed.). (1984). *Information Systems for Patient Care.* New York: Springer-Verlag.

Blum, B. I. (1986). *Clinical Information Systems.* New York: Springer-Verlag.

Boulding, K. E. (1956). General systems theory—the skeleton of science. *Management Science, 2,* 197–208.

Brookshear, J. G. (1991). *Computer Science: An Overview* (3d ed.). New York: Benjamin/Cummings.

College of American Pathologists. (1993). *SNOMED International: The Systematized Nomenclature of Human and Veterinary Medicine.* Northfield, IL.

Collen, M. F. (1983). The function of a HIS: An overview. In O. Fokkens et al. (Eds.), *MEDINFO 83 Seminars* (pp. 61–64). Amsterdam, Netherlands: North-Holland.

Collen, M. F. (1994). The origins of informatics. *Journal of the American Medical Informatics Association 1*(2), 91–107.

Computer-Based Patient Record Institute. (1993). *Appendix B: Vision, Mission and Goals.* In Report of the Work Group on Computerization of Patient Records, *Toward a National Health Information Infrastructure.* Washington, DC.

Cote, R. A., Rothwell, D. J., Palotay, J. L., and Beckett, R. S. (1993). *SNOMED International.* Northfield, IL: College of American Pathologists.

Dick, R. S., and Steen, E. B. (Eds.). (1991). *The Computer-Based Patient Record: An Essential Technology for Health Care* (p. 11). Washington, DC: National Academy Press.

Donnelly, G. F., Mengel, A., and Sutterley, D. C. (1980). *The Nursing System: Issues, Ethics and Politics.* New York: John Wiley.

Dorenfest, S. (1987, January). Despite interest, nation's hospitals slow to buy patient care systems. *Modern Healthcare,* 1–3.

Dorenfest, S. (1987, 1992). *The Dorenfest 3000+ Database and the Dorenfest Guide to the Hospital Information Systems Market.* Chicago: Published by the author.

Elmer-Dewitt, P. (1993, April 12). Take a trip into the future on the electronic superhighway. *Time,* 51–58.

Falk, B. (1994). *The Internet Roadmap.* Alameda, CA: SYBEX.

Fitzmaurice, J. M. (1994). *Putting the Information Infrastructure to Work: Health Care in the NII.* Rockville, MD: Agency for Health Care Policy and Research, PHS, US DHHS.

Gabrieli, E. R., and Hieb, B. R. (1994). *ASTM Committee E31: Fourth Draft: Guide for the Development of a Universal Health Care Identifier.* Philadelphia: American Society for Testing and Materials.

General Accounting Office. (1991). Report to the Chairman, Committee on Governmental Affairs, U.S. Senate. *Medical ADP Systems: Automated Medical Records Hold Promise to Improve Patient Care.* Washington, DC: U.S. General Accounting Office.

Graham, N. (1986). *The Mind Tool: Computers and Their Impact on Society.* New York: West.

Griffith, H. M., and Robinson, K. R. (1993). Current procedure terminology (CPT) coded services provided by nurse specialists. *Image, 25*(3), 178–186.

Hart, A. (1992). *Knowledge Acquisition for Expert Systems* (2d ed.). New York: McGraw-Hill.

Health Care Financing Administration. (1983). *Common Procedure Coding System.* Baltimore, MD: HCFA.

Henry, S. B., Holzemer, W. L., Reilly, C. A., and Campbell, K. E. (1994). Terms used by nurses to describe patient problems: Can SNOMED represent nursing concepts in the patient record? *Journal of the American Medical Informatics Association, 1*(1), 61–74.

Humphreys, B. L., and Lindberg, D. A. B. (1992). The unified medical language system project: A distributed experiment in improving access to biomedical information. In K. C. Lun, P. DeGoulet, T. E. Piemme, and O. Rienhoff (Eds.), *MEDINFO 92* (pp. 1496–1500). Amsterdam, Netherlands: North-Holland.

Krol, E. (1993). *The Whole Internet: User's Guide and Catalog.* Sebastopol, CA: O'Reilly & Associates.

Lamberts, H., and Wood, M. (Eds.). (1987). *International Classification of Primary Care* (ICPC). New York: Oxford.

Little, D. (1992). *Telecommunication: Can't Help Solve America's Health Care Problems?* Cambridge, MA: Arthur D. Little.

Massengill, S. (1993). The four technologies of the electronic patient record. In *Conference Proceedings: Toward an Electronic Patient Record '93* (pp. 92–94). Newton, MA: Medical Records Institute.

Masys, D. R., and Humphreys, B. L. (1992). Structure and function of the UMLS information sources map. In K. C. Lun, P. DeGoulet, T. E. Piemme, and O. Rienhoff (Eds.), *MEDINFO 92* (pp. 1518–1521). Amsterdam, Netherlands: North-Holland.

McDonald, C. J., and Hirpcsak, G. H. (1992). Data exchange standards for computer-based patient records. In M. J. Ball, and M. F. Collen (Eds.). *Aspects of the Computer-Based Patient Record* (pp. 157–164). New York: Springer-Verlag.

Medical Records Institute. (1993). Concepts models of patient identification: Issues surrounding the use of Social Security numbers for patient identification. In *Analysis Number 2: Toward an Electronic Record.* Newton, MA.

Milholland, D. K., and Heller, B. R. (1992). Computer-based patient record: From pipe dream to reality. *Computers in Nursing, 10*(5), 191.

Murphy, G. (1993). *ASTM Committee E31.12 Standard Guide for Description for Content and Structure of an Automated Primary Care Record of Care.* Philadelphia: American Society for Testing and Materials.

Office of Science and Data Development. (1994). *Current Activities of Selected Healthcare Informatics Standards Organizations.* Bethesda, MD: Agency for Health Care Policy and Research.

Office of Science and Technology Policy. (1993). *Grand Challenges 1993: High Performance Computing and Communications.* Washington, DC: Federal Coordinating Council for Science, Engineering, and Technology.

Optner, S. L. (1975). *Systems Analysis for Business Management* (2d ed.). Englewood Cliffs, NJ: Prentice-Hall.

Perreault, L. E., and Wiederhold, G. (1990a). Essential concepts for medical computing. In E. H. Shortliffe and L. E. Perreault (Eds.), *Medical Informatics: Computer Applications in Health Care* (pp. 117–150). Reading, MA: Addison-Wesley.

Perreault, L. E., and Wiederhold, G. (1990b). System design and evaluation. In E. H. Shortliffe, and L. E. Perreault (Eds.), *Medical Informatics: Computer Applications in Health Care* (pp. 151–178). Reading, MA: Addison-Wesley.

Report of the Work Group on Computerization of Patient Records: To the Secretary of the U.S. Department of Health and Human Services. (1993). *Toward a National Health Information Infrastructure.* Washington, DC.

Saba, V. K. (1974). Basic consideration in management information systems for public health/community health agencies. In National League for Nursing (Ed.), *Management Information for Public Health/Community Health Agencies: Report of the Conference* (pp. 3–13). New York: National League for Nursing.

Schneider, D. (1993). Internet: Linking nurses, scholars, libraries. *Reflections, 19*(1), 9.

Shortliffe, E. H. (1990). Clinical decision-support systems. In E. H. Shortliffe and
L. E. Perreault (Eds.), *Medical Informatics: Computer Applications in Health
Care* (pp. 466–502). Reading, MA: Addison-Wesley.

Shortliffe, E. H., and Perreault, L. E. (Eds.). (1990). *Medical Informatics: Computer Applications in Health Care.* Reading, MA: Addison-Wesley.

White House Council on Domestic Policy. (1993). *The Clinton Blueprint: The President's Health Security Plan.* Washington, DC: The White House.

Wiederhold, G., and Perreault, L. E. (1990). Hospital information systems. In E. H.
Shortliffe and L. E. Perreault (Eds.), *Medical Informatics: Computer Applications in Health Care* (pp. 219–243). Reading, MA: Addison–Wesley.

Workgroup for Electronic Data Interchange (1992). *WEDI Report to Secretary of
U.S. Department of Health and Human Services.* Washington, DC.

Workgroup for Electronic Data Interchange (1993). *WEDI Report.* Washington, DC.

Work Group on Computerization of Patient Records. (1993). *Toward a National
Health Information Infrastructure.* Washington, DC.

World Health Organization. (1980a). *International Classification of Diseases: 9th
Revision: Clinical Modifications* (ICD-9-CM). Geneva, Switzerland.

World Health Organization. (1980b). *International Classification of Diseases: 9th
Revision: Clinical Modifications: Volume 3* (ICD-9-CM: Vol.3). Geneva,
Switzerland.

World Health Organization. (1980c). *International Classification of Impairments,
Disabilities, and Handicaps.* Geneva, Switzerland.

World Health Organization. (1992). *International Statistical Classification of Diseases and Related Health Problems* (ICD-10). Geneva, Switzerland.

World Organization of National Colleges, Academies and Academic Associations of
General Practitioners/Family Physicians. (1987). *International Classification
of Primary Care.* Oxford, U.K.: Oxford University Press.

## BIBLIOGRAPHY

Ackoff, R. L. (1971). Toward a system of systems concepts. *Management Science,
17*(11), 661–671.

Anthony, R. N. (1965). *Planning and Control Systems: A Framework for Analysis.*
Cambridge: Harvard University Press.

Ball, M. (1973). Fifteen hospital information systems available. In M. Ball (Ed.),
*How to Select a Computerized Hospital Information System* (pp. 10–27). Basel,
Switzerland: S. Karger.

Ball, M. J. (1974). Medical data processing in the United States. *Hospital Financing Management, 28*(1), 10–30.

Ball, M. J., and Collen, M. F. (Eds.). (1992). *Aspects of the Computer-Based Patient
Record.* New York: Springer-Verlag.

Blum, B. I. (Ed.). (1984). *Information Systems for Patient Care.* New York: Springer-
Verlag.

Bocchino, W. A. (1972). *Management Information Systems: Tools and Techniques.*
Englewood Cliffs, NJ: Prentice-Hall.

Bronzino, J. D. (1982). *Computer Applications for Patient Care.* Reading, MA:
Addison-Wesley.

Capron, H. L. (1990). *Computers: Tools for the Information Age* (2d ed.). Menlo Park, CA: Benjamin/Cummings.

Capron, H. L., and Williams, B. K. (1984). *Computer and Data Processing* (2d ed.). Menlo Park, CA: Benjamin/Cummings.

Collen, M. F. (1974). *Hospital Computer Systems.* New York: John Wiley.

Collen, M. F. (1983). General requirements for clinical departmental systems. In J. H. Van Bemmel, M. J. Ball, and O. Wigertz (Eds.), *MEDINFO 83* (pp. 736–739). Amsterdam, Netherlands: North-Holland.

Covvey, H. D., Craven, N. H., and McAlister, N. H. (1985). *Concepts and Issues in Health Care Computing* (Vol. 1). St. Louis: Mosby.

Covvey, H. D., and McAlister, N. H. (1980). *Computers in the Practice of Medicine:* Vol. 2. *Issues in Medical Computing.* Reading, MA: Addison-Wesley.

Davis, G. A. (1983). Management information systems. In A. Ralston and E. D. Reilly, Jr. (Eds.), *Encyclopedia of Computer Science and Engineering* (2d ed.) (pp. 910–915). New York: Van Nostrand Reinhold.

Dayhoff, R. E. (Ed.). (1983). *Proceedings: The Seventh Annual Symposium on Computer Applications in Medical Care.* New York: IEEE Computer Society Press.

Donnelley, G. F., Mangel, A., and Sutterley, D. C. (1980). *The Nursing System: Issues, Ethics, and Politics.* New York: John Wiley.

Dorenfest, S. H. (1991, January). Hospitals move to multiple computer suppliers. *Computers in Healthcare.* Reprint.

Editors of Time-Life Books. (1986). *Understanding Computers: Artificial Intelligence.* Chicago: Time-Life Books.

Field, M. J., Lohr, K. N., and Yordy, K. D. (Eds.). Assessing health care reform. Washington, DC: Institute of Medicine, National Academy Press.

Fitzgerald, J., Fitzgerald, A. F., and Stalling, W. D., Jr. (1981). *Fundamentals of Systems Analysis* (2d ed.). New York: John Wiley.

Fokkens, O. (Ed.). (1983). *MEDINFO 83 Seminars.* Amsterdam: North-Holland.

Giebink, G. A., and Hurst, L. L. (1975). *Computer Projects in Health Care.* Ann Arbor, MI: Health Administration Press.

Gillies, D. A. (1982). *Nursing Management: A Systems Approach.* Philadelphia: Saunders.

Griffith, H. G., and Robinson, K. R. (1993). Current Procedural Terminology (CPT) coded services provided by nurse specialists. *Image 25*(3), 178–186.

Gugerty, B., Occhino, S., Ventura, M., and Haley, M. (1993). The interaction of information technology and nursing quality improvement: Important trends. *Journal of Nursing Care Quality 7*(4), 19–25.

Hamilton, D. L. (1992). Identification and evaluation of the security requirements in medical applications. In *Proceedings of the Fifth Annual IEEE Symposium on Computer-Based Medical Systems* (pp. 129–177). New York: IEEE Computer Society Press.

Hannah, K. J. (1976). The computer and nursing practice. *Nursing Outlook, 24*(9), 555–558.

Hart, A. (1992). *Knowledge Acquisition for Expert Systems* (2d ed.). New York: McGraw-Hill.

Hazzard, M. E. (1971). An overview of systems theory. *Nursing Clinics of North America, 6,* 385.

Hellerman, H., and Smith, I. A. (1983). Computer systems. In A. Ralston and E. D. Reilly, Jr. (Eds.), *Encyclopedia of Computer Science and Engineering* (2d ed.) (pp. 370–375). New York: Van Nostrand Reinhold.

Hopper, G. M., and Mandell, S. L. (1987). *Understanding Computers* (2d ed.). New York: West.

Information Infrastructure Task Force. (1993). *National Information Infrastructure: Agenda for Action.* Washington, DC: Department of Commerce.

Joos, I., Whitman, N. I., Smith, M. J., and Nelson, R. (1992). *Computers in Small Bytes: The Computer Workbook.* New York: National League for Nursing.

Kaufman, R. A. (1972). *Educational System Planning.* Englewood Cliffs, NJ: Prentice-Hall.

Kennevan, W. J. (1970, September). Management information systems—MIS universe. *Data Management.*

Kiley, M., Halloran, E. J., Weston, J. L., et al. (1983). Computerized nursing information systems (NIS). *Nursing Management, 14*(7), 26–29.

Lindberg, D. (1979). *The Growth of Medical Information Systems in the United States.* Lexington, MA: D. C. Heath, Lexington Books.

MacEachern, M. T. (1946). *Hospital Organization and Management.* Chicago: Physicians' Record.

Mandell, S. L. (1985). *Introduction to Computers Using the IBM PC.* New York: West.

Mandell, S. L. (1986). *Computers and Data Processing Today: With Basic* (2d ed.). New York: West.

McDonald, C. J., and Barnett, G. O. (1990). Medical-record systems. In E. H. Shortliffe and L. E. Perreault (Eds.), *Medical Informatics: Computer Applications in Health Care* (pp. 181–218). Reading, MA: Addison-Wesley.

McDonald, M. D., and Blum, H. L. (1992). *Health in the Information Age.* Berkeley, CA: Environmental Science and Policy Institute.

McWilliams, P. A. (1982). *The Word Processing Book.* Los Angeles: Prelude Press.

Mintzberg, H. (1979). *The Structuring of Organizations.* Englewood Cliffs, NJ: Prentice-Hall.

National League for Nursing. (1974). *Management Information System for Public Health/Community Health Agencies: Report of the Conference.* New York.

Orthner, H. F. (1992). New communication technologies for integrating hospital information systems and their computer-based patient records. In M. J. Ball and M. F. Collen (Eds.), *Aspects of the Computer-Based Patient Record* (pp. 176–200). New York: Springer-Verlag.

Owens, D. K., and Sox, H. C., Jr. (1990). Medical decision-making: Probabilistic medical reasoning. In E. H. Shortliffe and L. E. Perreault (Eds.), *Medical Informatics: Computer Applications in Health Care* (pp. 70–116). Reading, MA: Addison-Wesley.

Pfaffenberger, B. (1991). *Que's Computer User's Dictionary.* Carmel, IN: Que Corp.

Ralston, A., and Reilly, E. D., Jr. (Eds.). (1983). *Encyclopedia of Computer Science and Engineering* (2d ed.). New York: Van Nostrand Reinhold.

Salton, G. (1983). Information retrieval. In A. Ralston and E. D. Reilly, Jr. (Eds.), *Encyclopedia of Computer Science and Engineering* (2d ed.) (pp. 719–725). New York: Van Nostrand Reinhold.

Shoderbek, C. G., Shoderbek, P. P., and Lefales, A. G. (1980). *Management Systems: Conceptual Considerations.* Dallas: Business Publishers.

Siegel, E. R., Cummings, M. M., and Woodsmall, R. M. (1990). Bibliographic-retrieval systems. In E. H. Shortliffe and L. E. Perreault (Eds.), *Medical Informatics: Computer Applications in Health Care* (pp. 434–465). Reading, MA: Addison-Wesley.

Sullivan, D. R., Lewis, T. G., and Cook, C. R. (1985). *Computing Today: Microcomputer Concepts and Applications.* Boston: Houghton Mifflin.

Teichroew, D. (1983). Information systems. In A. Ralston and E. D. Reilly, Jr. (Eds.), *Encyclopedia of Computer Science and Engineering* (2d ed.) (pp. 726–729). New York: Van Nostrand Reinhold.

U.S. DHHS. (1973). *Records, Computers and the Rights of Citizens.* Washington, DC.

Van Bemmel, J., Ball, M. J., and Wigertz, O. (Eds.). (1983). *MEDINFO 83* (Vols. 1–2). Amsterdam, Netherlands: North-Holland.

Walsh, M. E. (1982). *Understanding Computers: What Managers and Users Need to Know.* New York: John Wiley.

Wiederhold, G. (1983). Hospital information systems. In A. Ralston and E. D. Reilly, Jr. (Eds.), *Encyclopedia of Computer Science and Engineering* (2d ed.) (pp. 686–688). New York: Van Nostrand Reinhold.

Work Group on Computerization of Patient Records. (1993). Appendix D: Computer-based patient records: Confidentiality, privacy and security concerns. In *Toward a National Health Information Infrastructure.* Washington, DC: US DHHS.

Workgroup for Electronic Data Interchange. (1992). Report to the Secretary of the U.S. Department of Health and Human Services. Appendix 4. *Confidentiality and Antitrust Issues.* Washington, DC.

Young, E. M. (1980). *Automated Hospital Information Systems:* Vol. 2. *Guide to AHIS Suppliers.* Los Angeles: Center Publications.

Yovits, M. C. (1983). Information and data. In A. Ralston and E. D. Reilly, Jr. (Eds.), *Encyclopedia of Computer Science and Engineering* (2d ed.) (pp. 714–717). New York: Van Nostrand Reinhold.

# 7

. . . . . . . . . . . . . . . . . . . . . . . .

# NURSING INFORMATICS

## OBJECTIVES

- Understand nursing informatics.
- Describe nursing data, nursing data standards, and nursing practice standards.
- Discuss nursing classification schemes.
- Describe nursing information systems models.
- Identify nursing information systems in nursing administration.
- Identify nursing information systems in nursing practice.
- Identify nursing information systems in nursing education.
- Identify nursing information systems in nursing research.

The evolution of nursing informatics began with the introduction of computers into nursing more than four decades ago. However, the term "nursing informatics" has appeared in the literature only within the last decade. Nursing informatics is a new nursing specialty which expands the scope of computers and nursing to include information sciences. Nursing informatics requires an understanding of systems theory, computer systems, and information systems as well as computers in nursing, nursing systems, nursing applications, and nursing information systems.

Nursing informatics is intrinsic to nursing. It is concerned with the legitimate access to and use of data, information, and knowledge to standardize documentation, improve communication, and support the decision-making process. It is also concerned with the design, development, and dissemination of new knowledge. It is used to enhance the quality, effectiveness, and efficiency of health care, and to empower clients to make health care choices. Nursing informatics is used to advance the science of nursing.

This chapter concentrates on all the above aspects of nursing informatics. It provides an overview of nursing informatics and nursing information systems (NISs). It discusses nursing data, nursing data standards, and nursing practice standards. Nursing classification schemes are described, including nursing data needs for the computer-based patient record (CPR) using the nursing process. The chapter provides an overview of NISs and NIS models and outlines the NIS applications found in hospitals, community health agencies, research centers, and educational institutions where nurses function. This chapter includes the following:

- Nursing informatics
- Nursing data
- Classification schemes for the nursing process
- Nursing information system models
- Overview of NIS applications

## NURSING INFORMATICS

Informatics is derived from the French word *informatique*, which refers to the computer milieu. It is a new science that encompasses computers and their application in all the health sciences and professions. Nursing informatics is a branch of informatics particularly concerned with nurses' use of computer technology and the management of information that facilitates nursing practice and enhances nursing knowledge. It focuses on this field of technology as it affects the nursing profession.

Nursing informatics describes the use of information technology to study and design NISs. It encompasses computer systems, information management, and nursing science and refers to the technology of tools and methods, whereas nursing information systems (NISs) operationalize the technology (computer systems) to manage and process nursing data and information. The terms "nursing informatics" and "nursing information systems" are often used interchangeably, and they will also be used interchangeably in this book. Nursing informatics has also emerged as a new nursing specialty. A discussion of nursing informatics follows. It includes:

- Evolution of nursing informatics
- Nursing informatics definitions

- Nursing informatics frameworks
- Scope of nursing informatics

## Evolution of Nursing Informatics

Nursing informatics began as early as the 1950s, when computers were introduced into the health care industry. As the computer industry grew, computer use in the health care industry and in nursing also grew. In the early hospital information systems, selected nursing applications were developed. As a result, NISs emerged which were designed to support selected nursing functions.

In the 1980s, nursing informatics evolved as advances in computers and technology affected the management of nursing practice information. The term "nursing informatics" is related to the term "medical informatics." In 1979, the International Medical Informatics Association (IMIA) was formed as a special interest group of the International Federation of Information Processing (IFIP). Although IMIA uses "medical informatics" to encompass all health fields, nursing informatics emerged as a separate entity and was first described by several British authorities. As early as 1980, Scholes and Barber discussed nursing informatics at the MEDINFO-1980 conference held in Tokyo.

In 1982 other authorities discussed the topic at the IFIP-IMIA Workshop on the Impact of Computers on Nursing, held in London, England (Anderson, 1983; Barber, 1983; Scholes and Barber, 1980). In 1986, informatics became visible in the United States, when a Medical Informatics Planning Panel, convened by the National Library of Medicine (NLM), focused on medical informatics as one of its long-range research initiatives. The report prepared by the NLM panel provided the impetus for several nursing experts in this country to begin to apply informatics to nursing (National Library of Medicine, 1986). Thus, the term "nursing informatics" began to appear in the nursing literature.

In 1985 Hannah described the impact of nursing informatics (NI) on nursing education (Hannah, 1985). In 1986 Schwirian designed the NI pyramid as a research model for nursing informatics (Schwirian, 1986). And in 1989 Graves and Corcoran developed a conceptual framework for nursing informatics based on their working definition of nursing knowledge (Graves and Corcoran, 1989).

By the late 1980s nursing informatics appeared as a new nursing concept to be applied to the computer systems being developed for processing nursing information. It became an integral part of nursing knowledge and is widely used today. Other events are noteworthy. In 1988, the National Center for Nursing Research (NCNR) initiated the Priority Expert Panel on Nursing Informatics. This group was one of seven panels identified at a conference conducted by the NCNR that were to develop a National Nursing Research Agenda (NNRA). Nursing informatics was selected as a critical research priority that addressed a "current or future health care need." As a result, this nursing informatics panel which consisted of leaders in the field was formed. It subsequently provided an overview of the field and made recommendations for the NCNR research agenda (National Center for Nursing Research Priority Expert Panel on Nursing Informatics, 1993).

In 1989 the National League for Nursing (NLN) renamed its special-interest computer council the Council for Nursing Informatics. That same year the NLN also published the recommended informatics competencies identified by the IMIA Working Group Eight Task Force on Education (Peterson and Gerdin-Jelger, 1989). In 1991 the American Medical Informatics Association renamed its nursing special-interest group the Nursing Informatics Working Group. Then in 1992 nursing informatics was recognized as an approved nursing specialty of the American Nurses Association (ANA) (Council on Computer Applications in Nursing, 1992). The ANA is now involved in the creation of a certification program for nursing informatics.

### Growth Trends

The growth of nursing informatics in the United States has been dramatic. In 1991 there were approximately 5,000 registered nurses who identified nursing informatics and/or NISs as their area of interest and expertise, in contrast to 15 nurses who first met as a group in 1981 during the Fifth Annual Symposium of Computer Applications on Medical Care (SCAMC). The growth in a ten-year period was over 500 percent (Fig. 7.1) (Fishman, 1994; Saba, 1994).

## Nursing Informatics Definitions

Definitions of nursing informatics, including definitions of NISs, emerged as nursing became involved in computer technology. The two terms are used interchangeably. The specialty became clearly delineated as described in this section. In 1980, two British professionals, Scholes and Barber, were the first to define nursing informatics. They provided a basic definition that still applies today. They defined nursing informatics as "the application of computer technology to all fields of nursing—nursing service, nurse education, and nursing research" (Scholes and Barber, 1980).

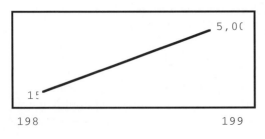

**Figure 7.1** Growth of nursing informatics specialists. (Saba, 1994.)

In 1982 the Study Group on Nursing Information Systems convened to discuss issues surrounding the design of systems of nursing data. They described an NIS as

A system that applies to the automated processing of the data needed to plan, give, evaluate, and document patient care, as well as to collect the data necessary to support the delivery of nursing care, such as staffing and cost (Study Group on Nursing Information Systems, 1983).

In 1985 Hannah also described and provided a definition of nursing informatics. She indicated that nursing informatics supported the entire gamut of nursing functions, including the information nurses use to make patient care decisions (Ball and Hannah, 1988; Hannah et al., 1994). She continues to use her definition, which follows: "The use of information technologies in relation to any functions which are within the purview of nursing and which are carried out by nurses in the performance of their duties" (Hannah, 1985).

In 1989 the IMIA Working Group Eight Task Force on Education not only defined broad competencies of nursing informatics, but also put forth its definition of nursing informatics as "the application of information science to nursing and patient care" (Peterson and Gerdin-Jelger, 1989, p. 117). Also in 1989 Graves and Corcoran proposed their definition. They made a distinction between their definition as a theoretical framework and their model, which illustrates their working definition. Their model illustrates the relationship between the management and processing of data, information, and knowledge. Their definition of nursing informatics is "a combination of computer science, information science, and nursing science designed to assist with the management and processing of data, information, and knowledge to support the practice of nursing and the delivery of nursing care" (Graves and Corcoran, 1989, p. 227).

In 1992 the ANA's Council on Computer Applications in Nursing (CCAN) provided one of the most significant definitions of nursing informatics. In its designation of nursing informatics as a nursing specialty in nursing practice, the CCAN defined nursing informatics as:

A specialty that integrates nursing science, computer science, and information science in identifying, collecting, processing, and managing data and information to support nursing practice, administration, education, and research; and to expand nursing knowledge. The purpose of nursing informatics is to: analyze information requirements; design, implement and evaluate information systems and data structures that support nursing; and identify and apply computer technologies for nursing (Council on Computer Applications in Nursing, 1992).

The authors of this book are proposing a working definition which can not only be used to define nursing informatics but also be applied to NISs. This definition modifies the one presented in the 1986 edition. It focuses on the use of technology, namely a computer system, to process nursing data into information.

Therefore, we define nursing informatics as:

The use of technology and/or a computer system to collect, store, process, display, retrieve, and communicate timely data and information in and across health care facilities that:

- Administer nursing services and resources
- Manage the delivery of patient and nursing care
- Link research resources and findings to nursing practice
- Apply educational resources to nursing education

This definition addresses the four major areas of nursing in which computer systems are found. Nursing informatics is also described and defined by several other experts and groups in the field. They reflect the way this new specialty affects nursing. As the technology expands and nursing practice advances, other definitions for this new specialty will continue to appear (Fishman, 1994). Nursing informatics, as defined by several authorities, encompasses concepts from three sciences: computer science, information science, and nursing science. A discussion of what each of these sciences provides follows.

## Computer Science

Computer science primarily refers to computer hardware—its configuration and architecture. The configuration refers to the computer system and all its hardware components—the size, type, and storage capacity of the computer system—whereas the architecture refers to the type of microprocessor (arithmetic logic and control unit) used to process data and determine memory size and processing speed.

## Information Science

Information science refers to computer software (computer programs). It encompasses how the data or tasks are processed, problems are solved, and products are produced. It refers to the algorithms, which are sets of well-defined, simple, and logical instructions or procedures that are followed to solve a problem or direct the execution of a task. Algorithms are essentially computer programs stored in the computer. Computer software is needed for computer hardware to work and computer systems to function. How a computer processes data is fundamental to its use.

## Nursing Science

Nursing science refers to the practice of nursing. It provides the basis for documenting nursing practice. Nursing science includes the integration of nursing data, information, and knowledge using computers. With the use of computer technology, nursing models and frameworks have become extremely complex and sophisticated. The models that are used in health care facilities provide not only the focus for nursing practice, but also the basis for the design of the computer-based NISs.

As the basis for the nursing profession, nursing science is responsive to the changing needs of society, patient care, and the nursing profession itself. Conceptualizing the phenomena of concern is critical to knowledge building and the scientific development of nursing science. Thus, nursing informatics is assisting in the enhancement of nursing practice, the improvement of nursing education, and the advancement of nursing science (Fitzpatrick, 1988).

## Nursing Informatics Frameworks

Nursing informatics models emerged with the introduction of computer applications in nursing. These models are generally graphic illustrations of conceptual frameworks and/or structures used for the design of nursing informatics, including identifying the data elements (inputs), processes, and products (outputs) of the NIS. Generally, they are a guide for the design of NISs. They illustrate the interrelationships of nursing data elements, which vary according to the different nursing applications, practice requirements, types of settings, clients, and nursing theories. They also illustrate the requirements that need to be considered regarding the structure, presentation, and means of generating nursing data, information, and knowledge for the users of the system.

### Conceptual Framework for the Study of Nursing Knowledge

A nursing informatics model—Conceptual Framework for the Study of Nursing Knowledge—has been proposed by Graves and Corcoran (1989). Their model is based on their definition of nursing informatics and illustrates the relationship between the concepts of management processing of nursing data, information, and knowledge. The model provides a framework for nursing information, which they describe as encompassing computer science, information science, and nursing science, which is also used in the ANA definition of nursing informatics (Council on Computer Applications in Nursing, 1992) (Fig. 7.2).

### Predicting Adoption of Innovative Technologies

Another nursing informatics model which demonstrates the factors that predict the adoption of innovative technologies, namely nursing technologies, was recently introduced by Romano (Romano, 1993). The Predicting Adoption of Innovative Technologies model suggests that multiple factors from at least three categories of predictors influence the adoption of computerized information systems in a health care organization. These categories

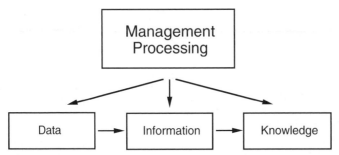

**Figure 7.2**   Conceptual framework for the study of nursing knowledge. [Courtesy Graves, J., and Corcoran, S. (1989). The Study of Nursing Informatics. *Image: Journal of Nursing Scholarship.* (Sigma Theta Tau International), 21(4), p. 228.]

are individual adopter characteristics, technology characteristics, and organization characteristics.

The individual adopter characteristics refer to selected characteristics, including communication behavior, of the nurse adopter. The technology characteristics refer to the perceived advantage, complexity, and need for the information technology. The organizational characteristics refer to the adoption behavior of peers and supervisors and the role an organizational member plays; organizational factors include the structural, political, and psychosocial aspects of an organizational system, which are interrelated and illustrate the complexity of the implementation of any computerized information system.

The technology and organization characteristics are directly related to adoption. The model illustrates that to encourage the adoption of computerized information technologies, strategies need to be developed that focus beyond the individual nurse adopter to include the characteristics of the technological innovation and the social system into which it is introduced (Fig. 7.3).

## Scope of Nursing Informatics

Nursing informatics encompasses a full range of activities that focuses on information management and processing of nursing data. This includes the use of technological tools or methods to identify, name, organize, categorize, collect, process, analyze, store, retrieve, or manage data and information. These technological tools include classification schemes, data collection tools, care protocols, and other special materials required to document, communicate, and process the nursing data. These nursing informatics technologies are used to design NISs for clinical nursing practice, administration, and support of nursing education and research. These four major nursing areas are described below and throughout this text.

## Proposed Model

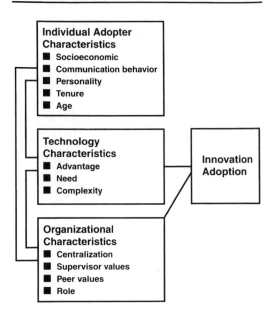

**Figure 7.3**   Predicting adoption of innovative technologies model. (Courtesy C. Romano, 1993.)

Nursing informatics focuses on how computer-based NISs are used to administer nursing services—that is, how the NISs ensure the efficiency of nursing resources; assist in the effective information management of nursing services; monitor the quality, effectiveness, and outcomes of nursing care; and protect the confidentiality and privacy of patient data. Such systems provide the information needed to support the area of nursing.

The aspects of nursing informatics that focus on the development of NISs support nursing practice and the delivery of patient care. NISs generally are components or subsystems of larger computer-based information systems in hospitals and other health care facilities. Such systems contain their own unique nursing databases, from which nursing data are integrated with the other patient data in the larger systems. However, NISs can also be stand-alone systems dedicated to specific applications, such as patient classification, nurse staffing, or nursing personnel management.

Nursing informatics addresses computer-based information systems found in community, public, and home health agencies. Such agencies use NISs in a manner similar to hospitals; that is, they have their own unique community health nursing databases which are integrated with other patient and service data within the agency, city, county, or state system. As part of their organizational structure, some of these systems have also developed communication networks linking the units throughout an agency, city, or state.

Nursing informatics supports nursing educational processes. It supports the NISs developed to manage nursing student and faculty data, as well as the use of technology to support innovative teaching strategies. Generally, schools of nursing have established learning resource centers which include technological resources. They include computer laboratories which are connected to the university computer systems and/or function as free-standing local area networks (LAN). Microcomputers are used by students to prepare papers, take examinations, or review new content. Resource centers usually have multimedia and interactive video (IAV) computer systems to "run" the new educational media and other generic software programs.

Additionally, nursing informatics supports the research process through several different technological approaches. It encompasses vocabularies, tools, and materials, as well as the bibliographic, informational, and knowledge databases needed to conduct nursing research. It encompasses the processing and statistical methods of analyzing research findings. And finally, it addresses the development of knowledge databases of aggregated data needed to develop and design clinical decision support systems, expert systems, and artificial intelligence. Thus, nursing informatics using NISs will enhance and advance the science of nursing.

## Computer Configurations

Nursing informatics adapts to the configuration of the computer-based systems used to process nursing data into nursing information. The size and purpose of computer systems vary. Mainframe systems are generally used to store and process large patient care databases and are generally located in large hospitals. Minicomputers are frequently dedicated to a specific application in specialty departments in hospitals. Microcomputers, on the other hand, are used by individual nurses to manage their own applications. Nurses no longer need programmers to prepare a program for a specific nursing application, but instead can adapt word-processing, spreadsheet, database management, and graphic software packages to facilitate their work.

## Informatics Nurse Specialist

A nurse who specializes in the field of nursing informatics and NISs is called an informatics nurse specialist. Others have used the term "nursing informatician"; however, either term implies that the person is not only a nurse, but also a specialist with a broad expertise in nursing informatics. Other terms used in the field vary. They include "nursing information specialist," "computer nurse," "systems nurse," "nursing systems analyst," and "information specialist." A nurse can be credentialed by the ANA in this new nursing speciality.

The title given to this specialist is important; however, the level of the specialist in the health care organization is equally critical. Other critical concerns include whether the position is a staff or line one and the description of duties, responsibilities, and functions. It is also important to ascertain who the informatician reports to, what his or her degree of authority is, and whether a budget is available. These are only a few of the characteristics that will affect the activities performed and decision-making capabilities of the nurse informatician.

## NURSING DATA

Basic to an understanding of nursing informatics is an understanding of nursing data, nursing data standards, and nursing practice standards. These concepts are influenced by the nursing classification schemes, taxonomies, and/or vocabularies that exist and influence the management of nursing information. The areas that are described include

- Nursing data standards
- Nursing practice standards

Nursing data form the basis and foundation of nursing informatics. Nursing data are needed for documenting nursing care and the information management of nursing practice. Nursing data are defined and coded terms or elements needed for the development of computer-based information systems, or NISs. Nursing data, once processed, produce nursing information, and nursing information, once analyzed, interpreted, and aggregated, produces nursing knowledge.

## Data versus Information versus Knowledge

### Data

Data are distinguished from information and knowledge, their end products. The term "data" is derived from the Latin verb *do, dare,* meaning "to give," and refers to unstructured raw facts. Data are discrete entities (facts) that have not been interpreted. These facts, even though they lack interpretation, are accepted by the computer as input in preparation for processing.

### Information

The term "information" is derived from the Latin verb *informo, informare,* meaning, "to give form to." Information is data that have been given form and interpreted. Unstructured data (facts) are processed by a computer to produce a structured form (information). Thus, an information system refers to the processing into information of data elements which are stored in a database. Information is interpreted by different users and is relative, whereas knowledge is needed to utilize information.

### Knowledge

Knowledge is described as aggregates of information derived from multiple databases. Knowledge also refers to synthesized information derived from the interpretation of data processed by an information system.

Knowledge is based on a set of rules or formulas which represent the management of aggregated information. Knowledge representation can form a knowledge base and provide the logical basis for making nursing decisions (Blum, 1990; Chang and Hirsch, 1991; Graves, 1993; Graves and Corcoran, 1989; Joos et al., 1992).

## Nursing Data Standards

Nursing data standards are needed to manage, document, and communicate nursing data for the CPR. Nursing data standards differ from nursing practice standards in that they refer to the structure, organization, and composition of the data elements used to implement the parameters of nursing practice. Nursing data standards are being developed by the professional nursing groups. The ANA Database Steering Committee has taken on this mandate and is the primary professional organization involved in the selection of nursing vocabularies and/or classification schemes.

Data standards for computer-based systems are also being established by recognized standards groups (national and international), professional organizations, health care institutions, and other special-interest groups. These organizations are addressing the physical structure of electronic media, as well as how they are used for automation. Data standards include the structure, definitions, and coded values of the data; procedures for automated processing, such as indexing, video display, storage, protection, transmission, selective retrieval, analysis, and manipulation of the information; and the security, protection, and confidentiality of the data.

## Nursing Practice Standards

Until recently, professional nursing practice standards that were proposed were primarily conceptual and not measurable. That is, they were theoretical standards that did not include measurable data approved by the profession that could be included in computer-based NISs. Additionally, the nursing profession did not have any standardized vocabularies, taxonomies, and/or classification schemes that could be used to accommodate all aspects of nursing practice. Thus nurses could not communicate with one another and with other members of the health care delivery system using a unified nursing language. As a result, most of the early NISs that were developed were based on the interpretation of practice standards using a vocabulary selected by a given health care facility and/or developer of a system.

### Nursing Classification Schemes

Nursing classification schemes, taxonomies, and/or vocabularies have come to the forefront with the evolution of nursing informatics. They emerged because of the need for standardized nursing vocabularies to name and communicate why and what nurses do.

## ANA Initiatives

The need to standardize nursing practice data has long been recognized by the ANA board of directors as critical to the profession. The ANA, over the past twenty years, has taken several actions to promote the development of practice standards and vocabularies for nursing. In 1970, the ANA recommended that the nursing process be used as the standard for documenting nursing practice. This was a practice standard based on a theoretical framework. At that time, because there were no approved standardized vocabularies for documenting the nursing process components, it could not be automated. As a result, the nursing process could not be implemented in computer-based NISs that were being developed.

In 1980 the ANA produced its social policy statement, which stated that "Nursing is the diagnosis and treatment of human responses to actual or potential health problems" (American Nurses Association, 1980). This definition was based on the definitions of nursing diagnoses which were being developed and approved by the North American Nursing Diagnosis Association (NANDA) during the late 1970s. In 1986, the ANA approved policies related to, and made a commitment for, the development of a classification system designed for all nursing practice settings. However, it was not until 1988 that the ANA board of directors accepted the NANDA Taxonomy I Revised as an approved nomenclature for the nursing profession (Fitzpatrick et al., 1989).

*Conference on Research Priorities in Nursing Science* In 1988, the ANA endorsed a Conference on Research Priorities in Nursing Science to delineate the basic research priority areas for the National Institute of Nursing Research (NINR) (previously the NCNR). The steering committee identified two major issues for nursing information systems that needed to be addressed, namely "the need for standardized data sets which document nursing care process across settings, and a taxonomy to classify nursing phenomena and allow the common use of terms" (NCNR Priority Expert Panel on Nursing Informatics, 1993).

*Nursing Minimum Data Set* In 1990 another action passed by the ANA House of Delegates was the recognition of the nursing minimum data set (NMDS), those data elements that should be included in any CPR system or national database. This nursing data set has become the place holder for nursing data in several national databases, including the CPR (Werley, 1988; Werley and Lang, 1988).

The NMDS was developed in 1985 by consensus of 64 experts at a three-day invitational conference. It consists of a set of 16 information items and categories of nursing data used throughout the health care system, with uniform definitions. The purposes of the NMDS are to (1) describe the nursing care of patients/clients and their families in a variety of settings, both institutional and noninstitutional; (2) establish comparability of nursing data across clinical populations, settings, geographic areas, and time; (3) demonstrate or project trends regarding nursing care provided and allocation of nursing resources to patients/ clients according to their health problems or nursing diagnoses; (4) stimulate nursing research through linkages of detailed data existing in NISs and in other health care information systems; and (5) provide data about nursing care to influence health policy and decision making (Prophet, 1994).

The NMDS is designed to be a tool for collecting uniform, standard, comparable, minimum nursing data needed by and for nurses to document care in any health care delivery setting. It is also designed to collect the set of information that is essential to meet the diverse information needs of nurses and other health professionals. The NMDS variables are envisioned as being used in computer systems to describe nursing care, measure its quality, and determine its cost.

The 16 data elements in the NMDS fall into three broad categories: (1) four nursing care elements, (2) five patient and client demographics elements, and (3) seven service elements. The NMDS data elements are listed in Table 7.1.

**TABLE 7.1**     NURSING MINIMUM DATA SET (NMDS) DATA ELEMENTS*

| **Nursing Care Elements** |
| --- |
| 1.  Nursing Diagnosis |
| 2.  Nursing Intervention (for initial testing) |
| 3.  Nursing Outcome |
| 4.  Intensity of Nursing Care |

| **Patient or Client Demographic Elements** |
| --- |
| 5.*  Personal Identification |
| 6.*  Date of Birth |
| 7.*  Sex |
| 8.*  Race and Ethnicity |
| 9.*  Residence |

| **Service Elements** |
| --- |
| 10.*  Unique Facility or Service Agency Number |
| 11.   Unique Health Record Number of Patient or Chart |
| 12.   Unique Number of Principal Registered Nurse Provider |
| 13.*  Episode Admission or Encounter Date |
| 14.*  Discharge or Termination Date |
| 15.*  Disposition of Patient or Chart |
| 16.*  Expected Payer for Most of the Bill |

*Elements comparable to those in the Uniform Hospital Discharge Data Set.
*Source:* Werley, 1988.

In 1991, the ANA published its revised social policy statement and introduced new nursing standards. The ANA *Standards of Clinical Nursing Practice* currently outline the nursing service delivery patterns and the process of patient care. With this document, the ANA reinforced its recommendation to use the nursing process to document clinical nursing practice, which was expanded to include six competent levels or phases of nursing care: assessment, diagnosis, outcome identification, planning, implementation, and evaluation (American Nurses Association, 1991).

This 1991 ANA publication also delineated the care that is provided to all clients of nursing services and the scope of clinical nursing practice standards as follows:

> The nursing process encompasses all significant actions taken by nurses in providing care to all clients, and forms the foundation of clinical decision making. Additional nursing responsibilities for all clients (such as providing culturally and ethnically relevant care; maintaining a safe environment; educating clients about their illness, treatment, health promotion, or self-care activities; and planning for continuity of care) are subsumed within these standards (American Nurses Association, 1991, p. 3).

These ANA standards serve as a basis for the computer-based NISs developed for hospitals, community health agencies, and other settings where nursing services are provided. With the introduction of several vocabularies approved by the ANA, the phases of the nursing process became not only theoretical but also measurable, making it possible to use them in CPR systems. The standards also serve as the basis for nursing applications for quality assurance systems, regulatory systems, prospective payment systems, research studies, and educational offerings. They are influencing the need for a unified nursing language to the approved standard for documenting the nursing process.

## ANA Database Steering Committee

The ANA Congress of Nursing Practice also mandated the formation of a Steering Committee on Databases to Support Clinical Nursing Practice. In 1991 this ANA committee was formed, with the responsibility for developing clinical nursing practice standards. The initial goals of the committee were as follows:

- Propose policy and program initiatives regarding nursing classification schemes, uniform nursing data sets, and the inclusion of nursing data elements in national databases.
- Build national data sets for clinical nursing practice based on elements contained in standards and criteria, and identify guidelines.
- Coordinate the ANA's initiatives related to all public and private efforts regarding development of databases and the relationship to the development and maintenance of standards on practice and guidelines and payment reform for nursing services (Lang et al., 1995).

The ANA Database Steering Committee has been involved in identifying and recognizing the vocabularies, taxonomies, and/or classification schemes designed to document nursing practice data. It complied with the ANA practice standards focusing on the nursing process as the framework for documenting care. The committee viewed the NMDS as the umbrella for the nursing process schemes; however, it determined that there is no one classification scheme that is considered to be the standard for documenting nursing care. In 1992 the ANA Database Steering Committee formally "recognized" four nursing vocabularies and taxonomies as usable classification schemes for documenting clinical nursing practice using the nursing process (McCormick et al., 1994; Zielstorff et al., 1995) (Table 7.2).

The four classification schemes, taxonomies, or nursing vocabularies that have been recognized by the ANA Database Steering Committee address not only clinical nursing practice standards but also the data standards required for a unified nursing language system. They are: (1) North American Nursing Diagnosis Association: NANDA Taxonomy I Revised, (2) Visiting Nurse Association of Omaha: The Omaha System, (3) Saba: Home Health Care Classification, and (4) University of Iowa: Nursing Intervention Classification.

Each of these schemes has been developed from different research processes, and by itself is usable for computer-based NISs. These classification schemes address different phases of the nursing process, and several of them are used to categorize a previously existing scheme. Each of the four schemes also addresses one or more of the four data elements in the nursing care category of the NMDS.

***NANDA Taxonomy I Revised***   Since 1937, the North American Nursing Diagnosis Association (NANDA) has been developing and evolving a list of nursing diagnoses. The initial list of 37 nursing diagnoses was developed by consensus to enable practicing nurses to determine health conditions which require nursing interventions. The original NANDA list of nursing diagnoses was expanded to 50 nursing diagnoses in 1982, subsequently to 114 in 1992 and 133 in 1995/1996. The list continues to be expanded with each NANDA convention, which is held biennially (North American Nursing Diagnosis Association, 1992; 1995/1996).

**TABLE 7.2**   FOUR ANA RECOGNIZED NURSING
CLASSIFICATION SCHEMES

- North American Nursing Diagnosis Association: **NANDA Taxonomy I Revised**
- Visiting Nurse Association of Omaha: **The Omaha System**
- Saba: **Home Health Care Classification (HHCC)**
- University of Iowa: **Nursing Intervention Classification (NIC)**

*Source:* McCormick et al., 1994; Lang et al., 1995.

In 1988 the NANDA Taxonomy Committee developed the first classification of nursing diagnoses, NANDA Taxonomy I. The list of 104 nursing diagnoses, labeled "conditions that necessitate nursing care," was categorized according to NANDA's Nine Human Response Patterns. The Nine Human Response Patterns constitute the most abstract level or Level I concepts, and provide the approved organizing framework for the nursing diagnoses. An example of a pattern is "Moving" (North American Nursing Diagnosis Association, 1990; 1992).

The Taxonomy I Revised is considered to be the initial classification of nursing diagnoses. It employs two different coding schemes. The first uses one to five levels for each of the Nine Human Response Patterns. For example, "activity intolerance" is coded as 6.1.1.2. In this scheme, the first digit, six, represents the pattern "Moving" and the other three digits represent additional coding levels.

The second coding scheme is the classification that was designed for the submission in 1989 of Taxonomy I to the World Health Organization (WHO). It is the same coding strategy used by WHO for the *International Statistical Classification of Diseases and Health Related Problems: Tenth Revision* (ICD-10). That scheme consists of a four-alphanumeric-character code: an alphabetical character in the first position followed by two numeric characters, and if needed a decimal point with a third numeric character. For example, "activity intolerance" is coded as Y50.0 (Fitzpatrick et al., 1989).

Nursing diagnoses have been also categorized by other authorities. The two significant ones are Gordon and Carpenito. Gordon identified eleven functional health patterns, each of which focuses on the assessment criteria needed to determine the specific nursing diagnoses for the patient (Gordon, 1982). In 1989 Carpenito expanded Gordon's eleven functional health patterns and added nine physiological conditions, resulting in twenty groups. The nine physiological conditions are physical body systems, such as the circulatory system. They were developed specifically to address collaborative problems resulting from the assessment of a disease, medical condition, or other condition requiring collaborative assessment (Carpenito, 1989).

*The Omaha System* The Omaha System originated as the Problem Classification Scheme at the Visiting Nurse Association (VNA) of Omaha, Nebraska. Beginning in 1975 and continuing into 1986, the VNA conducted three research studies which were funded by the Division of Nursing, Public Health Service, U.S. Department of Health and Human Services. The Omaha System is a taxonomy designed for the documentation of interdisciplinary practice and data management in community-focused settings. The taxonomy consists of three classification schemes: (1) Problem Classification Scheme, (2) Intervention Scheme, and (3) Problem Rating Scale for Outcomes.

*PROBLEM CLASSIFICATION SCHEME:* This scheme currently consists of a list of 40 client problems addressed by community health nurses. The problems are categorized into four domains—environmental, psychosocial, physiological, and health-related behaviors—each with five problem modifiers as well as clusters of problem-specific signs and symptoms. The problems are coded from 1 to 44, and the signs and symptoms are coded as a subset for each problem (Visiting Nurse Association of Omaha, 1986; Martin and Scheet, 1992).

*INTERVENTION SCHEME:* This scheme was developed to provide organized language that community health professionals could use to address activities involved in community health nursing practice, including health promotion and disease prevention. It currently consists of 62 intervention target labels organized into four categories: (1) health teaching, guidance, and counseling, (2) treatments and procedures, (3) case management, and (4) surveillance.

*PROBLEM RATING SCALE FOR OUTCOMES:* This scale consists of three concepts: (1) knowledge, (2) behavior, and (3) status. It is also used to score outcomes to measure progress on the clients' identified problems. Each is scored using five degrees of intensity.

***Saba: Home Health Care Classification*** The Home Health Care Classification (HHCC): Nursing Diagnoses and Interventions was developed by Saba et al. to classify, code for computer processing, and analyze the data for the Georgetown University (GU) HHCC Project (1988–1991). The HHCC is used to assess, document, code, and classify home health nursing diagnoses, their expected outcomes, nursing interventions, and types of nursing intervention actions according to their components of care (see Chap. 12).

*HHCC: NURSING DIAGNOSES:* The HHCC of Nursing Diagnoses currently consists of 145 Home Health Nursing Diagnoses (50 two-digit major categories and 95 three-digit subcategories) and a modifier of three possible expected outcomes/goals: (1) improved, (2) stabilized, and (3) deteriorated. This classification was developed from empirical data; approximately 40,000 nursing diagnostic or patient problem statements were collected for the HHCC project. It expands and enhances the NANDA list of nursing diagnoses. Each nursing diagnosis is coded using one expected outcome or goal of the care process as determined by the planned interventions. Each nursing diagnosis is also evaluated on discharge or at discrete time periods during an episode of care.

*HHCC: NURSING INTERVENTIONS:* This currently consists of 160 Home Health Nursing Interventions (60 two-digit major categories and 100 three-digit subcategories) and a modifier of four possible nursing intervention actions: (1) assess, (2) direct care, (3) teach, and (4) manage. Each nursing intervention is identified with the appropriate nursing diagnosis. The HHCC of Nursing Interventions was also developed from empirical data; approximately 80,000 nursing activities, services, treatments, and/or procedures statements were collected for the HHCC project.

**HOME HEALTH CARE COMPONENTS:** Twenty components of home health care are currently used for classifying in the HHCC. These components are also based on empirical data. Each of the components represents a cluster of functional, behavioral, physiological, and psychological home health care patterns which were based on Gordon's eleven functional health patterns. They provide the framework for assessing patients/clients and classifying and coding nursing diagnoses and nursing interventions in the HHCC; that is, they cover the assessment phase of the nursing process as applied to home health nursing (Saba 1992a; Saba, 1992b; Saba and Zuckerman, 1992; Saba et al., 1991).

**HHCC CODING STRUCTURE:** The coding structure of the HHCC follows the structure used to code the ICD-10. It consists of a five-character alphanumeric code (World Health Organization, 1992). The first position is an alphabetic character for the home health component category, followed by two decimal digits for the major category, followed by a decimal point and another digit for a subcategory, and still another digit for the modifier (Figs. 7.4 and 7.5).

***Nursing Intervention Classification*** In 1992, a scheme for documenting nursing practice was developed by McCloskey and Bulechek at the University of Iowa (McCloskey and Bulechek, 1992). The Nursing Intervention Classification (NIC) consists of a list of interventions that nurses perform primarily

**Figure 7.4** Coded examples of nursing diagnoses with and without expected outcome modifiers. (Saba, 1992a.)

| Nursing Diagnosis | Final Code | Expected Outcome | Sub-Category* | Diagnostic Category | HHC Component |
|---|---|---|---|---|---|
| Activity Alteration Improved | A01.01 | ►Improved ►None | | Activity ►Alternation | ►ACTIVITY |
| Acute Pain Stabilized | Q45.12 | ►Stabilized | ►Acute Pain | Comfort ► Alteration | ►SENSORY |
| Breathing Pattern Impairment | L26.2 | | Breathing ►Pattern Impairment | Respiration ►Alteration | ►RESPIRATORY |

* Insert zero for none or blank

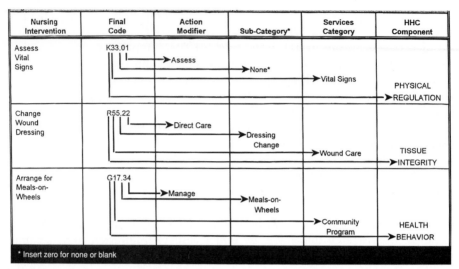

| Nursing Intervention | Final Code | Action Modifier | Sub-Category* | Services Category | HHC Component |
|---|---|---|---|---|---|
| Assess Vital Signs | K33.01 | ►Assess | ►None* | ►Vital Signs | PHYSICAL ►REGULATION |
| Change Wound Dressing | R55.22 | ►Direct Care | ►Dressing Change | ►Wound Care | TISSUE ►INTEGRITY |
| Arrange for Meals-on-Wheels | G17.34 | ►Manage | ►Meals-on-Wheels | ►Community Program | HEALTH ►BEHAVIOR |

\* Insert zero for none or blank

**Figure 7.5**   Coded examples of nursing interventions with types of action modifiers. (Saba, 1992a.)

in hospitals and acute care settings. It is a standardized list of direct care treatments designed to allow practitioners to document their care and assess their impact on patient outcomes. It currently includes 336 nursing intervention labels, which are alphabetized and grouped into six domains: (1) Physiological: Basic, (2) Physiological: Complex, (3) Behavioral, (4) Family, (5) Health System, and (6) Safety. NIC provides nurses with a standardized language to describe nursing treatments and to document care (Prophet, 1994).

### Other Nursing Practice Standards Initiatives
Other initiatives are being conducted nationally and internationally which affect the classification of nursing practice. Each has attempted to develop taxonomies for different aspects of nursing. One group developed a taxonomy for nursing-related dissertations and stated that a taxonomy should (1) be theoretically meaningful and reflect nursing's phenomena, (2) be comprehensive and realistic, and (3) be easy to use (Germain and Dodd, 1993). Another group, Henry, Holzmer, and Reilly (1991), produced a scheme for documenting the care of persons with AIDS. The list of research descriptors developed by Sigma Theta Tau for coding research studies can also be considered a research taxonomy (Watts, 1993). Two other major projects are now discussed.

***Nursing Intervention Lexicon and Taxonomy Study***   The Nursing Intervention Lexicon and Taxonomy (NILT), developed by Grobe, is another scheme; it consists of eight groups that can be used to code nursing interventions. These eight groups resulted from a study using content analysis and natural language-based methods to delineate categories for classifying interventions. The eight NILT categories are: (1) Care Need Determination, (CND); (2) Care Vigilance (CV); (3) Care Environment Management (CEM); (4) Therapeutic Care General (CG); (5) Therapeutic Care Specific (TCS); (6) Therapeutic Care Psychosocial (TCP); (7) Therapeutic Care Cognitive Understanding and Control (TCCD and CO; and (8) Care Information Provision (CIP) (Grobe and Hughes, 1993).

## Patient Care Database Project

A Patient Care Database Project is being developed by Ozbolt at the University of Virginia, Thomas Jefferson University Hospital, and The University Hospital Consortium. The goal of the project is to develop standard coded statements for documenting nursing care in a patient record from which selected data could be abstracted for a database to be used for effectiveness research. The data to be recorded will include nursing diagnoses, interventions, and patient outcomes. Standardized terms are being developed which can be coded and used to abstract relevant nursing data from a patient record. They are being categorized and coded according to the Saba HHCC (Ozbolt et al., 1994).

## International Nursing Practice Standards Initiatives

Many international activities have been initiated that are affecting nursing practice standards. These activities are also directed toward developing an international nursing vocabulary. Within the European region, two initiatives took place in 1993. The Dutch Institute, LEO Nursing Management, and the Danish Institute for Health and Nursing Research organized the First European Conference on Nursing Diagnoses. The aim was to enable nursing leaders, teachers, and researchers to share and exchange information across languages and countries about the need for a common language and, more specifically, nursing diagnoses. Several other conferences have been and continue to be held. The Second European Conference on Nursing Diagnoses and Interventions is planned for 1995.

The Danish Institute also conducted a study, TELENURSING, of several European countries. TELENURSING is a European concerted action to promote the standardization of definitions, classifications, and coding of nursing data to further the development of international efforts to develop a uniform nursing language. Concepts were collected related to the nursing process and health care informatics, namely the nursing process steps, nursing problems/diagnoses, interventions, and outcomes. This ongoing study provides and supports the efforts toward the International Classification of Nursing Practice (ICNP)(Nielsen and Mortensen, 1994).

*International Classification of Nursing Practice* In 1993, the International Council of Nurses (ICN) proposed a beginning draft of the ICNP. The ICN indicated that an international common nursing language is needed for the nursing profession because "if we cannot name it, we cannot control it, finance it, research it or put it into public policy" (International Council of Nurses, 1993).

The ICNP emerged from a 1989 initiative of the ICN Council of Representatives' meeting in Seoul, Korea, where the Professional Services Committee agreed that it would initiate a project to develop the ICNP. The ICNP is divided into three elements of nursing practice: (1) nursing problems/nursing diagnoses, (2) nursing interventions, and (3) outcomes. Each of the ICNP elements consists of an alphabetized data dictionary of several schemes that have been merged. The ICNP will provide nursing with a nomenclature or classification that can be used to describe and organize nursing data in order to provide a tool for documenting nursing practice.

The ICN plans to collect all schemes that document nursing practice from around the world and integrate them into the ICNP. The major goals are to (1) develop specified process and product components, (2) achieve recognition by the national and international nursing communities, (3) ensure compatibility with and complement the WHO International Classification of Diseases (ICD) and the WHO Family of Classifications, (4) support the development and utilization of national databases, and (5) establish an international minimum data set (Fig. 7.6). Once the process is completed and the goals achieved, ICN plans to submit the ICNP to WHO for approval and endorsement (Clark and Lang, 1992; International Council of Nurses, 1993).

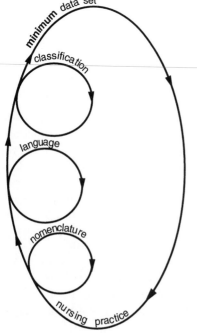

**Figure 7.6**   ICNP model. (Clark and Lang, 1992.) (Courtesy International Nursing Review/ICN.)

## Unified Nursing Language System

The ANA Database Steering Committee is also involved in the development of a common nursing language called the Unified Nursing Language System (UNLS). The committee believes that a UNLS is essential for the information technology age, and the development of a language critical and timely. The ANA Database Steering Committee established criteria for the selection of the schemes to be included in the UNLS (Lang et al., 1995; McCormick et al., 1994; Milholland, 1992). The selection of classification schemes and vocabularies for clinical practice should be based on the following criteria:

- They should be clinically useful for making diagnostic and intervention and outcome decisions.
- They should be stated clearly and unambiguously, with terms defined precisely.
- They should have been tested for reliability of the vocabulary terms.
- They should have been validated as useful for clinical purposes.
- They should be accompanied by documentation of a systematic methodology for development.
- They should be accompanied by evidence of a process for periodic review and provision for adding, revision, or deleting terms.
- Terms should be associated with a unique identifier or code.

The ANA Database Steering Committee, to date, has recommended the four nursing taxonomies or classification schemes for nursing practice listed above, which met their criteria and form the basis for the UNLS.

## Unified Medical Language System

In 1986 the NLM initiated the Unified Medical Language System (UMLS). The goal of the UMLS is to develop a computer-based information resource for health professionals. It is designed to link information sources to one another, namely scientific literature and computer-based patient care records, factual databases, expert systems, and other health-related databases. Three new knowledge sources were identified as part of the UMLS: (1) a Metathesaurus, which is a set ef terms and concepts from several biomedical vocabularies, (2) a semantic network, which links the Metathesaurus vocabularies together using broad categories or semantic concepts; and (3) an information sources map, which provides a description of the available databases (Humphreys and Lindberg, 1992). An example of a semantic network linking nursing concepts to the nursing vocabularies is shown in Fig. 7.7.

Using the same design, the NLM is linking several nursing vocabularies and their concepts together in an attempt to develop a UNLS. The ANA Database Steering committee is collaborating with the NLM to incorporate the four ANA-recognized vocabularies, taxonomies, and classification schemes into the UMLS (McCormick et al., 1994). As vocabularies are "recognized," they will be added to the UNLS.

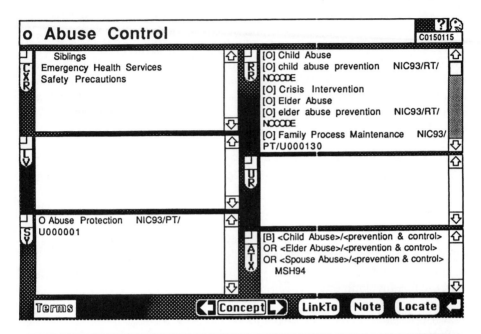

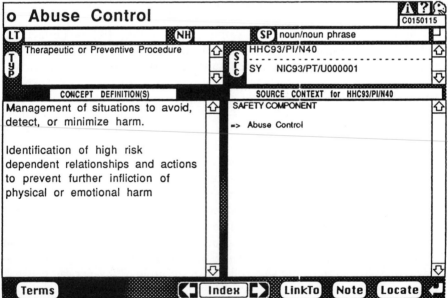

**Figure 7.7** UMLS semantic nursing network map. (Information from the National Library of Medicine's UMLS Metathesaurus, as displayed in MetaCard, a browser application developed by Lexical Technology, Inc.)

The UNLS will allow for the integration of patient data, scientific data, and bibliographic literature data and, once these data are integrated, will bring the information to the bedside to improve the decision making of practicing nurses. It will identify linkages and associations across classification systems, and at the same time allow each classification system to remain a unique entity. It will also facilitate other linkages across databases, such as linking clinical practice data, cost data, and educational case simulation data (McCormick, 1988; McCormick and Zielstorff, 1993).

## CLASSIFICATION SCHEMES FOR THE NURSING PROCESS

To standardize nursing practice, classification schemes need to be developed that not only address the six phases of the nursing process but also can be an integral part of the CPR. That is, they need to be structured and coded to meet both nursing practice standards and data standards. Once integrated into the CPR, they can be used for cost-effective decision support/expert systems and thus become visible in the care process and travel on the information highway (Prophet, 1994; Saba, 1995).

### Computer-Based Patient Record

The CPR will require an electronic structure for three major types of health-related information: (1) common coding strategies, (2) content and structure of the CPR, and (3) structure of the message exchange (see Chap. 6) (Computer-Based Patient Record Institute, 1993). The common coding strategy refers to the utilization of standard patient, provider, and site of care identifiers. Identifiers for patients and facilities are essential for sharing data across settings and care givers (Hammond, 1994). The content and structure of the CPR requires the use of classification and coding schemes. A common language that combines data structures and grammar for clinical care is needed so that meaningful coded messages can be transmitted between CPR systems. The major domains identified, thus far, as needing a common language include nursing; however, the content and structure still have not been identified. The message standards for communication and electronic interchange of data within an organization and from one organization to another are also critical. They will differ according to subject matter and kind of communication.

### Nursing Process Phases

Several schemes have been developed which can be used for documenting the nursing process in computer-based NISs and are affecting the nursing profession and nursing informatics (Henry et al., 1994; Milholland, 1992).

**TABLE 7.3** STANDARDS OF CLINICAL NURSING PRACTICE:
NURSING PROCESS SIX PHASES

- **Assessment:** Collects client health data.
- **Diagnosis:** Analyzes assessment data to determine diagnosis.
- **Outcome Identification:** Identifies expected outcomes of client for nursing diagnoses.
- **Planning:** Develops plan of care and prescribes interventions to attain expected outcomes.
- **Implementation:** Implements the interventions (types) in the plan of care.
- **Evaluation:** Evaluates client's attainment of outcomes.

*Source:* American Nurses Association, 1991, p. 3.

At this time, different schemes are described according to the six phases of the nursing process: (1) assessment, (2) diagnosis, (3) outcome identification, (4) planning, (5) implementation, and (6) evaluation (American Nurses Association, 1991). They are described in Table 7.3.

The six phases of the nursing process can be used to structure an algorithm of care, a protocol of care, and/or a care map. In an algorithm, each phase is linked and related to the other phases. It is similar to a system in which each element is separate but an integral part of the whole. Algorithms need to be developed for the major diagnoses and/or care patterns.

An overview of the nursing process follows.

## Assessment Phase

The assessment phase is the first phase of the nursing process and is viewed as the basic focus for organizing the diagnostic categories of a specific taxonomy. Assessment refers to the collection of client health data needed to evaluate the health status of a patient.

Assessment categories are generally dictated by the conceptual framework of the diagnostic scheme and vary in name and scope. They are used to identify the basic root for the data tree for the CPR and information systems used to document patient care.

## Diagnosis Phase

The diagnosis phase is the second phase of the nursing process. It is the analysis of the assessment data to determine a diagnosis. Diagnosis represents a pattern of one or more related cues derived from the analysis of the assessment data. It is also used to facilitate a plan of care including outcomes. The diagnosis provides a label, which can be coded, for documenting patient care. According to NANDA, a nursing diagnosis is

A clinical judgment about individual, family, or community responses to actual and potential health problems/life processes. Nursing diagnoses provide the basis for selection of nursing interventions to achieve outcomes for which the nurse is accountable (North American Nursing Diagnosis Association, 1992, p. 5).

**Outcome Identification Phase**
This phase identifies the expected outcomes for the client, given a nursing diagnosis. The outcomes are the goals of the care process. Identified outcomes can also be compared to the actual outcomes at the termination of the care process.

**Planning Phase**
This phase develops the plan of care and prescribes interventions to attain the expected outcomes. The plan of care is developed by a nurse and/or a physician and outlines the care and interventions needed to address the identified diagnosis.

**Implementation Phase**
In this phase the interventions, services, significant treatments, or activities identified in the client's plan of care are implemented. The plan of care and interventions can be linked to the identified diagnoses being addressed to attain the desired outcomes.

**Evaluation Phase**
In this phase the client's attainment of outcomes is evaluated. The evaluation phase represents the attainment of the actual outcome of care, and can be compared to the identified goal of the diagnosis and care process.

## NURSING INFORMATION SYSTEM MODELS

There are many NIS models which illustrate different concepts of NISs and nursing informatics. Many have been developed as the framework for the four major areas of nursing—administration, practice, education, research—as well as nursing informatics. Selected examples of these models are presented below.

## Design of NIS Models

Two models to guide in the design of NISs were developed by Graves and Corcoran (1989). One focuses on the flow of information and the second on the conceptual and practice components of nursing data. The flow of information model illustrates an NIS by (1) its symbolic content, which is represented by data, information, and knowledge, (2) how the content is organized, and (3) how the content flows through the system. An example of how the model can be operationalized is "A Research Knowledge System" (ARKS), which is designed to present research knowledge from scientific literature to users in the form of concept maps. The purpose of the concept maps is to restructure knowledge into a more useful form in order to assist nurses in the design of research strategies. ARKS can be used to develop nursing research knowledge databases (Fig. 7.8) (Graves, 1991; Graves and Corcoran, 1988).

The second model which, represents the conceptual and practice elements required for the design of an NIS was also developed by Graves and Corcoran (1989). They identify the conceptual design of an NIS as due to

**Figure 7.8**   Flow of information model. [Courtesy J. Graves and S. Corcoran, 1988. (Permission W. B. Saunders/Health Profession Journal).]

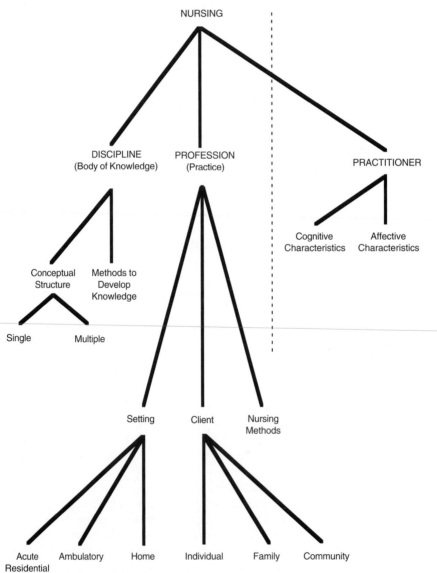

nursing orientation or definitions of nursing. Nursing can use multiple conceptual models based on their orientation to patients, settings, health status, and nursing actions, whereas the complexity of the NISs varies according to different nursing practice elements—different types of settings, clients, and nursing methods. This model provides another guide for the design of an NIS. It provides the requirements that should be considered regarding the structure, presentation, and means of delivering nursing data, information, and knowledge to the users of the systems.

## Linked Model

The linked model developed by Gassert (1989) is a graphic model for defining NIS requirements (MDNISR). The MDNISR consists of five elements: (1) nurse users, (2) information processing, (3) NISs, (4) nursing information, and (5) nursing system goals. The model is used to describe a process of determining the data elements for inputs, processing, constraints, and outputs for each of the five model elements. The model delineates and assists developers in defining the elements and outputs for an NIS in a hospital setting. It is considered to be not only valid but also complete, useful, and clear (Fig. 7.9) (Gassert, 1989, 1991).

**Figure 7.9**   Linked model. (Courtesy C. Gassert, 1989, University of Maryland/ SCAMC/AMIA.)

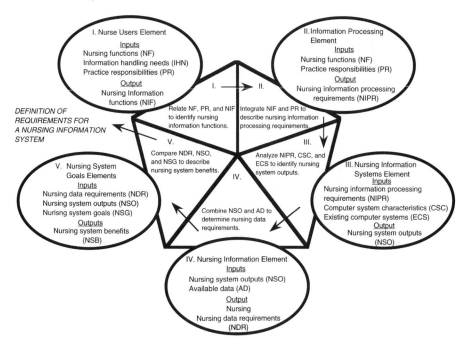

## Nursing Administration Models

There are many NIS models for the administration of nursing services. They generally outline the design specifications for the NIS component or subsystem of a larger hospital information system.

### Military Nursing Model for Patient Care

This model is a nursing administrative model developed by a Tri-Service Nursing Requirements Committee under the direction of Karen Rieder (NNC) which identified the information requirements for the military computer-based NIS. The military model for patient care addressed the nursing requirements for patient care unit management and nursing administration for the inpatient, outpatient, and critical care areas, such as the operating room and intensive care units. It also provided the blueprint for improving nursing care to patients through the proposed computer-based system (Fig. 7.10) (Rieder and Norton, 1989).

### Computer Effectiveness Model

This model addresses the impact of computer technology on the job to be done and focuses on the organizational side of computer technology. This model, introduced by Guttman and Pocklington, illustrates a hierarchy of effectiveness reflecting the degree to which a task is accomplished or not accomplished, ranging from task failure to task creativity (Pocklington, 1983).

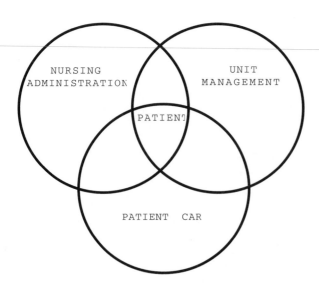

**Figure 7.10** Military nursing model for patient care. (Rieder and Norton, 1989, with permission of Springer-Verlag.)

## Nursing Practice Models

Nursing practice models focus primarily on patient care and the nursing care planning process. Generally, the nursing practice models reflect the nursing theory that provides the basis for the care philosophy in a given hospital. For example, a hospital that bases patient care on the Orem theory will structure its NIS differently from one that bases patient care on Maslow's hierarchy of needs.

### Nursing Practice Data Base Model

One of the first nursing practice models was developed in 1978 for the nursing component of the Technicon Medical Information System (TMIS). It was designed as the framework for documenting nursing care planning at the National Institutes of Health (NIH) in order to outline the NIS requirements for its TMIS hospitalwide computerized system.

The NIH Nursing Practice Data Base Model includes three major components of nursing data: (1) interdependent nursing interventions (physician orders), (2) independent nursing interventions (nursing orders), and (3) interaction of interdependent and independent nursing functions (involvement of both providers). Each of these components incorporates different nursing data elements required for the development of an NIS that was designed to document nursing care and generate nursing care plans. The independent nursing interventions component encompasses a nursing assessment cluster which is based on thirteen categories of patient needs based on Maslow's hierarchy of needs. This model offers a dynamic approach to the process of nursing care (Romano et al., 1982).

### Patient Care Integration Nursing Model

Another model depicting the interactive function of nursing in a patient care information system was proposed by Cook (1982). The Patient Care Integration Nursing Model identifies the interactions between the various components of a patient care information system and their interrelationships with nursing. Such a comprehensive information system can not only enhance the professional practice of nursing but also improve patient care. It can facilitate the planning, managing, implementing, and documenting of patient care.

### General Model of the Nursing Process

Another model for documenting nursing care is the model for the nursing process designed by Goodwin and Edwards. They demonstrated that the nursing process was a systems model that could be computerized (Ozbolt, 1983). The General Model for the Nursing Process is a model that depicts a problem-solving process for providing patient care. The model provides a simplified representation of nursing practice and depicts the process that nurses use to deliver care. It is an open system with a feedback loop. As new data are collected and new diagnoses identified from the outcomes of the interventions, they are redirected into the feedback loop as new inputs into the system. Thus, this model represents an expert system or a decision support system (Ozbolt et al., 1985).

## Educational Models

Models have been developed that assist nurse educators to view different aspects of nursing informatics and focus on the educational processes. Some models focus on innovative teaching strategies, others on the use of different educational media, and still others on evaluating the teaching process.

Several models of interest include the following: (1) Nursing Informatics Educational Model developed by Riley and Saba, (2) General Curriculum Development Model developed by Ronald and Skiba (1987), (3) the Ronald Collaborative Education Model (1991), and (4) the Evaluation Model of Computer-Assisted Instruction by Billings (1984). These are described in detail in Chap. 14.

## Research Models

Many models have been developed for computer-based nursing research applications. Models are used to depict the conceptual framework and the data variables needed for the research method.

### Nursing Informatics (NI) Pyramid Model

One of the first computer-based clinical nursing research models was developed by Schwirian. The Schwirian cube, as it was called, illustrated what nurse researchers could do with computers. The Schwirian cube was expanded to provide the NI pyramid, a model for research in nursing informatics. It provides a framework that depicts the information nursing informatics experts need to conduct research. This model contains four elements arranged to form a pyramid: (1) nursing information or raw material, (2) computer system or technology, (3) users, and (4) the goal of the system. Three of these elements—information, computer system, and users—form the base needed to achieve the fourth element, which is the goal of the system and is illustrated on the apex of the pyramid (Schwirian, 1986).

## Conceptual Design Models

Conceptual models have also been developed that illustrate a computer-based patient care system, expert system, decision support system, and a multitude of other different NIS processes. Nurses use decision-modeling systems to solve a decision problem when more analysis is needed instead of more data. Modeling is primarily one approach to providing decision support. There are several models and software packages that build models to provide nurses and clinical practitioners with decision support capabilities. Decision support systems generally use one of two models: (1) decision analytic model or (2) expert system model. These models are used to construct the decision problem designed to determine a course of action that will achieve a specific outcome.

### Decision Analytic Model

This model relies on rules to determine the outcome with the greatest probability of achievement, whereas the multiple criteria model dictates the best course of action based on choices. This computerized decision support system, developed by Brennan, links computer technology with decision-making algorithms to support decisions made by nurses providing clinical care (Brennan, 1988).

### Expert System Model

This model outlining the components of an expert system was developed by Chang. An expert system is a computer program that uses artificial intelligence technology to represent human logic, knowledge, experience, and judgment for a specific domain. Chang's model illustrates the relationships between three modules with an optional fourth and/or fifth: (1) a conceptual base with factual and procedural data, (2) an inference engine controlling the rules of the knowledge base for clinical decision making, and (3) a user interface which allows the nurse (user) to communicate with the expert system (Fig. 7.11). Optional explanation and learning modules

**Figure 7.11**  Components of an expert system. (Courtesy B. Chang, 1990, with permission of Mosby-Year Book, Inc.)

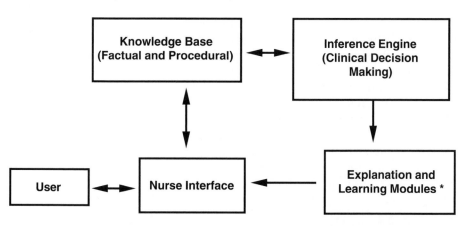

\* Additional modules that may be operational.

explain the reasons for the decisions proposed by the program. Expert systems are used in health care to address a clinical, educational, or research problem (Chang, 1990).

## OVERVIEW OF NIS APPLICATIONS

Nursing informatics applied to the design of computer systems is an NIS. As stated previously, information systems are computer systems described according to their purpose, focus, use, and service; when they encompass nursing applications, components, or functions, they are considered to be NISs. An NIS is an invaluable aid for processing nursing information. NISs are used to administer hospital and community health agencies, assist in delivering nursing practice, support the educational process, and retrieve information and analyze data for research.

The early NISs developed by vendors or health care facilities primarily computerized existing paper-based methods of documenting nursing. They were generally based on standardized nursing care protocols for a medical diagnosis, surgical procedure, specific diagnosis related group (DRG), or research protocol. Others were designed using standardized protocols for care of a specific patient condition, such as pain, incontinence, decubiti, or colostomy.

Generally, most hospitals implement some type of hospital information system (HIS) or medical information system (MIS), sometimes called a patient care system (PCS). Such systems generally include subsystems or components specifically developed for nursing, and hence called NISs. Such NISs are designed to assist nurses in managing information needed to provide patient care. NISs may also be found in hospitals as stand-alone systems specifically designed for the nursing department and specifically implemented to process special nursing applications such as patient classification systems for nurse staffing.

Hospitals can also have many different types of information systems, including NISs, all dedicated to specific applications. Hospitals are beginning to establish communication networks to share information with other hospitals for certain applications. The emerging NIS stand-alone systems, which use minicomputers or microcomputers for specific nursing applications, are designed to generate timely statistics for managing and allocating nursing personnel and resources.

NISs help nurses to administer nursing departments, deliver patient care, and support nursing education and nursing research. The state of the art of NISs for these and other related applications is described in the remaining chapters of this book.

### Nursing Administration

In the area of nursing administration, NISs are generally found in hospitals as subsystems of larger mainframe systems that are dedicated primarily to administering nursing services and nursing unit management. NISs that address nursing practice in hospitals focus on nursing information management systems for patient care. They utilize several innovative technologies such as staffing scheduling systems, decision support (expert) systems, imaging/vital signs systems, discharge care planning systems, bedside terminals, and workstations/LANs (local area networks).

## Nursing Practice

Nursing practice applications focus on the computer-based nursing documentation systems that address patient care. They include basic categories and those that address the nursing process, and often use bedside terminals and/or integrated workstations. There is a need for a UNLS.

### Critical Care

Critical care focuses on the care of patients located in intensive care units, emergency rooms, and operating rooms. These systems include arrhythmia monitors, physiologic monitors, special-purpose systems, and patient data management systems. Such systems may be stand-alone or be connected to an NIS that integrates the information from the monitors into a patient data management system (PDMS). Special-purpose systems, also found in the area on nursing practice, are generally stand-alone systems for processing information from specific technological equipment.

### Outcomes and Guidelines

The integration of administrative and practice documentation encompasses the new area of monitoring outcomes, integrating clinical practice guidelines, and managing care. The focus is on outcomes of care, efficiency, and effectiveness in delivering quality care at reasonable costs. This component of nursing information describes new tools in case management for tracking patients' progress, as well as using the information and profiles of care.

### Community Health Nursing

Community health nursing agencies employ both administrative and practice NISs, either subsystems in larger agencies or stand-alone systems in small agencies. Such systems, called community health nursing management information systems, focus on financial applications and billing, statistical reporting, and patient care. They also encompass ambulatory care and special-purpose applications. Documentation systems also address patient assessment, nursing care planning, protocols of care, the critical path method, and discharge/outcomes, which includes evaluating the outcomes of the care process on discharge. These systems use standardized computer-based protocols or hand-held computers to collect the visit data.

## Nursing Education

In the area of nursing education, NISs address the educational process, including computer-assisted instruction and interactive video instruction. Educational applications also include those which address the management of nursing education, including management of students, courses, and faculty. Computer support systems and student computer-based services are provided in computer resources centers. The services include practice for exams and tests, authoring systems, and decision support systems. The expert systems offer a form of artificial intelligence and act as knowledge synthesizers and nurse extenders.

## Nursing Research

Systems used to support the nursing research process include document retrieval systems and other databases that allow for searching the nursing literature. Document retrieval systems include nursing literature databases, informational databases, and knowledge databases for searching the literature and other sources of information on the research topic. They also include tools used for conducting research: statistical software packages, file managers, graphic displays, text editors, and database management systems. They focus on computing and communication of research using high-speed networks, including the Internet and other on-line networks.

## SUMMARY

This chapter provided an overview of nursing informatics and NISs. It described the emergence of nursing informatics and how it interrelated with computers and nursing and with NISs. It provided an overview of the development, definitions, scope, and dimensions of nursing informatics. It included a discussion on nursing data, including nursing data standards and nursing practice standards. Nursing classification schemes were presented using the nursing process to illustrate how they can be used in the computer-based patient systems. An overview of nursing informatics was presented with examples of the different applications that exist.

Finally, an overview of the various NISs found in nursing were presented. The four areas in which NISs are found—namely, nursing administration, practice, research, and education—were described. This section also included a discussion of the new integration of administration and practice and other information systems that nurses use in providing patient care and carrying out nursing activities. A model of the scope of NISs for nursing was also presented.

# REFERENCES

American Nurses Association. (1980). *Nursing: A Social Policy Statement* (p. 9). Kansas City, MO.

American Nurses Association. (1991). *Standards of Clinical Nursing Practice* (p. 3). Kansas City, MO.

Anderson, J. (1983). Informatics and clinical nursing records. In M. Scholes, Y. Bryant, and B. Barber (Eds.), *The Impact of Computers on Nursing: An International Review* (pp. 126–132). Amsterdam, Netherlands: North-Holland.

Ball, M. J., and Hannah, K. J. (1988). What is informatics and what does in mean for nursing? In M. J. Ball, K. J. Hannah, U. Gerdin-Jelger, and H. Peterson (Eds.), *Nursing Informatics: Where Caring and Technology Meet* (pp. 81–87). New York: Springer-Verlag.

Barber, B. (1983). Computers need nursing. In M. Scholes, Y. Bryant, and B. Barber (Eds.), *The Impact of Computers on Nursing: An International Review* (pp. 24–33). Amsterdam, Netherlands: North-Holland.

Billings, D. M. (1984). Evaluating computer-assisted instruction. *Nursing Outlook, 32*(1), 50–53.

Blum, B. L. (1990). Medical informatics in the United States, 1950–1975. In B. I. Blum, and K. Duncan (Eds.), *A History of Medical Informatics* (pp. xvii–xxx). Reading, MA: Addison-Wesley.

Brennan, P. F. (1988). Modeling for decision support. In M. J. Ball, K. J. Hannah, U. Gerdin-Jelger, and H. Peterson (Eds.), *Nursing Informatics: Where Caring and Technology Meet* (pp. 267–273). New York: Springer-Verlag.

Carpenito, L. J. (1989). *Nursing Diagnosis: Application to Clinical Practice*. New York: Lippincott.

Chang, B. L. (1990). Potential and pitfalls of expert systems in nursing. In J. C. McClosky and H. K. Grace (Eds.), *Current Issues in Nursing* (pp. 71–76). St. Louis: Mosby.

Chang, B. L., and Hirsch, M. (1991). Knowledge acquisition and knowledge representation in a rule-based expert system. *Computers in Nursing, 9*(5), 174–178.

Clark, J., and Lang, N. (1992). Nursing's next advance: An international classification for nursing practice. *International Nursing Review, 39*(4), 109–112.

Computer-Based Patient Record Institute, Inc. (1993). *Position Paper: Computer-Based Patient Record Standards*. Chicago.

Cook, M. (1982). Using computers to enhance professional practice. In B. Blum (Ed.), *Proceedings: The Sixth Annual Symposium on Computer Applications in Medical Care* (pp. 583–586). Washington, DC: IEEE Computer Society Press.

Council on Computer Applications in Nursing (1992). *Report on the Designation of Nursing Informatics as a Nursing Specialty* (Congress of Nursing Practice unpublished report). Washington, DC: American Nurses Association.

Fishman, D. J. (1994). Nursing informatics: The electronic information revolution in education and practice. In O. L. Strickland and D. J. Fishman (Eds.), *Nursing Issues in the 1990s* (pp. 471–488). Albany, NY: Delmar.

Fitzpatrick, J. J. (1988). Nursing: How do we know; what do we do; and how can we enhance nursing knowledge and practice. In N. Daly and K. J. Hannah (Eds.), *Nursing and Computers: Proceedings of Third International Symposium on Nursing Use of Computers and Information Science* (pp. 58–65). St. Louis: Mosby.

Fitzpatrick, J. J., Kerr, M. E., Saba, V. K., et al. (1989). Nursing diagnosis: Translating nursing diagnosis into ICD code. *American Journal of Nursing, 89*(40), 493–495.

Gassert, C. A. (1989). Defining nursing information system requirements: A linked model. In L. C. Kingsland III (Ed.), *Proceedings of the Thirteenth Annual Symposium on Computer Applications in Medical Care* (pp. 779–782). Washington, DC: IEEE Computer Society Press.

Gassert, C. A. (1991). Validating a model for defining nursing information system requirements. In E. S. Hovenga, K. J. Hannah, K. A. McCormick, and J. S. Ronald (Eds.), *Nursing Informatics '91* (pp. 214–219). New York: Springer-Verlag.

Germain, C. P., and Dodd, M. J. (Eds.). (1993). *Developing Taxonomies for Nursing Research.* Washington, DC: American Nurses Publishing.

Gordon, M. (1982). *Nursing Diagnosis: Process and Application.* New York: McGraw-Hill.

Graves, J. R. (1991). ARKS: A Research-Knowledge System. In E. S. Hovenga, K. J. Hannah, K. A. McCormick, and J. S. Ronald (Eds.), *Nursing Informatics '91* (p. 811). New York: Springer-Verlag.

Graves, J. R. (1993). Data versus information versus knowledge. *Reflections, 19*(1), 4–5.

Graves, J. R., and Corcoran, S. (1988). Design of nursing information systems: Conceptual and practice elements. *Journal of Professional Nursing, 4,* 168–177.

Graves, J. R., and Corcoran, S. (1989). The study of nursing informatics. *Image: Journal of Nursing Scholarship, 21*(4), 227–231.

Grobe, S. J., and Hughes, L. A. (1993). The conceptual validity of a taxonomy of nursing interventions. *Journal of Advanced Nursing, 18*(12), 1942–1961.

Hammond, W. E. (1994). The role of standards in creating a health information infrastructure. *International Journal of Bio-Medical Computing, 34,* 29–44.

Hannah, K. J. (1985). Current trends in nursing in informatics: Implications for curriculum planning. In K. J. Hannah, E. J. Guillemin, and D. N. Conklin (Eds.), *Nursing Uses of Computers and Information Science* (pp. 181–187). Amsterdam, Netherlands: North-Holland.

Hannah, K. J., Ball, M. J., and Edwards, M. J. A. (1994). *Introduction to Nursing Informatics.* New York: SpringerVerlag.

Henry, S. B., Holzmer, W. L., and Reilly, C. A. (1991). Nurses' perspectives on problems of hospitalized patients: Implications for the development of a nursing taxonomy. In P. D. Clayton (Ed.), *Proceedings of the Fifteenth Annual Symposium on Computer Applications in Medical Care* (pp. 177–181). New York: McGraw-Hill.

Henry, S. B., Holzmer, W. L., Reilly, C. A., and Campbell, K. E. (1994). Terms used by nurses to describe patient problems: Can SNOMED III represent nursing concepts in the patient record? *Journal of the American Medical Informatics Association, 1*(1), 61–74.

Humphreys, B. L., and Lindberg, D. B. (1992). The unified medical language system project: A distributed experiment in improving access to biomedical information. In K. C. Lun, P. DeGoulet, T. E. Piemme, and O. Rienhoff (Eds.), *MEDINFO '90* (pp. 1496–1500). Amsterdam, Netherlands: North-Holland.

International Council of Nurses. (1993). *Nursing's Next Advance: An International Classification for Nursing Practice (ICNP). A Working Paper* (p. 3). Geneva, Switzerland.

Joos, I., Whitman, N. I., Smith, M. J., and Nelson, R. (1992). *Computers in Small Bytes: The Computer Workbook* (Pub. No. 14-2496). New York: National League for Nursing.

Lang, N. M., Hudgings, C., Jacox, A., et al. (1995). Toward a national database for nursing practice. In *An Emerging Framework for the Profession: Data System Advances for Clinical Nursing Practice.* Washington, DC: American Nurses Association.

Martin, K. S., and Scheet, N. J. (1992). *The Omaha System.* Philadelphia: Saunders.

McCloskey, J. C., and Bulechek, G. M. (Eds.). (1992). *Nursing Interventions Classification (NIC): Iowa Intervention Project.* St. Louis: Mosby.

McCormick, K. A. (1988). A unified nursing language system. In M. J. Ball, K. J. Hannah, U. Gerdin-Jelger, and H. Peterson (Eds.), *Nursing Informatics: Where Caring and Technology Meet* (pp. 168–178). New York: Springer-Verlag.

McCormick, K. A., Lang, N., Zielstorff, R., et al. (1994). Toward standard classification schemes for nursing language: Recommendations of the American Nurses Association Steering Committee on Databases to Support Nursing Practice. *Journal of the American Medical Informatics Association, 1*(6), 421–427.

McCormick, K. A., and Zielstorff, R. (1993). Building a unified nursing language system. In *Papers: Nursing Minimum Data Set Conference, Edmonton, Alberta* (pp. 127–133). 1993 Alberta, Canada: Canadian Nurses Association.

Milholland, D. K. (1992). Naming what we do—Nursing vocabularies and databases. *Journal of American Health Information Management Association, 63*(10), 58–61.

National Center for Nursing Research Priority Expert Panel on Nursing Informatics. (1993). *Nursing informatics: Enhancing patient care* (p. 11). Bethesda, MD: National Center for Nursing Research, NIH, PHS, US DHHS.

National Library of Medicine. (1986). *Medical Informatics: Report of Panel 4: Long Range Plan.* Rockville, MD: NLM, NIH, PHS, US DHHS.

Nielsen, G. H., and Mortensen, R. A. (1994). *TELENURSING: Documentation of the Nursing Process in Hospitals by Computers in Europe* (Vol. I). Copenhagen, Denmark: The Danish Institute for Health and Nursing Research.

North American Nursing Diagnosis Association (1990). *Taxonomy I: Revised 1990.* St. Louis.

North American Nursing Diagnosis Association. (1992). *NANDA nursing diagnoses: Definitions and Classification 1992* (p. 5); 1995/1996. St. Louis, MO.

Ozbolt, J. (1983). A prototype information system to aid nursing decision. In B. Blum (Ed.), *Proceedings: The Sixth Annual Symposium on Computer Applications in Medical Care* (pp. 653–657). New York: IEEE Computer Society Press.

Ozbolt, J. G., Fruchnicht, J. N., and Hayden, J. R. (1994). Toward data standards for clinical nursing information. *Journal of the American Medical Informatics Association, 2*(2), 171–185.

Ozbolt, J. G., Schultz II, S., Swain, M. A., and Abraham. I. L. (1985). A proposed expert system for nursing practice: A springboard to nursing science. *Journal of Medical Systems, 9,* 57–68.

Peterson, H. E., and Gerdin-Jelger, U. (Eds.). (1989). *Preparing Nurses for Using Information Systems: Recommended Informatics Competencies* (Pub No. 14-22334) (p. 117). New York: National League for Nursing.

Pocklington, D. B. (1983). Models for evaluating faculty/student acceptance and effectiveness of computer technology in schools of nursing. In R. Dayhoff (Ed.), *Proceedings: The Seventh Annual Symposium on Computer Applications in Medical Care* (p. 495). New York: IEEE Computer Society Press.

Prophet, C. M. (1994). Nursing interventions classifications. In S. J. Grobe and E. S. P. Pluyter-Wenting (Eds.). *Nursing Informatics: An International Overview for Nursing in a Technological Era* (pp. 692–696). New York: Elsevier.

Rieder, K. A., and Norton, D. A. (1989). An integrated nursing information system: A planning model. In V. K. Saba, K. A. Rieder, and D. B. Pocklington (Eds.). *Nursing and Computers: An Anthology* (pp. 15–27). New York: Springer-Verlag.

Romano, C. (1993). *Predictors of Nurse Adoption of a Computerized Information System as an Innovation* (doctoral dissertation). Baltimore, MD: University of Maryland.

Romano, C., McCormick, K. A., and McNeely, L. D. (1982). Nursing documentation: A model for a computerized data base. *Advances in Nursing Science, 4*(2), 43–56.

Ronald, J. S. (1991). A collaborative model for specializing in nursing informatics. In. E. V. Hovenga, K. J. Hannah, K. A. McCormick, and J. S. Ronald (Eds.), *Nursing Informatics '91: Proceedings of the Fourth International Conference on Nursing Use of Computers and Information Science.* (pp. 662–666). New York: Springer-Verlag.

Ronald, J. S. and Skiba, D. J. (1987). *Guidelines for Basic Computer Education in Nursing* (Pub. No. 41-2177). New York: National League for Nursing.

Saba, V. K. (1992a). The classification of home health care nursing diagnoses and interventions. *CARING Magazine, 11*(3), 50–57.

Saba, V. K. (1992b). Home health care classification. *CARING Magazine, 12*(5), 58–60.

Saba, V. K. (1994). Nursing informatics: An overview. In M. O. Mundinger (Ed.) *Phizer Guide: Nursing Career Opportunities* (pp. 288–293). Old Saybrook, CT: Merritt Communications.

Saba, V. K. (1995). A new nursing vision: The information highway. *Nursing Leadership Forum,* accepted for publication.

Saba, V. K., O'Hare, A., Zuckerman, A. E., et al. (1991). A nursing intervention taxonomy for home health care. *Nursing and Health Care, 12*(6), 296–299.

Saba, V. K., and Zuckerman, A. E. (1992). A new home health classification method. *CARING Magazine, 12*(10), 27–34.

Scholes, M., and Barber, B. (1980). Towards nursing informatics. In D. A. D. Lindberg and S. Kaihara (Eds.), *MEDINFO: 1980* (pp. 70–73). Amsterdam, Netherlands: North-Holland.

Schwirian, P. A. (1986). The NI pyramid: A model for research in nursing informatics. *Computers in Nursing, 4*(3), 134–136.

Study Group on Nursing Information Systems. (1983). Special report: Computerized nursing information systems: An urgent need. *Research in Nursing and Health, 6*(3), 101–105.

Visiting Nurse Association of Omaha. (1986). *Client Management Information System for Community Health Nursing Agencies.* (NTIS Pub. No. HRP-0907023). Rockville, MD: Division of Nursing, BHP, HRSA, PHS, US DHHS.

Watts, M. (1993). *1993 Directory of Nurse Researchers* (4th ed.). Indianapolis, IN: Sigma Theta Tau International, Honor Society of Nursing.

Werley, H. H. (1988). Introduction to the nursing minimum data set and its development. In H. H. Werley and N. M. Lang (Eds.), *Identification of the Nursing Minimum Data Set* (pp. 1–17). New York: Springer.

Werley, H. H., and Lang, N. M. (Eds.). (1988). *Identification of the Nursing Minimum Data Set.* New York: Springer.

World Health Organization. (1992). *International Statistical Classification of Diseases and Health Related Problems: Tenth Revision* (ICD-10). Geneva, Switzerland.

Zielstorff, R. D., Lang, N. M., Saba, K. A., and Milholland, D. K. (1995). *Toward a Uniform Language for Nursing in the U.S.: Work of the American Nurses Association Steering Committee on Databases to Support Clinical Practice.* Amsterdam, Netherlands: Elsevier.


# BIBLIOGRAPHY

Arnold, J. M., and Pearson, G. A. (Eds.). (1992). *Computer Applications in Nursing Education and Practice* (Pub. No. 14-2406). New York: National League for Nursing.

Ball, M. J. and Collen, M. F. (1992). *Aspects of the Computer-Based Patient Record.* New York: Springer-Verlag.

Ball, M. J., and Hannah, K. J. (1984). *Using Computers in Nursing.* Reston, VA: Reston Publishing.

Ball, M. J., Hannah, K. J., Gerdin-Jelger, U., and Peterson, H. (Eds.). *Nursing Informatics: Where Caring and Technology Meet.* New York: Springer-Verlag.

Bronzino, J. D. (1982). *Computer Applications for Patient Care.* Reading, MA: Addison-Wesley.

Canadian Nurses Association. (1992). *Papers from Nursing Minimum Data Set Conference, 27–29 October 1992: Edmonton, Alberta.* Ottawa, Ontario: Canadian Nurses Association.

Chang, B. L. (1990). Potential and pitfalls of expert systems in nursing. In J. C. McClosky and H. K. Grace (Eds.), *Current Issues in Nursing.* St. Louis: Mosby.

Chang, B. L., and Gilbert, J. (1990). Reliability and validity of an assessment guide for nursing diagnoses. *Australian Journal of Advanced Nursing,* 5, 16–22.

Collen, M. F. (1994). The origins of informatics. *Journal of American Medical Informatics Association,* 1(2), 91–107.

Daly, N., and Hannah, K. J. (Eds.). *Proceedings of Nursing and Computers: Third International Symposium on Nursing Use of Computers and Information Science.* Washington, DC: Mosby.

Devine, E. C., and Werley, H. H. (1988). Test of the nursing minimum data set: Availability of data and reliability. *Research in Nursing and Health,* 11, 97–104.

Dick, R. S., and Steen, E. B. (Eds.). (1991). *The Computer-Based Patient Record: An Essential Technology for Health Care.* Washington, DC: National Academy Press.

Edmunds, L. (1983). Making the most of a message function for nursing services. In R. Dayhoff (Ed.), *Proceedings: The Seventh Annual Symposium on Computer Applications in Medical Care* (pp. 511–513). New York: IEEE Computer Society Press.

Flynn, J. B., Foerst, H., and Heffron, P. B. (1984). Nursing: Past and present. In J. B. McCann/Flynn and P. B. Heffron (Eds.), *Nursing: From Concept to Practice* (pp. 31–88). Bowie, MD: Robert J. Brady.

Gillis, P. A., Booth, H., Graves, J. R., et al. (1994). Translating traditional principles of system development into a process for designing clinical information systems. *International Journal of Technology Assessment in Health Care, 10*(2), 235–248.

Goodwin, J. O., and Edwards, B. S. (1975). Developing a computer program to assist the nursing process. *Nursing Research, 24*(4), 299–305.

Gordon, M. (1985). Practice-based data set for a nursing information system. *Journal of Medical Systems, 9*, 43–56.

Grobe, S. J. (1984). *Computer Primer and Resource Guide for Nurses.* Philadelphia: Lippincott.

Grobe, S. J. (1994). Nursing informatics: State of the science. In J. H. van Bemmel and A. T. McCray (Eds.). *Yearbook of Medical Informatics: 94, Advanced Communications in Healthcare* (pp. 85–94). Geneva, Switzerland: Schattauer Verlag.

Grobe, S. J., and Pluyter-Wenting, E. S. P. (Eds.). *Nursing Informatics: An International Overview for Nursing in a Technological Era.* New York: Elsevier.

Hannah, K. J., Guillemin, E. J., and Conklin, D. N. (Eds.). (1985). *Nursing Uses of Computers and Information Science.* Amsterdam, Netherlands: North-Holland.

Hovenga, E. J. S., Hannah, K. J., McCormick, K. A., and Ronald, J. S. (Eds.). *Nursing Informatics '91: Proceedings of the Fourth International Conference on Nursing Use of Computers and Information Science.* New York: Springer-Verlag.

Kiley, M., Halloran, E. J., Weston, J. L., et al. (1983). Computerized nursing information systems (NIS). *Nursing Management, 14*(7), 26–29.

Marek, K. D., and Lang, N. M. (1992). Nursing standards outcomes. In Canadian Nurses Association, *Papers from Nursing Minimum Data Set Conference, 27–29 October 1992: Edmonton, Alberta* (pp. 100–120). Ottawa, Ontario: Canadian Nurses Association.

Marr, P. B., Axford, R. L., and Newbold, S. K. (Eds.). *Nursing Informatics '91: Proceedings of the Post Conference on Health Care Information Technology: Implications for Change.* New York: Springer-Verlag.

McCann/Flynn, J. B., and Heffron, P. B. (Eds.). (1984). *Nursing: From Concept to Practice.* Bowie, MD: Robert J. Brady.

Milholland, D. K., and Heller, B. R. (1992). Computer-based patient record: From pipe dream to reality. *Computers in Nursing, 10*(5), 189–190.

Nielsen, G. H., and Mortensen, R. A. (1994). *TELENURSING: Definition, Classification, and Coding of the Nursing Process in Hospitals in Europe* (Vol. II). Copenhagen, Denmark: The Danish Institute for Health and Nursing Research.

Nielsen, G. H., and Mortensen, R. A. (1994). *TELENURSING: Nursing and Standardization Efforts in Health Care Informatics in Europe* (Vol. III). Copenhagen, Denmark: The Danish Institute for Health and Nursing Research.

Nielsen, G. H., and Mortensen, R. A. (1994). *TELENURSING: Nursing Minimun Data Sets in Europe* (Vol. IV). Copenhagen, Denmark: The Danish Institute 2for Health and Nursing Research.

Orem, D. E. (1971). *Nursing: Concepts of Practice.* New York: McGraw-Hill.

Pocklington, D. B., and Guttman, L. (1984). *Nursing Reference for Computer Literature.* Philadelphia: Lippincott.

Rogers, M. E. (1970). *An Introduction to the Theoretical Basis of Nursing.* Philadelphia: F. A. Davis.

Roy, C. (1975). A diagnostic classification system for nursing. *Nursing Outlook, 23*(2), 90–94.

Ryan, S. A. (1985). An expert system for nursing practice: Clinical decision support. *Computers in Nursing, 3*(2), 77–84.

Saba, V. K., Rieder, K. A., and Pocklington, D. B. (Eds.). (1989). *Nursing and Computers: An Anthology.* New York: Springer-Verlag.

Schneider, D. (1993). Internet: Linking nurses, scholars, libraries. *Reflections, 19*(1), 9.

Scholes, M., Bryant, Y., and Barber, B. (Eds.). (1983). *The Impact of Computers on Nursing: An International Review.* Amsterdam, Netherlands: North-Holland.

Sparks, S. M., and Taylor, C. M. (1993). *Nursing Diagnosis Reference Manual.* Springhouse, PA: Springhouse Corp.

Sweeney, M. A. (1985). *The Nurses' Guide to Computers.* New York: Macmillan.

Sweeney, M. A., and Olivieri, P. (1981). *An Introduction to Nursing Research.* Philadelphia: Lippincott.

Thompson, C., Ryan, S. A., and Baggs, J. G. (1991). Testing of a computer-based support system in an acute care hospital. In E. S. Hovenga, K. J. Hannah, K. A. McCormick, and J. S. Ronald (Eds.), *Nursing Informatics '91: Proceedings of the Fourth International Conference on Nursing Use of Computers and Information Science* (pp. 769–779). New York: Springer-Verlag.

Turley, J. P. (1992). A framework for the transition from nursing records to nursing information system. *Nursing Outlook, 40*(4), 177–181.

Turley, J. P., and Newbold, S. K. (Eds.). *Nursing Informatics '91: Pre-Conference Proceedings.* New York: Springer-Verlag.

Werley, H., and Grier, M. (Eds.). (1981). *Nursing Information Systems.* New York: Springer.

Young, E. M. (Ed.). (1980). *Automated Hospital Information Systems Workbook:* Vol. 2. *Guide to AHIS Suppliers.* Los Angeles: Center Publications.

Yura, H., and Walsh, M. B. (1973). *The Nursing Process: Assessing, Planning, Implementing, Evaluating* (2d ed.). New York: Appleton-Century-Crofts.

Zielstorff, R. D. (Ed.). (1980). *Computers in Nursing.* Wakefield, MA: Nursing Resources.

Zielstorff, R. D., Hudgings, C., and Grobe, S. and the National Commission on Nursing Implementation Project (NCNIP) Task Force on Nursing Information Systems. (1993). *Next-Generation Nursing Information Systems: Essential Characteristics for Clinical Practice.* Washington, DC: American Nurses Association.

Zielstorff, R. D., Jette, A. M., and Barnett, G. O. (1990). Issues in designing an automated records system for clinical care and research. *Advances in Nursing Science, 13*(2), 75–88.

Zielstorff, R. D., McHugh, M. L., and Clinton, J. (1988). *Computer Design Criteria: For Systems That Support the Nursing Process.* Kansas City, MO: American Nurses Association.

# 8

• • • • • • • • • • • • • • • • • • • • • • •

# IMPLEMENTING AND UPGRADING NURSING INFORMATION SYSTEMS

## OBJECTIVES

- Describe the seven phases in developing, implementing, or upgrading a nursing information system.
- Describe the personnel responsible for implementing or upgrading a nursing information system.
- Identify the various tools of the trade used in developing, implementing, and upgrading a nursing information system.
- Describe the methods of evaluating a nursing information system.
- Describe new challenges in implementing and upgrading nursing information systems.

A computerized nursing information system (NIS), which assists nurses with decision making and problem solving, may be designed for different purposes: to (1) administer a nursing department, (2) assist the management of nursing practice, (3) assist nursing education, or (4) support nursing research. However, the NIS described in this chapter is designed primarily for a nursing department of a health care facility that provides patient care.

An NIS can be designed as a stand-alone system, a subsystem of a larger system, or an integral part of the health care organization's overall information system (Simpson, 1993a). It can be programmed for processing by a mainframe, a minicomputer, or a microcomputer, and it may share the same equipment that other systems in the facility use.

Because of the increasingly complex technology and information requirements, few hospitals and nursing departments develop or build their own NISs. Nevertheless, guidelines for implementing and upgrading a system generally apply to any situation in which nurses must evaluate an existing system, particularly since most systems serve as a "base" system which each nursing department or health care institution customizes or adapts to its unique and special needs.

In today's health care environment there are many hospitals that have implemented NISs, maintained them, and even completed an evaluation of their NISs. From the evaluation, new uses of the system have been demonstrated or suggested. Because of new legislation, new regulations, and new professional standards, NISs that are 10, 15, or even 20 years old must be upgraded. A discussion of the issues involved in upgrading an already existing NIS are a new feature of this chapter.

Regardless of what type of system is designed or what size computer it runs on, implementing and upgrading any NIS for a health care facility generally follows the seven phases listed below and adheres to the problem-solving approach or the scientific method. However, the terminology in this chapter has been updated to be consistent with proposed American Society for Testing and Materials language (ASTM, 1993). ASTM is a nonprofit organization whose technical committees establish standards for medical computer systems, among other things. The seven phases of implementing and upgrading an NIS are:

1. Planning phase
2. Analysis phase
3. Design phase
4. Development phase
5. Implementation phase
6. Evaluation phase
7. Upgrade phase

Nurse administrators are key to the successful implementation or upgrading of an NIS. They need to have a "vision" that accepts the importance of the information these systems can provide: (1) a business vision of the impact on the nursing department's resources, (2) a management vision of the policies and action plans that support the planning, implementation, and maintenance of these systems, and (3) a nursing vision of how the system can enhance the administration of clinical nursing practice (AONE and CHIM, 1993). Nurse administrators need to be involved in system selection, implementation, evaluation, and upgrading. In 1991 their involvement and participation in the selection process was mandated by the Joint Commission on Accreditation of Health Care Organizations

(JCAHO) (Simpson, 1991). JCAHO guidelines require that nurses be involved in evaluating, selecting, and integrating all systems that affect patient care and that this participation be documented as part of the Commission's accreditation reviews.

## NURSE EXECUTIVES' PREPLANNING REQUIREMENTS

Successful implementation of an NIS has been accomplished by many nurse administrators. In retrospect, recommendations to other nurse administrators have also been developed. They recommend that a preplanning business plan with the following features be included:

- An executive summary that "sells" the idea of information.
- An introduction that includes the purpose and objectives of the system.
- An environmental assessment of the NISs currently in use in similar hospitals.
- A design and implementation plan that includes the objectives, identification of test sites, listing of equipment needs, staffing projections, time resources, potential costs, and evaluation methodologies.
- A financial plan that projects staffing, budget, expenses, capital expenditures, and miscellaneous expenditures.
- A systems analysis of the nursing department culture, infrastructure, policies, and information needs.

All of these concepts are expanded in the seven phases of implementing a system that are described in this chapter.

## NIS Committee and Project Staff

Before an NIS is developed or selected, administrators must appoint an NIS committee and a project staff (Fig. 8.1). The NIS committee generally includes the following:

- A nursing representative from administration to uphold the nursing department's commitments
- A nursing representative from each of the major health care departments, programs, or units in the hospital
- A clinical nurse specialist/advanced practice nurse
- A systems nurse
- A staff physician
- A computer consultant
- A systems analyst
- Other appointed members

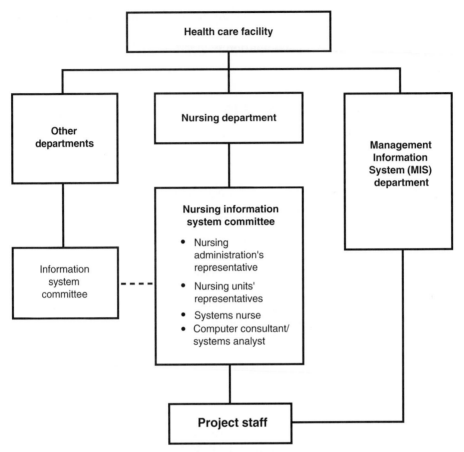

**Figure 8.1**   Organizational chart depicting an NIS committee.

The NIS committee needs to agree on the problem to be solved or the stated goal to be accomplished. If the system will affect nursing interactions or communications with physicians or other departments, then representatives from each should also be on the committee and involved in order to ensure acceptance at an early stage of the system plan and its phases. A clinical nurse specialist/advanced practice nurse should be on the committee in order to represent the patient-centered perspective because of his or her expert knowledge and familiarity with the care process (Simpson and Somers, 1991). Because of this patient-centered perspective, this specialist should have not only voting but also veto power on the committee.

The systems nurse must have had academic as well as hands-on practical training in computer technology; that is, the nurse must be both knowledgeable about computer technology and computer literate. He or she must also thoroughly understand the facility's nursing department and be authorized to act on its behalf. The computer consultant and systems analyst should have experience in developing information systems for the particular type of problem or particular goal in question. They may be staff members or may be contracted from outside.

The NIS committee has the responsibility for coordinating the entire project. Committee members must be responsive and assure that all activities are performed; they are responsible for obtaining needed resources. They must look after the nursing department's interests and those of the system's potential users. The committee must also collaborate with any other information system committees functioning in the facility. The committee, once established, initiates the system phases.

A project staff should also be established. This team should include at least the key members of the committee—the systems nurse, the clinical nurse specialist, and the computer department's systems analyst. The project staff is responsible to the NIS committee but also reports to the computer department in the facility. They are responsible for carrying out the seven phases and determining how the project is proceeding. Project staff size will vary depending on the size and scope of the system being selected, implemented, or upgraded. This staff must coordinate their activities with any other information system committee in the facility.

## PLANNING PHASE

A planning phase is critical, since during this initial phase the information required to solve the problem or accomplish the goal needs to be assessed. The information needs for the selection, implementation, or upgrading of an NIS, including implications for nursing services, nursing practice, and quality care, must also be identified. In the new proposed ASTM standards, the planning phase is referred to as the Project Definition. Computer vendors consider this phase the most critical factor in the selection of a system, even more important than the system itself (Zinn, 1989). Excellent planning is time-consuming and costly. It is estimated that the process of selecting a system can take up to 2 years and involves meetings that take from several hours to all day (Ginsburg and Browning, 1989). This phase is critical whether a system is actually being developed or existing vendor systems are being evaluated for selection fit. Either way, the same principles apply. The planning phase involves the following steps:

- Define problem and/or stated goal
- Conduct feasibility study
  - State objectives
  - Determine scope

     — Determine information needs
     — Decide whether to proceed
     — Negotiate the project definition agreement
     — Write the project definition document
- Allocate resources

## Define Problem

The first step in planning, to define the problem and/or stated goal precisely, is critical. It may not be easy because the stated problem and/or stated goal and the "real" problem and/or goal may differ. Not until the information requirements and outcomes of the problem and/or stated goal are determined are the real characteristics revealed (Fitzgerald et al., 1981).

     For example:

- Unfair nurse staff assignments may relate to an invalid patient classification tool (inaccurate grouping of patients) rather than to workload measurements and/or acuity scores.
- Duplicate health department reports may result from inappropriate statistics being collected instead of unique atomic-level data elements.

     The project definition should also include a description of how the system will be evaluated, so that when the evaluation phase is entered, several of the components being evaluated will have been documented. The results and improvements expected from installing the system need to be realistically described. These might include increased processing capabilities, savings in time, decreased costs, or increased personnel productivity. In updated or expanded NISs, the project definition should also include the identification of equipment currently available, its age, the degree of amortization, and the need for hardware or software upgrades.

## Conduct Feasibility Study

The feasibility study analyzes the problem and/or stated goal to determine how either and if the development of an NIS will solve the problem or achieve the goal. The feasibility study not only clarifies the problem and/or stated goal but helps to identify the objectives, scope, and information needs. The feasibility study helps the NIS committee understand the real problem and/or goal by analyzing all the parameters and presenting possible solutions. It highlights whether the system is worth what it costs and whether it will produce usable products. Thus, the study addresses the critical elements for developing a system and is, in a sense, a model of a "minisystem." It includes a description of the human resources required and how the selected system will be developed and implemented.

The feasibility study should describe the procedures and the process needed to obtain administrative, financial, and technical approvals to proceed with each phase of the project. It is critical to consider relevant organizational and statutory requirements.

## State Objectives

The first step in the feasibility study is to state the objectives for the proposed system, which constitute the purpose(s) of the system. All objectives and outcomes should be stated in terms appropriate for computer processing. They should identify the "end product" and what the NIS will do for the nurses.

For example:

- An objective relating to nurse assignments might be stated as follows: "Develop a nurse staffing and scheduling NIS that uses a valid and reliable patient classification system.
- An objective relating to statistical reporting in a community health agency might be stated as follows: "Develop a system for reporting atomic-level statistical data as required by local, state, and federal authorities."

## Determine Scope

The scope of the proposed system establishes system constraints, including its controls and parameters, and outlines what the proposed system will and will not produce.

For example:

- The scope of a nurse staffing system might be stated as follows: "The system should provide nurse staffing only for the medical and surgical units, and not for specialty units."
- The scope of a system relating to community health statistical reporting might be stated as follows: "The system should collect only data needed for routine and ongoing, not one-time, reports."

## Determine Information Needs

In this step, sometimes called a needs assessment, the information that system users will require is outlined. Identifying the information needed helps clarify what users will expect from the system. Such knowledge is essential in designing system output, input, and processing needs.

For example:

- A nurse staffing and scheduling system based on patient classification would need the following information:
  — A valid patient classification tool for determining staffing requirements
  — The number of nursing personnel required to staff each medical and surgical unit
  — Types of nursing personnel required to staff the units

- A statistical reporting system designed to meet local, state, and federal reporting would require the following information:
  — Time personnel spend making visits
  — Cost of visits by type of provider
  — Number of clients per program
  — Number of services provided to clients by nurses
  — Sites where services are provided

## Decide Whether to Proceed with the Project

Committees often forget that they can not only decide to proceed but also decide not to proceed with a project. In considering the upgrading or expansion of a system, improvements in the management and coordination of existing systems must be implemented before new systems are procured. It is critical to consider whether more personnel or equipment rather than more computerization is what is required. Besides identifying potential hardware and software improvements, the costs and benefits are also weighed at this time.

## Negotiate the Project Definition Agreement

A project definition agreement that has been accepted by the full committee and has administrative and financial approvals is needed. The agreement should also include technical management and personnel who will maintain the equipment. The agreement should cover the following issues:

- What is the real problem to be solved and/or stated goal to be achieved?
- Why is the project to be accomplished?
- What specific outcomes are expected from the project?
- What is to be accomplished in the project?
- What are the measurable benefits from the above outcomes?
- What are the estimated costs?
- What is the justification for the project, including the relationship between costs and benefits?
- What are the assumptions that support the project?
- What are the known constraints on the project?
- What are the boundaries/limitations of the project?
- What are the project risks and their causes?
- What is the timing of the remaining phases of the project?
- Who will be committed to implementing the project, and what positions do they hold?

## Write the Project Definition Document

The project proposal is a written document that includes the feasibility of the project, formal project requests and approvals, and the project definition agreement (above). If the project includes several subprojects, a separate project definition should be written for each.

## Allocate Resources

The last step in the planning phase is determining what resources are needed to make the NIS work. A firm commitment of resources for development of the entire NIS is needed before the system can fulfill its stated objectives. The following points should be considered: present workload; human resources, with numbers, experience, and abilities; present cost of operation; space available; and current equipment available.

## ANALYSIS PHASE

The analysis phase, the second phase of developing an NIS, is the fact-finding phase. All data related to the problem are collected and analyzed in order to understand what exists and what is needed. This analysis is essential to the actual system design. Also examined are the objectives and scope as written in the feasibility study, the informational and functional requirements, the data flow procedures, and the scope (boundaries, interfaces, and decision points). Current costs and resources required for processing the data are compared with estimates for a new system. If a system is being upgraded or expanded, it is during this phase that the current equipment and functions are described. Depreciation of available equipment and budget for projected future expansion are also described.

The analysis phase consists of the following four steps:

- Collect data
- Analyze data
- Review data
- Identify benefits

## Collect Data

Collecting data is a fact-finding activity. In the analysis of the existing nursing problem or goal, data collection reveals the full scope of the project. The major sources of data essential for this activity are as follows:

- Written documents
- Questionnaires
- Interviews
- Observations

## Written Documents

Written documents, collected to ascertain different aspects of the nursing problem or stated goal, must be carefully reviewed. They include standards, orders, procedures, operating manuals, routine reports, and forms used to collect data. Further, the raw facts (data elements) themselves must be analyzed, including their processing, a flowchart of the process, and the resultant reports.

## Questionnaires

Questionnaires, another source of information, provide useful information without being too time-consuming. Questionnaires sent to the potential users can ascertain the needs of the different types of system users and collect the opinions of the potential users as to what should be computerized, what the turnaround-time requirements should be, and what products should be produced.

## Interviews

Interviews are one of the best sources of information on an existing nursing problem or stated goal. Interviews with selected personnel at all organizational levels can elicit very specific information on how, when, where, and in what kinds of situations data are processed. Moreover, standard interviews help to document, in a logical sequence, the kinds of information requested.

## Observations

Observations are another excellent way to understand staff views. They can reveal how staff members relate to one another, how they manage the information they handle, and how they use that information. For example, this may include a time study to determine the time spent on various nursing activities.

## Analyze Data

The proposed analysis of the data is critical. This process provides a complete overview of the nursing problem and/or stated goal in order to better understand its scope. Several tools and methods of documentation are necessary to help review and gain perspective on all collected data. Some of the more common tools are as follows:

- Data flowchart
- Grid chart
- Decision table
- Organizational chart
- Model

## Data Flowchart

A data flowchart, one of the most important tools in data analysis, graphically illustrates the sequential steps in processing the nursing problem or accomplishing the stated goal. It provides a "road map" of the flow of information. A flowchart of the data is an excellent tool for tracing where and when the flow of information begins and where it goes.

## Grid Chart

A grid chart, also called a data analysis chart, analyzes the interrelationships of the data used to process the nursing problem and/or achieve the stated goal. It generally includes a listing of all the data elements collected as input that are processed and generated as output. A grid chart can also be used to list the kinds of information generated as output, including purpose and recipient.

## Decision Table

A decision table, sometimes called a decision-logic table, illustrates the logical decisions and possible alternatives for solving the nursing problem and/or achieving the stated goal. It provides a tabular display of all relevant data, lists all possible choices, and highlights the logical rules used for processing the data.

## Organizational Chart

An organizational chart depicts the levels of authority and the formal lines of interorganizational communication. The chart also helps to distinguish line personnel from staff personnel, depicts the reporting relationships among various positions, and shows various jobs. It helps clarify who is responsible for what and how current data are processed.

## Model

A model provides an abstraction of a real situation, thus helping to analyze circumstances that are too complex for actual presentation. Moreover, it is far more economical to develop a model that graphically displays the proposed system than to present the real-life situation.

For example:

- A model can outline the various nurse staffing patterns for the different care units.
- A model can display the flow process of statistical data from origin to termination.

The two major types of models relevant to data analysis are forecasting and simulation. Forecasting helps with decision making. For example, it may be used to predict future staffing needs based on certain assumptions.

Simulation, on the other hand, presents an abstraction of reality. Simulations can be used to present how different staffing needs will vary based on different ground rules. Both models can be used to determine the best method of predicting staffing.

Other types of models are available. Network planning models can highlight the resources, time, materials, and major activities relevant to a given process. Both the program evaluation review technique (PERT) and the critical path method (CPM) are network models for planning, scheduling, and controlling a system's activities. The latter generally highlights a time frame and sometimes the cost for completing a project.

## Review Data

The next step in the analysis phase is to review all the data. All pertinent information on the nursing problem and/or stated goal is summarized in a report that is sent to the NIS committee. This final review furnishes the basis for recommendations concerning the proposed NIS and raises the question: "How well will the proposed NIS correct or eliminate the existing nursing problem or accomplish the stated goal?"

Carefully managed, data review can be beneficial. In a sense, it clarifies what can be done and what should be done. It can help develop better standards, documentation, and procedures for better management control, and it sets forth the requirements for the new system design. As a result of this review, a model that graphically displays the major components of the proposed system is produced. In addition to displaying the major components, the model outlines what information is required and what resources (functional requirements) are needed to carry out the stated objectives. In addition, the model shows system controls. Finally, the model presents the actual time and costs needed to make the system work.

## Identify Benefits

There are many benefits of a careful structured analysis. The major benefit is an early understanding of the design and a focus on user-friendliness; the users are able to evaluate the system's potential capability and begin to plan for training and for the implementation of the system.

The benefits to the technicians on the team are in determining the feasibility of their design, determining if the time estimates are accurate, promoting better understanding, and focusing on efficiency and flexibility in design.

The major benefits for staff include the following:

- Users: A careful analysis allows review of information and input, helps them to understand what implementation plans need to be designed, and helps them to coordinate with the client code.

- Management: The careful design allows monitoring of the vendors' ability to deliver products on time and within budget, and determining the level of potential user satisfaction.
- Sales and marketing personnel: The analysis provides valuable information for marketing.

The benefits for services include the following: (1) for documentation, the facility can start early pilots and sequence screens appropriate to data needs, and (2) for quality assurance, it can establish early standards for review and begin to test the content.

## DESIGN PHASE

The design phase is divided into two parts: (1) functional design and (2) implementation design. In the functional design phase, the existing nursing problem is solved and/or the stated goal is achieved with a better system. It is possible to design a new system because the problem and/or goal has been defined, analyzed, and reviewed.

## Functional Design

Functional requirements for an NIS include a detailed description of the system inputs, outputs, and transfer functions that are needed. In short, the functional design highlights what the proposed system will encompass and provides the framework for its operation. A functional design study identifies the types of information that are relevant to solving the problem and the types of computer resources that are essential for developing the system. It provides a cost estimate and presents ways to manage and maintain the system; it also gives a projected time frame for completion. A functional design is a detailed description of a system that includes all flows of information, timing diagrams, and state transition diagrams, and is independent of particular hardware and software. The functional design is an exact, concise description of the functions required in a proposed computerized system. It describes how the computer will accomplish its task.

Nurse administrators or project staff should require that each vendor produce a detailed functional specifications document that includes an introduction, a section for each pathway, and a technical section. Also included in the functional design phase are the definitions of technical and nontechnical considerations. They include:

- Personnel
- Time frame
- Cost and budget
- Facilities and equipment
- Data manipulation and output

- Operational considerations
- Human–computer interactions
- System validation plan

## Personnel

The additional staff needed to implement the system may be drawn from several sources, including the nursing department, an existing management information system unit, or a consulting firm or computer vendor. Three types of personnel should be hired or contracted for consultation: the systems analyst, the functional designer, and the business expert (Edmunds, 1992). These personnel act as translators between the users and the programmers so that before any line of code is created, there is a detailed understanding of what the application will do and how it will work. It is recommended that the group communicate via verbal agreements, text documents, prototypes, detailed functional specifications, models, and case tools.

The project staff appointed at the beginning of the investigation should, if possible, be retained for the duration of the project. These persons, especially the systems nurse and the computer consultant or systems analyst, have worked closely with NIS committee members through the planning phase and the decision to proceed.

In all nursing matters related to developing an NIS, the systems nurse assumes leadership. He or she is directly responsible to the nursing department administrator and the nursing committee. The "key person" who understands the functions of the nursing department, the systems nurse has the clinical expertise to implement the nursing requirements of the NIS and the ability to implement the training programs to educate nursing personnel about the system.

A successful NIS requires a capable systems analyst, one who has been vital in developing the information system for nurses. He or she must be able to design, develop, and implement an information system. The systems manager may be selected from any of the above sources but must be a capable administrator. Such a person not only supervises the development of the system but administers project staff personnel, time, budget control, and cost activities. This person is responsible to the NIS committee.

## Time Frame

A time frame for outlining and synchronizing all the steps in developing the NIS is needed. The functional design phase includes a detailed description of a system, which provides all flows of information, timing diagrams, and state transition diagrams, and which is independent of particular hardware and software. A milestone chart or a Gantt chart can be useful for plotting, in sequence, the major tasks and accomplishments required in developing the NIS. The milestone chart consists of lines; the Gantt chart uses bar graphs to highlight activities and the time of their completion (Fig. 8.2).

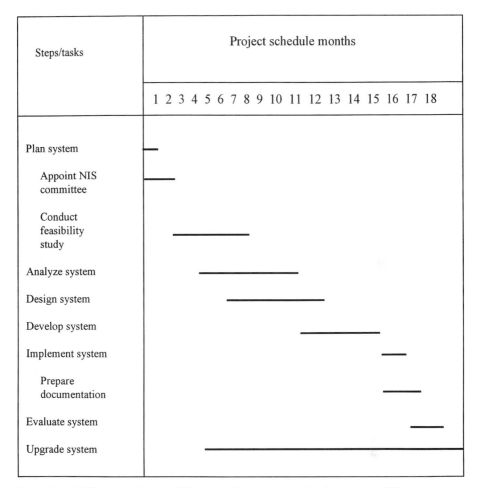

**Figure 8.2**    Milestone chart outlining major steps in developing an NIS.

## Cost and Budget

The cost and budget for developing an NIS must be established and approved "up front," since without them the system cannot be completed in a timely, cost-effective manner. It is critical that funds be set aside for developing, managing, maintaining, and evaluating the system. Funds are also needed for ongoing staff training. The budget for the system must be approved by the NIS committee, but continued budget control and auditing are the project manager's responsibility.

## Facilities and Equipment

All computerized systems require facilities and equipment, that is, hardware, software, and peripheral equipment. A computer–information system unit may be needed to house the basic hardware and its components, especially if a mainframe or large minicomputer system is being considered. Such a unit must be large enough to store all relevant working materials and equipment. The computer unit staff must also be organized, with lines of authority and established formal communication channels.

## Data Manipulation and Output

There are several considerations for handling data manipulation and output (ASTM Proposed Standards, 1993). The detailed functional specifications are critical to the designer, since they analyze every screen, every flow, every print, and every report that the user can expect to see. The designer can provide this level of detail with sketches, explanations, and/or examples. With a sketch the designer can show the project team that standards have been incorporated into the design to minimize ambiguity in communication features. From a designer's perspective, these sketches also decrease required programming time. The explanation specification provides a drawing to show what the system will look like and clarify how the system will work. The examples incorporate real data into the explanations and drawings.

During this phase the designers and users have to determine what the actual raw data will look like and whether they need to be transformed. Are slopes or maximum and minimum values required? What is the length of time that the data need to remain in a file? What are the procedures for converting raw data into transformed information? Finally, the accuracy and precision of the transformed data need to be stated and determined.

## Operational Considerations

The operational considerations include detailed information related to when the system would be scheduled for routine maintenance, plans for operations during system failures, and acceptable time for the system to be out of service. Additional requirements for data reliability and availability are stated for planned and unplanned system failures. Another important feature is to define data recovery procedures after a system has failed.

## Human–Computer Interactions

The team must take into account the level of education and training expected for each person who will interact with the computer, that person's ability to query the system or designers and operators, and the access that person will have to individual sections of the system.

## System Validation Plan

For each element in the functional requirements, criteria should be set for measuring system validity. Included in these criteria are accuracy, precision, production rate, and "throughput." Regulations and recommendations emerging from standard setting groups suggest that a validation plan be in place for meeting formal quality and accreditation requirements.

## Implementation Design

The second part of the systems design phase is the implementation design. This design produces the complete detailed specifications of the proposed system. The outline indicates how the system functions and explains how it will look and what it will offer its users. An implementation design puts together the goals, constraints, and functional requirements to determine a strategy for implementation. During this phase, inconsistencies are found and the earlier documents have to be corrected. This phase considers the important steps in the efficient implementation of a computerized system. Whereas the functional design focuses on system constraints, such as time, costs, and personnel, the implementation design phase focuses on experience, professional judgment, and good craftsmanship. The major steps leading to such a design include the following:

- Design inputs
- Design outputs
- Design files and databases
- Design controls

### Design Inputs

Designing the inputs is a major step in system design. Inputs (data) make up the computer files and databases. What type of inputs to design depends largely on how data will be processed (e.g., on-line, real-time/interactive, or batch processing) and on the required outputs. Input and output designs require the following factors: content, data source, scope, format, medium, coding scheme, editing rules, testing, estimates of volumes, and frequency.

The content of each input (data element) must be specified in detail to meet output requirements. Each data element that is an input should be processed for an output. The source, definitions, rules, and codes of the data elements must be fully spelled out. Data that are collected repeatedly, such as patient identification information, should be entered only once.

The scope of the data inputs should always be the smallest definable data elements. For example, the birth date and not the age of a patient should be entered as an input. Each input must also be in a format that users will readily understand. For example, temperature, pulse, and respirations, when collected, should be entered in that order.

All types of input must be tested to ensure that essential data elements needed for outputs are logical and have been collected. They should be revised and retested, if necessary, to guarantee that they are correct. Also, both estimated volume and frequency must be addressed. The number of input forms that will be completed establishes certain input requirements. Likewise, how often nurses use a cathode ray tube (CRT) terminal determines how many terminals the system will require.

## Design Outputs

Designing the NIS outputs is concurrent with designing the inputs. They must be completed when or before the inputs are designed because they identify the data required as input. The outputs provide the information the users need and basically justify the system. The design of the outputs is critical to the success of the NIS. Good output design requires an understanding of users' (i.e., nurses') needs. The following factors must be considered: content, format, medium, estimated volume, frequency, and distribution.

The content and purpose of each output must be specified in detail, and each output should be in a meaningful and easy-to-understand format. For example, the format of a report may increase its effectiveness if numbers appear with clarifiers such as percentages. Also to be considered is what type of medium will best present the output. An output can be a report produced on paper, microfilm, or microfiche; a display on a CRT terminal; or a graphic representation from a graphic output device. Sometimes output may be a product from any of the other computer output media.

The estimated volume, frequency, and distribution of the outputs should be based on potential users' expected needs. Who the users are, what outputs they require, and at what time must be spelled out in detail.

## Design Files and Databases

Files and databases must be designed to ensure efficient data processing and to help ensure prompt responses to users' informational needs. Several areas of concern must be explored: content, record format, file organization, file access, and storage requirements. The size of each file and database, including the content and format of records, must be specified in detail. Both are essential to avoid redundancy in filed data. Also, the data elements themselves must be organized in the records, files, and databases to enhance processing.

File organization is also important, since it determines whether files and databases will be developed according to the "top-down" or "bottom-up" approach. The top-down approach starts with the end product and proceeds to analyze its data elements. The bottom-up approach starts with the data elements and builds them up for processing into the end product. For example, a patient classified by one number (level) reflects the top-down approach. However, a patient classified by combining activities reflects the bottom-up approach.

Storage requirements are also affected by users' needs. Files that must be accessed by on-line or real-time/interactive processing will require random access storage devices. However, files that are accessed off-line for batch processing, for example, can use off-line storage devices. Storage is also affected by file size and volume and frequency of use. Another aspect of file storage is the updating and purging of files. Special rules for retaining and destroying data are required. What data are stored and for how long are questions that must be resolved. The use of data for analysis, such as audit, quality assurance, and research, will also affect storage requirements.

### Design Controls

Design controls ensure that input data are duly processed, that output information is complete and accurate, and that no data have been lost or stolen. System controls help minimize and eliminate system errors. Adequate controls can be established by several different methods. It is possible, for example, to determine the accuracy of the source documents being input by balancing the input totals against the output totals. Controls of data input may be achieved through automatic checking of data limits to ascertain that the data are within normal ranges. Audit trails can also be used to check and trace transactions from input to output. The matching of computer-processed outputs with manually processed ones can help to ascertain that data are being processed correctly.

Still another type of system control calls for backup files. They allow the NIS to remain intact even if its current data files are damaged or destroyed. System controls also imply that the files are secure and protected. The security of the files must be maintained, and every effort must be made to protect the privacy of patients' files. Procedures must be followed to ensure system integrity and security.

## Functional Design Phase Criteria

In 1988, the American Nurses Association (ANA) published a booklet that described the design of computer systems that support the nursing process (Zielstorff et al., 1988). Four categories of criteria to consider are described: (1) NIS capabilities, (2) user–machine interface, (3) hardware requirements, and (4) data security and integrity.

## DEVELOPMENT PHASE

In the development phase, the design is completed and the system is ready for preparation. Generally, whether a system is developed in-house or through a contract with a computer vendor or system supplier, contract services will be required for maintenance. Selecting contract services is time-consuming. It requires the following activities:

- Request for proposal
- Evaluate responses
- Negotiate contract

## Request for Proposal

The results of the planning phase are generally summarized in a report for review by the NIS committee. The report should contain the planning phase findings as outlined in the earlier section and should make recommendations concerning whether the existing information system should be upgraded, a new system instituted, or the proposed system incorporated into an existing larger system. It recommends the kind of system, subsystem, or components appropriate for solving the problem and whether the system should be developed in-house or through contract services. It also needs to estimate both costs and benefits. This report must be approved by the NIS committee before the project staff can develop the NIS.

If a system is being purchased from a vendor or outside developer, the organization must clearly spell out its objectives, functional requirements, budgetary constraints, and schedules in the request for proposal (RFP). An RFP, sometimes called a solicitation bid, is circulated among prospective bidders. A formal statement of the specifications of the system, it is a standard document that outlines the system objectives and design requirements and provides the basis for judging the vendor's ability to meet all requirements using weighted values and proper term definitions to identify general requirements.

The RFP should include the following points:

- Introduce the vendor or contractor to the overall environment in the organization and in which the system will be used.
- Identify general requirements and describe how information will be supplied.
- Describe any performance bond or equivalent requirement.
- State conditions of an equipment demonstration.
- Outline the method of financing.
- Specify training and orientation for the products.
- Cite criteria for evaluating proposals.
- State the standards of performance that will be used in deciding system acceptability.
- State specific hardware and software requirements.

Initially, as mentioned earlier, an RFP is circulated among the prospective bidders. The prospective bidders generally respond with a response called a request for contract (RFC).

## Evaluate Responses

The bidders' RFCs are evaluated by the NIS committee and the financial and contract officers and/or lawyers from the agency. An evaluation form is used to score the vendors' capabilities for fulfilling the system requirements (Fig. 8.3). The evaluation scores help to identify the eligible system suppliers. Once a bidder's proposal has been selected, the NIS committee

Reviewer Name: _____

Reviewer Name: _____   Date: _____

Application: _____

| SYSTEM ATTRIBUTES | CIRCLE SCORE |
|---|---|
| Availability of Required Features | 1   2   3   4   5 |
| Ease of Use | 1   2   3   4   5 |
| System Flexibility | 1   2   3   4   5 |
| Appearance of Screens | 1   2   3   4   5 |
| Appearance of Reports | 1   2   3   4   5 |
| Confidence That System Will Meet Expectations | 1   2   3   4   5 |
| Response Time | 1   2   3   4   5 |
| Availability of Health Features | 1   2   3   4   5 |
| Quality of Documentation | 1   2   3   4   5 |
| Impression of Vendor | 1   2   3   4   5 |
| Overall System Desirability | 1   2   3   4   5 |
| **TOTAL AVERAGE RATING** | 1   2   3   4   5 |

LEGEND:       POOR (1)       AVERAGE (2-3)       GOOD (4-5)

COMMENTS: _____

_____

**Figure 8.3**   Vendor demonstration evaluation form.

should make site visits to view the proposed system in operation and check out other facilities that use the supplier's systems. Such visits allow the committee members not only to see the system but also to question nurses using the system. Issues that might be addressed on a site visit are included in Fig. 8.4. Questions that might be asked on the site visit are included in Table 8.1. The vendors' costs should be compared and ranked prior to negotiating the contract (Tables 8.2 and 8.3).

## Negotiate Contract

The final step in this process is to select the supplier and negotiate a contract. The successful bidder is contracted to develop a system, provide an already developed system, or adapt another facility's system to meet the NIS committee's specifications. The system that is chosen for purchase must be described in the negotiated contract between the supplier and the buyer. Recommended negotiation strategies include ten principles for making the contract process less cumbersome (Ciotti & Bogutski, 1994):

- Negotiate with several "finalists" because this allows hospitals to make concessions outside of competitive negotiations.
- Start making concession statements a part of the RFP, and make the RFP checklist a part of the contract as the "product definition."

Reviewer Name: _____
Application: _____

| SYSTEM ATTRIBUTES | VENDOR #1 | VENDOR #2 | VENDOR #3 |
|---|---|---|---|
| Availability of this system to support the operation | 1 2 3 4 5 | 1 2 3 4 5 | 1 2 3 4 5 |
| Ease with which the customer learned to use the system | 1 2 3 4 5 | 1 2 3 4 5 | 1 2 3 4 5 |
| Least amount of difficulty implementing the system | 1 2 3 4 5 | 1 2 3 4 5 | 1 2 3 4 5 |
| Vendor support of the customer | 1 2 3 4 5 | 1 2 3 4 5 | 1 2 3 4 5 |
| Overall customer satisfaction with the vendor | 1 2 3 4 5 | 1 2 3 4 5 | 1 2 3 4 5 |
| Least resources necessary to support the system | 1 2 3 4 5 | 1 2 3 4 5 | 1 2 3 4 5 |
| Overall system desirability for hospital | 1 2 3 4 5 | 1 2 3 4 5 | 1 2 3 4 5 |
| TOTAL AVERAGE RATING | | 1   2   3   4   5 | |

| LEGEND: | POOR (1) | AVERAGE (2-3) | GOOD (4-5) |
|---|---|---|---|
| | Vendor #1 | Vendor #2 | Vendor #3 |
| Advantages | | | |
| Disadvantages | | | |
| Critical Changes (necessary to use this system) | | | |

**Figure 8.4**   Vendor site visit evaluation form.

**TABLE 8.1**     SITE VISIT QUESTIONNAIRE

Departmental Questions

Vendor name _____ Date ___/___/___

Institution _____

Contact name _____

Contact title _____

Department director _____

Phone number/extension ___(___  ___)_____

What is your length of employment with this facility? _____yrs

Were you involved in the selection of the system?   Yes _____No _____

What is your opinion of the vendor personnel who assisted you in the:

Training _____
_____

Installation _____
_____

Conversion _____
_____

Support _____
_____

**TABLE 8.2**    WORKSHEET COMPARING VENDOR COSTS

| Information System Application | Vendor/Supplier Costs | | | | | |
|---|---|---|---|---|---|---|
| | **A** | **B** | **C** | **D** | **E** | **F** |
| Admission/patient registration | $ | $ | $ | $ | $ | $ |
| Master patient census | $ | $ | $ | $ | $ | $ |
| Order-entry network | $ | $ | $ | $ | $ | $ |
| Patient care plans/protocols | $ | $ | $ | $ | $ | $ |
| Patient accounts | $ | $ | $ | $ | $ | $ |
| Patient classification | $ | $ | $ | $ | $ | $ |
| Nurse staffing | $ | $ | $ | $ | $ | $ |
| Nurse scheduling | $ | $ | $ | $ | $ | $ |
| Nurse personnel payroll | $ | $ | $ | $ | $ | $ |
| Total | $ | $ | $ | $ | $ | $ |

- Insist on having draft copies of proposed contracts in advance of contract signing, and change contract language until it is acceptable.
- Request staggered payments, for example, 10 percent with contract, 30 percent upon delivery of hardware and software, 20 percent upon successful implementation, 20 percent upon full implementation, and 20 percent 30 days after the first month-end and the corrections of any discrepancies that have been noticed. It is usually not until after implementation that problems are found in systems.
- Understand when final acceptance occurs, i.e., when the development and implementation phases end and the maintenance phase begins.
- Extend payments of invoices beyond 45 to 60 days to reflect the ability of the hospital accountants to check for accuracies.
- Negotiate the interest rate paid on payments beyond the specified due date to what Medicare, Medicaid, and Blue Cross pay in your state for remittances older than one month.

**TABLE 8.3**    WORKSHEET RANKING VENDORS

| System Vendor/ Supplier Name | Vendor/Supplier Functional Requirements | |
|---|---|---|
| | Total Points (100 Maximum) | Rank |
| A | 72 | 5 |
| B | 65 | 6 |
| C | 80 | 2 |
| D | 85 | 1 |
| E | 77 | 3 |
| F | 75 | 4 |

- Insist on taking several months after the system has been implemented to determine if the product matches the vendor's positive performance responses in the vendor's proposal.
- Insist on response time guarantees.
- Require installers to walk through your facility before contract negotiations are signed, and/or negotiate an installation plan the same way that the system negotiations were carried out.

On the other hand, if the NIS committee decides to develop its own system, the project staff must proceed with the development phase of the system, which includes the following:

- Select hardware
- Develop software
- Test system
- Document system

## Select Hardware

Selecting the correct hardware for the system depends on the system's design, application, and software requirements. These conditions dictate whether to select a mainframe, a minicomputer, a microcomputer, or a combination. Computer hardware is obtained in several different ways. Mainframes and minicomputers may be purchased or leased from a vendor for in-house use. However, if cost is a factor, then timesharing with other facilities should be considered. Since microcomputers are small, they may be the most economical for network applications. Input, output, and processing media, including secondary storage, must also be selected, and all hardware must be installed and able to test the computer programs at the appropriate time.

## Develop Software

Developing software requires careful consideration of the system design. Software must suit the hardware and the specific application, making it necessary to choose the correct software programs and/or the correct programming language in which to write the computer programs. If programs are to be written, the composition of the computer hardware and the programming needs of the NIS must be examined before an appropriate programming language can be selected. A programmer must write the computer program, which is generally done in the following logical sequence: (1) prepare a narrative description of the system, (2) develop flowcharts showing program codes, (3) write the actual programs needed to process all inputs, design the files and databases, and generate all outputs, and (4) test and debug the computer programs until they are considered free of errors.

## Test System

The system must be tested to ensure that all data are processed correctly and generate the desired outputs. Testing helps verify that the computer programs are written correctly and ensures that, when implemented, the system will run as planned.

The computer programs are tested first to determine whether the programming protocols are used correctly and then to determine if they are correct. Use live data (real facts) to test the overall computer programs, and revise and retest the programs until they are proved to be reliable and valid. This process provides a review of all test inputs, test files, and test outputs to ensure that all data are entered, stored, and processed correctly. The procedures needed to implement the system are also tested, including all procedures that users will follow to "run" the system.

## Document System

Documentation, the preparation of documents to describe the system for all users, must be an ongoing activity as the various system phases and steps are developed. Documentation should begin with the initial description of the project and continue through the system design, implementation, evaluation, and upgrading. It must give detailed specifications on what information the system requires and what makes the system function, and it must include detailed information on the design and coding structure of inputs, outputs, and flowcharts and file layouts.

Several manuals are usually prepared, the major ones being a user's manual, an operator's manual, and a maintenance manual. These manuals provide guides to the system components and outline how the entire system has been put together.

### User's Manual
The user's manual discusses how to use the system and describes what outputs the system can produce.

### Operator's Manual
The operator's manual instructs operators on how to run the system. It describes what data are input, how they are processed, and the way in which particular outputs are generated.

### Maintenance Manual
The maintenance manual enables operators to keep the system "live" by providing the specifications needed to upgrade, revise, and correct it.

Proper documentation is directed to the system users and operators who will maintain it. Manuals must be written in sufficient detail to help all of these people understand how the system was developed, how it operates, and how it can be maintained, updated, and repaired.

# IMPLEMENTATION PHASE

The implementation phase, often called the "go-live phase," ensures that once the system is installed, it will run smoothly. The implementation design includes a detailed description of the system that specifies not only all hardware and software components but implementation, training, operation, and maintenance procedures as well. To implement the system, the project staff and NIS committee must coordinate their efforts and conduct the following steps:

- Train users
- Install system
- Manage and maintain system

## Train Users

It is essential to train nurses how to use the system properly. Usually the systems nurse does this training. An NIS will function only as well as its users understand its operation. Nurses must understand the capabilities of the system. Training should take place before, during, and, as needed, after system implementation.

Training generally consists of lectures on system use. Training guides or manuals can explain the system. Computer-assisted instruction (CAI) in a special training room or on the units and/or an integral part of the system can be used to provide hands-on experience. Training should be offered at two levels: one to provide a general overview of the system, and another to explain the system in detail. The first presentation is aimed at NIS committee members or others needing an introduction to system objectives and capabilities. The second presentation, directed at nursing personnel using the system, must explain the system in detail and provide in-depth information on how to use it. These users will also require on-the-job assistance. The user's manual, described above, should be retained for all users.

## Install System

Implementation means installing the system and then getting it to operate correctly after the computer programs have been tested, debugged, revised, and retested; users trained, procedures established; and the total system rechecked. The conversion from the old method to the new depends on available personnel and equipment, system complexity and size, and users' needs.

Four approaches are possible: (1) parallel, (2) pilot, (3) phased-in, and (4) crash. In the parallel approach, the new system runs in parallel with the existing method until users can adjust. In the pilot approach, a few users try out the new system to see how it works and help others to use it. In the phased-in approach, the system is implemented one unit at a time. In the crash approach, the old system is stopped abruptly and the new one is installed.

System installation includes establishing procedures for operating the system, including time frames and deadlines for entering data and generating outputs and reports. Accepted procedures for correcting errors and checking data also are important. Decisions on how long data files will be stored and when they will be purged or destroyed must be resolved. In short, all procedural activities must be put in final form.

## Manage and Maintain System

System success depends on management and maintenance. Management of an NIS is a continuous process. A separate unit in the agency may be needed to administer the system. Such a unit requires not only a clear line of authority but adequate staffing, an office, and a budget. Special procedures and operating policies must be established to guide the unit. The unit staff, generally consisting of the project staff, oversees the management of the system and ensures that the operating procedures are followed. They must be able to respond properly and assist system users.

The system also needs continuous maintenance and monitoring by the unit staff. Maintenance activities include keeping the hardware in working order, monitoring system security, updating and revising computer programs as needed, and instituting cost-saving measures.

## EVALUATION PHASE

Evaluating the system is the final step in implementation. The system must be assessed to determine whether it meets the stated objectives satisfactorily. An evaluation study attempts to describe and assess, in detail, system performance. It summarizes the entire system, thus identifying any weaknesses. A sound evaluation study can sometimes lead to a revised, and better, system.

During this phase the system is evaluated to determine whether it has accomplished the stated objectives. A system evaluation involves a comparison of a working system with its requirements to determine how well the requirements are met, to determine possibilities for growth and improvement, and to preserve the lessons of a computerization project in preparation for future efforts. A collection of system documents can facilitate the evaluation phase if appropriate parts of the planning and design phases of the project were kept.

This evaluation component becomes a continuous phase in total quality management. The totally implemented system will require continuous

evaluation to determine if upgrading is appropriate or what enhancements could be added to the current system. Evaluation also helps to identify components of the implemented system that are obsolete.

Evaluation generally takes place not less than 6 months after the system has been implemented and routinely every 2 to 4 years thereafter.
The evaluation should be conducted by an outside evaluation team so that
it will be objective.

## Review Entire System

The evaluation process involves a review of the entire system. This includes
the hardware, software, and products. In essence, a study has to be conducted that not only provides an overview of the system, but also evaluates
its results. The entire computer operation, including users, procedures,
quality of equipment, and the scope and validity of databases, are examined. Functional performance and technical performance are evaluated thoroughly, and system costs and benefits are assessed (McCormick, 1983).

The following criteria are considered essential in selecting a nursing
information system and can be used as a basis for evaluation (Hewlett-
Packard, 1993):

- Applications
- Overall system performance
- Evaluation features
- Ease of system use
- Configuration or program-
  ming performance
- Security

- Simplification of reports
- Database access
- Hardware and software
  reliability
- Connectivity
- System cost

Evaluation of the functional performance of the system requires
methods and tools that compare operations before and after system
implementation. Such tools should be designed to identify the effects the
NIS has on the nursing components of patient care. For example:

- Did nurses improve their documentation of patient care by system use?
- Did their documentation take less time than previously and thus leave
  more time for providing patient care?
- Did system use increase their awareness of patients' problems?

If so, the system may be considered an aid to improving the quality of
patient care. In addition, nurse administrators should also be concerned
with "high-level" benefits such as nursing satisfaction (which can be ascer-
tained by retention levels and questionnaires), patient satisfaction, decreased
lengths of stay, reduced errors of omission, and improved quality of care
(Simpson, 1993b).

In evaluating an implemented NIS, many other principles are also important. One authority suggests evaluating duplication, fragmentation, misplaced work, complexity, bottlenecks, review/approval process, error reporting (or the amount of reworking of content), movement, wait time, delays, setup, low-importance outputs, and unimportant outputs (Young, 1981).

The recommended solutions to some of these problems are to eliminate the activity, combine activities, transfer activities, simplify the flow of work, change methods or add resources to eliminate the bottleneck, self-inspect, eliminate causes, combine steps or move personnel, change the flow or balance the loads, change methods of doing things, prepare fewer output reports or print them less frequently, and eliminate unused or useless parts of the medical record that are not required for legal or regulatory documentation.

Various methods and tools for evaluating a system's functional performance include

- Record review
- Time study
- User satisfaction
- Cost-benefit analysis

## Record Review

A record review assesses how comprehensive the documentation of nursing care activities is. The manual record or the output of the old system can be compared with the output of the new system to determine if there is a difference. Other variables can also be evaluated, such as (1) completeness of the database as measured by the nursing audit, (2) progress notes, (3) statement of types of patient problems, (4) nursing orders, (5) listed interventions, (6) interdisciplinary communications, and (7) teaching plans.

## Time Study

A time study can be conducted both before and after system implementation to compare the time staff take to provide specific patient care activities under the old and new systems. Such a study can also include the time nursing staff spend in other activities required in the old versus the new system. Time studies can also be conducted, once the computer system is in place, to determine system use by nursing staff. For example, a time study can show how often nursing personnel use the CRT (i.e., document patient care). It can highlight whether the system increased or decreased the time spent in providing patient care. Time studies can also help estimate the cost of resources as well as other factors needed to run the system.

## User Satisfaction

A questionnaire or a checklist can assess users' reactions to and perceptions of the system. A questionnaire can assess the degree to which a user is satisfied with overall system performance. A checklist can identify system strengths and weaknesses. It can measure whether the system improves the nurses' understanding of patient problems and thus affects patient care, and it can assess the usefulness and contributions of the system. Some specific questions to assist in this evaluation and criteria for appraising the system's technical performance are listed in Table 8.4.

Other approaches to evaluating the functional performance of a system also exist. Such functions as administrative control, medical/nursing orders, charting and documentation, and retrieval and management reports can be appraised through time observations, work sampling, operational audits, and surveys. Also, system functional performance can be assessed by examining patient care, nurses' morale, and nursing department operations (McCormick, 1983).

Documentation of care must be assessed if patient care benefits are to be evaluated. The following questions (on page 295) must be answered:

**TABLE 8.4**　　USER SATISFACTION CHECKLIST

| Performance Area | Satisfaction Level | | | | |
|---|---|---|---|---|---|
| | Very Satisfied | Satisfied | Neutral | Dissatisfied | Very Dissatisfied |
| Accuracy | 1 | 2 | 3 | 4 | 5 |
| Timeliness | 1 | 2 | 3 | 4 | 5 |
| Reliability | 1 | 2 | 3 | 4 | 5 |
| Training | 1 | 2 | 3 | 4 | 5 |
| Routine task | 1 | 2 | 3 | 4 | 5 |
| Full system potential | 1 | 2 | 3 | 4 | 5 |
| Manuals | 1 | 2 | 3 | 4 | 5 |
| Ease of use | 1 | 2 | 3 | 4 | 5 |
| Data entry | 1 | 2 | 3 | 4 | 5 |
| Information retrieval | 1 | 2 | 3 | 4 | 5 |
| Legibility | 1 | 2 | 3 | 4 | 5 |
| Completeness | 1 | 2 | 3 | 4 | 5 |
| Data entry | 1 | 2 | 3 | 4 | 5 |
| Information retrieval | 1 | 2 | 3 | 4 | 5 |
| Flexibility | 1 | 2 | 3 | 4 | 5 |
| Data entry | 1 | 2 | 3 | 4 | 5 |
| Information retrieval | 1 | 2 | 3 | 4 | 5 |
| Conciseness | 1 | 2 | 3 | 4 | 5 |
| Data entry | 1 | 2 | 3 | 4 | 5 |
| Information retrieval | 1 | 2 | 3 | 4 | 5 |
| Overall performance | 1 | 2 | 3 | 4 | 5 |

- Does the system assist in improving the documentation of patient care?
- Does the system reduce patient care costs?
- Does the system prevent errors and save lives?

Evaluating nurses' morale requires appraising nurses' satisfaction with the system. The following questions must be answered:

- Does the system facilitate nurses' documentation of patient care?
- Does it reduce the time spent in such documentation?
- Is it easy to use?
- Is it readily accessible?
- Are the video display screens easy to use?
- Do the video displays capture patient care?
- Does the system enhance the work situation and contribute to work satisfaction?

Evaluating the nursing department's benefits requires determining if the NIS helps improve administrative activities. The following questions must be answered:

- Does the new system enhance the goals of the nursing department?
- Does it improve department efficiency?
- Does it help reduce the range of administrative activities?
- Does it reduce clerical work?

Other criteria are necessary to evaluate technical performance, including reliability, maintainability, use, responsiveness, accessibility, availability, and ability to meet changing needs. These areas must be examined from several different angles; the technical performance of the software as well as the hardware must be appraised. The following questions must be answered:

- Is the system accurate and reliable?
- Is it easy to maintain at a reasonable cost?
- Is it flexible?
- Is the information consistent?
- Is the information timely?
- Is it responsive to users' needs?
- Do users find its inputs and outputs satisfactory?
- Are input devices accessible and generally available to users?

## Cost-Benefit Analysis

A cost-benefit analysis is necessary to determine if the system is "worth" its price. The cost-benefit analysis relates system costs and benefits to system design, level of use, time frame, and equipment costs. Each of these costs must be assessed in relation to benefits derived. Such an evaluation can help determine the future of the system.

## UPGRADE PHASE

Existing NISs may have been developed so many years ago that they need upgrading in order to keep up with new technologies that were not available when the original systems were implemented. To upgrade a system, one essentially goes through the same phases and activities as in developing and implementing a system. However, in upgrading, one considers the use of new technologies. Some of the important considerations in upgrading a system include the following new technologies:

- Bedside/point-of-care terminals
- Workstations
- Multimedia presentations
- Decision support systems
- Artificial intelligence
- Neural networks
- Integrated systems architecture
- Interfaced networks
- Open architecture

All of these are discussed in other chapters of this book, except for the concepts of integrating, interfacing, and open architecture. These three important concepts are related to upgrading because they approach the potential of upgrading with different resources.

## Interfaced Systems versus Integrated Systems

The principles of interfaced versus integrated systems need to be considered (Bleich and Slack, 1992). An interfaced system is a system in which each department is responsible for its own database, e.g., the laboratory, radiology, nursing, and medicine. The computer hardware may be shared, but the departments' databases are not. If data are shared by departments, they are usually duplicated and transmitted to another department. These systems can be run on different hardware and different operating systems that are not necessarily able to communicate with one another. Department heads usually prefer interfaced systems because they have more authority over the type of system purchased and because it is custom-tailored for their department.

An integrated system is a system in which all hospital departments share a common database. All information is stored in the same computer file. There is no need to interface, since all data captured are essentially available to any department. When an integrated system is developed and implemented, all personnel are aware of the type of computer hardware and software that is available.

Hardware and software are interchangeable between departments, so a large backup of equipment and software is not necessary. The major advantage of integrated systems is the functionality of the system for sharing common data. Most of the new systems are integrated. Most hospitals that have integrated systems have built their own, e.g., Latter-Day Saints Hospital in Salt Lake City, Beth Israel Hospital in Boston, and the University of Iowa Medical Center.

## Open Systems

Today, as we look at wide area networks, the concepts of interfacing and integrating are being challenged by the open architecture (Clayton et al., 1992). The concept of open architecture as an approach to computing systems assumes a heterogeneous mixture of applications, host computers, systems, and databases. Usually they are interfaced, or minimally interfaced, with one another by means of de facto conventions and standards. The network is an important architectural component that integrates the heterogeneous components. When all departments move onto a network, the ring is broken on access, but the heterogeneity of hosts and workstations is maintained.

### Workstations

The workstation becomes the means of gaining access to multiple applications. Users do not have to know or understand what type of hardware or software they are accessing, only that they have access to a broad array of information from the point of care or the point of management. Practice applications using workstations are discussed in Chap. 10.

However, workstations are discussed in this chapter as something to consider during the upgrading or enhancing of existing systems. As an example, a nurse using the system can go into the Physicians' Desk Reference database to check on side effects of a medication prescribed for the patient, enter H*STAR to determine the new guideline related to the use of this medication, enter MEDLINE to search for new uses of this therapy, send electronic mail to colleagues about the drug, and enter the patient documentation system to chart that the medication was given. The security and confidentiality issues that these new open architecture systems raise are being handled by the installation of security servers, registration centers to register use of information, or protocols requiring authorization.

According to Clayton et al., the advantages of updating using open architectures are modularity, rapid implementation, simultaneous existence of old and new systems running side by side, redundant pathways, and vendor and platform independence. The major disadvantage of the open architecture is the lack of national standards that allow all machines to communicate using a common communication language.

## System Issues

As new technologies are evaluated and upgrading is considered, the design team should reassess the original functional requirements to determine whether they were too limiting for the new modification. If the system has not been used to its limit, there may be some reserve capacity to expand the original functional requirements with the existing hardware. Insofar as possible, the team needs to determine if a subsystem can be added to the working system. Some options that exist are to expand and elaborate the initial functions or to add functions similar to the initial functions.

New functions might be required that entail procuring additional hardware. To determine if hardware or software tradeoffs should be considered, the following questions might be raised:

- Which hardware subsystems will be most difficult to implement?
- Can this new function be performed with existing software?
- Is the throughput of the rate-limiting feature of the system improved by changing from software to hardware or vice versa?
- Can alterations of current hardware or software improve the feature without compromising capabilities?
- Are additional mechanical or electrical devices required to make the change?
- Are some functions better handled by remote or local processors?

## FUTURE TRENDS

The introduction of the computer-based patient record (CPR) has been recommended by the IOM report, which states that the designs of the 1990s should expand to improve the fundamental resource in health care beyond the automating of patient records (Dick and Steen, 1991).

The CPR designs of the next decade will be more useful if they provide practical and accurate data, practitioner reminders and alerts, clinical decision support systems, links to bodies of medical knowledge, and other aids in expanding knowledge needed in clinical decision making. Within this definition is the concept of broadening the CPR from its origin as an "automated patient record" to a resource in the management of data in a lifelong health care record and in the extension of knowledge.

Many of the already implemented systems will have to be upgraded in line with these future trends. The next decade will require expanded system capabilities. They will include (Edmunds, 1992)

- Databases and database management systems
- Workstations
- Data acquisition and retrieval
- Text processing
- Advanced image processing and storage
- Data-exchange and vocabulary standards
- System communications and network infrastructure
- System reliability and security
- Linkages to secondary databases

The fully configured workstations will require new windowing applications, accelerated processors, graphical user interfaces (GUI), and large storage capabilities in order to retrieve and process data transactionally for case management, clinical pathways, and outcomes of care analysis. This may necessitate a change from traditional interfaces to high-powered workstations with user-oriented graphical, object-oriented, and metaphoric interfaces; intuitive, consistent, and forgiving software, the user in control; and relational databases that support ad hoc querying and allow multiprocessing.

In upgrading and expanding systems, the trends to watch will be the use of interfacing, integrating, or open architectures for attaining maximum advantages, cost-benefit, and ease in communication. The challenge for the decade ahead will be to upgrade systems so that communication exists between the hospital, the health care provider's office, and the patient's home. The use of large regional networks, linked to the superhighway, provides the greatest potential to accomplish these goals. The issues of standards and confidentiality of data must be recognized before these upgrades can move ahead with great speed.

## SUMMARY

This chapter described the process of implementing an NIS for nursing departments in health care facilities. It outlined and described the seven phases of the process—planning (project definition), analysis, design (functional requirements and implementation design), development (system assembly), implementation, evaluation, and upgrading. The phases recommended by ASTM were incorporated into this new edition since many consultants will be using those terms in contracts to help nursing departments implement systems.

The planning phase determines the problem scope and outlines the entire project to determine whether the system is feasible and worth developing, given the allocated resources. The analysis phase assesses the problem being studied. The design phase produces detailed specifications of the proposed system. Development involves the actual preparation of the system. Implementation involves system installation, assessment, and documentation, including training users and managing and maintaining the system. Evaluation determines the need to change the implemented content or to add to or upgrade the system. Upgrading the system involves expansion or elaboration of initial functions by expanding capability or function or by adding entirely new roles.

## REFERENCES

American Association of Nurse Executives (AONE), in cooperation with the Center for Healthcare Information Management (CHIM). (1993). *Informatics: Issues and Strategies for the 21st Century Health Care Executive* (Resource Book and Video Set). Chicago: American Hospital Association Services.

ASTM Proposed Standards (E622) (1993). *Standard Guide for Developing Computerized Systems*. Philadelphia.

Bleich, H. L., and Slack, W. V. (1992). Designing a hospital information system: A comparison of interfaced and integrated systems. *MD Computing, 9*(5), 293–296.

Ciotti, V., and Bogutski, B. (1994, July). 10 Commandments: Negotiating HIS contracts. *Healthcare Informatics, 11*(7), 16–20.

Clayton, P. D., Sideli, R. B., and Sengupta, S. (1992). Open architecture and integrated information at Columbia-Presbyterian Medical Center. *MD Computing, 9*(5), 297–303.

Dick, R. S., and Steen, E. B. (Eds). (1991). *The Computer-Based Record—An Essential Technology for Health Care*. Washington, DC: National Academy Press.

Edmunds, L. (1992). Methodologies for defining system requirements. Part 1. Methodology Overview. *MEDINFO-92* (unpublished report from workshop handouts). Geneva, Switzerland.

Fitzgerald, J., Fitzgerald, A. F., and Stallings, W. D. (1981). *Fundamentals of Systems Analysis* (2d ed). New York: John Wiley.

Ginsburg, D. A., and Browning, S. J. (1989). Selecting automated patient care systems. In V. K. Saba, K. A. Rider, and D. B. Pocklington (Eds.), *Nursing and Computers: An Anthology* (pp. 229–237). New York: Springer-Verlag.

Hewlett-Packard. (1993). *Choosing a Clinical Information System: A Blueprint for Your Success*. Waltham, MA.

McCormick, K. A. (1983). Monitoring and evaluating implemented HIS. In R. E. Dayhoff (Ed.), *Proceedings of the Seventh Annual Symposium on Computer Applications in Medical Care* (pp. 507–510). New York: IEEE Computer Society Press.

Simpson, R. L. (1991). The Joint Commission did what you wouldn't. *Nursing Management, 22*(1), 26–27.

Simpson, R. L. (1993a). *The Nurse Executive's Guide to Directing and Managing Nurse Information Systems*. Ann Arbor, MI: The Center for Healthcare Information Management.

Simpson, R. L. (1993b). Creating a paradigm shift in benefits realizations. *Nursing Management, 24*(6), 14–16.

Simpson, R. L., and Somers, J. B. (1991). The role of the clinical nurse specialist in information systems selection. *Clinical Nurse Specialist, 5*(3), 159–163.

Young, E. M. (Ed.). (1981). *Automated Hospital Information, Vol. 1, Guide to Planning, Selecting, Acquiring, Implementing and Managing an HIS.* Los Angeles: Center Publications.

Zielstorff, R., McHugh, M., and Clinton, J. (1988). *Computer Design Criteria for Systems That Support the Nursing Process* (pp. 1–40). Kansas City, MO: American Nurses Association.

Zinn, T. K. (1989, September/October). Automated systems selection. *Health Care,* 45–46.

# BIBLIOGRAPHY

American Nurses Association. (1980). *Nursing: A Social Policy Statement.* Kansas City, MO.

American Nurses Association (1991). *Standards of Clinical Nursing Practice.* Kansas City, MO.

Anser Analytic Services. (1982). *Evaluation of the Medical Information System at the NIH Clinical Center,* Vol. 1, *Summary of the Findings and Recommendations* (contract no. NO1-CL-0-2117). Arlington, VA: Anser Analytic Services.

Arnold, J., and Pearson, G. (1992). *Computers Applications in Nursing Education and Practice* (Pub. No. 14-2406). New York: National League for Nursing.

Austin, C. J. (1983). *Information Systems for Health Services Administration.* Ann Arbor, MI: Health Administration Press.

Ball, M. J., and Collen, M. F. (Eds.). (1992). *Aspects of the Computer-Based Patient Record.* New York: Springer-Verlag.

Burnard, P. (1991). Computing: An aid to studying nursing. *Nursing Standard, 5*(17), 16–22.

Campbell, B. (1990). The clinical director's role in selecting a computer system. *Caring, 9*(6), 36–38.

Capron, H. L., and Williams, B. K. (1984). *Computers and Data Processing* (2d ed.). Menlo Park, CA: Benjamin/Cummings.

Center for Healthcare Information Management (CHIM). (1991). *Guide to Making Effective H.I.S. Purchase Decisions.* Ann Arbor, MI.

Evans Paganelli, B. (1989). Criteria for the selection of a bedside information system for acute care units. *Computers in Nursing, 7*(5), 214–221.

Gassert, C. A. (1989). Defining nursing information system requirements: A linked model. In L. C. Kingsland (Ed.), *Proceedings of the Thirteenth Annual Symposium on Computer Applications in Medical Care* (pp. 779–783). Washington, DC: IEEE Computer Society Press.

Gillis, P. A., Booth, H., Graves, J. R., et al. (1994). Translating traditional principles of system development into a process for designing clinical information systems. *International Journal of Technology Assessment in Health Care, 10*(2), 235–248.

HCIA. (1994). *100 Top Hospitals: Benchmarks for Success.* Baltimore, MD.

Holzemer, W. L., and Henry, S. B. (1992). Computer-supported versus manually-generated nursing care plans: A comparison of patient problems, nursing interventions and AIDS patient outcomes. *Computers in Nursing, 10*(1), 19–24.

Hopper, G. M., and Mandell, S. L. (1984). *Understanding Computers.* New York: West.

Jenkins, S. (1988). Nurses' responsibilities in implementation of information systems. In M. Ball, K. Hannah, U. Gerdin-Jelger, and H. Peterson (Eds.), *Nursing Informatics: Where Caring and Technology Meet* (pp. 216–231). New York: Springer-Verlag.

Jones, K. (1991). Computer systems in labor and delivery units: Critical issues. *Journal of Obstetric, Gynecologic and Neonatal Nursing, 20*(5), 371–375.

Kelly, P. A., and Hanchett, E. S. (1977). *The Impact of the Computerized Problem-oriented Record on the Nursing Components of Patient Care* (contract no. NO1-NU-44126). Hyattsville, MD, Division of Nursing, PHS, US DHHS.

Mitchell, M. (1993). Systems design and management. *Capsules & Comments in Nursing Leadership & Management, 1*(3), 1.

Saba, V. K. (1974). Basic considerations in management information systems for public health/community health agencies. In National League for Nursing (Ed.). *Management Information Systems for Public Health/Community Health Agencies: A Report of a Conference* (pp. 3–13). New York.

Salois-Swallow, D. (1991). Formal process for the acquisition of an automated nurse scheduling system. In E. J. S. Hovenga, K. Hannah, K. A. McCormick, and J. S. Ronald (Eds.), *Proceedings of the Fourth International Conference on Nursing Use of Computers and Information Science* (pp. 358–360). New York: Springer-Verlag.

Shelly, G. B., and Cashman, T. J. (1980). *Introduction to Computers and Data Processing.* Brea, CA: Anaheim Publishing.

Shortliffe, E. H., Tank, P. C., Amatayakul, M., et al. (1992). In M. J. Ball and M. Collen (Eds.), *Aspects of the Computer-Based Patient Record* (pp. 273–293). New York: Springer-Verlag.

Silva, J. S., and Zawilski, R. J. (1992). The health care professional's workstation: Its functional components and user impact. In M. J. Ball and M. F. Collen (Eds.), *Aspects of the Computer-Based Patient Record* (pp. 102–124). New York: Springer-Verlag.

Simpson, R. (1992). What nursing leaders are saying about technology. *Nursing Management, 23*(7), 28–32.

Sorrentino, E. A. (1991). Overcoming barriers to automation. *Nursing Forum, 26*(3), 21–23.

Young, E. M. (Ed.). (1981). *Automated Hospital Information,* Vol. 2, *Guide to AHIS Suppliers.* Los Angeles: Center Publications.

Warnock-Matheron, A., and Plummer, C. (1988). Introducing nursing information systems in the clinical setting. In M. Ball, K. Hannah, U. Gerdin-Jelger, and H. Peterson (Eds.), *Nursing Informatics: Where Caring and Technology Meet* (pp. 115–127). New York: Springer-Verlag.

Wegner, E. L., and Hayashida, C. T. (1990). Implementing a multipurpose information management system: Some lessons and a model. *Journal of Long Term Care Administration, 18*(1), 15–20.

Zielstorff, R., Grobe, S., and Hudgins, C. (1992). *Nursing Information Systems: Essential Characteristics for Professional Practice.* Kansas City, MO: American Nurses Association.

# NURSING
# APPLICATIONS

# *9*

· · · · · · · · · · · · · · · · · · · · · · ·

# ADMINISTRATIVE APPLICATIONS

## OBJECTIVES

- Describe new uses of computers for nurse administrators.
- Understand administrative costs of data.
- Identify the standards for nurse administrators.
- Describe the benefits of computers for nurse administrators.
- Discuss nursing services administration systems.
- Describe nursing unit management systems.

Today nurse administrators and managers are experiencing major changes in health care delivery in the environment of health care reform. Cost control, managed competition, increasing regulation, quality monitoring, and efficient management are becoming increasingly important. The message of this chapter was headlined in the October 1993 *Wall Street Journal*: "Hospitals Wake Up to the Power of Computers" (Winslow, R., Oct. 8, 1993. *Wall Street Journal*, col. 6, p. 4). This chapter describes how computerized nursing systems can help the nurse administrator obtain, manage, and utilize information to enhance and improve individual patient care, organizational performance, staff productivity, governance, management, and support processes.

This chapter presents an overview of administrative applications of computers. Specifically, this chapter will discuss the uses of computerized information for the following two administrative levels:

- Nursing service administration
- Nursing unit management

In this chapter the director of a nursing service is considered an administrator or chief executive officer or vice president who requires nursing services information to run a nursing department. A head nurse or supervisor of several nursing units or workstations is considered a manager who requires nursing unit management information. Classification schemes are also included in this chapter; however, the tools that administrators in community health and educational settings use are described in other chapters.

## NEW USES OF COMPUTERS FOR NURSE ADMINISTRATORS

In today's new environment it is critical that administrators have data that will enable them to measure, monitor, and manage services in terms of incidence, cost, intensity, resource utilization, and outcomes of care. Chapter 13 integrates the concepts of nursing administrative support and practice documentation to describe in more detail the data used to support outcomes management.

Nurse administrators are increasingly responsible for more effective financial management and patient care data management for

- Meeting the requirements of voluntary accreditation standards set by the Joint Commission on Accreditation of Health Care Organizations (JCAHO) and documenting voluntary compliance with standard-setting organizations.
- Documenting conformity to state and federal government regulations.
- Compiling nursing qualification files.
- Organizing risk management programs to reduce liabilities of the institution, identify legal risks, and limit financial losses in legal matters.
- Creating an internal organization that constructively engages all types and levels of staff.
- Assuring the presence of the personnel, information, and technologic infrastructure to accomplish the goals of the organization.
- Assuring the satisfaction of the consumer (patient).
- Evaluating prospective and retrospective quality of patient care through review and analysis of patterns of care, benchmarking, and sharing outcomes of care.

- Promoting effective and efficient use of facilities, equipment, services, and financial resources.
- Determining the hospital's case mix in terms of patient diagnosis, age, and other variables required for reimbursement from third-party payers.
- Assuring follow-up care of patients with long-term illnesses and assessment of the efficiency of the care given.
- Providing new data for managed care contracts.
- Responding to new financial demands as a result of competition to demonstrate that the facility is efficient, effective, and has high performance standards (Shortliffe et al., 1992; American Association of Nurse Executives and Center for Healthcare Information Management, 1993).

In the decade ahead, the nurse administrator will want to focus on outcomes of care (Ullian, 1992). This would channel patients to particular facilities where outcomes reflect the quality of care and services. Presuming that all outcomes are satisfactory and consistent with good clinical care, having these monitors permits individual hospital administrators to measure performance.

## ADMINISTRATIVE COSTS OF DATA

The control of administrative data, and documentation to be used in monitoring quality and assessing cost and value, is consuming as much as 20 percent of the total health care spending in the United States. This is at least twice and possibly ten times the costs in other countries, including countries with national health care (e.g., Canada and the United Kingdom).

Because hospitals create, move, store, and retrieve billions of patient record documents per year, nurse administrators can better control this information through computerization. It is known that at least 30 percent of the information required to make decisions about diagnosis and treatment of patients is not available at the time the decision needs to be made (Dick and Steen, 1991). Much of this information is nursing information. One deficiency in documentation for administration of medication is adverse drug events, which add roughly $3 billion per year to hospital bills (Melmon, 1971). In Canada, hospitals estimate that 30 to 40 percent of all hospital admissions are due to adverse drug reactions in the aged. Hospital bills could be reduced by $140 million a year through better control. In the Latter-Day Saints Hospital in Salt Lake City, Utah, a computerized system monitoring medication changes, abnormal laboratory results, and incidents was 60 times better than reliance on practitioners alone. The Latter-Day Saints Hospital estimates that a $471.1 million reduction in costs was realized by controlling medication errors (Classen et al., 1991).

Direct care providers will remain the primary user of future computerized patient records; however, the future systems will allow administrators to synthesize information for research, policy, and reimbursement. JCAHO has proposed 1996 as the target date for requiring on-line hospital monitoring of clinical quality indicators to reduce the time and effort required for performance review.

The annual savings in labor costs through on-line medical records have been estimated at $14.3 million (Wasden, 1991).

Overall, the reductions in health care costs that health care administrators can contribute to through four applications of computers are estimated to be $36 billion per year: $30 billion saved by managing and transporting patient information by computer, $6 billion by electronic processing of health care claims, $600 million by using electronic inventory management systems, and $200 million through videoconferences for professional training.

Specifically, through automation, the nurse administrator can help reduce annual costs to hospitals by at least $12.7 billion by

- Reducing costs associated with adverse medical reactions.
- Decreasing nursing clerical time.
- Reducing costs associated with record maintenance.
- Curtailing malpractice costs.
- Hastening retrieval of valid and reliable information.
- Easing aggregation of medical information for research.
- Improving internal and external review of records (Little, 1992).

But what of the cost of computerizing? The cost of automating a nursing office for nursing administrative purposes has decreased from an estimated $4 million in 1972 to less than $5,000 in 1992 for a computer with the same power (Hannah, 1993).

## STANDARDS FOR NURSE ADMINISTRATORS

In recent years, professional nursing standards have urged nurse administrators to focus on effective and efficient administration. Since 1988 the American Nurses Association (ANA) has described standards for professional nurses which make them responsible for planning strategy and determining nursing goals for allocating human, material, and financial resources. The standards define two levels of administration: the nurse administrator and the nurse manager. The nurse administrator is charged with providing leadership in setting goals for the effective and efficient care for patients and evaluating the quality of the nursing services that are provided. The administrator is further responsible to the organization as a whole, the community, and the nursing profession and the health care delivery system (American Nurses Association, 1988).

In the 1988 ANA standards, the nurse manager, who is accountable for controlling the nursing services and reports sent to nurse administrators, is charged with coordinating nursing activities, participating in resource utilization decisions, and serving as the link between nursing services staff both internally and externally in the organization. Nurse managers implement a strategic plan for the organization and participate in policy formation, as well as develop staffing, scheduling, and evaluation performance standards.

The activities of both nurse administrators and nurse managers involve the collection and analysis of large amounts of data. Such data need to be supported by management information systems. Since computers can make the delivery of care more efficient and effective, they are an essential ingredient in fulfilling that goal. Five types of computer programs that nurse administrators need in order to integrate the information needs in their environment are (1) bibliographic databases, (2) word processing, (3) database programs, (4) decision analysis programs and spreadsheets, and (5) project management programs (Anderson et al., 1992).

The essential computer systems for nursing administration and nursing management include a measurement of patient dependence, patient classification schemes, nursing workload management, a scheduling system, and a business and accounting system. Nursing participation in the selection of patient care systems is now mandated by JCAHO.

Also as a result of JCAHO initiatives, the focus in the 1990s has shifted to outcome-oriented computer systems rather than process-oriented systems. JCAHO also recommends accreditation based on tracking clinical indicators by computer. The proposed JCAHO standards of information management will require new combinations of data from different sources, linkages of clinical and administrative data, and the use of external databases to monitor hospital performance (American Association of Nurse Executives and Center for Healthcare Information Management, 1993). Critical areas in information management that may be important to JCAHO in its new survey (Porter, 1994) include:

- External comparison databases
- Data security and confidentiality
- Knowledge-based systems
- Physicians' information systems
- Continuous quality improvement projects
- Data integrity
- Standards and procedures in place related to documentation requirements
- Needs assessments

In addition, the Institute of Medicine's report on the automated patient record recommends the use of computer-based patient medical records by the end of the 1990s (Simpson, 1991a–d).

# BENEFITS OF COMPUTERS TO NURSE ADMINISTRATORS

In general, the benefits of computers to nurse administrators are improved communication, order entry, and continuity of care; availability of more time for patients; access to guided critical thinking; availability of expert resources; and the ability to evaluate care. Specifically, nurse administrators have identified several other benefits to using computers in nursing management (American Association of Nurse Executives and Center for Healthcare Information Management, 1993).

- More complete utilization of nursing staff resources
- Improved quality of patient care monitoring
- Improved documentation
- Improved communication
- Improved planning systems
- More standardization of nursing practice
- Capability to define the practice, the problems, and the issues
- Defined methods to track patient care delivered, outcomes achieved, and revenue generated
- Enhanced recruitment and retention
- Improved evaluation of care provided
- Ability to become a dynamic organization, capable of change

# COMPUTER APPLICATIONS FOR NURSING ADMINISTRATION

Approximately 26 administrative information functions for nurse administrators and managers are available on computers. Table 9.1 summarizes the available administrative applications, of which 12 relate to the nursing services administrators and the remaining 14 relate to the nursing unit managers.

# NURSING SERVICES ADMINISTRATION SYSTEMS

The essential applications of a nursing services administration information system have expanded over the past five years. In general, they are concerned with the information needed for planning, budgeting, and reporting to ensure quality care. The major applications concern the following:

- Quality assurance
- Personnel files
- Communication networks

**TABLE 9.1**   COMPUTER APPLICATIONS FOR ADMINISTRATIVE
INFORMATION MANAGEMENT

- Quality assurance
- Personnel files
- Communication networks within the nursing department and outside the nursing department
- Budgeting and payrolls
- Census
- Summary reports for state, federal, and hospital regulations
- Forecasting and planning
- Claims processing (reimbursement)
- Risk pooling
- Costing nursing care
- Case-mix management
- Consumer surveys
- Nursing intensity
- Patient classification
- Acuity systems
- Staffing and scheduling
- Inventory
- Patient billing
- Incident and other reports
- Poison control
- Allergy and drug reactions
- Error reports
- Infection control
- Unit reports
- Utilization review
- Shift summary reports

- Budgeting and payrolls
- Census
- Regulatory reports
- Forecasting and planning
- Claims processing and reimbursement
- Risk pooling
- Costing nursing care
- Case-mix management
- Consumer surveys

## Quality Assurance

Quality assurance concepts related to nursing services administration are described here, whereas those concepts that integrate quality assurance with outcomes of care are highlighted in Chap. 13. The key words for measuring quality in the decade ahead are effectiveness, efficiency, and outcomes. A key concept for reporting quality in the future is "report cards."

The nursing profession evaluates the impact of the health care it delivers to the consumer. Since health care encompasses many variables, an assessment method for evaluating structure, actions, outcomes, process, and competency levels of the nurse provider and patient consumer is considered a monitor of quality assurance. Nursing has dedicated more than a decade to the issue of quality assurance; many frameworks and methods have been described. Potentially all quality assurance worksheet forms can be set up to be computerized.

In 1989 the ANA, the National Commission on Nursing Implementation Project (NCNIP), and the National League for Nursing (NLN) sponsored an invitational conference to identify what was needed to assess the quality of nursing care. Participants agreed that establishing nursing information systems (NISs) would facilitate a quality assurance system and that establishing a taxonomy or classification nomenclature system such as nursing diagnosis would facilitate the standardized database for nursing. Continued studies on the impact of nursing on patient outcome and the structural variables affecting the nursing process and outcomes of nursing care were also deemed necessary.

However, computer systems have not solved the problem of identifying valid and reliable criteria on which to input information. These systems have the potential for producing the same information with the same problems as the manual mechanism of monitoring quality assurance.

Even the JCAHO uses computers to monitor adherence to its quality assurance standards. The only difference is that the commission uses computers to analyze the volumes of data that standard compliance reviews accumulate annually. A goal of JCAHO in the future is to make these databases available to describe the quality of institutions compared to one another.

Ensuring quality care that is efficient and cost-effective is of importance in today's health care environment. A decision support system for clinical management, utilization review credentialing, and quality assurance, including clinical indicators and peer review criteria, and report adherence to professional/hospital standards and performance measures will be the goal of administrative systems as we turn into the twenty-first century (Simpson, 1992). There will be a need for complete information on recommendations from the national and local level, and hospitals will need to include individual provider policies and guidance. Resource allocation decisions that have previously been based on best guesses in health care will be derived from quantitative data and profiles of professional performance and utilization of resources (Silva and Zawilski, 1992).

Increasingly the decade ahead will require quality management that ensures the value of purchased care (Sennett, 1992). Computer support attempts to identify care that is inappropriate or inefficient or excessive, and to identify the care that is the lowest-cost possible alternative. Such programs are marketed as health care management systems.

In evaluating care, computerized patient record documentation is used to understand the logic of diagnosis, planning, interventions, and outcomes achieved. Trends toward prospective management or point-of-service management are emerging, since retrospective management offers less opportunity to rationally manage care.

Identification of patterns of care and providers who are high performers or low performers implies that data are needed over time and in relation to the outcomes achieved. The medical record becomes the site for recording clinically relevant events, describing the persons served, and summarizing these events. This type of analysis is becoming especially important to profile managers or case managers. The desired characteristics of the record are accessibility, standardization, simplicity, accuracy, completeness, and cost-effectiveness.

Advantages to nurse administrators of the computer-based patient record system for the twenty-first century are its ability to

- Provide accessible clinical data that characterize patients' conditions, prior management, and current treatment.
- Provide clear and defined databases to permit epidemiologic assessment of patient outcomes and patterns of practice, revealing the merits of management strategies that are highly desirable and identifying strategies that are not desirable.
- Provide interactive decision support tools on information derived from large groups of patients.
- Decrease administrative record keeping and standardize forms for reimbursement.

Figure 9.1 is a model for computerization of quality assurance with expanded nursing input, and new outputs, for the total information management of quality in a nursing department.

## Personnel Files

Because computers can help organize information, they are being used to assist administrators in personnel planning and productivity analysis. Such systems maintain and update employees' permanent files, provide ready access to personnel profiles, and allow for employee quality control. These systems generate reminders for various personnel actions, such as license renewal or position change, and they produce reports on labor costs, employee analysis, and forecast requirements (Austin, 1979).

A personnel file can be used to do the following:

- Generate mailing lists.
- Plan educational programs.
- Determine promotion eligibility.
- Provide a census of personnel.

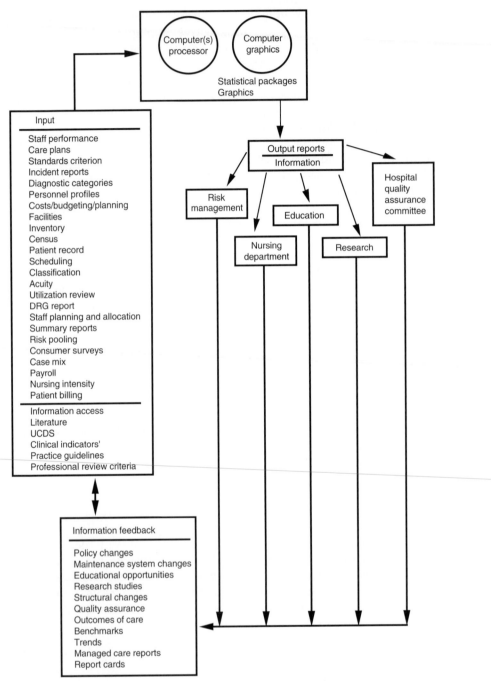

**Figure 9.1**    A model for computerization of quality assurance.

- Generate budget expenditures for personnel.
- Identify personnel with special preparation.
- Validate registered licenses.
- Validate certification updates.
- Prepare profile analysis of nursing personnel.

A relatively new system that has been described in the literature is the "recruitment manager" for nurse administrators (Garre, 1990). This software accurately and rapidly tracks and monitors recruiting efforts. The author describes it as a necessary tool to maintain a competitive advantage, to facilitate policy, and to enhance predictability in the market.

## Communication Networks

Computer systems that facilitate communication are designed to transmit information from point to point in a computer terminal network. In these systems, messages are not usually processed but are transmitted from one terminal (entry) to another (receiver). The computer is a communication integrator, which is also an integral part of any hospital information system (HIS) or management information system (MIS). The computerized communication system affects work patterns, thus reducing nurses' clerical functions. These systems also enhance interhospital communication networks (Schmitz et al., 1976).

Communication systems have many functions. A common communication network has the following features (Filosa, 1978):

- Send notices of patient appointments, admissions notification, discharges, and hospital census.
- Provide summary information on laboratory tests, medications, and other orders.
- Locate patients.
- Identify current charges and patient needs.
- Provide accurate billing.

Computer communication systems eliminate searches through procedure manuals and expedite delivery of requisitions for services and procedures, thus reducing clerical tasks. Such systems reduce the need for couriers to hand-carry reports and forms from the nursing department to the nursing unit, thus serving as efficient message centers.

More recent communication systems link nurse administrators through networks to nursing departments outside the hospital or agency to profile comparisons between facilities. Network links broaden the range of information to which nurse administrators can have access.

## Budgeting and Payrolls

One of the greatest advantages of computers for nurse administrators is in budgeting, a complex process that includes many layers of cost analysis. Included below is a list of financial functions which computer systems provide for nurse administrators. They can be derived from the hospital cost accounting systems or downloaded from spreadsheet software into nursing administration systems.

- Accounts receivable
- Patients' accounts
- Accounts payable
- General ledger
- Property ledger accounting
- Debts
- Collections
- Preventive maintenance costs
- Medicare/Medicaid patient profiles
- Private insurance profiles
- Cost allocation
- Cash control

Intimately related to the central budget are the information reports that come from payroll systems, inventory records, incident reports, length of stay reports, the nursing record, and quality care information.

Because nursing is a central activity in the delivery of health care, the ability to assess the adequacy of care and determine the cost of care is vital. Criteria frequently used in evaluating nursing productivity include nursing hours per patient day, staff-to-patient ratios, the number of full-time and part-time employees, and cost per patient day. Formulas for analyzing the cost of nursing care have also been developed. Since these reports require information, computers have been used to process summary reports.

Computer systems can be used for several types of budgeting. The three most common are (1) a fixed budget, where an absolute dollar amount is specified and no provision for variance is allowed because an absolute volume throughout the year is assumed; (2) a flexible budget, which assumes the expected procedures, with monthly variance reports that reflect actual volume, since the manager cannot control volume; and (3) a case-based budget, which is built around a product line structure and assumes that department managers control neither volume, procedures, nor revenue. Budget assumptions flow from demand forecasts by product, bills of sources by product, and case-based reimbursement. Variance reports are adjusted for variations in actual versus expected volume.

## Census

Census systems provide users with the capability of entering information on patient admission, discharge, birth, death, or transfers. A master file of available beds and bassinets is maintained with the appropriate legal information on occupancy. A census is a registration of inpatients and the beds they occupy. Many hospitals do the census on a microcomputer. The census application is also the heart of most HISs; newer HISs usually allow on-line control of the census function. The census report is needed at all times in order to account for patients in the hospital, emergency room, or outpatient clinics. All hospital areas must have continuous access to the computer system in order to determine a patient's status related to preadmission, admission, transfer, discharge, or death. The census systems usually provide immediate information on bed availability. Standard reports, usually a part of a census system, can provide statistical analysis and forecasting information, such as which units have reduced census between April and July or September and December.

The census system is the cornerstone of an administrative system. It provides daily, weekly, or monthly statistical analysis of patient admissions by hospital service, sex, and age. The detailed census statistics include patient days for each sex and age category for each hospital service and are used to analyze hospital services and to determine variations in patient mix over time for each hospital service.

## Regulatory Reports

Several types of summary reports can facilitate meeting the requirements of state and federal regulators, as well as JCAHO accreditation standards. If a hospital has an HIS or a microcomputer, summary reports might include incident reports; poison control; allergy and drug reactions; error reports; infection control reports; unit reports, including census, patient status, activities, procedures, and patients at risk; and utilization review information. Most of these reports originate on the nursing unit and are prepared by staff nurses, head nurses, unit managers, or supervisors. If a nursing service administrator neglects to include the regulation reports into nursing service information, however, this important information may not receive adequate attention.

## Forecasting and Planning

Systems have been designed to predict staff needs, determine trends in patients' nursing care needs, and forecast departmental budgetary compliance. They can also make predictions for effective management of float personnel and interunit exchange of personnel. Nurse administrators can use computers to define monitoring tasks and to establish what variables nurses must monitor in patients requiring different care patterns.

Many types of systems are available for planning schedules, planning hospital expansions, financial planning, and preventive maintenance planning. An on-line patient scheduling system can provide accuracy, flexibility, and timeliness for outpatient and inpatient scheduling. Visit codes can be described, and length of visits and the number of assigned professional staff can be controlled. Summary reports can facilitate planning for clinic and inpatient staffing.

Hospital expansion can be facilitated with data from other systems, including census, staffing, scheduling, and financial information. Similarly, hospital programs that need to be eliminated can be identified. Financial planning can be done with many available systems. Currently, prospective financial information has replaced retrospective planning.

Preventive maintenance planning includes systems that aid in organizing and scheduling maintenance. This type of planning system provides for more reliable equipment and reduces equipment failure. Even the computer needs a maintenance planning system to determine downtime as well as scheduled maintenance.

## Planning Systems

Planning systems can also be used to determine what information is needed for what services. When special services are audited periodically, particular services may prove to be unnecessary or may need to be used by different groups of patients. For example, an audit of the use of lodging for parents of pediatric patients with terminal cancer may show that the services are underused. However, spouses and relatives of geriatric patients may need such a facility. Computerized planning systems can provide the information to accommodate these decisions.

Planning systems can also help administrators determine where space is available both within the hospital and on hospital grounds. These advantageous systems can also categorize space by type, location, amount, and other criteria.

An important aspect of directing a service is being able to define the service's mission and scope, define the objectives that follow the mission, and specify the desired outcome of a department. Another important resource for today's administrator is a business plan that includes (1) an organization plan, (2) a market/competition analysis, (3) a production or operations plan, (4) a marketing/distribution plan, (5) a management/personnel organizational plan, (6) a development timeline or schedule, and (7) a financial plan. The preparation of each of these plans can be facilitated by computerized software. For example, an organization plan can be prepared with one of the new graphics software packages that allow the development of flowcharts or organizational plans. There are several graphics software packages that could accomplish this.

Additional plans can be supported with spreadsheets for the production of development schedules. Gantt charts can be used to graphically depict blocks of time, such as the number of weeks (or months or years) required to complete tasks. They are useful for displaying critical and noncritical tasks in attaining goals or programs. Several software products are now available to prepare Gantt charts. Figure 9.2 shows how a Gantt chart can be used for schedule development and project monitoring. This example was developed by an administrator proposing a new outpatient clinic (Johnson, 1988).

Program evaluation review technique (PERT) is a model used to develop operations analysis and project management tasks also related to scheduling. Projects with "critical paths" can be monitored using PERT charts. An illustration of a simple critical path is shown in Fig. 9.3. There are many new software products that can facilitate the development of PERT project charts.

## Financial Plan

The financial plan should include at least two levels of planning: (1) a strategic level and (2) an operational level. The time frame of a strategic-level plan may be five to ten years. However, the operational-level plan usually covers a shorter time period, such as a year, broken down into quarters or months. The projections included in the operational plan include the volume, revenue, rates, expenses, inflation, growth, assets required, financing of those assets (capital structure), net income, and cash flow. Most software packages today allow the user to prepare three basic financial statements: (1) income statement, (2) cash flow statement, and (3) balance sheet. Examples of these statements are shown in Tables 9.2, 9.3, and 9.4.

An income statement is generated from specifications of the charge units, payer mix, reimbursement type, expenses, profit margin, revenues/ rates, and market limits for prices.

The cash flow statement can be generated from the income statement data and the cash sources.

The balance sheet defines the equipment, cash, and other assets and the business liabilities and financing structure. To prepare the balance sheet, it is necessary to define cash, accounts receivable, inventory, capital assets, accumulated depreciation, accounts payable, long-term debt, and equity.

Before using the software to prepare financial statements, financial specialists may have to be consulted. Definitions of the terms used are found in nursing management textbooks and are not given in this chapter.

Putting the financial plans in place is shown in Tables 9.5, 9.6, and 9.7, which outline the income statement, revenue projections, and salary projections for establishing a gerontologic care unit. The break-even

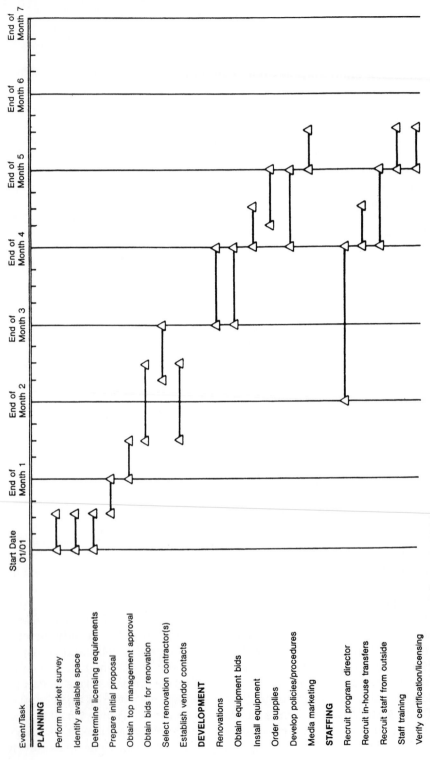

**Figure 9.2** Gantt chart. (Johnson, 1988.)

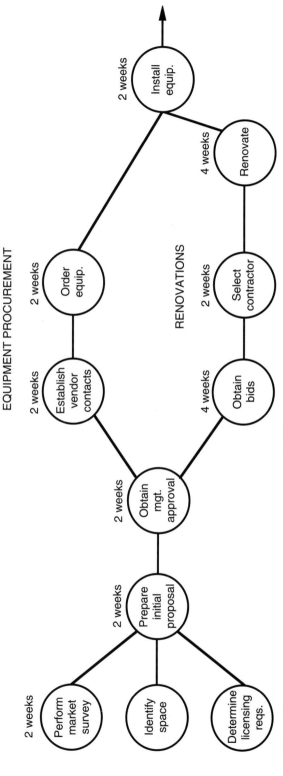

EQUIPMENT PROCUREMENT

RENOVATIONS

**Figure 9.3** PERT chart showing a critical path. (Johnson, 1988.)

**TABLE 9.2** EXAMPLE OF AN INCOME STATEMENT

**Business ABC**
**Income Statement**

| | |
|---|---|
| Gross revenues | $XXX,XXX.XX |
| Less: Allowances and bad debts | XX,XXX.XX |
| Net revenues | $XXX,XXX.XX |
| Other revenues | X,XXX.XX |
| Operating expenses | $XXX,XXX.XX |
| Interest expenses | XX,XXX.XX |
| Depreciation and amortization | XX,XXX.XX |
| Total expenses | $XXX,XXX.XX |
| Net income (loss) pretax | $ X,XXX.XX |
| Taxes | XXX.XX |
| Net income (loss) | $ X,XXX.XX |

*Source:* Johnson, 1988.

analysis for different occupancy rates for two different years is depicted in Figs. 9.4 and 9.5. The break-even analysis shows that a unit would be profitable at a minimum of 62.1 percent occupancy for 1978 and 53.1 percent occupancy in 1988.

**TABLE 9.3** EXAMPLE OF A CASH FLOW STATEMENT

**Business ABC**
**Statement of Cash Flows**

| | |
|---|---|
| Beginning cash balance | $XXX,XXX.XX |
| Net income | X,XXX.XX |
| Depreciation and amortization | XX,XXX.XX |
| Increase to debt | XX,XXX.XX |
| Accounts payable: Current | X,XXX.XX |
| Accounts payable: Prior | (X,XXX.XX) |
| Total cash sources | $XXX,XXX.XX |
| Uses of cash | |
| Accounts receivable: Current | $ X,XXX.XX |
| Accounts receivable: Prior | (X,XXX.XX) |
| Inventory: Current | X,XXX.XX |
| Inventory: Prior | (X,XXX.XX) |
| Payment of debt | XX,XXX.XX |
| Capital expenditures | XX,XXX.XX |
| Total uses of funds | $ XX,XXX.XX |
| Ending cash balance | $XXX,XXX.XX |

*Source:* Johnson, 1988.

**TABLE 9.4**   EXAMPLE OF A BALANCE SHEET

**Business ABC**
**Example of a Balance Sheet**

| | |
|---|---|
| Assets | |
| Cash | $XXX,XXX.XX |
| Accounts receivable | XX,XXX.XX |
| Inventory | XX,XXX.XX |
| Total current assets | $XXX,XXX.XX |
| Capital equipment | XXX,XXX.XX |
| Less accumulated depreciation | XX,XXX.XX |
| Net fixed assets | XXX,XXX.XX |
| Total assets | $XXX,XXX.XX |
| Liabilities and equity | |
| Accounts payable | $XXX,XXX.XX |
| Long-term debt | XX,XXX.XX |
| Equity | |
| Paid-in capital | XXX,XXX.XX |
| Retained earnings | XX,XXX.XX |
| Total equity | XXX,XXX.XX |
| Total liabilities and equity | $XXX,XXX.XX |

*Source:* Johnson, 1988.

## Claims Processing and Reimbursement

Claims information for third-party payers relies upon accurate and reliable documentation. The most important information to be captured is the type of services that were provided, the agent (provider) to be reimbursed for those services, the amount charged for the services, and sufficient information about the patient to permit linkage to the type of health insurance policy that is reimbursing the patient. The patient record can be the source of this information provided that it is accurate, accessible at low cost, and timely, and that it is possible to extract the critical review criteria or indicators, and in sufficient detail to capture the medical and nursing elements.

## Risk Pooling

Risk pooling or risk adjustment is the process of describing the relative risks of populations by age, sex, race, and clinical condition to manage the resources required to serve them. To minimize the risks of population differences, most administrators focus on the process of care delivery (e.g., number of pregnant women seen during their first trimester) rather than

**TABLE 9.5** INCOME STATEMENT FOR GCU

| Category | Sept–Dec 1987 | 1988 | 1989 | 1990 |
|---|---|---|---|---|
| Gross patient revenue | $410,200 | $1,328,600 | $1,560,375 | $1,799,450 |
| Deductions from revenue | 75,800 | 245,800 | 288,700 | 332,900 |
| Net patient revenue | 334,400 | 1,082,800 | 1,271,675 | 1,466,550 |
| Direct expenses | | | | |
| Salaries | 148,909 | 459,777 | 548,444 | 647,959 |
| Benefits—15% salaries | 22,336 | 68,967 | 82,267 | 97,197 |
| Office supplies | 735 | 2,205 | 2,293 | 2,408 |
| Medical supplies | 2,435 | 7,305 | 7,670 | 8,130 |
| Equipment depreciation | 4,367 | 13,100 | 13,100 | 500 |
| Misc. expense | 625 | 1,875 | 1,931 | 1,989 |
| Renovation | 5,375 | — | — | — |
| Totals | 184,782 | 553,229 | 655,705 | 758,203 |
| Indirect expense | 146,329 | 438,102 | 519,253 | 600,421 |
| Total expense | 331,111 | 991,331 | 1,174,958 | 1,358,624 |
| Gain/loss | 3,289 | 91,469 | 96,717 | 107,926 |
| Statistics | | | | |
| Patient days | 1,465 | 4,745 | 5,475 | 6,205 |
| % of occupancy | 57.2 | 61.9 | 71.4 | 81.0 |
| Break-even patient days | 1,439 | 4,071 | 4,763 | 5,372 |
| Break-even % occupancy | 56.2 | 53.1 | 62.1 | 70.1 |

*Source:* Johnson, 1988.

the outcomes (number of low-birth-weight infants, hospital readmission rates). Interpretation of outcome measures can be affected by characteristics of the patient population. Health services research in this area needs to be expanded to refine this serious limitation on interpreting and comparing outcomes.

**TABLE 9.6** REVENUE PROJECTIONS FOR GCU

| Source | 1987 | 1988 | 1989 | 1990 |
|---|---|---|---|---|
| Patient service revenues | | | | |
| Charge per patient day | $280 | $280 | $285 | $290 |
| Projected occupancy | 57.2% | 61.9% | 71.4% | 81.0% |
| Patient days | 1,465 | 4,745 | 5,475 | 6,205 |
| Gross revenue | $410,200 | $1,328,600 | $1,560,375 | $1,799,450 |

Expressed as a percentage of gross revenue; calculated using appropriate patient mix and payer reimbursement methods: PPS for Medicare, per diem for Medicaid, and percentage of charges for Blue Cross, HMOs, and commercial insurers.
Note: Patient day charges will increase in 1989 and 1990 based upon hospital rate increases.
*Source:* Johnson, 1988.

**TABLE 9.7**     SALARY PROJECTIONS FOR GCU

|                          | 1987       | 1988       | 1989       | 1990       |
|--------------------------|------------|------------|------------|------------|
| RNs                      |            |            |            |            |
| Patient days             | 1,465      | 4,745      | 5,475      | 6,205      |
| Standard                 | 6.2        | 6.2        | 6.2        | 6.2        |
| Man-hours                | 9,083      | 29,419     | 33,945     | 38,471     |
| Average hourly rate      | $12.46     | $13.08     | $13.81     | $14.64     |
| Salaries                 | $113,174   | $384,801   | $468,780   | $563,215   |
| Unit secretaries         |            |            |            |            |
| Man-hours                | 1,738      | 5,200      | 5,200      | 5,200      |
| Average hourly rate      | $7.50      | $7.88      | $8.32      | $8.32      |
| Salaries                 | $13,035    | $40,976    | $43,264    | $45,864    |
| Coordinator              |            |            |            |            |
| Man-hours                | 1,396      | 2,080      | 2,080      | 2,080      |
| Salaries                 | $22,700    | $34,000    | $36,400    | $38,900    |
| Total manhours           | 12,217     | 36,699     | 41,225     | 45,751     |
| FTEs                     | 16.23      | 15.39      | 19.82      | 22.00      |
| Total salaries           | $148,909   | $459,777   | $548,444   | $647,979   |
| Increases                |            |            |            |            |
| RN and unit secretary    | 0          | 5%         | 5.6%       | 6%         |
| Coordinator              | 0          | 0          | 7%         | 7%         |

Source: Johnson, 1988.

Risk pooling also depends on the ability to aggregate data on the expected health care costs of distinct populations. These can be based upon individual risks or group risks. The patient record can provide this information if the data stored go beyond morbidity and mortality and address functional status, health status, satisfaction, and other quality indicators of care. Current patient records have too much superfluous information to contain specific risk factors, but they could include those data elements. Many of the indicators of complications of care, safety, and incidents will be found within the nursing record and should be considered a source of those data elements.

According to Sennett (1992), an impediment to risk pooling is the lack of standardization of vocabulary within current patient records. Similarly, confidentiality requirements for data must be assured. Finally, explicit guidelines for use that describe the specific data elements need to be specified, and systems developed to assure compliance with those guidelines (Sennett, 1992).

## Costing Nursing Care

In 1981, it was estimated by Thompson that nursing services account for 35 percent of total hospital costs (Thompson, 1981). In a country with na-

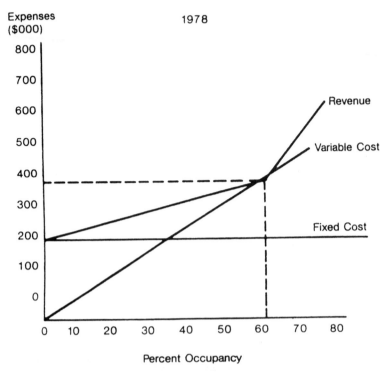

**Figure 9.4**　Break-even analysis for GCU occupancy. (Johnson, 1988.)

tional health care, like Australia, where costs have been examined, nursing service has been identified as the largest single component of a hospital's expenditure (Picone, 1987). In the United States, Halloran estimates that hospital nursing costs average 25 percent of total hospital costs, with the range going from 20 percent in large hospitals to 50 percent in small hospitals (Halloran, 1994). With hospital costs at 40 percent of health care costs, citizens of the United States pay about $100 billion per year for hospital nursing.

The cost identification of nursing services is but one system in a series of systems, independent and interdependent, that need to be available. (Van Slyck, 1991a–g). Room and board rates have been used traditionally instead of services rates as the basis of costs.

In order to cost out nursing services today, a logical and sequential series of activities needs to occur. Several functions of nursing care are required, including a classification and staffing system. Systems to collect classification and staffing information based upon acuity will be discussed later in the chapter when nursing unit management concepts are described, since these data are collected at the unit level. However, they are

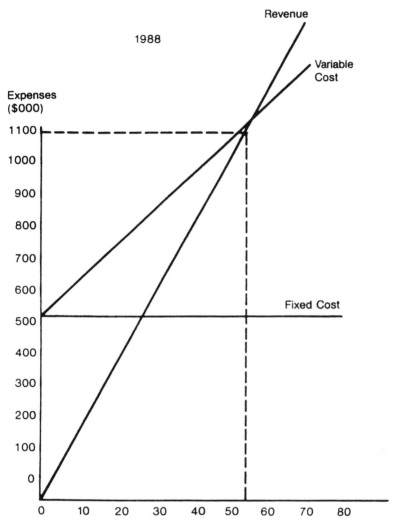

**Figure 9.5**   Break-even analysis for GCU occupancy. (Johnson, 1988.)

mentioned here because nurse administrators need to integrate these unit tools to cost out nursing care.

In order to cost out nursing services, Van Slyck states, systems and subsystems that are independent and interrelated need to be identified. She states that systems that need to be in place to cost out nursing care are (1) a belief system that identifies the organization's statements on patient cost identification, pricing policy, and nursing care, (2) a patient classification system in which patients are categorized into distinct groups based on preestablished criteria, (3) a staffing system that identifies patients, nursing staff requirements, and allocation based on the quantifiable needs (acuity) of the patients, (4) a costing system or method by which nursing care costs can be identified within a facility for each patient for each hospital day, and (5) an audit system for formal and systematic verification of patient acuity levels.

Halloran identifies other factors besides patients' dependence on nursing care as contributing to hospital costs of nursing (Halloran, 1994). They are tradition, budgetary constraints, the effects of physical facilities, and the staff nurse organization. Tradition involves how nurses perceive their job—as procedural or helping doctors cure patients, for example. Budgetary constraints are inherent in hospital organization, since fundamental changes in budget are difficult to make at best. The effect of physical size and layout is important because some ward sizes may be inefficient with only one head nurse, one evening nurse, and secretarial support. An organization factor that causes variation in nursing costs is whether nurses perceive their role as professional or technical.

Inherent in the above systems is a need to explore a number of other premises. The first is the statement that patient charges should be based on the cost of providing the services. The second is the statement that patients should pay for the services they receive and not subsidize other patients and other services. The third premise is that the costs for each service can be identified, defined, and measured, and revenue assigned to the departments, service centers, or product lines that incur the cost of providing the service. The fourth is that hospitals believe that patients have a right to know what they are paying for. The fifth is that charges make a contribution to the organization.

Inherent in a costing system is a classification system as a method of sorting the patient population within a given hospital into homogeneous groups based on established criteria. To be used for costing, a patient classification system needs to be simple and practical at the staff-nurse level. The system would include the patient's significant others that nurses teach and counsel. The system cannot use zeros, because even if the patient does not require a procedure (e.g., ambulation), the nurse is still accountable for monitoring and evaluating the appropriateness of that decision (to ambulate or not to ambulate). The system should emphasize process, which involves assessing, planning, interventions, and evaluation of outcomes, rather than just tasks alone.

The classification system needs to be integrated with the patient record because entries in the patient record are more accurate than a survey tool. The classification system obtains legitimacy by keeping the outlier patients to a minimum. Including a classification system in the patient record also allows for archival retrieval of critical information. The system should be based on services delivered instead of perceived patient need. Patients need to be charged for nursing care delivered.

Staffing systems identify and allocate nursing resources. This system needs to be flexible enough to include direct care, indirect care, and general unit activities.

In the costing system, data taken from the classification, staffing, and belief systems are used to identify the cost of delivering nursing services. In order to accomplish this, the nursing and financial management systems must be integrated, and costs and cost accounting methodologies defined similarly.

The final system is the audit system. It is most important for the long-term integrity of the data. The audit system verifies the patient acuity level. Since patient acuity drives nursing staffing, and thus directly affects the costs of nursing, the design and implementation of the audit system are critical to the overall success.

Three models are currently used for costing nursing: (1) charge codes are specified for services or track (e.g., nursing education, third-party coverage for nursing care), (2) an acuity-based cost is placed on the patient bill without an associated charge, and (3) nursing and nonnursing components of room and board charges are separated using acuity-based nursing costs.

## Nursing Resource Use

A study of nursing resource usage and costs in Australia defined the elements of a valid and reliable workload measurement in the acute care environment (Hovenga, 1994). The workload is necessary as an indicator of resource usage and how nursing service hospital costs can be captured. The many variables that go into determining case mix, resource usage, and inpatient costs are shown in Fig. 9.6. Hovenga describes the monitoring system for workload as using either individual activities or a patient classification method (patient groups) as its basis.

Nursing classification schemes are needed to classify nursing resource usage for patients in defined groups in order to cost out nursing services. Three ways of classifying patient groups have been defined: patient nurse dependency, diagnosis related groups (DRGs), and severity of illness.

The problem with classifying patients to determine costs is that because of their different perspectives, different persons in the health care environment require different information on patient care and resources. For example, the nursing administrator needs to know the amount and type of nursing services required to care for patients, the health provider is more interested in defining the health care condition and its concurrent diagnoses and therapeutic procedures, and the hospital administrator wants to identify patients in different classes in order to determine total resources to be provided to meet patient requirements.

In an unpublished study of predicting nursing care costs with nursing diagnoses, Halloran predicts that the cost of caring for one nursing diagnosis in a large university hospital in the United States is $8.90 (in 1987

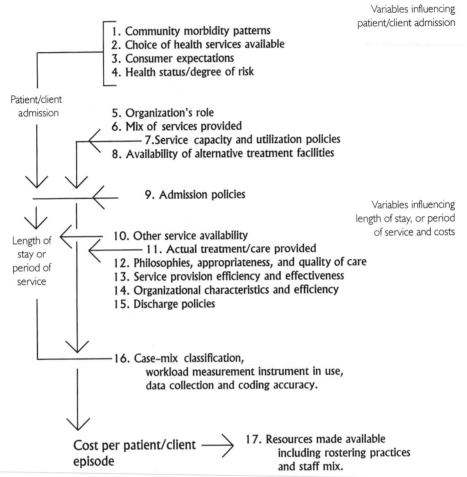

**Figure 9.6**  Conceptual framework of variables influencing case-mix, resource usage, and in-patient costs. (Hovenga, Ph.D. thesis, 1994.)

dollars). This figure comes from calculated hours of nursing care to take care of a patient with one nursing diagnosis. To cost out nursing diagnoses, Halloran did not distinguish one nursing diagnosis as more costly than another. He used nursing diagnoses instead of classification instruments alone to cost out nursing, since nursing diagnoses include the physical and functional status of patients in addition to their psychological and social characteristics. On average, in an acute care hospital, a patient has 13 nursing diagnoses per day and 22 nursing diagnoses observed during a typical hospital stay. In examining the relationship between nursing diagnoses and DRGs in terms of nursing time, Halloran found that 45 percent of the variation in time nurses spent with patients related to their nursing diagnoses, 15 percent to their DRGs, and less than 2 percent to demographics. In addition, in previous publications, he found that nursing diagnoses explained 50 to 60 percent of the variation in length of stay except in maternity and newborn nursery environments (Halloran et al., 1988). In this study, the nursing staff manually entered the nursing diagnoses for each patient at 3 P.M. every day, and these data were entered into the HIS. When aggregated nursing diagnoses were examined, the nurses' management of patient discomfort was the most frequently found nursing diagnosis (altered comfort: discomfort) (Table 9.8).

## Case-Mix Management

Case-mix management includes integrated application of several systems to determine the patient's demographics, financial payers with cost and charges, and general administrative information, including

- Discharge status
- Length of stay
- DRG classification
- Department usage
- Utilization of services
- Severity of illness
- ICD diagnoses and procedures
- Nursing diagnoses and procedures
- Attending M.D. and primary nurse
- Readmission status

In addition, nursing-specific data include acuity, nursing hours, and the patient classification to determine the patient intensity. The name of the case manager is also important to case mix.

In 1987, Halloran described a nursing management information system based on case-mix and nurse capability. This nursing case mix complemented the DRG medical system and the social data system. Together they were found to be highly predictive of patient resource use, cost, and length of stay. The cost implications were derived from patient classification (patient demand) and nurse assignment (capability). Patient dependency was examined using nursing diagnoses (Halloran, 1987).

In January 1990 Tong and Jones described the advantages of case-mix management on patient care. They analyzed the differences in case-mix-managed care versus usual care. The differences in tracking patient care in terms of patient outcomes, length of stay, and costs are shown in Table 9.9. They concluded that case-mix management is more cost-effective in profiling patient care, practice patterns, and budgeting product lines. Case-mix management is designed to maintain optimum quality while conserving resources.

**TABLE 9.8**  NURSING HOURS AND COST PER PATIENT CONDITION BY DIVISION USING NURSING DIAGNOSES

| Nursing Diagnoses Areas | Total Patient Days Reported | Mean Number Nsg. Dx for Patient Day | Total Number Nsg. Dx for Time Interval | Nursing Hours (a) Worked per Nursing Dx | | | Nursing Hours Paid (b) per Nursing Dx | | | Cost (c) Worked Hours per Nursing Dx | | | Cost (d) Paid Hours per Nursing Dx | | |
|---|---|---|---|---|---|---|---|---|---|---|---|---|---|---|---|
| | | | | * | ** | *** | * | ** | *** | * | ** | *** | * | ** | *** |
| MATERNITY/PERINATAL NURSING | | | | | | | | | | | | | | | |
| M4 | 4685 | 8.807 | 41,263 | 0.99 | 1.60 | 1.60 | 1.12 | 1.82 | 1.82 | 13.95 | 20.02 | 20.02 | 16.37 | 23.47 | 23.47 |
| MA5 | 8476 | 13.379 | 188,643 (e) | 0.33 | 0.59 | 0.59 | 0.37 | 0.67 | 0.67 | 4.34 | 7.27 | 7.27 | 5.09 | 8.49 | 8.49 |
| MN5 | 6017 | 12.505 | | | | | | | | | | | | | |
| MA6 | 1709 | 12.852 | 26,010 (e) | 2.32 | 3.43 | 3.43 | 2.60 | 3.91 | 3.91 | 30.98 | 41.01 | 41.01 | 35.71 | 47.83 | 47.83 |
| MN6 | 438 | 9.2371 | | | | | | | | | | | | | |
| Total & Mean MacDonald | 21325 | 12.001 | 255,916 | 0.63 | 1.04 | 1.04 | 0.72 | 1.19 | 1.19 | 8.60 | 12.76 | 12.76 | 10.02 | 14.91 | 14.91 |

(a) Total nursing hours worked for time interval ÷ total number of nursing diagnoses for time interval
(b) Total nursing hours paid for time interval including benefits ÷ total number of nursing diagnoses for time interval
(c) Total nursing dollars paid for worked hours for time interval ÷ total number of nursing diagnoses for time interval
(d) Total nursing dollars paid for time interval including benefits ÷ total number of nursing diagnoses for time interval
* Category of worker includes head nurse, assistant head nurse, advanced clinical nurse, staff nurse I and II, PRN nurse, LPN I and II, or tech I and II.
** All categories of workers as defined on attachment.
*** All categories of workers as defined on attachment except for Hemo, PES, AES, OR/RR.

Source: Halloran, 1994.

**TABLE 9.9**   FINANCIAL EFFECTS OF TWO TREATMENT PLANS

| Case as managed | Alternative treatment |
|---|---|
| **Tuesday** | **Tuesday** |
| Admission for severe anemia, chronic rectal bleeding, lower abdominal pain | Admission for severe anemia, chronic rectal bleeding, lower abdominal cramps |
| Workup for anemia | Consultation by gastroenterologist |
| Transfusions | Workup for anemia |
| **Wednesday** | Transfusions |
| Consultation by gastroenterologist | **Wednesday** |
| **Thursday** | Upper endoscopy of stomach and duodenum |
| Upper endoscopy of stomach and duodenum | **Thursday** |
| **Friday** | Barium enema (large bowel x-ray study) |
| Barium enema (large bowel x-ray study) | Attending physician checks results: cancer of the cecum |
| **Saturday** | Call surgeon |
| Attending physician checks results: cancer of the cecum | Coordinate colonoscopy and surgery |
| **Monday** | **Friday and Saturday (Sunday)** |
| Surgical consultation | Bowel preparation with laxatives and antibiotics |
| **Tuesday** | |
| Colonoscopy | **Monday** |
| **Wednesday** | Colonoscopy followed by resection of right colon |
| Bowel preparation with laxatives and antibiotics | Eight-day postoperative management |
| **Friday** | |
| Resection of right colon | |
| Eight-day postoperative management | |

|              |          |       |              |          |
|--------------|----------|-------|--------------|----------|
| Total length of stay: | 18 days |  | Total length of stay: | 14 days |
| Total cost:  | $12,405  |       | Cost savings: |          |
|              |          |       | Four hospital days | $2,180.00 |
|              |          |       | One bowel preparation | 11.17 |
|              |          |       | Total savings: | $2,191.17 |

18 percent of total cost

*Source:* Tong and Jones, 1990. (Reprinted by permission, from Healthcare Financial Management, January 1990. Copyright 1990 by the Healthcare Financial Management Association.)

## Consumer Surveys

The administrative applications of the 1990s require more information on performance measures, including surveys of the elements of the health care, the providers of the health care, and the consumers or purchasers of the health care services. These measures are important in order to effectively utilize data to better understand health care services and to improve the health care services provided. One element of performance measures is consumers' satisfaction with care. Managed care systems are including patient survey information in the minimum data standards, since consumer satisfaction can be used to market the services of an organization. However, the variability in tools for collecting satisfaction information is limiting the comparability of data from different health plans. The principal advantage of standardizing the consumer response is the ability to make comparisons among the multiple sites of hospital chains. Standardization may also have a benefit in terms of aggregating data to develop state-of-the-art survey instruments. A number of survey tools have been recently developed for use in the managed care industry (Allen, 1993; Davies and Ware, 1991; Ware and Sherbourne, 1992).

### Patient Satisfaction

Patient satisfaction information is more important in the outcomes-oriented health care of today, since the health care outcomes may be positive and the patient's satisfaction with care negative. The corollary might also be true, that the consumer's health outcome is negative (even death), but the consumer or significant other was very satisfied with the care. In addition to satisfaction surveys, the consumers need to be queried regarding their decisions about purchasing health care, their attitudes toward products, and their perceptions of convenience, location, price, reputation, and quality. Demographic patient data need to be collected in relation to the survey; these include socioeconomic level, age, sex, race, and address.

### Access to Care

Another element covered by consumer surveys is access to care. A recent Institute of Medicine report defines access as "a shorthand term for a broad set of concerns that center on the degree to which individuals and groups are able to obtain needed services from the medical care system" (Millman, 1993). This same report describes specific indicators to measure access, including prenatal care and breast and cervical cancer screening. The number of patients who have encounters with the health care system, the amount of time they wait, the availability of primary care or specialty physicians, and the availability of nurse practitioners to triage patients will become more important in the new computer systems responsive to managed care. The provision of access standards and actual performance at patient visits or from telephone responses will also become important patient survey information.

## NURSING UNIT MANAGEMENT SYSTEMS

Nursing unit management computer systems facilitate nursing unit management. The essential applications of nursing unit management systems have also expanded over the past five years. The essential ones include the following:

- Nursing intensity
- Patient classification systems

- Acuity systems
- Staffing and scheduling systems
- Inventory
- Patient billing
- Other unit management reports

## Nursing Intensity

Nursing intensity includes measures of nursing hours per patient day derived from census data, cost data, and patient classification or workload measures. It combines patient acuity and patient classification or workload measurements to determine the nursing resources required (Thompson and Diers, 1991). To date, there is no single system that allows comparisons between units within a hospital or between hospitals. An administrator comparing intensity per case could not currently discern whether differences are due to differences in patient acuity or to the bias introduced by using different classifications or workload measurements. Comparing hospitals, one could not determine whether differences in intensity are due to different levels of personnel, sicker patients, or poor administrative management. Until systems are developed that weight or risk-adjust the many variables involved in assessing intensity, cross-site comparisons will be based upon several underlying assumptions.

Nursing intensity refers to the amount and type of nursing resources used to care for an individual patient over the entire hospital stay or episode of care (O'Brien-Pallas and Giovanetti, 1993). Further, nursing resources are defined as the nursing care time (in hours) required to deliver both direct and indirect care, and the mix or level of nursing staff involved in the delivery of that care (Giovanetti, 1978).

The Patient Intensity of Nursing Index (PINI) includes the amount of care measured in hours, the complexity of care, the clinical judgment necessary to care for a patient in specific clinical settings, and the medical severity (Prescott, 1991). This is one of the models that includes a risk adjustment in the acquisition of data.

Recently, intensity was expanded to include hours of care, complexity of patient conditions, medical severity, and the environment (O'Brien-Pallas et al., 1994).

Halloran (1987) and Reitz (1985) have also developed approaches to measuring patient classification based on nursing intensity which incorporate nursing's critical thinking associated with assessment and management of patient care. These systems have been developed and tested mostly in adult medical and surgical patients.

In a recent validation study of nursing intensity measures, Rosenthal et al. (1992) described the use of a nursing severity index based upon nursing diagnoses. The finding that the nursing severity index was related to mortality rates and had prognostic accuracy similar to that of other nursing intensity scores makes this tool potentially useful in case-mix management, outcomes assessment, quality assurance, and care management. The prognostic accuracy of this system was similar to that of a commercially available and widely used severity of illness measure (Medigroups). This system needs to be tested in a variety of hospitals to determine if hospital comparability and variance can be explained by nursing diagnoses.

## Patient Classification Systems

An approach to management efficiency is the patient classification system, a scheme by which patients' needs for nursing services can be assessed (Jelinek et al., 1973, 1974). Patient classification is defined as the "identification and classification of patients into groups or categories, and the quantification of these categories as a measure of the nursing effort required (in caregiving)" (Giovanetti, 1979). Such systems are ultimately used to plan nurse staffing assignments based upon patient needs. To date, over 200 different systems have been identified (Aydelotte, 1973; Giovanetti, 1978). This development of patient classification systems was stimulated in the early 1980s by JCAHO (then JCAH), recommending that all hospitals use a documented method to allocate and distribute nurses based on patient care requirements so that nursing resources and nurse staffing could be more effective.

Currently, the JCAHO states that for accreditation of health care organizations, the following standards must be met (Joint Commission on Accreditation of Health Care Organizations, 1993): "The nurse executive and other appropriate registered nurses develop hospital wide patient care programs, policies, and procedures that describe how the nursing care needs of patients or patient populations are assessed, evaluated, and met. . . . The hospital's plan for providing nursing care is designed to support improvement and innovations in nursing practice and is based on both the needs of the patients to be served and the hospital's mission."

There are three types of patient classification systems that rely on task determinations: (1) the system identifies patient profiles and predicts the need for nursing, (2) the system identifies all nursing care tasks associated with patient care and standard times used to conduct each task, which are then summed to produce hours of care needed, and (3) the system uses a critical indicator approach, basing total nursing care time on a few indicators of care, which are weighted to reflect relative nursing effort.

In 1978, the federal government published reports on methods for studying nurse staffing in a patient unit. The project recommended that staffing needs be established by comparing the service level with care estimates based on patient classification and the head nurse's perception of adequate care. The model also provided a conceptual framework for evaluating personnel skills or different staffing patterns (Division of Nursing, Department of Health and Human Services, 1978).

Today, however, many issues still exist in choosing a patient classification system, including whether a staffing formula based on patient classification is reliable and which method of patient classification is best for a particular institution. The major classification systems are Medicus, Grasp, Atwork, and Exelcare.

A stated aim of patient classification and its methodology is to match staffing to patient requirements, resulting in the following:

- Optimum use of personnel
- Improved quality of care
- Savings from prevention of overstaffing

Further, the patient classification systems represent a methodological approach unique to the nursing profession. By devising a method to assess patients' needs for nursing care and thus the hours of care required during each 24-h period and the category of personnel needed, a quantitative statement of patients' requirements for nursing care can be established. The better classification systems include measures of functional status, patterns of dependency, and quality-of-life measures to support clinical nursing decisions.

The settings using computers in administration have expanded from hospitals to long-term care facilities, community and home health agencies, ambulatory care centers, and independent nursing practices (Sennett, 1992). These settings will also require quality management that ensures the value of purchased care.

A disadvantage of having approximately 200 classification systems currently available is that estimating overall time, complexity of patient care, and nursing involvement in attaining patient outcomes is not possible. Unless one classification system is used, nursing use of time, skills, and complexities cannot be compared from setting to setting. There are three possible solutions: (1) develop a national model for a patient classification system for all hospitals to use, (2) let each site use its own system and never use classification in outcomes research, or (3) reduce all systems to a common denominator which then would be used to study variability of nursing time, complexity, and costs across different patient conditions. This was done by Thompson and Diers (1988), who described nursing care costs across different DRGs in a study of eight hospitals with different patient classification systems. They converted all classification systems to the common denominator of time of patient care. If some form of hours of nursing care could be added to a national database, one would be able to see trends in nursing care per patient condition (Prescott, 1994). According to Prescott, the major disadvantage to using hours of nursing care as a measure of nursing intensity is the lack of inclusion of complexity in the definition and the fact that many hospitals do not store their patient classifications in a computerized system from which they can be retrieved.

One of the disadvantages of using the classification systems available to date is that the concept of risk adjustment for patients' age, sex, socioeconomic status, and numbers of conditions has not been incorporated, nor has the concept of risk adjustment for level of nurse providing care, e.g., MSN, BNS, ADN, or diploma, with licensed or not licensed assistive personnel. The skill or years' experience of the nurse also confounds the measurement of hours of care given (McHugh, 1994). Therefore, there is a risk that comparisons of one hospital against another do not reflect the sicker, older, or more disadvantaged patients in one group or the level and/or experience of the nurse provider. Since most current measures arrive at a number of nurses per patient medical or nursing diagnosis, they do not take into account the role of clinical nurse specialists, case managers, or consultants in care. With the move away from acute care environments, and with patients receiving care in day-care centers or urgent care environments for day surgery, the concept of the unit of time versus episode of care has not been resolved. Should the classification be based on time per day, episode of care, or encounter of care? Nurse administrators should understand these basic limitations when interpreting and comparing certain outcome measures. Further refinements of measurement will be needed in the future.

### Decision Support System

A decision support system for patient classification will include components of more than patient classification for nursing staffing. An example of a variance report based on acuity level derived from a decision support system is shown in Table 9.10. It should integrate costing of nursing services, budgeting, program assessment, quality screens, activity tracking, communication with departments, and the development of nursing charges per patient. The resultant reports needed in today's environment will give average values per patient and per skill mix per shift, and hours or units of classification by day or stay. These types of decision support systems become the engines needed by the critical path manager or the case manager for integrating costs with resources and outcomes of care. The advantage to these systems is that they can identify high-volume cases; develop treatment profiles; build profiles of baseline data for usual lengths of stay, costs, outcomes, and staffing requirements; review the patient distribution across nursing units; and identify providers associated with high or low outcomes for special patient conditions. Nurse case managers can build treatment profiles by day or stay; separate normative patients from outliers; select model providers who attain outcomes; compare alternative treatment patterns with outcomes based on nursing services, skill mix, experience mix, or units; and identify the cost per case. The advantages to the integrated system are discussed in Chap. 13.

**TABLE 9.10**   VARIANCE REPORT BASED ON ACUITY LEVEL*

| Products in Product Field E | (REF) Cases | (REF) Budget Cases | Actual Variable Costs | Budgeted Variable Costs | Variance | Percent Variance | (REF) Units |
|---|---|---|---|---|---|---|---|
| 1 Acuity Level 1 | 85 | 81 | 129,276 | 115,510 | 13,766 | 10.65% | 11,553 |
| 2 Acuity Level 2 | 76 | 69 | 208,959 | 177,755 | 31,204 | 14.93% | 17,709 |
| 3 Acuity Level 3 | 53 | 55 | 237,078 | 213,005 | 24,073 | 10.15% | 21,128 |
| 4 Acuity Level 4 | 29 | 21 | 272,907 | 175,788 | 97,120 | 35.59% | 25,882 |
| 1 Medical | 243 | 225 | $848,221 | $682,058 | $166,163 | 19.59% | 76,272 |
| DRG 89 SIMP PNEUM/PLEUR AGE >17 W | 268 | 244 | $953,567 | $793,311 | $160,256 | 16.81% | 85,120 |
| REPORT TOTAL | 446 | 439 | $1,484,072 | $1,282,659 | $201,413 | 13.57% | 130,944 |

*Amherst Regional Hospital Nursing Acuity Budget Variance Report (Detailed 3 Feb 95 11:18 AM) DRG 89 SIMP PNEUM/PLEUR AGE>17 W/ 1 Medical.

Source: HBO & Company's Amherst Product Group, 1995.

A classification scheme called the Patient Assessment and Information System (PAIS), which was developed in Australia by Hovenga (1994), began to be used in 1983 in many Australian hospitals. The system has been extended for use in allocating nursing services and costing nursing services per DRG. One of the difficulties in adapting PAIS for many hospitals in Australia was the lack of a uniform nursing language system to classify and describe consistently how nurses describe their practice and what they do. When examining and analyzing nursing work, Hovenga finds the elements in Table 9.11 important. She further classifies nursing work into direct patient/nurse interactions (medication administration), indirect patient-related interactions (documentation), and indirect non-patient-related interactions (education and committee attendance).

## Acuity Systems

Acuity values reflect the relative proportion of nursing time required for each classified patient type. Classification translated into workload equals acuity. Staffing is based on patient types. Newer computer systems integrate acuity with nursing care planning or cost out nursing based on acuity needs.

Software programs, interchangeable with programmable calculators, can compute staffing needs, allocate staff, and construct management reports. In addition, they provide a unit profile that adjusts for staff illness and absences, overtime, and other factors.

**TABLE 9.11**    ELEMENTS IMPORTANT WHEN ANALYZING NURSING WORK

- Time required to perform the job
- Organization and methods employed, including the availability and use of labor-saving devices
- Cost of providing the nursing service
- Numbers of patients cared for
- Education, skills, experience, and physical attributes required to perform the job
- Boundaries of nursing practice and relationship with other health professionals
- Philosophical basis of work performed and its relationship to objectives to be achieved
- Working conditions relative to award requirements or other health workers
- The value of the job
- Level of agreement of actual job to job description
- Level of job satisfaction
- Opportunity for staff development and career advancement
- The quality of the product in terms of:
    Meeting organizational objectives
    Meeting professional standards of practice
    Compliance with legal and statutory regulations
    Meeting consumer expectations
    Meeting other health workers' expectations
    Meeting accreditation requirements

*Source:* Adapted from Hovenga, 1994.

In 1989, Weitzman and Clapham described the use of the HBO Clinical Cost Accounting System to integrate acuity into a clinical cost accounting–decision support system at Northwestern University. It is based upon the system developed at Northwestern, which classifies patients into five levels of acuity. In addition, this newer decision analysis system incorporates 60 other factors in 14 categories that are used to classify patients into groups according to level of illness and nursing care requirements. The two major components are patient attributes and nursing staffing data. The 14 categories of nursing activities assign a weight to care in areas such as patient status, medication and I.V., irrigation, special treatments, emotional support, diet, hygiene needs, and observations. The system requires a patient to have at least one overnight stay in order to be useful. The data are entered for days, evenings, and nights. A clinical nurse manager, who is not included in the staffing score, oversees the validity of the scores. Three levels of nursing skills are identified: registered, licensed or graduate, and nursing assistants in 2-, 4-, and 8-h time frames. Nursing acuity scores reflect charge codes that are unit-specific and acuity-level-specific.

A study by Kuhn (1980) indicated that 69 percent of the variation in estimating nursing activity and the needs for staffing could be predicted by assessing hygiene, nutrition, elimination, body fluids, patient sex, and whether the patient was quadriplegic, paraplegic, or terminally ill. Halloran (1985) found that the patient's ability to perform activities of daily living (ADL), the degree of mobility, and the presence of pain were predictive of the nursing care needs.

Finnegan et al. (1993) describe the need to link acuity systems with cost and care and quality measurement with patient outcomes. The resulting system enables a more complete picture of the nursing role in the attainment of outcomes. In the decade ahead, acuity, classification, and intensity systems with better control of variables and standardization for comparison between sites will have to be developed.

## Staffing and Scheduling Systems

Computer systems for staffing and scheduling have existed for almost 25 years. An early description of computer systems for nursing staffing rosters was written in 1970. Computers were used to allow objective and consistent staffing assignments (Dominick, 1970).

Staff rosters and scheduling systems are available on mainframes, minicomputers, and microcomputers. A staff roster can operate on the hospital's patient acuity system or census. Daily staffing worksheets, productivity sheets, assignments based on qualifications, unit preference, and skills are available through these systems. These systems boast of saving 90 percent time in staffing and scheduling and six full-time equivalents (FTEs) or more in improved staff control. The scheduler systems create customized schedules and automatically incorporate workload, work preferences in nursing, special requisitions, and assignments to continuing education programs.

The success of a nurse scheduling system will depend on its being able to accommodate many of the constraints involved in adequately staffing a hospital (Okada, 1992). These include

- Recognizing day-to-day sequencing of the varied roles a nurse may assume. For example, the system may include hospital policy concerning how many consecutive days a person must remain on the night shift.
- Satisfying individual preferences for days off or for particular role tasks. For example, some nurses need every Monday off for child care, or they prefer to treat only patients with particular conditions.
- Requiring an equality of workload. For example, weekend/holiday services should be distributed equally among nurses either monthly or annually.
- Constraining team member composition. For example, nurses have special skills, and a hospital requirement may be that at least two leadership nurses must be available on each shift or that the team must be composed of one nurse from each skill category.

Administrative systems help administrators to manage patient data, staff data, and financial data. A full system includes acuity, staffing, scheduling, staff profiles, assignments, and management reports.

McHugh (1987) studied four staffing patterns using computer simulation to examine differences in wage costs and in overstaffing and understaffing produced by the four patterns. The patterns that she studied were fixed distributed, float pool, controlled variable, and skill center staffing. The study modeled three types of hospitals: a small community hospital, a large community hospital, and a large Veterans Administration hospital. She found that fixed distributed staffing produced the highest wage costs, followed by float pool staffing. There were no differences between controlled variable and skill staffing in terms of mean yearly wage costs. With regard to the incidence of overstaffing, fixed distributed staffing performed poorly compared with the other three staffing patterns.

A nurse scheduling decision support system available on microcomputers has been described by Randahawa and Sitompul (1993). The system includes algorithms and databases for developing weekly work and shift patterns and for combining these patterns to produce nurse schedules. It also includes heuristic modeling to generate patterns and output schedules for many hospital environments.

## Inventory

An inventory is a record of pharmacy items and other supplies that have been received and disbursed; it shows what is in stock on nursing units.

These applications provide necessary information for auditing and analyzing use of unit stock and maintenance files on unit stock activity. Nursing unit managers are often accountable for records related to storeroom and sterile supplies. Computerized supply inventories provide them with the capability to account for stock items, track expired lots, and bill patients for supplies used.

A special type of inventory is the narcotic usage inventory, which produces special records that describe the receipt, disbursement, and amount of narcotic drugs on a nursing unit. These systems can produce summary reports acceptable for legal documentation of narcotic usage.

Inventory systems using bar codes have become the primary mechanism for billing patients, measuring utilization, and automatically tracking resource consumption.

## Patient Billing

Computers allow nurse managers to enter charges for services rendered or supplies used. More important, computers can record charges and transmit them to patient files to be compiled and entered into the patient's overall bill. Two stages of compilers are common: (1) recording the charges for compilations and changing incorrect charges to correct ones, and (2) transmitting unit charges to a central automated record that is compiled with the patient's total hospital bill.

## Other Unit Management Reports

Many nursing unit management reports can be recorded and transmitted to the appropriate hospital department. Such reports cover the following:

- Incident reports
- Poison control
- Allergy and drug reactions
- Error reports
- Infection control reports
- Unit activity reports
- Utilization review
- Shift summary reports

### Incident Reports

Incident reports identify patient, visitor, or personnel accidents. A documented record of incidents can be summarized regularly, and corrective policies, education, or research programs can be initiated. When incident reports are printed in the risk management office as they occur, corrective actions may be taken. For example, if a nurse receives a needle puncture, the nurse administrator might inform that nurse to seek corrective treatment immediately, assign a float nurse to cover, and inform the head nurse of an emergency sick leave request.

When incident report summaries indicate statistically significant occurrences of particular problems (e.g., patient falls and medication errors), the incidents may precipitate policy changes, new documentation requirements, or in-service education programs. If patients fall frequently on geriatric services, nurse administrators may want to determine if the nursing assessment for documentation on the computer includes a category for "mobility" or "potential for trauma." If nursing personnel are not using that category either before or after an incident, in-service education, policy changes, and documentation requirements might be considered.

### Poison Control

Poison control report systems have also been described. Capable of maintaining files that report accidental poisoning, these systems also include information on the most common toxic substances and appropriate antidotes or therapy.

### Allergy and Drug Reactions

Allergy and drug reaction reports include not only patients with particular allergies but those patients receiving medications known to have incompatibilities. These reports can be produced regularly, and logs can be compiled indicating the number of patients who have come in contact with drugs they are allergic to or medications that are incompatible with other drugs.

### Error Reports

Error reports may include medication or documentation errors. They can be summarized and transmitted to a nurse administrator for review on a regular basis. Some error systems track errors on line, allowing nurse managers to take quick corrective action. Modern error systems include the inappropriate assignment of DRG codes to patients, inappropriate use of procedures and tests, undocumented follow-up on abnormal procedures, delays in scheduling tests and procedures, and closer monitoring of errors related to the achievement of outcomes.

### Infection Control Reports

Infection control reports recognize patterns of bacterial or viral spread throughout a hospital or nursing unit. These systems integrate infection reports, incident reports, and laboratory culture screening reports over time to describe patterns of probable infection in the hospital. Often the area of contamination can be recognized from these reports. Computerized monitoring provides summary information.

The HELP system has automated an antibiotic consultant so that when pathogens are reported, the appropriate antibiotic regimen would be chosen for the patient (Evans et al., 1993). The Antibiotic Assistant also helps to identify patients who are receiving inappropriate antibiotic therapy as soon as the results of the antibiotic susceptibility tests are known. Early results show that the clinician was influenced by the knowledge within the antibiotic consultant system 66 percent of the time.

## Unit Activity Reports

Unit activity reports include census, patient status, shift reports, identification of patients at risk, and other unit activities and procedures. They have been computerized in several hospitals nationwide. They provide timely information that the unit nurse can enter into the terminal and send to the nurse administrator's office. In some hospitals, shift reports are no longer collected, photocopied, and distributed by the evening and night supervisors; these supervisory personnel have been relieved of this secretarial function. Since the secretarial function is no longer required, many hospitals have eliminated this level of supervision.

Patients at risk can be automatically and rapidly identified through computer systems. In addition, when special procedures or medications are ordered for patients at risk, alert notices are printed at the nursing station. If emergencies occur, emergency procedures can be printed on the unit.

## Utilization Review

Utilization review summary reports include information on the concurrent review of all patients. Information is available to certify each patient for admission and length of stay. Patient demographic information is combined with the diagnosis and operative information to determine length of stay data. Daily summary reports may then be produced for the utilization review. The summary report lists all patients who must be reviewed for admission certification and extension of length of stay.

Utilization review subsystems are available. Reports are available 5 days a week to identify patients who are near the end of their certified stay and who need continued stay review. The report includes up-to-date patient information, including diagnoses, procedures, previous certification detail, and reviewer comments. The utilization review is sequenced by the nursing station, identified hospital service and bed, or last review coordinator and bed review. Daily summaries are provided when needed, and current and future review loads are predicted. To indicate future staffing needs, the system provides summaries of future patient loads. Each month the summary reports review each patient's admitting diagnosis to provide information to establish cost rates for each diagnosis, to examine the effectiveness of the review mechanism, and to support more effective discharge scheduling. These systems can provide either diagnosis or procedure reviews.

New utilization review software pools information about successful procedures and tests to attain outcomes, includes documents and reference literature that support the appropriate use of the procedures and tests, and provides boundaries of practice for the health care provider. These new systems are often cited as including "clinical practice guidelines"; however, the process of producing these systems and the results are distinctly different from the clinical practice guidelines described in Chap. 13. The success of these products is related to the establishment of boundaries of practice that are predetermined for managed care.

### Shift Summary Reports

Shift summary reports allow a summary of patient classifications, acuity/ staffing information, and nursing personnel information to be computerized. These cumulative shift reports integrate the information of other nursing unit reports and are then transmitted to the nursing administrator to integrate with nursing service information. These records are also integrated with the hospital or nursing department budgeting system.

## SUMMARY

This chapter presented a broadened description of the expanded responsibilities of the nurse administrator of today. Because of these increased responsibilities, this chapter also described the expanded systems which serve as tools for nursing services administration and nursing unit management. Especially expanded were the discussions of costing of nursing care and classification systems. Because the obligations of nursing administration have been expanded, computer applications that facilitate efficient capture of financial data have been augmented. Today's nurse administrator has moved into the role of corporate executive officer who has obligations to report to the institution, to society, and to national accrediting bodies. These responsibilities are also imposed by the professional practice of nursing. Today's nurse administrator needs more than a basic understanding of word processing and mail systems. The nurse administrator has a moral obligation to help reduce health care costs through better management of nursing information.

## REFERENCES

Allen, N. A., and Davies, A. R. (1993). *Employee Health Care Value Survey* (unpublished). Boston: New England Medical Center Hospitals.

American Association of Nurse Executives (The) (AONE) in Cooperation with the Center for Healthcare Information Management (CHIM). (1993). *Informatics: Issues and Strategies for the 21st Century Health Care Executive. Resource Book and Video Set.* Chicago: American Hospital Association Services.

American Nurses Association Task Force on Standards for Organized Nursing Services. (1988). *Standards for Organized Nursing Services and Responsibilities of Nurse Administrators across All Settings.* Kansas City, MO: American Nurses Association.

Anderson, R. A., Dobal, M. T., and Blessing, B. B. (1992). Theory-based approach to skill development in nursing administration. *Computers in Nursing, 10*(4):152–157.

Austin, C. (1979). *Information Systems for Hospital Administration.* Ann Arbor, MI: Health Administration Press.

Aydelotte, M. (1973). *Nursing Staffing Methodology: A Review and Critique of Selected Literature* (DHEW Pub. No. 73-433). Washington, DC: U.S. Government Printing Office.

Classen, D. C., Pestotnik, S. L., Evans, R. S., and Burke, J. P. (1991). Computerized surveillance of adverse drug events in hospital patients. *Journal of the American Medical Association, 266*(20), 2847–2851. (Published erratum appears in *Journal of the American Medical Association, 267*(14), April 8, 1992).

Davies, A. R., and Ware, J. E. (1991). *Customer Satisfaction Survey and User's Manual* (2d ed.) (unpublished). Washington, DC: Group Health Association of America.

Division of Nursing, Department of Health and Human Services. (1978). *Methods for Studying Nurse Staffing in a Patient Unit: A Manual to Aid Hospitals in Making Use of Personnel* (DHHS Pub. No. 78-3). Washington, DC: U.S. Government Printing Office.

Dick, R. S., and Steen, E. B. (Eds.). (1991). *The Computer-Based Patient Record: An Essential Technology for Health Care.* Institute of Medicine, Washington, DC: National Academy Press.

Dominick, V. (1970). Automation of nursing staff allocation. *Supervisor Nurse,* 43,209.

Evans, R. S., Pestotnik, S. L., Classen, D. C., and Burke, J. P. (1993). Development of an automated antibiotic consultant. *M.D. Computing, 10*(10), 17–22.

Filosa, L. (1978). Automated communication saves time, money. *Hospital Progress,* 49, 115–118.

Finnegan, S. A., Abel, M., Dobler, T., et al. (1993). Automated patient acuity: Linking nursing systems and quality measurement with patient outcomes. *Journal of Nursing Administration, 23*(5), 62–71.

Garre, P. P. (1990). A computerized recruitment program. *Journal of Nursing Administration, 20*(1), 24–27.

Giovanetti, P. (1978). *Patient Classification Systems in Nursing: A Description and Analysis* (DHEW Pub. No. HRA 78-22). Hyattsville, MD: U.S. Government Printing Office.

Giovanetti, P. (1979). Understanding patient classification systems. *Journal of Nursing Management, 15*(8), 31–34.

Halloran, E. (1987). Case-mix: Matching patient need with nursing resource. *Nursing Management, 18*(3), 27–42.

Halloran, E. (1994). Predicting nursing care costs with nursing diagnoses. Personal communication.

Halloran, E., Kiley, M. L., and England, M. (1988). Nursing diagnosis, DRGs and length of stay. *Applied Nursing Research, 1*(1), 22–26.

Halloran, E., Patterson, C., and Kiley, M. (1985). Nursing workload, medical diagnosis related groups, and nursing diagnoses. *Research in Nursing and Health,* 8, 421–433.

Hannah, K. J. (1993). Nursing management of information. In M. Ogilvie and
    E. Sawyer (Eds.), *Managing Information in Canadian Health Care Facilities.*
    Ottawa, Canada: Canadian Hospital Association Press.

Hovenga, E. (1994). *Casemix, Hospital Nursing Resource Usage and Costs: The
    Basis for a Nursing Utilization Review System.* Ph.D. dissertation. Sydney,
    Australia: University New South Wales.

Jelinek, R., Haussman, D., Hegyvary, S., and Newman, J. (1974). *A Methodology
    for Monitoring Quality of Nursing Care* (DHEW Pub. No. HRA 74-25). Wash-
    ington, DC: U.S. Government Printing Office.

Jelinek, R., Zinn, T., and Brya, J. (1973). Tell the computer how sick the patients
    are and it will tell how many nurses they need. *Modern Hospital,* 121, 81–85.

Johnson, J. (Ed.). (1988). *The Nurse Executive's Business Plan.* Rockville, MD:
    Aspen Publishers.

Joint Commission on Accreditation of Health Care Organizations. (1993). *Accredi-
    tation Manual for Hospitals* (AMH). Oakbrook Terrace, IL.

Kuhn, B. G. (1980). Prediction of nursing requirements from patient characteris-
    tics (Parts I and II). *International Journal of Nursing Studies, 17,* 5–12;
    69–78.

Little, A. D. (1992). *Telecommunications: Can It Help Solve America's Health Care
    Problems* (Reference No. 91810-98). Cambridge, MA.

McHugh, M. (1987). *Comparison of Four Nurse Staffing Patterns for Wage Costs
    and Staffing Adequacy Using Computer Simulation.* Doctoral dissertation,
    Ann Arbor, MI: University of Michigan.

McHugh, M. (1994). Issues in defining "intensity of nursing care" as an element of
    the nursing minimum dataset (unpublished). Report to the Database Steering
    Committee, American Nurses Association, March 1–2, 1994.

Melmon, K. (1971). Preventable drug reaction—Causes and cures. *New England
    Journal of Medicine, 284*(24), 1, 361.

Millman, M. (Ed.). (1993). *Access to Health Care in America* (Institute of Medicine
    Report). Washington, DC: National Academy Press.

O'Brien-Pallas, L., and Giovanetti, P. (1993). Nursing intensity. In *Papers from
    Nursing Minimum Data Set Conference, 27–29 October 1992: Edmonton,
    Alberta, Canada* (pp. 68–76). Ottawa, Ontario: Canadian Nurses Association.

O'Brien-Pallas, L., Giovanetti, P. and Peerboom, E. (1994). *Care Costing and
    Nursing Workload: Past, Present and Future, A Review of the Literature.*
    Toronto, Canada: University of Toronto Quality of Nursing Worklife Mono-
    graph Series.

Okada, M. (1992). An approach to the generalized nurse scheduling problem—
    Generation of a declarative program to represent institution-specific knowl-
    edge. *Computers and Biomedical Research, 25*(5), 417–434.

Picone, D. M. (1991). *Casemix Funding: Professional and Industrial Impacts on
    Nursing.* National Casemix Conference.

Porter, S. (1994). Complying with JCAHO's IM Standards. *Healthcare Informatics,
    11*(7), 62, 64, 66.

Prescott, P. (1991). Nursing intensity: Needed today for more than nurse staffing.
    *Nursing Economics, 9*(6), 409–414.

Prescott, P. (1994). Personal communication.

Randahawa, S. U., and Sitompul, D. (1993). A heuristic-based computerized nurse
    scheduling system. *Computer Operations Research, 20*(8), 837–844.

Reitz, J. (1985). Toward a comprehensive nursing intensity index. Part I, Development, and Part II Testing. *Nursing Management, 16,* 21–42.

Rosenthal, G. E., Halloran, E. J, Kiley, M., Pinkley, C., and Landefeld, C. S. (1992). Development and validation of the nursing severity index: A new method for measuring severity of illness using nursing diagnoses. *Medical Care, 30*(12), 1127–1141.

Schmitz, H., Ellerbrake, R., and Williams, T. (1976). Study evaluates effects of new communication system. *Hospitals, 50,* 129.

Sennett, C. (1992). The computer-based patient record: The third party payer's perspective. In M. J. Ball and M. F. Morris (Eds.), *Aspects of the Computer-Based Patient Record* (pp. 40–45). New York: Springer-Verlag.

Shortliffe, E. H., Tang, P. C., Amatayakul, M. K., et al. (1992). Future vision and dissemination of computer-based patient records. In M. J. Ball, and M. F. Collen (Eds.), *Aspects of the Computer-Based Patient Record* (pp. 273–293). New York: Springer-Verlag.

Silva, J. S., and Zawilski, A. J. (1992). The health care professional's workstation: Its functional components and user impacts. In M. J. Ball, and M. F. Collen (Eds.), *Aspects of the Computer-Based Patient Record* (pp. 102–124). New York: Springer-Verlag.

Simpson, R. (1991a). The role of the clinical nurse specialist in information systems selection. *Clinical Nurse Specialist, 5*(3), 159–163.

Simpson, R. (1991b). The Joint Commission did what you wouldn't. *Nursing Management, 22*(1), 26–27.

Simpson, R. (1991c). Technology: Nursing the system, Computer-based patient records, Part I: The Institute of Medicine's vision. *Nursing Management, 22*(10), 24–25.

Simpson, R. (1991d). Technology: Nursing the system, Computer-based patient records, Part II: IOM's 12 requisites. *Nursing Management, 22*(11), 26–27.

Simpson, R. (1992). *Decision Support for Product Line Management in Technology: Nursing the System.* Atlanta, GA: HBO.

Thompson, J. D. (1981). Prediction of nurse resource use in treatment of diagnosis related groups. In H. Werley and M. R. Grier (Eds.), *Nursing Information Systems* (pp. 60–75). New York: Springer.

Thompson, J. D., and Diers, D. (1988). Management of nursing intensity. *Nursing Clinics of North America, 23*(2), 473–491.

Thompson, J. D., and Diers, D. (1991). *Nursing Resources: DRG Their Design and Development* (pp. 121–122). Ann Arbor, MI: Health Administration Press.

Tong, D. A., Jones, P. L. (1990, January). Physicians, financial managers join forces to control costs. *Healthcare Financial Management, 44*(1), 21–22, 24, 26 passim.

Ullian, E. (1992). Hospital administrators' needs for computer-based patient records. In M. J. Ball and M. F. Collen (Eds.), *Aspects of the Computer-Based Patient Record* (pp. 30–35). New York: Springer-Verlag.

Van Slyck, A. (1991a). A systems approach to the management of nursing services, Part I: Introduction. *Nursing Management, 22*(3), 16–19.

Van Slyck, A. (1991b). A systems approach to the management of nursing services, Part II: Patient classification system. *Nursing Management, 22*(4), 23–25.

Van Slyck, A. (1991c). A systems approach to the management of nursing services, Part III: Staffing system. *Nursing Management, 22*(5), 30–34.

Van Slyck, A. (1991d). A systems approach to the management of nursing services, Part IV: Productivity monitoring system. *Nursing Management, 22*(6), 18–20.

Van Slyck, A. (1991e). A systems approach to the management of nursing services, Part V: The audit system. *Nursing Management, 22*(7), 14–15.

Van Slyck, A. (1991f). A systems approach to the management of nursing services, Part VI: Costing system. *Nursing Management, 22*(8), 14–16.

Van Slyck, A. (1991g). A systems approach to the management of nursing services, Part VII: Billing system. *Nursing Management, 22*(9), 18–21.

Ware, J. E., and Sherbourne, C. D. (1992). The MOS 36-item short-form health survey (SF-36): Conceptual framework and item selection. *Medical Care, 30,* 473–483.

Wasden, W. (1991). Quality assessment: From paper shuffle to paperless review. *Computers in Healthcare,* p. 30.

Weitzman, L. J., and Clapham, K. T. (1989). Nursing acuity sensitive decision support system. In L. Kingsland (Ed.), *Proceedings from the Thirteenth Annual Symposium on Computer Applications in Medical Care* (pp. 844–847). Washington, DC: IEEE Computer Society Press.

Winslow, R. (Oct. 8, 1993). Hospitals wake up to the power of computers. *Wall Street Journal,* p. 4.

# BIBLIOGRAPHY

Ball, M. J., and Collen, M. F. (Eds.). (1992). *Aspects of the Computer-Based Patient Record.* New York: Springer-Verlag.

Connor, R., et al. (1961). Effective use of nursing resources: A research report. *Hospital, 35,* 30–39.

Davies, A. R. (1992). Health care researchers' needs for computer-based patient records. In M. J. Ball and M. F. Collen (Eds.), *Aspects of the Computer-Based Patient Record* (pp. 46–56). New York: Springer-Verlag.

Diers, D. (1992). Diagnosis related groups and the measurement of nursing. In L. Aiken and C. Fagin (Eds.), *Charting Nursing's Future.* Philadelphia: Lippincott.

Finkler, S. A. (1991). Variance analysis: Extending flexible budget variance analysis to acuity (Parts I and II). *Journal of Nursing Administration, 21*(7–8), 19–25.

Fralic, M. F. (1992). Into the future: Nurse executives and the world of information technology. *The Journal of Nursing Administration, 22*(4), 111–112.

Giovanetti, P., and Mayer, G. (1984). Building confidences in patient classification systems. *Nursing Management, 15*(8), 31–34.

Halloran, E. (1988). Nursing workload, medical diagnosis related groups, and nursing diagnosis. *Research Nursing Management, 18*(3), 27–30; 32–36.

Health Department of Western Australia (1991, September). *Nursing Staffing Methodology.* Report, 1–86.

Health Management Technology. (1995, February 15). 1995 Market Directory Issue. *Health Management Technology,* 15–81.

Lewis, E. N. (1988). *Manual of Patient Classification.* Rockville, MD: Aspen Publishers.

O'Connor, F. (1983). Nurse management systems and budget control. In O. Fokkens, A. Haro, and A. Vanderwerff et al. (Eds.), *MEDINFO 83 Seminars.* Amsterdam, Netherlands: North-Holland.

Prescott, P. A. (1986). DRG prospective reimbursement: The nursing intensity factor. *Nursing Management, 17*(1), 43–48.

Prescott, P., and Phillips, C. (1988). Gauging nursing intensity to bring costs to light. *Nursing and Health Care, 9*(1), 17–22.

Prescott, P. A., Ryan, J. A., Soeken, K. L, et al. (1991). The patient intensity for nursing index: A validity assessment. *Research in Nursing and Health, 14,* 213–221.

Saba, V. (1988). Classification schemes for nursing information systems. In N. Daly and K. Hannah (Eds.), *Proceedings of Nursing Computers, Third International Symposium on Nursing Use of Computers in Information Science* (pp. 184–193). St. Louis: Mosby.

Saba, V., Johnson, J., Halloran, E., and Simpson, R. (1994). *Computers in Nursing Management.* Washington, DC: American Nurses Publishing.

Saba, V., Reider, K., and Pocklington, D. (Eds.). *Nursing and Computers: An Anthology.* New York: Springer-Verlag.

Simpson, R., and Waite, R. (1989). NCNIP's system for the future: A call for accountability, revenue control, and national data sets. *Nursing Administration Quarterly, 14*(1), 72–77.

Software guide. (1993). *Nursing Management, 24*(7), 70–98.

Sovie, M. D., Tarcunale, M. A., Vanputte, A. W., and Stunden, A. E. (1985). Amalgam of nursing acuity, DRGs and costs. *Nursing Management, 16*(3), 22–42.

Thibault, C., David, N., O'Brien-Pallas, L., and Vinet, A. (1990). *Workload Measurement Systems in Nursing.* Montreal: Quebec Hospital Association.

Thompson, J. D. (1984). The measurement of nursing intensity. *Health Care Financing Review,* Suppl: 47–55.

# *10*

• • • • • • • • • • • • • • • • • • • • • • •

# PRACTICE
# APPLICATIONS

## OBJECTIVES

- Understand enhanced nursing documentation systems trends.
- Understand standards for computerized documentation of nursing practice.
- Define the advantages of nursing documentation systems.
- Understand the basic categories of nursing documentation systems.
- Describe a proposed documentation system.
- Describe the issues involved in using bedside terminals.
- Describe the integrated professional workstation networks.
- Identify decision support systems available for nursing practice.
- Describe U.S. initiatives toward a unified nursing language system.
- Describe international initiatives toward a unified nursing language system.

It has been estimated that nurses spend 30 percent of their time documenting direct care (Shortliffe et al., 1992). The computerized nursing record gives nurses in practice settings access to patient information through computer systems. But the nurse needs access to other information that supports patient care, including patient diagnostic data such as laboratory tests, information for processing medication orders, information for monitoring quality of care, and professional literature and standards (Martin, 1990). The computer provides accurate and accessible information that is important to determine the quality and costs of nursing care.

This chapter presents new concepts in computer applications for nursing practice documentation. It highlights the different types of computers that are available to document direct patient care. It also describes new trends related to computerized nursing documentation, current standards, and possible future uses of computers in nursing practice. This chapter has been expanded to also include such new directions as the professional workstation, case management, decision support systems for nursing practice, and bedside terminals. Advances in nursing information systems (NISs) to document nursing practice cannot take place without standards and uniform language systems. Advances toward a nursing unified language system are described, as well as an extended view of nursing documentation systems internationally. Chapter 13 more fully integrates the concept of nursing documentation from admission to discharge, including critical paths, the use of guidelines, and the use of information for determining patient outcomes, with the financial management of patient care so that costs can be determined and predicted.

## ENHANCED NURSING DOCUMENTATION SYSTEMS TRENDS

Because nurses are requested to assess patient-centered problems on which patient care decisions are based, the methods employed in collecting and recording data have changed. As early as the 1950s health care agencies began using computers to facilitate financial information. In the 1960s the agencies expanded usage of computers to handle patient laboratory data. In the 1970s nurses began to ask how computer usage could be expanded to document practice. By the 1980s the computer was being used for more integrated functions in practice, and applications of computers in decision support were being challenged. The use of practice applications for monitoring and measuring quality performance was being tested, and computers were being brought to the bedside. The use of documentation to look at patient trends, variability in practice, and research was being initiated.

For the next decade, workstations and integrated documentation systems for patient care and nursing practice must be provided. Practice applications need to provide feedback on patient and nursing performance profiles and monitor outcomes of care. Computer systems must be used to provide improved quality, efficacy, and effectiveness of care at lower cost. These systems will need to be expanded to include patient preference, patient outcomes, and patient satisfaction. In addition, during the 1990s nurses will be more conscious of the documentation of other health professionals in the patient record related to the outcomes of care that they are expected to achieve (e.g., respiratory therapy, physical therapy, pharmacy, etc.).

The bedside terminal or even the notebook type computer, whose practicality was questioned in 1986, is becoming a reality for nursing practice. Computers are now being used more frequently to document nursing practice in both U.S. and foreign hospitals.

Currently, the computerized patient care record provides the nurse at the bedside or in the nursing unit with access to limited information. The point-of-care or bedside terminal is not able to give the nurse access to outside information that is needed to make patient decisions unless the terminal can be connected to a mainframe through a workstation.

Beyond that, the nurse routinely has new needs in health care, including access to guidelines and updated knowledge to enable prompt decisions regarding patient care (Spath, 1993). An estimated 70 percent of information needs are currently unmet during the patient's encounter with health professionals (Covell, 1985). There are approximately 360,000 new journal articles in health care published annually (National Library of Medicine, 1989). No nurse has the time to read and synthesize that amount of information. Even if the nurse read only the nursing information, it would be nearly impossible for the nurse to utilize that information in practice without someone else reading and synthesizing it.

Workstations can help in the immediate future; however, in the long term workstations connected to national networks will provide the high-speed capabilities to integrate the documentation systems with other computer systems outside of the hospital.

Among the major problems with patient care records have been the lack of integration of inpatient and outpatient records, lack of access to other computer systems outside of the hospital, and failure to share patient profile information related to quality and outcomes of patient care from one hospital to another.

Quality assurance requires that information needs be processed for the accreditation of the hospital by the Joint Commission on Accreditation of Health Care Organizations (JCAHO) (Joint Commission on Accreditation of Health Care Organizations, 1994). Quality assurance programs can be facilitated by computer processing only when the documentation of nursing practice includes nursing process and outcome information, and is complete, without missing data.

## Growth of Nursing Documentation in Hospital Information Systems

A 1993 telephone survey, of the top 100 U.S. hospitals that were determined to be most efficient in controlling costs (determined by an HCIA, Inc., survey), indicated that 15 have in-house-developed hospital information systems (HISs), 13 still use manual documentation, and 64 have one of 8 large information systems. The remaining 8 hospitals had other information systems (Healthcare Informatics, 1994). Figure 10.1 shows the top 10 patient care systems in those 100 hospitals.

Several hospitals are set up to share the same computers. Today, many systems are adapting software developed by a prototype hospital for new facilities. Each system has its own capabilities, which are described as the standards for those systems.

The existing systems have been predominantly developed in-house or by commercial vendors, are marketed as prototype systems, and are adapted as required for a specific facility. Many of the previous vendors have merged, been purchased by other companies, or changed their names. Such large vendors generally timeshare the hardware or provide dedicated equipment and have standard software packages that can be adapted to the needs of a specific hospital with minimal effort, time, and expense. The list of current vendors can be obtained annually from such sources as the *Nursing Management Software Guide* and the *Health Management Technology Market Directory* (1995, February issue). These two sources are published annually and should be referred to for a current listing of companies.

**Figure 10.1**   Top 10 patient care systems at 100 of the best U.S. hospitals. (Courtesy Healthcare Informatics, 1994.)

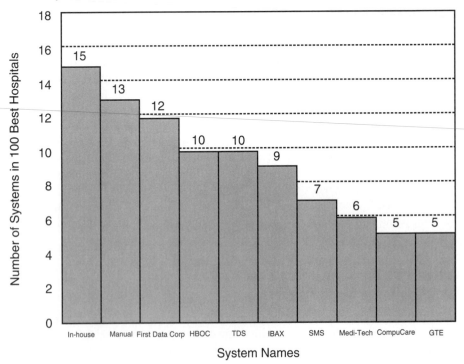

HISs are being increasingly replaced by a constellation of delivery network groups. Through the network groups, the currently closed proprietary systems have the capability of being integrated at the network level into an accessible, open system. This architecture will require several years of engineering, and will be difficult to totally implement without national standards and some uniform language and content structure.

## Standards for Computerized Documentation

Historically, nursing documentation has been consistent with hospital standards, nurse practice acts, and legal definitions of clinical nursing practice. These concepts have not changed with the new computerization of nursing documentation. As these controls grew, the amount and quality of nursing documentation also increased. Nursing documentation in the patient record has become more complex as nursing practice has expanded to encompass care of critically ill and specialty patients. However, nursing documentation, whether manual or computerized, must adhere to certain professional standards and state laws. Nurses should refer to the current standards governing computerized documentation before its application.

While much of the technology may be changing and improving, the standards that govern nurses' documentation of patient care have only become more clearly articulated. Practice acts establish regulatory and statutory rules, JCAHO and the American Nurses Association (ANA) set standards required for hospital accreditation and professional practice, and hospitals establish policies on which malpractice negligence rules are supported. A computer system only automates what other forces mandate; it cannot improve nursing practice or patient care. Computer systems should only facilitate documentation of nurses' actions, patients' conditions, and outcomes of care planning.

Legally, an undisputed independent area of professional nursing is the recording and reporting of a nursing note. Legal definitions of nursing include necessary documentation requirements. Documentation is also clearly a nursing function recognized equally by judicial decisions (Lesnik and Anderson, 1955). Nurses can be found negligent in a malpractice case with supporting evidence from a nursing note. In a legal defense, if the hospital or staff are not legally responsible for a negligent act, conclusions to this effect may be drawn from the records. A court faced with a conflict between the record of an event made at the time and the evidence of a witness relying on several years' memory is hard pressed to accept the witness's evidence. A witness is preferable only when the records are "inaccurate, illegible, or obviously unreliable" (Rozovsky, 1978).

Despite legal arguments, nursing research studies have shown that nurses have not always recorded in the nursing notes. As early as the 1950s standards of recording and reporting were found wanting (Lesnik and Anderson, 1955). Even two recent studies of nurses' documentation in long-term care facilities demonstrate that manually recording patient information leads to inaccurate and incomplete information (Petrucci et al., 1987; Palmer et al., 1992).

The discrepancy between what is required by law, standards, the profession, and nurse practice acts and actual documentation is great. Documentation should reflect an expanding profession's numerous independent and interdependent functions, particularly when evidence of assessment, planning, implementation, and evaluations is required by JCAHO and ANA standards (Joint Commission on Accreditation of Health Care Organizations, 1994; American Nurses Association, 1991).

## ADVANTAGES OF DOCUMENTATION SYSTEMS

There are in 1994 a substantial number of hospitals and nurses who have experience with computerized documentation systems. Surveys have now been completed on their perceived satisfaction with those systems. In a 1991 survey of 750 nurse executives, 340 responded. Of these, 38 percent said they had computerized NISs (Simpson, 1992). Of 129 respondents who had computers, only 29 percent said that they had bedside capabilities, and only 3 percent were dissatisfied with their system. The 340 respondents were asked to indicate the most essential functions which the computer performed; the 20 considered most essential are ranked in Table 10.1.

With the exception of bedside capability and case management, these data replicate findings of over a decade ago with nurses who were using computerized patient records (McCormick, 1983). The survey done by Simpson confirms that nurses need information on the physician's diagnosis and treatment plan. The systems have made the flow of information between the doctor and the nurse more accessible and easier to read, and have put nurses in control of the information that they need in order to observe, assess, and document complications or outcomes of medical and surgical care.

In the decade ahead, however, nurses will need different order/entry data, since the monitoring of outcomes requires information on why the physician/practitioner chose one particular intervention over another, whether the patient's preference was considered in selecting an intervention, whether the efficacy of a diagnostic procedure or intervention is documented, and whether the benefits of a procedure or intervention outweigh the risks.

Only 30 percent of the respondents in Simpson's survey thought that more functions were needed in an NIS. Of the 340 who rated the benefit of computerizing nursing process, the most important benefits were:

- Increased time nurses spend with patients
- Access to information
- Improved quality of documentation
- Improved quality of patient care
- Increased nursing productivity

- Improved communications
- Reduced errors of omissions
- Reduced medication errors
- Reduced hospital costs
- Increased nurse job satisfaction
- Compliance with JCAHO regulations
- Development of a common clinical database
- Improved patient's perception of care
- Enhanced ability to track patient's record
- Enhanced ability to recruit/retain staff
- Improved hospital image

Of the 16 listed items, benefits related to the direct care of patients ranked highest. Benefits that could be ascribed or related to hospital administration and personnel management were ranked lowest. Additionally, in 1988 the ANA described the benefits of automating nursing documentation (Zielstorff et al., 1988). The benefits of automated systems that support the nursing process described in that report were as follows:

- Help structure the care planning process.
- Support the nurses' clinical decision-making skills.

**TABLE 10.1**   THE 20 MOST ESSENTIAL FUNCTIONS THE COMPUTER PERFORMS AS FOUND FROM A SURVEY OF 340 NURSE EXECUTIVES

1. Order/entry
2. Integrate care plans with charting functions
3. Prepared patient care plans
4. Track medication administration
5. Discharge planning
6. Determine patient acuity level
7. Hospital's ability to customize system
8. Report generator capability
9. Prepare nursing assessments
10. Patient education
11. Quality assurance
12. Ancillary department access
13. Admission interview
14. Patient acuity list
15. Cost tracking and reporting
16. On-line interdepartmental communications
17. Graphical display of patient data
18. Automated medical record
19. Bedside capability
20. Case management of critical pathways

*Source:* Simpson, 1992.

- Analyze aggregated data from the care outcomes of many clients in order to guide future nursing decisions.
- Help detect or prevent certain types of nursing errors.
- Automate the retrieval of computer-stored clinical information to expand the capabilities of the quality assurance efforts.
- Facilitate access to data for nursing research. Availability of an electronically retrievable information resource will increase the number of retrospective investigations, thereby increasing the body of nursing knowledge.
- Increase the availability of information to nursing administration systems to improve the quality of nursing management decisions.
- Support the nursing process to facilitate efforts to define nursing care costs by client.
- Automate nursing care plan systems to automatically produce the patient acuity/classification report.

## BASIC CATEGORIES OF NURSING DOCUMENTATION SYSTEMS

The documentation of patient care that falls within the capability of computers includes the following categories:

- Care planning systems
- Direct patient care systems
- Discharge care planning systems
- Case management systems

The computer facilitates the documentation of nursing care activities. It is used not only for documenting care planning, which is one of the professional areas of nursing documentation, but also for documenting direct patient care, such as vital signs and intake and output records. The discharge planning component of nursing documentation provides the continuity of communication from the hospital environment to community settings. In nursing case management reports, the computer facilitates the documentation of critical paths.

### Care Planning Systems

Since 1980 the ANA has approved the nursing process and more recently approved nursing diagnosis as one of the classification schemes for a patient problem list. The care planning systems of today use the nursing process and are based on nursing diagnostic schemes or patient problem lists in North America and on patient problem lists in Europe (Saba, 1993). These systems include assessment, diagnosis, intervention, and outcome components of care.

With the advent of the computer-based patient record, the nursing care planning process can be automated. These systems enhance the quality of information, reduce documentation, reduce errors, and increase communication between nurses and other health care professionals within a hospital. An example of a computerized patient care planning system based on the nursing process that uses the nursing diagnoses is shown in Fig. 10.2.

## Direct Patient Care Systems

There are three components of direct patient care systems: those resulting from processes of care delivery that are interdependent with medical care, those that are independent, and those that are dependent on medical care (Romano et al., 1982). Some of the interdependent and dependent care processes that are facilitated by the computer are order entry of procedures and medications, retrieval of test results or historical information, scheduling procedures and services, tracking patients, and providing background information on patients' medical and physical condition. The use of computers for these functions has produced remarkable improvements over manual documentation because computers provide an infrastructure for managing a hospital and also increase communication within hospitals.

The components of the direct patient care system for documenting nursing practice that are independent of medical care, listed below, are based on the nursing process as defined by the ANA *Standards of Clinical Nursing Practice* (1991). Both in the United States and abroad, the organization of nursing documentation has used nursing process designs since 1983 (Ashton, 1983). However, since that time, ANA nursing standards defining the nursing process have expanded to incorporate assessment, diagnosis, outcome identification, planning, implementation, and evaluation (ANA, 1991). Figure 10.3 is a model of the new ANA standards for the nursing process.

No one system currently contains all the following components, which were derived from several nursing evaluation studies (Edmunds, 1984; Lang et al., 1995; Lombard and Light, 1983; McCormick, 1981; Rieder and Norton, 1984; Saba, 1993; Scholes et al., 1983).

    **I.** Nursing process

        **A.** Assessment

            **1.** Admission assessment

                **(a)** Defining characteristics

                **(b)** Nursing examination: physiological, psychological, behavioral, functional

                **(c)** Vital signs, height and weight, and other flow sheets

        **B.** Diagnosis

            **(a)** Cluster defining characteristics

        **C.** Outcome identification

            **(a)** Linkage to diagnoses

```
17WES-0236            NYUMC HOSPITAL# 4
07/06/95 06:21 PM               PAGE 001
(QAT$$P)
```

```
JUAN DON                    1713
4970290 77996 02/14/44  51  M
AMOROSI EDWARD MD
```
                                                        **JUAN DON**

```
          REPORT PERIOD:07/06/95 12:00 MN TO 06:21 PM
```

```
VITAL SIGNS:              T-O   T-R   P-R   P-A  R    BP
07/05 12:00MN                   98.0        68      120/70      RN#4
07/06 06:00AM                               66      120/70      RN#4
      06:00AM             99                                    RN#4
07/06 12:00NN                   98.7        74      122/68      RN#4
07/06 06:00PM                   99.2        72      118/70      RN#4
```

**ADL ASSESSMENTS/OBSERVATIONS:**
```
07/06 06:00AM NG, DRAINING BILE, IRRIGATED W/30CC NS, RETURNS
  CLEAR, CONNECTED TO INTERMITTENT SUCTION                     RN#4
07/06 10:00AM PT REMAINS NPO FOR OR                            RN#4
 PASSING FLATUS                                                RN#4
 NO BM                                                         RN#4
 VOIDING W/O DIFFICULTY                                        RN#4
 URINE: CLEAR, YELLOW                                          RN#4
 OOB AD LIB                                                    RN#4
 HYGIENE SELF ADMINISTERED                                     RN#4
 PT DENIES ABDOMINAL PAIN                                      RN#4
 PRE-OP TEACHING REINFORCED WITH PATIENT; INSTRUCTED IN, COUGHING
  & DEEP BREATHING, PREP, OR/RR COURSE, TUBES & DRAINS, ROOM
  CHANGES, DIET, PRE-OPERATIVE MEDICATION, ANESTHESIOLOGIST VISIT,
  EXPLANATION OF SURGERY, POST SURGERY INSTRUCTIONS            RN#4
 PATIENT DEMONSTRATES ABILITY TO PREFORM COUGHING & DEEP BREATHING RN#4
 PATIENT VERBALIZES UNDERSTANDING OF ALL OF THE ABOVE          RN#4
 NG, DRAINING BILE, IRRIGATED W/30CC NS, RETURNED CLEAR,
  CONNECTED TO INTERMITTENT SUCTION                            RN#4
07/06 06:00PM NG, DRAINING BILE, IRRIGATED W/30CC NS, RETURNED
  CLEAR, CONNECTED TO INTERMITTENT SUCTION                     RN#4
```

**PHYSICAL ASSESSMENTS/OBSERVATIONS:**
```
07/06 06:00AM
 PT'S PHYSICAL ASSESSMENT IS UNCHANGED                         RN#4
07/06 06:00PM
 TELEMETRY MAINTAINED                                          RN#4
 TELEMETRY #32                                                 RN#4
 PT'S PHYSICAL ASSESSMENT IS UNCHANGED                         RN#4
07/06 10:00AM
 NEURO ASSESSMENT: NO CHANGE IN NEURO STATUS                   RN#4
 RESPIRATORY ASSESSMENT: LUNGS CLEAR THROUGHOUT ALL FIELDS, LUNGS
  EXPANSION NORMAL, COUGH NON-PRODUCTIVE                       RN#4
 CARDIOVASCULAR ASSESSMENT: APICAL PULSE EQUALS RADIAL PULSE,
  RHYTHM REG                                                   RN#4
 RHY/ARRHY: NORMAL SINUS RHY WITH RARE PVCS                    RN#4
 PERIPHERAL VASCULAR ASSESSMENT: PEDAL PULSES POSITIVE, NO PEDAL
  EDEMA, EXTREMITIES WARM TO TOUCH                             RN#4
```

```
                        CONTINUED
```

```
JUAN DON                                      PATIENT RECORD
```

**Figure 10.2**  An example of a computerized patient care planning system based on the nursing process that uses the nursing diagnoses. (Courtesy NYUMC Hospital.)

```
07/06/95 06:21 PM              PAGE 002
(QAT$$P)
```

JUAN DON                       1713
4970290 77996  02/14/44   51   M
AMOROSI EDWARD MD

JUAN DON

REPORT PERIOD:07/06/95 12:00 MN TO 06:21 PM

GASTRO INTESTINAL ASSESSMENT: BOWEL SOUNDS POSITIVE, ABDOMEN SOFT RN#4
GENITO-URINARY ASSESSMENT: BLADDER NON-DISTENDED, NO PAIN ON
  SUPRA PUBIC PALPATION, GENITALIA NORMAL                      RN#4
SKIN ASSESSMENT: ON-GOING SKIN SURVEY                          RN#4
SKIN INTACT                                                    RN#4
NO EVIDENCE OF SKIN COLOR CHANGE INDICATIVE OF PRESSURE DAMAGE. RN#4

UNIT TESTS:
07/06 06:00AM GASTRIC DRAINAGE, GUAIAC NEG, PH 5-7            RN#4
07/06 10:00AM GASTRIC DRAINAGE, GUAIAC NEG, PH 5-7            RN#4
07/06 02:00PM GASTRIC DRAINAGE, GUAIAC NEG, PH 5-7            RN#4
07/06 06:00PM GASTRIC DRAINAGE, GUAIAC NEG, PH 5-7            RN#4

MEDICATIONS:
HEPARIN SOD INJ (5,000U/ML) 5,000U,
07/06 10:00AM   SC,GIV,ABDOMEN          REGISTERED NURSE
INDERAL,PROPRANOLOL HCL TAB
07/05 12:00MN   20MG, PO,GIV,--CRUSHED VIA NGT
                                        REGISTERED NURSE
07/06 06:00AM   20MG, PO,GIV,--CRUSHED VIA NGT
                                        REGISTERED NURSE
07/06 12:00NN   20MG, PO,GIV,--CRUSHED VIA NGT
                                        REGISTERED NURSE
07/06 06:00PM   20MG, PO,GIV,--CRUSHED VIA NGT
                                        REGISTERED NURSE

IV'S,BLOOD:

3 PERIPHERAL LINE #1 D5/.33% NACL,1000CC KCL 20MEQ RATE 125CC/HR
07/06 10:00AM  ,OBSV,SITE:,RIGHT,PVL,LINE PATENT,
               INFUSING AS ORDERED,CLEAN & DRY,
               NO SWELLING NOTED,NO REDNESS NOTED            RN#4
07/06 06:00PM  ,OBSV,SITE:,RIGHT,PVL,LINE PATENT,
               INFUSING AS ORDERED,CLEAN & DRY,
               NO SWELLING NOTED,NO REDNESS NOTED            RN#4

INTERDISCIPLINARY NOTES:

*NURSING:*

          SEE PATIENT CARE NOTES

*COMPUTER SIGNATURES:*
               REGISTERED NURSE              RN#4

                    LAST PAGE

JUAN DON                                PATIENT RECORD
-*-

**Figure 10.2**  *Continued*

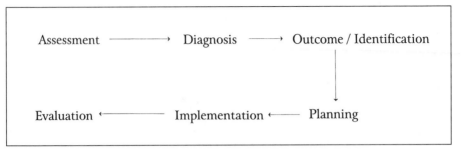

**Figure 10.3**   A model of the revised American Nurses Association standards of care: Nursing process. (From *Standards of Clinical Nursing Practice*, American Nurses Association, 1991.)

    **D.** Planning
        **(a)** Linkage between diagnoses, outcomes, and interventions
        **(b)** New nursing diagnosis
    **E.** Implementation
        **1.** Nursing interventions responsive to plans of care
            **(a)** Nursing order entry and transmission
            **(b)** Risk management
        **2.** Nursing actions responsive to nurse's or physician's orders and/or risk management to satisfy a diagnosis
            **(a)** Medication administration, intravenous medications, and blood
            **(b)** Vital signs and graphic flow sheets
            **(c)** Intake and output
            **(d)** Diet
        **3.** Nursing actions responsive to procedures and unit tests and/or risk management
            **(a)** Automatic patient order reminders
        **4.** Patient's actions
        **5.** New actions
    **F.** Evaluation
        **1.** Patient's response and actual outcomes resulting from nursing actions in relation to the diagnoses
        **2.** Patient's response and expected outcomes resulting from physicians' orders
        **3.** Patient's response and expected outcomes resulting from procedures and tests
        **4.** Patient's response and expected outcomes resulting from patient's expectations
        **5.** Patient's response and expected outcomes resulting from care delivered by other allied health professionals
  **II.** Transfer note
 **III.** Discharge care plan and summary

The following reports could result from a direct patient care system:

- Admission assessment
- Nursing care plan, including nursing diagnosis or Kardex
- Daily nursing progress note, including documentation of every problem or potential problem identified in the initial admission assessment and a reassessment or analysis of new nursing diagnoses, nursing actions, and evaluations
- Medical administration sheets, including regularly scheduled medications, intravenous medications, and blood administration
- Vital signs and other flow sheets, including intake and output, height and weight, and diet
- Nursing order summary sheets
- Automatic schedule summaries for special procedures and unit tests
- Transfer note and care plan
- Discharge care plan and summary

## Discharge Care Planning Systems

The documentation of patient care usually begins with the admission assessment and ends with the discharge care plan. Discharge care planning systems provide for continuity of care from the home to the hospital and back to the community, another care facility, an outpatient department, or the home. The computer facilitates this communication network and can provide for this continuity when computer systems within hospitals and other care facilities can communicate with each other. An advantage of open network systems is that communication between settings can be better facilitated and continuity of care improved.

Computer systems within a single hospital are being used to generate a discharge care plan for each patient. In such computerized systems, the discharge plan includes five components (Romano et al., 1982):

- A summary of the admission assessment
- A summary of the learning needs that the patient had at discharge
- A multidisciplinary plan covering problems that are still unresolved and outcomes that were not met during hospitalization
- Medication and procedures that the patient must continue
- A summary of selected patient outcomes that a multidisciplinary team desired as minimal criteria for the patient to have achieved during hospitalization

Computerized discharge care plans have the potential to be used for quality assurance, audit, research data, and information necessary for categorizing persons at discharge for prospective payment. Patients can be sent home with printed discharge plans if the content of the computerized nursing interventions or those outcomes that were not met while the patient was hospitalized are used. The problem list can also be sent with patients who are transferred to different institutions or to different wards within the same hospital (Wessling, 1972).

## Case Management Systems

Case management systems include the concepts of the nursing process. If nurses are truly using the nursing process, all components of care, outcomes management, and evaluation are in place.

One reason nursing personnel need to become more conscientious in their documentation of patient care is the use of documentation for case management. Within the concept of primary care, many hospitals are moving toward case management, or professional nursing networks, or managed care in leveled practice (Etheridge and Lamb, 1989; DiJerome, 1992; Lamb and Stempel, 1994; Loveridge et al., 1988). This chapter discusses case management from the perspective of the nursing documentation required for it. Chapter 13 describes the integration of nursing documentation with quality monitoring.

Within case management, the level of accountability shifts from the individual patient to the management of care for entire patient caseloads, allowing profiles of patients and critical paths that patients take from admission to discharge to be defined. The critical path focuses on the patient outcome and/or the patient outcome time line, rather than on the assessments and intervention strategies.

These systems provide further monitoring of the care process being completed, integration of patient care with community and home health services, and linking of patterns of care and associated costs. These systems are not designed to track all patients but only (1) those with high recidivism, (2) those with medical co-morbidities, (3) the frail elderly, (4) the chronically ill, (5) the terminally ill, or (6) "outliers" in terms of cost or length of stay. This is becoming a demographic profile of most patients who are admitted to hospitals.

Evaluation of the impact of the systems has suggested as outcomes (1) increased client satisfaction, (2) decreased hospital admissions and emergency room visits, (3) decreased costs and acuity of hospital stay, (4) minimized hospital revenue loss, (5) increased job satisfaction for nurses, and (6) decreased job stress.

Care plans are an integral part of operationalizing case management systems. In addition, patient care plans help to assure that appropriate nursing diagnoses and interventions have been selected, admission assessment requirements are completed, discharge planning and social service needs are assessed, focused utilization/quality review is done, and patient education needs are identified. At the management level, coverage is verified, benefits are identified, certification requirements are verified, second opinion requirements are verified, and potential billing problems are identified.

These functions can occur preadmission, concurrent with care, or back-end after discharge from chart reviews. From chart reviews, the managed care coordinator must rely on expert documentation, which implies the presence of information systems to audit the occurrence of these events.

# A PROPOSED DOCUMENTATION SYSTEM

An ideal computer system could operate as follows to document nurses' notes, care plans, and other traditional documentation requirements.

## Assessment/Reassessment

On admission the nurse could complete a nursing assessment covering the patient's history; this includes physical characteristics, signs, and symptoms. The assessment is made 24 to 72 h after admission, depending on the hospital's policy. The nurse would enter the information into the computer through a terminal at the nursing station, a workstation at the nursing station, a pocket terminal, a notebook brought to the bedside, or a bedside terminal.

If the computer can accept order entry from the practitioner, other patient problems (e.g., allergies) could be added to the nursing assessment. Orders for special procedures and medications could also become a part of the nursing implementation profile. The system could then prompt nurses to identify nursing care orders resulting from new practitioners' orders. The computer output generated from physicians' orders that nurses would need includes medication administration sheets, vital signs and other flow sheets, and additional physician-ordered actions on the nursing order summary sheet.

## Diagnosis

Either potential or confirmed nursing diagnoses and/or patient problems are then listed by the nurse manually, or if the nurse is interacting with an expert decision support system, the computer would suggest the probable diagnoses that exist. The nurse could select from predefined screens or enter these nursing and other patient problems into the computer through a terminal, or the expert system would generate a list of potential diagnoses.

## Outcomes Identification

A list of outcomes related to the nursing diagnoses could be generated by the computer for the nurse to select from, or with a decision support system, the known outcomes related to the particular nursing diagnoses could be presented to the nurse.

# Plan/Interventions

The computer could prompt the nurse to describe interventions (actions), observations, further assessments, or teaching that the nurse determines to be necessary for patient care. Included in these interventions are actions that the nurse takes because the patient has nursing care problems and actions that are taken in response to a physician's order. From the list of nursing actions, the computer could print automatic schedule reminders as needed. Included in these interventions are the patient's actions. However, if the nurse is interacting with a decision support system, the preprogrammed logic would list the potential nursing interventions, the expected percent improvement in outcomes based upon these interventions, and the side effects or complications associated with these interventions. In addition, this decision support system could display the costs of selecting alternative interventions.

# Implementation

The case manager or clinical nurse specialist now has the basic ingredients needed from the primary care nurse in order to generate a critical path or implementation strategy for the patient.

# Evaluation

The nurse could enter evaluation information into the computer, including the patient's response to actions, expected outcomes, and dates of expected outcomes. An expected outcome could be established for every patient, every nursing or medical problem, or every action. The nurse would sign his or her name and the date. If the nurse is interacting with a decision support system, a profile of other patients' response to this same condition could be displayed to facilitate the nurse's decision. For a single patient who has a long length of stay, e.g., beyond 3 days, the computer screen can display a graphic profile of the patient's progress toward reaching the expected outcomes. This type of profile is similar to the physiologic monitoring capabilities in the current intensive care environment. However, even on acute medical wards, trends in patients' blood pressure, temperature, pulse, respirations, and other variables could be followed.

Later, the nursing progress note could contain:

- New observations, signs, and symptoms.
- Current nursing and other problems; the computer could then prompt the nurse to comment if problems have changed or new problems have occurred.
- The previously ordered actions are documented as done/not done or given/not given, and new orders are prompted or summarized.
- The patient's response to all actions is documented (e.g., ability to learn a certain principle of hygiene).

- The patient's desires in selecting interventions are documented, as well as his or her preference for outcomes.
- The patient's satisfaction with care is summarized.

The transfer note could summarize most of the above information when the patient is transferred. The nurse determines what information will be processed. The discharge care plan and summary are similar; the nurse determines the content from the patient's hospitalization—current problems, procedures, and nursing actions. In decision support systems, a profile of the patient's problems, interventions, outcomes, and satisfaction is entered into aggregate information to profile groups of patients with the same problems (see Chap. 13 for more detail on profiles).

In 1992 the ANA published a booklet that described the criteria for and principles of a good documentation system within an NIS (Zielstorff et al., 1992). The booklet includes recommendations for the capabilities of hardware and software, including overall characteristics and highlights for user interfaces.

### Critical Paths

The critical path is mentioned here so that the nurse who is documenting practice can envision the documentation needed for the critical path. The critical path form is a summarized worksheet that can be computerized for case management (Arnold and Pearson, 1992; Marriner-Tomey, 1992; Rowland and Rowland, 1992; Swansburg, 1990; Wood et al., 1992; Zander, 1990; Zander et al., 1993). The concept of critical paths is discussed more completely in Chap. 13 as it relates to outcomes.

The nurse case manager designs the patient's care plan and monitors the progress of the actions and interventions. The computerized form allows for flexibility and individualized care, while monitoring what actions were done and what interventions were performed, and determining if the patient's expected outcomes were met. The computerized format makes it easy to make revisions to increase quality of patient care if the pathway is analyzed concurrently with the patient's hospitalization. Computerized case management assists in providing comprehensive, coordinated, and cost-effective patient care.

Figure 10.4 illustrates a critical path for patients with congestive heart failure. This path has been developed by clinical nurse specialists as a means of fulfilling managed care requirements. Clinical events are listed for each day to meet patient and family needs as well as the requirements of the utilization review, third-party payer, and accrediting agencies. Events on the path that are not completed are listed as exceptions or variances for follow-up and quality improvement activities.

A computerized system of critical pathways has been designed by DiJerome using an IBM PC with dBase software at the New England Medical Center Hospital (DiJerome, 1992).

McLAREN REGIONAL MEDICAL CENTER

## CHF CLINICAL PATH

PATIENT_____ PHYSICIAN_____ CASE TYPE_____ DRG_____ WITHOUT COMPLICATIONS_____ WITH COMPLICATIONS_____ LOS_____

- Not on Titrating vasopressors
- No endotracheal tube, vent. or CPAP

- VSS for patient
- Alert, follows commands

- Patient or S.O. is a candidate for teaching

| | DAY 1 | DAY 2 | DAY 3 | DAY 4 | DAY 5 |
|---|---|---|---|---|---|
| TEACHING | - Family/patient support; explanation of care given<br>- Anti-anxiety methods<br>- Pacing of activities | - CHF booklet<br>- Dietary booklet<br>- "Feeling Good"<br>- Medication teaching<br>- Weight monitoring<br>- Diet teaching | - With family -<br>  ADL/restrictions<br>- Activity/medications | - Teach pulse taking, signs & sx of hypokalemia, dig. tox., importance of daily wt. | - Discharge instructions (include family) |
| DISCHARGE PLANNING | - Screen for discharge planning & social services ———————————————————→ | | | | |
| CONSULTS | - Cardiology<br>- Dietary<br>- Discharge planning<br>- Social services | | | | |
| TESTS | - CXR  EKG<br>- ABG  CPK/CPKMB every 8° X3<br>- Lytes<br>- Bun  CBC<br>- Creat | - Chem profile | - CXR<br>- Lytes<br>- Bun<br>- Creat<br>- Pulse ox room air | | |
| ACTIVITY | - Dangling<br>- BSC with assist | - Up in chair | - Up in room | - Fully ambulatory ———————→ | |
| TREATMENTS | - Daily weight<br>- O₂ as ordered<br>- IV<br>- I & O<br>- Fluid restriction | - Saline lock ————→ | O₂ prn | | - D/C Saline lock |
| MEDS | - As ordered ———————————————————————→ | | | | |
| DIET | - 2 Gm Na ↓ Chol. ———————————————————→ | | | | |

Clinical Pathway (Courtesy McLaren Regional Medical Center, Flint, MI, 1993)

**Figure 10.4**  A critical path for patients with congestive heart failure. (Courtesy McLaren Regional Medical Center, Flint, MI, 1993.)

## BEDSIDE TERMINALS

In a three-part study of the impact of bedside terminals on the quality of nursing documentation at New York University Medical Center, researchers differentiated the usefulness of bedside terminals from the benefit of computers in general (Marr et al., 1993). The Medical Center already had computerized documentation at the nursing terminal and added bedside terminals to measure the differences in medication administration, daily charting, which included a record of the patient's daily functional activities and physical assessment, and admission nursing notes. The variables measured were completeness of documentation, measured by the presence or absence of each component of the record, and timeliness of documentation, which was determined by comparing the time of actual entry to the time of the actual delivery of care. The investigators found "no significant relationship" between the presence of bedside terminals and the completeness and timeliness of medication administration, daily charting of physical activity, or admission nursing notes. In their study, the investigators found that the bedside terminal was used less often than a computer away from the patient's bedside. They conclude that nursing personnel actually may need time away from the patient to collaborate with colleagues and to have thoughtful time to make substantial documentation notes. An interesting finding was that absolutely no admission notes were charted at a patient's bedside terminal. Another interesting finding was the frequency with which nurses documented care for one patient at the bedside of another patient. An acknowledged limitation of the study was the placement of the bedside terminals in the patients' rooms. It was determined by "available space" rather than designed convenience. The authors acknowledge that more research needs to be carried out to substantiate the benefits of bedside terminals. The qualitative benefits discussed in the study are shown in Table 10.2 (Marr et al., 1993).

However, Marr et al. have reported other benefits from bedside terminals, including: (1) the integration of the care plans with the nursing interventions, (2) calculation of specific acuity, and (3) automatic billing for nursing services. Others have also reported that bedside terminals improve nursing efficiency (Korpman, 1991). Additional lessons learned from bedside terminals are that aides, nurses, and management need different access and content; clinical utilization is only as good as the design is for the users; and the benefits are realized only when the organization makes changes in policies that support the new technology.

In the July 1993 issue of *Nursing Management,* which publishes a software directory annually, there were approximately 32 companies listed as having bedside capability. By 1994 about 35 systems described bedside capabilities for nursing practice documentation. By a strict definition, bedside computers are data capture devices specifically intended to be used at the bedside. In several classification schemes, one may see home health

**TABLE 10.2**    QUALITATIVE BENEFITS OF THE BEDSIDE TERMINAL
FROM A STUDY OF NURSING USE.  DIFFERENCE
WAS COMPARED TO DOCUMENTATION AT THE
NURSING STATION

- Timeliness
  a. Medication administration—No difference
  b. Daily charting—No difference
  c. Physical assessment—No difference
  d. Admission nursing notes—No difference
- Completeness of documentation
  a. Medication administration—No difference
  b. Daily charting—No difference
  c. Physical assessment—No difference
  d. Admission nursing notes—No difference

*Source:* Marr et al., 1993.

care systems or surgical scheduling systems classified as bedside computers. They may be point-of-care systems, which is a broader term that
includes computerization capabilities at points where care is rendered or
where patients are tested. Capabilities of bedside terminals range from
full patient care systems integrated with larger HISs to stand-alone nursing systems using portable data terminals. The systems are available for
medical-surgical units, ICU/CCU systems, and emergency rooms. Bedside
terminals also include hand-held portable units, but these have given way
for the most part to fixed devices.

A relatively new device being tested is the "electronic clipboard" or
notebook. This type of computer can be used at the point of care, downloaded to a workstation, and the workstation made available to an open
network. Another innovative design that is currently in beta testing is the
use of an "electronic pen" with which the user writes on a clipboard rather
than typing onto a keyboard or keypad. The software clearly recognizes
handwriting (Donovan and Corrales, 1991).

Table 10.3 identifies some of the major benefits that have been
claimed by vendors of bedside terminal systems. These benefits are in
addition to the integration of the care plan with nurses' usual care activities, calculation of hospital specific acuity, and the ability to automate
nursing billing services (Hendrickson and Kovner, 1990; Herring and
Rockman, 1990; Kahl et al., 1991; Marr et al., 1993).

In a study using a bedside terminal in Milwaukee, Wisconsin, at St.
Joseph Hospital, the hours per patient day were calculated for nursing
activities related to shift-to-shift communication of the report, chart documentation, input and output (I/O) and vital signs, access travel time to computer, and care planning. When time logs were kept for the activities, the
researchers calculated the estimated potential savings from the implementation of bedside terminals in terms of hours per patient day and overtime.

**TABLE 10.3**   THE MAJOR BENEFITS THAT HAVE BEEN CLAIMED
BY VENDORS OF BEDSIDE TERMINAL SYSTEMS

---

- Accuracy of documentation
- Timeliness of documentation
- Completeness of documentation
- Few medication errors
- More time spent in the presence of the patient
- Improved communications between shifts
- Reduced time/costs for documentation function
- Better nursing morale
- More effective care plans/case management
- Improved quality of patient care

---

Supporting the concept of time spent with patients is a paper by Hendrickson et al. (1990) that states that nurses spend only 31 percent of their direct time with patients. Recommending solutions to reduce nonessential nursing functions, the authors recommend that nurses delegate responsibilities, shift some responsibilities to other hospital staff, and use computers.

Finally, some of the important characteristics of bedside systems are (1) their ergonomic design, i.e., how easy they are to use, where they are placed in the patient's room, how accessible they are, how quiet they are, how unobtrusive they are to access when the patient is asleep, (2) their ease of use, i.e., handwriting or pen usage, finding items to chart, and time to chart; (3) how much they eliminate the need for redundant data, i.e., does the information have to be reentered into the mainframe or workstation, (4) whether the system supports what the user needs at the bedside, (5) whether the system is fail-safe and available 24 h a day, (6) whether the system has current information, and (7) whether the system provides access to decision support such as expert shells or guidelines.

## INTEGRATED WORKSTATION NETWORKS

An integrated professional workstation (PWS) is a concept of information management at the point of care or the point where service is delivered. All utilities that enable the nurse to communicate within the point of care and outside the point of service are available. These might include access to hospital information, including policies, procedures, and guidelines, and E-mail. Additionally, nurses can access generic software such as spreadsheets, statistical calculators, graphics, flowcharts, file management, word processing, and other utilities. Also Internet or Bitnet communications may be accessed, or there may be direct on-line access to bibliographic citations and abstracts through CINAHL, the National Library of Medicine, GRATEFUL-MED, and/or H*STAR. These local work capabilities are in addition to access to HISs, or patient management information systems.

There are currently no known systems that offer all the requirements of a health care PWS (Silva and Zawilski, 1992). However, the vision of the need for such a system is driven by three major forces: (1) the rapid inflow of information and technology in patient care, (2) the need for quality assurance and medicolegal concerns about documentation required for audit trails, and (3) the new management initiatives to control costs and enhance effectiveness, efficiency, and productivity in health care.

The benefits of the PWS defined by Silva and Zawilski (1992) are listed in Table 10.4. Because many sources of information are available to the clinician at the point of service, time is saved by accessing information during documentation, integrated with documentation, or when the clinician has a question about a policy, a procedure, or a treatment intervention.

While the lessened risk of losing stored data and the ability to retrieve data that were not previously recoverable are potential advantages of a PWS, determining what types of data to use in the workstation and what to download to the HIS, or ultimately to the network, is the greatest administrative challenge. Similarly, areas of common interface or interaction, e.g., the nursing unit and the clinical laboratory, if both are working on a workstation, need to download essential information on a routine basis in order for other practitioners to have access to that information. Research on the interrelationships of data within a hospital will have to

**TABLE 10.4**    THE BENEFITS OF A PROFESSIONAL WORKSTATION (PWS)

1. Increased provider productivity by reducing data entry time and eliminating redundant data entry.
2. Standardized provider/system interface.
3. Completed documentation during the patient encounter.
4. Increased quality through integration with diagnosis and treatment clinical practice guidelines.
5. Increased provider awareness of exceptional conditions, information, or data through innovative displays.
6. Facilitated management of free text.
7. Expanded provider interaction between provider and system using voiced input/output, handwriting recognition, and diagnostic imaging files.
8. Integrated administrative (cost) and clinical data to determine patient outcomes and conduct management studies.
9. Increased accessibility to medical information through access to networks [e.g., MEDLINE, Clinical Practice Guidelines, PDQ (Physicians Data Query of diagnostic and treatment protocols for cancer), CINAHL, or Internet connections].
10. Provided output access to integrate various results into readily useful displays (e.g., statistical analysis or graphic displays of results).
11. Lessened risk of losing data through storage, or ability to retrieve data not previously recoverable after transmission to the HIS.

*Source:* Silva and Zawilski, 1992.

be conducted so that the common minimum data and the unique professional minimum data are refined.

## DECISION SUPPORT SYSTEMS

A decision support system facilitates nurse decisions at the point of care or at the point of service. The future of nursing documentation will require the decision support for development of several areas of nursing practice. For example, in a study by Petrucci et al. (1992), nursing personnel improved their decision making and the outcomes of patient care when decision support was offered to assess and intervene with patients who have urinary incontinence. This decision support system assisted the professional nurses, and the support staff, who frequently are primary care givers in long-term care, by describing signs and symptoms and providing preprogrammed nursing judgment that offers possible nursing diagnoses.

Other nursing systems have been developed in the areas of computer-aided diagnosis and intervention (CANDI) (Chang et al., 1988), AIDS (Larson, 1988), and pain management (Heriot et al., 1988). These systems may also include such areas as nursing knowledge, reimbursement criteria, and the cost of care. Each collection of facts is arranged in a series of logical statements that reflect the thinking process of experts in the appropriate field. Depending on the application, these experts include nurses, physicians, and others in health care. The logical statements are often called algorithms, protocols, or rules.

Expert systems are similar to artificial intelligence (AI) in that both technologies reproduce the human ability to select the relevant facts and draw logical conclusions. But there is an important difference between expert systems and the more experimental AI. One of the underlying principles of AI is that the system learns from previous situations. For example, if an AI system comes to a mistaken conclusion once, it can add information to its knowledge base that might help it avoid the same mistake in the future. In a system at the Latter-Day Saints Hospital in Salt Lake City, Utah, decision support comes from algorithms to assist health care decisions in the form of alerts, warnings, possible diagnoses, possible procedures, care plan outlines, drug alternatives, findings and interpretations, protocol implementation, physician standing orders, and identification of contraindications. This system gains the confidence of users by employing the same logic that they use in making decisions.

Two reviews that summarize the current decision support systems in health care have been published by Miller (1994) and Johnston et al. (1994). A nursing system that met all the criteria of a decision support system that could be used to facilitate patient outcomes was developed by Petrucci et al. (1992) and is described above.

# A UNIFIED NURSING LANGUAGE SYSTEM

## U.S. Initiatives toward a Unified Nursing Language System

Since 1988, nurses in the United States have been working toward the development of uniform classification schemes to incorporate into nursing documentation systems and a unified nursing language system (UNLS) to improve communication about nursing (McCormick et al., 1994). Forces driving these movements include the need to track outcomes of care, case management, policies regarding the quality of care, and the utilization of nursing resources. The ANA has taken positions on recognizing classification schemes that have been added to the Unified Medical Language System (UMLS) to provide a UNLS (McCormick et al., 1994). Several nurses are involved in research studies to determine from nursing documentation whether standard language is used in the nursing profession.

Zielstorff et al. (1992) conducted an analysis of nursing terminology in the UMLS. They found that direct matches with the North American Nursing Diagnosis Association (NANDA) Taxonomy and the Omaha System lists of terms were possible 10 percent of the time, but that 32 percent of the time terms were split.

Grobe (1992) developed research on processing methods to analyze and classify statements of nursing interventions in home health care. The statements reflect organizing concepts of the interventions that nurses prescribe in home health care.

Henry et al. (1994) described the feasibility of using SNOMED III to represent nursing terms in patients with AIDS. Nurses used NANDA terms for documentation of care. Direct matches with SNOMED III were 30 percent, but when subsets of terms were used, the match increased to 69 percent. This group has also classified nursing interventions for persons with AIDS (Holzemer et al., 1994). In a three-hospital study with 201 patients, 21,492 nursing activities were coded by nurses. The major nursing activities were patient interview, nursing interview, intershift report, and chart audit.

Another research project that is supported by the University of Virginia, Thomas Jefferson University Hospital, and the University Hospital Consortium is attempting to develop a set of terms to represent nursing diagnoses, nursing intervention, and patient outcomes (Ozbolt et al., 1994). It uses Saba's 20 Home Health Care Components (HHCCs) to classify 209 nursing diagnostic terms, 545 interventions, and 122 expected outcomes from 7 nursing units in 2 hospitals. The intent of the project is to determine what the most frequently occurring clinical problems are, what interventions nurses use to solve the problem, and what outcomes are attained. In addition, the group attempts to determine the relationships between productivity and quality, with the goal of linking these relationships to costs.

At Georgetown University School of Nursing, the faculty are teaching basic nursing assessment and care planning using Saba's 20 care components. The Home Health Care Classification: Nursing Diagnoses and Nursing Interventions has been added to the UMLS and has been found to map to the other nursing taxonomies with ease.

A group implementing an HIS, including nursing documentation, in a Texas–Mexico border hospital developed standard nursing data based on assessment, NANDA nursing diagnoses, patient outcomes, nursing interventions, evaluation of whether outcomes were met, and reassessment if necessary (Taylor et al., 1994). They found that the nursing process with the nursing minimum data set (NMDS) as a structure was missing the demographic component—the culture of poverty and issues of nationality and entitlement, as well as the elements of race and ethnicity. They also found that when evaluating care based on patient outcomes, it was clear that a classification or taxonomy of patient care standards or outcomes had to be developed so that the entire construct of the nursing process could be articulated. While their interventions did not follow the nursing intervention classification (NIC), they found in retrospect that there was remarkable consistency between the interventions stated by their hospital nurses (McCloskey and Bulechek, 1992).

## International Initiatives toward a Unified Nursing Language System

An update of activities related to the development of a UNLS system has been written (McCormick, 1995). It includes a more extensive examination of endeavors in the international arena because many of the countries that have had national health care for over 20 years have had to define the nursing data requirements. In addition, these countries have had to develop uniform standards for nursing language and have experience in implementing the NMDS. Information on international projects involving such countries as the United Kingdom, the Netherlands, Sweden, Belgium, Denmark, and Australia have been published.

### United Kingdom
The United Kingdom has established a Steering Group on Health Services Information through the National Health Service (NHS), the Department of Health and Social Security. It has produced seven volumes of recommendations for data collection in many areas of health care. These reports are called the Korner report. While it is focused primarily on organizing medical data, Wheeler (1991) recently indicated that the Korner data set has evolved to include nursing elements. The specific nursing elements that have been included are nursing episode, which describes incidents when nurses are totally responsible for care; right admission, since nurses in the United Kingdom have some admitting privileges; and nurs-

ing home operation plan, which describes facilities offered by nurses in units run by nurses.

The National Health System Information Management Center describes the development of the Common Basic Specification for information systems with the NHS. This is a conceptual model of health care activities using a business model of care rather than a professional patient-centered model. It has been tested in an application related to delivery of babies in maternity care (Currell, 1992).

There are about 30 different computerized NISs currently in use throughout the United Kingdom (GCL, 1993). Some support workload and rostering only, but others have care planning modules. Each of these systems has its own care plan library, and many have been locally developed. Casey (1994) relates that it is not uncommon to find a problem such as pressure sores included in the library several times, or for the library to include several ways of saying the same order, e.g., nothing by mouth, NIL, NPO, no fluids, etc.

Casey (1994) also reports on the terms project. The primary aim of this project is to produce a thesaurus of health care terms, coded (in Read codes) for use in computer systems and mapped to ICD-9. The project includes broad nursing terms, midwifery terms, and health visiting nurse terms. Currently over 20,000 terms have been identified as unique to nursing. A Strategic Advisory Group for Nursing Informatics (SAGNIS) is working to get information management, information competencies, and support of the standardized vocabulary into the mainstream of nursing education. As a step toward an agreed-upon language, the project will define terms and classify concepts, following the identification of terms.

### United European Efforts

A recent analysis of international systems indicates that while the United Kingdom preceded other European countries in the development of NISs, other European countries are now following. One large European effort is RICHE (Réseau d'Information et de Communication Hospitalier Européen), a project funded by the Commission of the European Community (CEC) under the European Strategic Programme for Research in Information Technology (ESPRIT). The mission of RICHE is to construct a framework for overall open information and communication systems for health care in Europe. The nursing components of that system are using BAZIS, which is a Dutch HIS-integrated NIS called VISY and the Universita Cattolica del Sacro Cuore (UCSC) together with the software house GESI from Rome, Italy. The Italian partners are developing the operational management activities for clinical wards, and the BAZIS system staff are generating the care planning components. VISY is in use in about 35 percent of all Dutch hospitals and has been developed on hospital wards from the Leiden University Hospital since 1987.

The NIS includes the following main functions: admission-discharge, vital signs, individual patient care plans, fluid balance, x-ray appointments, laboratory specimen collection, dietary function, information retrieval function, nursing work plan, patient agenda, medication, and doctors' visits. Other functions include the patient registration, nurse registration, and shift registration.

### Sweden

In Sweden, Ehnfors (1994) has extended research on uniform key words used to document nursing practice in a new model called VIPS. The Swedish authorities have described the utility of the patient record in supporting the health professionals in the delivery of care, to serve as a basis for quality care, to be the reference point for judgments and choice of interventions to be implemented by health providers, to be a tool in quality assurance, to be the basis for audit and control, and to give the patient insight into the treatment and care he or she has received.

The VIPS model was used for documentation of nursing care on seven wards in two hospitals in Sweden (Ehnfors, 1994). The process model went beyond the development of terms, including nursing history, nursing status, nursing diagnoses, goals, nursing interventions, nursing outcomes, and nursing discharge note. There are 10 key nursing interventions: participation, information, education, support environment, general care, training, observation, special care, continuity, and coordination. One hundred forty patient records were evaluated before and after structured nursing documentation with uniform key words and nursing educational seminars. Criteria were developed to measure changes in documentation before and after intervention on a Delphi scale ranging from (1) the problem is described in the problem list or intervention or outcome to (5) the problem is described with relevance to nursing. After the planned intervention, the number of records with notes and the number of notes per record increased for all parts of the nursing process except goals. The greatest increase was a fivefold increase in the discharge note, followed by a threefold increase in the use of nursing diagnoses and an almost doubling of the use of nursing outcomes. The numbers of notes per record increased for nursing interventions.

In another project initiated by SPRI in Sweden, Sahlstedt describes the results of common language in computers in 200 installations all over Sweden (1994). Ehnfors' key words (described above) with definitions served as the language, and nursing process served as the structure for nursing documentation. The project was initiated in acute care, psychiatric, geriatric, and primary community care environments. The key concepts used were (1) patient well-being, (2) respect for integrity, (3) prevention, and (4) safety. The nursing history component consisted of admission, health situation, hypersensitivity, previous health care, social history, and lifestyle. Nurs-

ing status was represented by terms such as communication, breathing/
circulation, nutrition, elimination, skin, activity, sleep, pain, sexuality, psychosocial, spiritual, and finally well-being. Nursing interventions were classified the same way as in the project described by Ehnfors (1994). Use,
satisfaction, and quality of notes were evaluated and shown to be improved
with the UNLS and computerized nursing process.

## Belgium

Collecting the NMDS four times per year has been required by law in
Belgian general hospitals since January 1, 1988 (Sermeus and Delesie,
1994). Inherent in the collection of the NMDS has been the need to generate uniform nursing language. In 1985 the Belgian Nurses Association
produced a list of 111 nursing interventions. This list has been decreased
to 23 nursing interventions for sampling purposes; these accommodate 80
percent of the statistical information in the whole list of 111. In Belgium,
the essential elements in defining patient population and variability are
identifying the diversity of the patient population (medical diagnosis, age,
degree of dependency on daily activities found in the nursing notes) and
variability of practice (23 nursing interventions, length of stay, number of
nursing staff, level of qualifications of the nursing staff) (Vandewal and
Vanden Boer, 1994). In the majority of Belgian hospitals, the reliability
of nursing intervention data collection is about 80 percent, with emotional support and patient teaching being slightly reliable. NMDS data in
Belgium have also been linked with the San Joaquin Patient Classification System (Vanden Boer and Vandewal, 1994). The four categories of
intensity that have become standard in the country are no help, average,
more than average, and intensive care. These four classifications of
patients coincide with the NMDS national map separating patients into
self-care, care-oriented needing complete help, and cure-oriented needing
complete help.

Data have been collected cross-sectionally rather than longitudinally
in Belgium. Two national presentations have been used to describe data:
the fingerprint and the national map. The fingerprint gives a picture of
individual ward data, and the national map depicts all nursing units in
the country. An important element of the Belgian data collection is the
feedback given in a booklet published by the Ministry of Public Health
entitled "National Statistics." Also, a computer diskette has been produced
for each hospital documenting its nursing units compared with the whole
country.

An educational program has been developed with seven Belgian universities to educate nursing directors and head nurses on how to work
with the program and read the fingerprints generated by their hospitals,
and how to read the national map. At a governmental level, there is a proposal to use the NMDS information to determine hospitals' budgets.

## TELENURSING

A European Union (EU) program called Advanced Informatics in Medicine (AIM) initiated a program called TELENURSING in 1991 "to promote standardization of definitions, classifications and codings of essential nursing care data in order to further the development of internationally comparable minimum data sets in nursing based upon uniform definitions of data items" (Nielson and Mortensen, 1994). The sole contractor for this project is the Danish Institute for Health and Nursing Research in Copenhagen, Denmark. A group of nurses in Europe aspire to create a Euro-Nursing Health Data Base. The three objectives of this project are to (1) distribute a questionnaire with three dimensions: (a) a professional dimension (including nursing process), (b) a technical dimension (including documentation, definition, coding, classification, standardization, and an NMDS), and (c) a decisional dimension (including from a national to a ward level); (2) develop a TELENURSING proposal to generate a European Standard Data Sheet for collecting essential nursing data on patient problems/nursing diagnoses, interventions, and patient outcomes; and (3) collect data and create a mini-computerized European Nursing Health Data Base (CAN—Computerized Availability of Nursing Care Data) in accordance with the European Standard Data Sheet (Mortensen et al., 1994). The first CAN project included a European Standard Data Set to collect data on feeding problems and verbal communications. Later the group will expand to sleep, elimination, pain, and emotion. From the pilot results of the CAN data sheet, a formal proposal will be made to the Telematics for Health Care in the EU.

The group envisions definitions in nursing as consisting of nursing terms (1) derived by the nursing process, (2) obtained from clinical practice, and (3) originating from literature of nursing theorists (Nielson and Mortensen, 1994). Overriding the nursing process are terms similar to those described earlier and endorsed by the ANA: assessment, problem/nursing diagnosis, goal, intervention, and outcome.

Nurses in Europe are committed to the nursing process. Additionally, there is a tendency to define nursing terms for problems/nursing diagnoses, interventions, and outcomes, with more definitions for patient problems/nursing diagnoses coming from theory rather than practice.

The application of such nursing standards is believed to improve the availability, quality, and comparability of nursing data. In addition, this group hopes to coordinate its efforts with those of the AIM committee that has been working on European standardization (CEN), the Technical Committee (TC251) that has been working since April 1990 to develop standards in health care informatics, and the International Council of Nurses.

In addition, WHO/EURO initiated a multinational study in 1981 called "Peoples Need for Nursing Care," which collected data to demonstrate nursing's contributions to physical, mental, and social well-being in care (Ashworth et al., 1987). More recently (1993), WHO/EURO has proposed a European strategy for continuous quality improvement to identify the specific physical, mental, and social well-being health indicators related to nursing (Mortensen et al., 1994). For each of these projects, a nursing data set has been indicated for adequate information systems.

### Australia

Standards for health information management in Australia are being taken in a new direction to make them compatible with diagnosis related group (DRG) requirements and to standardize content in HISs. The Australian Council of Healthcare Standards has been developing hospitalwide clinical indicators to measure the outcomes of care. These are being extended by medical colleges and the Royal College of Nursing, Australia. The goal is to integrate the patient data with uniform cost allocation methods. The nursing goals complement the Health Information Committee and other subcommittees of Standards Australia (Heemskerk and Niewman, 1992; Hovenga, 1992).

In Australia, a Community Nursing Minimum Data Set has been described and is being pilot-tested (Foster and Conrick, 1994; Gliddon and Weaver, 1994). This involves defining standard terms at a national level for a national minimum data set that includes four elements—(1) an Australian thesaurus, (2) an Australian taxonomy, (3) data definitions and classifications, and (4) data format—before developing an NMDS. The Australia NMDS for Community Health includes 18 nursing elements, and a recent book has been published containing the data dictionary and guidelines (Home and Community Care Program, 1994).

### Canada

In Canada, nurses in the province of Alberta are centering activities on a standardized format (NMDS) for purposes of ensuring entry, accessibility, and retrievability of nursing data. The Canadian Nurses Association held a conference in the fall of 1992 to address topics and issues related to developing an NMDS.

## SUMMARY

The use of the computer for nursing documentation was described in this chapter. New standards, uses, and criteria for documentation systems were included. In 1986 this chapter described the computer as a facilitator of nursing documentation. In this revision the new integration of computers into nursing decision making at the bedside was described. New tools to monitor patient outcomes and to integrate nursing decisions with information beyond the bedside were also highlighted.

The components of the nursing care system were discussed within the new definition of the nursing process, since nursing practice in the United States remains committed to this standard. The pros and cons of new hardware and software applications were described, including bedside terminals and critical paths. Beyond the microcomputer and mainframe is the concept of the networked integrated workstation, which was also discussed. Finally, the use of computers in the documentation of nursing practice was described within the national and international framework, since several excellent resources are available in Europe, Canada, and Australia.

## REFERENCES

American Nurses Association. (1991). *Standards of Clinical Nursing Practice.* Kansas City, MO.

Arnold, J., and Pearson, G. (1992). *Computers Applications in Nursing Education and Practice* (Pub. No. 14-2406). New York: National League for Nursing.

Ashton, C. (1983). Nursing care plans: Aspects of computer use in nurse-to-nurse communication. In O. Fokkens et al. (Eds.), *MEDINFO '83 Seminars* (pp. 332–336). Amsterdam, Netherlands: North-Holland.

Ashworth, P., et al. (1987). *People's Need for Nursing Care; A European Study.* Copenhagen, Denmark: World Health Organization.

Casey, A. (1994). Nursing, midwifery and health visiting terms project. In S. Grobe and E. S. P. Pluyter-Wenting (Eds.), *Nursing Informatics: An International Overview for Nursing in a Technological Era* (pp. 639–642). Amsterdam, Netherlands: Elsevier Science B.V.

Chang, B. L., Roth, K., Gonzales, E., et al. (1988). CANDI: A knowledge-based system for nursing diagnosis. *Computers in Nursing, 6*(1), 13–21.

Covell, D. G., Uman, G. C., and Manning, P. R. (1985). Information needs in office practice: Are they being met? *Annals of Internal Medicine, 103*, 596–599.

Currell, R. A. (1992). Models for nursing: The paradox of business activity modelling. In K. C. Lun, P. Degoulet, T. E. Piemme, and O. Rienhoff (Eds.), *MEDINFO '92* (pp. 964–969). Amsterdam, Netherlands: North Holland-Elsevier Science Publishers.

DiJerome, L. (1992). The nursing case management computerized system: Meeting the challenge of health care delivery through technology. *Computers in Nursing, 10*(6), 250–258.

Donovan, W., and Corrales, S. (1991). *The Book on Bedside Computing.* Long Beach, CA: Inside Healthcare Computing.

Edmunds, L. (1984). Computers for inpatient nursing care. *Computers in Nursing 2*, 102–108.

Ehnfors, M. (1994). Nursing information in patient records: Towards uniform key words for documentation of nursing practice. In S. J. Grobe and E. S. P. Pluyter-Wenting (Eds.), *Nursing Information: An International Overview for Nursing in a Technological Era* (pp. 643–647). Amsterdam, Netherlands: Elsevier Science B.V.

Etheridge, P., and Lamb, G. S. (1989). Professional nursing case management improves quality, access and costs. *Nursing Management, 20*(3), 30–35.

Foster, J., and Conrick, M. (1994). Nursing minimum data sets: Historical perspective and Australian development. In S. J. Grobe and E. S. P. Pluyter-Wenting (Eds.), *Nursing Information: An International Overview for Nursing in a Technological Era* (pp. 150–154). Amsterdam, Netherlands: Elsevier Science B.V.

GCL. (1993). *Nursing Management System: A Guide to Existing and Potential Products* (9th Release). Macclesfield, Clacshire, England: Greenhalgh and Co., Ltd.

Gliddon, T., and Weaver, C. (1994). The community nursing minimum data set Australia—From definition to the real world. In S. J. Grobe and E. S. P. Pluyter-Wenting (Eds.), *Nursing Information: An International Overview for Nursing in a Technological Era* (pp. 163–168). Amsterdam, Netherlands: Elsevier Science B.V.

Grobe, S. J. (1992). Nursing intervention lexicon and taxonomy. In K. C. Lun, P. DeGoulet, T. E. Piemme, and O. Rienhoff (Eds.), *MEDINFO '92* (pp. 981–986). Amsterdam, Netherlands: North Holland-Elsevier Science Publishers.

Healthcare Informatics. (1994, May). Top 100 Hospitals and Systems. *Healthcare Informatics, 11*(5), 13.

Health Management Technology. (1995, February). 1995 Market Directory Issue. *Health Management Technology*, pp. 14–98.

Heemskerk, P. R. B., and Niewman, H. B. J. (1992). Initiatives for NIS in Europe. In K. C. Lun, P. DeGoulet, T. E. Piemme, and O. Rienhoff (Eds.), *MEDINFO '92* (pp. 970–975). Amsterdam, Netherlands: North Holland-Elsevier Science Publishers.

Hendrickson, G., Doddato, T. M., and Kovner, C. T. (1990). How do nurses use their time? *Journal of Nursing Administration, 20*(3), 31–38.

Hendrickson, G., and Kovner, C. T. (1990). Effects of computers on nursing resource use: Do computers save nurses time? *Computers in Nursing, 8*(1), 16–22.

Henry, S. B., Holzemer, W. E., Reilly, C. A., and Campbell, K. E. (1994). Terms used by nurses to describe patient problems: Can SNOMED represent nursing concepts in the patient record? *Journal of the American Medical Informatics Association, 1*(1), 61–74.

Heriot, H., Graves, J., Bouhaddou, O., et al. (1988). A pain management decision support-system for nurses. In R. A. Greenes (Ed), *Proceedings of the Twelfth Annual Symposium on Computer Applications in Medical Care* (pp. 63–68). Washington, DC: IEEE Computer Society Press.

Herring, D., and Rockman, R. (1990). A closer look at bedside terminals. *Nursing Management, 21*(7), 554–561.

Holzemer, W. L., Henry, S. B., Reilly, C. A., and Miller, T. (1994). The classification of nursing interventions for persons living with AIDS. In S. J. Grobe and E. S. P. Pluyter-Wenting (Eds.), *Nursing Informatics: An International Overview for Nursing in a Technological Era* (pp. 687–691). Amsterdam, Netherlands: Elsevier Science B.V.

Home and Community Care Program (1994). *Community Nursing Minimum Data Set Australia, Version 1.0: Data Dictionary and Guidelines* (CNMDSA). Bayswater Nth, Victoria, Australia: Australian Council of Community Health Nursing Services.

Hovenga, E. (1992). The need for an Australian Nursing Data Dictionary. In K. C. Lun, P. DeGoulet, T. E. Piemme, and O. Rienhoff (Eds.), *MEDINFO '92* (pp. 987–991). Amsterdam, Netherlands: North Holland-Elsevier Science Publishers.

Johnston, M. E., Langton, K. B., Haynes, R. B., and Mathieu, A. (1994). Effects of computer-based clinical decision support systems on clinician performance and patient outcomes. *Annals of Internal Medicine,* 120, 135–142.

Joint Commission on Accreditation of Health Care Organizations. (1994). *1994 Accreditation Manual for Hospitals.* Oakbrook Terrace, IL.

Kahl, K., Ivancin, L., and Fuhrmann, M. (1991). Identifying the savings potential of bedside terminals. *Nursing Economics, 9*(6), 391–400.

Korpman, R. A. (1991). Patient care automation: The future is now. Part I: Introduction and historical perspective. *Nursing Economics, 8*(3), 191–193.

Lamb, G. S., and Stempel, J. E. (1994). Nurse case management from the client's view: Growing as insider-expert. *Nursing Outlook, 42*(1), 7–13.

Lang, N. M, Hudgins, C., Jacox, A., et al. (1995). Toward a national database for nursing practice. In *An Emerging Framework for the Profession: Data System Advances for Clinical Nursing Practice.* Washington, DC: American Nurses Association.

Larson, D. (1988). Development of a microcomputer-based expert system to provide support for nurses caring for AIDS patients. *Proceedings of Nursing and Computers: Third International Symposium on Nursing Use of Computers and Information Science* (pp. 682–690). St. Louis: Mosby.

Lesnik, M., and Anderson, B. (1955). *Nursing Practice and the Law* (2d ed.). Philadelphia: Lippincott.

Lombard, N., and Light, N. (1983). On-line nursing care plans by nursing diagnosis. *Computers in Healthcare, 4,* 22–23.

Loveridge, C. E., Cummings, S. H., and O'Malley, J. (1988). Developing care management in a primary nursing system. *Journal of Nursing Administration, 18*(1), 36–39.

Marr, P., Duthie, E., Glassman, K., et al. (1993). Bedside terminals and quality of nursing documentation. *Computers in Nursing, 11*(4), 176–182.

Marriner-Tomey, A. (1992). *Guide to Nursing Management* (4th Ed.). St. Louis: Mosby Year Book.

Martin, J. B. (1990). The environment and future of health information systems. *Journal of Health Administration Education,* 8, 11–24.

McCloskey, J. C., and Bulechek, G. M. (Eds.). (1992). *Nursing Interventions Classification* (NIC). St. Louis: Mosby Year Book.

McCormick, K. (1981). Nursing research using computerized data bases. In H. Heffernan (Ed.), *Proceedings of the Fifth Annual Symposium on Computer Applications in Medical Care* (pp. 738–743). Silver Spring, MD: IEEE Computer Society Press.

McCormick, K. A. (1983). Monitoring and evaluating implemented HIS. In R. Dayhoff (Ed.), *Proceedings of the 7th Annual Symposium on Computer Applications in Medical Care* (pp. 507–509). Silver Spring, MD: IEEE Computer Society Press.

McCormick, K. A. (1995). An update on nursing's unified language system. In M. J. Ball, K. J. Hannah, S. K. Newbold, and J. V. Douglas, *Nursing Informatics 2: Where Caring and Technology Meet.* New York: Springer-Verlag.

McCormick, K. A.. Lang, N., Zielstorff, R., et al. (1994). Toward standard classification schemes for nursing language: Recommendations of the American Nurses Association Steering Committee on Databases to Support Clinical Nursing Practice. *Journal of the American Medical Informatics Association, 1*(6), 421–427.

Miller, R. A. (1994). Medical diagnostic decision support systems—Past, present, and future. *Journal of the American Medical Informatics Association, 1*(8), 8–27.

Mortensen, R., Mantas, J., Manuaela, M., et al. (1994). Telematics for health care in the European Union. In S. J. Grobe and E. S. P. Pluyter-Wenting (Eds.), *Nursing Informatics: An International Overview for Nursing in a Technological Era* (pp. 750–752). Amsterdam, Netherlands: Elsevier Science B.V.

Mortensen, R., and Nielson, G. H. (in press). TELENURSING and CAN: Clinical Nursing Vocabulary as part of two European studies. *Proceedings of a Postconference on Informatics: The Infrastructure for Quality Assessment and Improvement in Nursing* (June 23, 1994). Austin, TX.

National Library of Medicine. (1989). *MEDLARS: The World of Medicine at Your Fingertips* (NIH Pub. No. 89-1286). Bethesda, MD: US DHHS.

Nielsen, G. H., and Mortensen, R. A. (1994). *TELENURSING: Documentation of the Nursing Process in Hospitals by Computers in Europe* (Vol. 1, pp. 10–11). Copenhagen, Denmark: The Danish Institute for Health and Nursing Research.

Nursing Management. (1993). *Software Guide, 24*(7), 70–98.

Ozbolt, J., Fruchtnight, J. N., and Hayden, J. R. (1994). Toward data standards for clinical nursing information. *Journal of the American Medical Informatics Association, 1,* 175–185.

Palmer, M. H., McCormick, K. A., Langford, A., et al. (1992). Continence outcomes: Documentation on medical records in the nursing home environment. *Journal of Nursing Care Quality, 6*(3), 36–433.

Petrucci, K. M., McCormick, K. A., and Scheve, A. (1987). Documenting patient care needs in the nursing home: Do nurses do it? *Journal of Gerontological Nursing, 13*(11), 34–38.

Petrucci, K. M., Jacox, A., McCormick, K. A., et al. (1992). Evaluating the appropriateness of a nurse expert system's patient assessment . . . Urological Nursing Information System (UNIS). *Computers in Nursing, 10*(6), 243–249.

Rieder, K, and Norton, D. (1984). An integrated nursing information system—A planning model. *Computers in Nursing, 2,* 73–79.

Romano, C., McCormick, K., and McNeely, L. (1982). Nursing documentation: A model for a computerized data base. *Advances in Nursing Science, 4,* 43–56.

Rowland, H., and Rowland, B. (1992). *Nursing Administration Handbook* (3d ed.). Gaithersburg, MD: Aspen Publishers.

Rozovsky, L. (1978). Medical records as evidence. *Dimensions in Health Services.* 55(7), 16–17.

Saba, V. (1993). Nursing diagnostic schemes. In *Papers from the Nursing Minimum Data Set Conference, Edmonton, Alberta* (pp. 54–63). Ottawa, Ontario: Canadian Nurses Association.

Sahlstedt, S. (1994). Computer support for nursing process and documentation. In S. J. Grobe and E. S. P. Pluyter-Wenting (Eds.), *Nursing Informatics: An International Overview for Nursing in a Technological Era* (pp. 648–652). Amsterdam, Netherlands: Elsevier Science B.V.

Scholes, M., Bryant, Y., and Barber, B. (1983). *The Impact of Computers on Nursing: An International Review.* Amsterdam, Netherlands: North-Holland.

Sermeus, W., and Delesie, L. (1994). The registration of a Nursing Minimum Data Set in Belgium: Six years of experience. In S. J. Grobe and E. S. P. Pluyter-Wenting (Eds.), *Nursing Informatics: An International Overview for Nursing in a Technological Era* (pp. 144–149). Amsterdam, Netherlands: Elsevier Science B.V.

Shortliffe, E. H., Tank, P. C., Amatayakul, M., et al. (1992). Future vision and dissemination of computer-based patient records. In M. J. Ball and M. F. Collen (Eds.), *Aspects of the Computer-Based Patient Record* (pp. 273–293). New York: Springer-Verlag.

Silva, J. S., and Zawilski, R. J. (1992). The health care professional's workstation: Its functional components and user impact. In M. J. Ball and M. F. Collen (Eds.), *Aspects of the Computer-Based Patient Record* (pp. 102–124). New York: Springer-Verlag.

Simpson, R. (1992). What nursing leaders are saying about technology. *Nursing Management, 23*(7), 28–32.

Spath, P. L. (1993). *Succeeding with Critical Paths.* Forest Grove, OR: Brown-Spath Associates.

Swansburg, R. C. (1990). *Management and Leadership for Nurse Managers.* Boston: Jones and Bartlett.

Taylor, M. E., Scholten, R., Cassidy, D. A., and Corona, D. F. (1994). Using nursing standards as a basis for reporting care using a computer. In S. J. Grobe and E. S. P. Pluyter-Wenting (Eds.), *Nursing Informatics: An International Overview for Nursing in a Technological Era* (pp. 625–629). Amsterdam, Netherlands: Elsevier Science B.V.

Vanden Boer, G., and Vandewal, D. (1994). Linkage of NMDS-information and patient classification systems. In S. J. Grobe and E. S. P. Pluyter-Wenting (Eds.), *Nursing Informatics: An International Overview for Nursing in a Technological Era* (pp. 158–162). Amsterdam, Netherlands: Elsevier Science B.V.

Vandewal, D., and Vanden Boer, G. (1994). Using NMDS-information for the allocation of budgets to nursing units. In S. J. Grobe and E. S. P. Pluyter-Wenting (Eds.), *Nursing Informatics: An International Overview for Nursing in a Technological Era* (pp. 129–133). Amsterdam, Netherlands: Elsevier Science B.V.

Wessling, E. (1972). Automating the nursing history and care plan. *Journal of Nursing Administration, 2,* 34–38.

Wheeler, M. (1991). Nurses do count. *Nursing Times, 87*(16), 64–65.

Winslow, R. (Oct. 8, 1993). Hospitals wake up to the power of computers. *Wall Street Journal,* p. 4.

Wood, R., Bailey, N., and Tilkemeier, D. (1992). Managed care: The missing link in quality improvement. *Journal of Nursing Care Quality, 6*(4), 55–65.

Zander, K. (1990). Managed care and nursing case management. In G. Mayer, M. Madden, and E. Lawrenz (Eds.), *Patient Care Delivery Models.* Rockville, MD: Aspen Publishers.

Zander, K., Etheredge, M., and Bower, K. (1993). *Case Management: Blueprints for Transformation.* Boston: New England Medical Center.

Zielstorff, R., McHugh, M., and Clinton, J. (1988). *Computer Design Criteria for Systems that Support the Nursing Process* (pp. 1–40). Kansas City, MO: American Nurses Association.

Zielstorff, R., Cimino, C., Barnett, G., et al. (1992). Representation of nursing terminology in the UMLS metathesaurus: A pilot study. In M. E. Frisse (Ed.), *Proceedings of the Sixteenth Annual Symposium on Computer Applications in Medical Care* (pp. 393–396). New York: McGraw-Hill.

# BIBLIOGRAPHY

Abrami, P., and Johnson, J. (1990). *Bringing Computers to the Hospital Bedside: An Emerging Technology.* New York: Springer.

American Nurses Association. (1980). *Nursing: A Social Policy Statement.* Kansas City, MO.

American Nurses Association. (1989). *Classification Systems Describing Nursing Practice: Working Papers* (pp. 55–61). Kansas City, MO.

Bauer, C. A. (1992). Information management in nursing care: One state's approach. In J. M. Arnold and G. A. Pearson (Eds.), *Computer Applications in Nursing Education and Practice* (pp. 48–52; Pub. No. 14-2406). New York: National League for Nursing.

Bower, K. (1992). *Case Management by Nurses.* Washington, DC: American Nurses Publishing.

Brennan, P. F., and McHugh, M. (1988). Clinical decision-making and computer support. *Applied Nursing Research, 1*(2), 89–93.

Canadian Nurses Association. (1993). *The Nursing Minimum Data Set Conference.* Edmonton, Alberta, Canada.

Casey, A. (in press). The UK clinical terms projects and quality improvement. *Proceedings of a Postconference on Informatics: The Infrastructure for Quality Assessment and Improvement in Nursing* (June 23, 1994). Austin, TX.

Clark, J. (in press). An international classification for nursing practice (ICNP). *Proceedings of a Postconference on Informatics: The Infrastructure for Quality Assessment and Improvement in Nursing* (June 23, 1994). Austin, TX.

Clark, J., and Lang, N. M. (1992). Nursing's next advance: An international classification for nursing practice. *International Nursing Review, 39,* 109–112, 128.

Danish Institute for Health and Nursing Research. (1991). *Information and Diagnosis.* Copenhagen, Denmark.

Dick, R. S., and Steen, E. B. (Eds.). (1991). *The Computer-Based Record: An Essential Technology for Health Care.* Washington, DC: National Academy Press.

Enfors, M. (1993). Quality of care from a nursing perspective. Methodological considerations and development of a model for nursing documentation (doctoral dissertation). *Acta Universitatis Upsalaiensis,* Uppsala.

Enfors, M., Thorel-Ekstrand, I., and Ehrenberg, A. S. (1991). Towards basic nursing information in patient records. *Vard I Norden, 21,* 12–21.

Ethridge, P. (1991). A nursing HMO: Carondelet St. Mary's experience. *Nurse Manager, 22,* 22–29.

Evans-Paganelli, B. (1989). Criteria for the selection of a bedside information system for acute care units. *Computers in Nursing, 7*(5), 214–221.

Fitzpatrick J. J., Kerr, M. E., Saba, V. K., et al., (1989). Translating nursing diagnosis into ICD code. *American Journal of Nursing, 89,* 493–495.

Halloran, E. J. (1988). Computerized nurse assessments. *Nursing & Health Care, 9*(9), 497–499.

Henderson, V. (1977). *Basic Principles of Nursing Care.* Geneva, Switzerland: International Council of Nurses.

Holzemer, W. L., and Henry, S. B. (1992). Computer-supported versus manually-generated nursing care plans: A comparison of patient problems, nursing interventions and AIDS patients outcomes. *Computers in Nursing, 10*(1), 19–24.

International Council of Nurses. (1993, October). *Nursing's Next Advance: An International Classification for Nursing Practice (ICNP). A working paper.* Geneva, Switzerland.

International Council of Nurses. (1994, February). *Report of Advisory Meeting on the Development of Information Tools to Support Community Based and Primary Health Care Nursing Systems.* Geneva, Switzerland.

Jones, F. M., Rice, V. E., and Plymat, K. R. (Eds.). (1992). *Nurses and Nursing in Primary Health Care: An Australian Database. Preliminary Report.* Sydney, Australia: WHO Collaborating Center for Nursing Development in Primary Health Care.

Korpman, R. A. (1990a). Patient care automation: The future is now. Part 2: The current paper system—Can it be made to work? *Nursing Economics, 8*(4), 263–267.

Korpman, R. A. (1990b). Patient care automation. The future is now. Part 3. The five rules of automation. *Nursing Economics, 8*(5), 345–349.

Korpman, R. A. (1991a). Patient care automation. The future is now. Part 6: Does reality live up to the promise. *Nursing Economics, 9*(3), 175–178.

Korpman, R. A. (1991b). *Integrated Nursing Systems. The Future Is Now.* Paper presented at the Fourth International Conference on Nursing Use of Computers and Information Science (pp. 1–4). Melbourne, Australia.

Korpman, R. A., and Lincoln, T. L. (1988). The computer-stored medical record: For whom? *Journal of the American Medical Association, 259,* 3454–3456.

Lamb, G. (1992). Conceptual and methodological issues in nurse case management research. *Advances in Nursing Science, 15,* 16–24.

Lang, N. M., and Marek, K. D. (1990). The politics of outcomes. *Journal of Professional Nursing, 6,* 158–163.

Lindberg, D. A., Humphreys, B. L., and McCray, A. T. (1993). The unified medical language system. *Methods of Information in Medicine, 32,* 281–291.

Lyon, J. C. (1993). Models of nursing care delivery and case management: Clarification of terms. *Nursing Economics, 11,* 163–169.

Martin, K. S., and Scheet, N. J. (1992). *The Omaha System: Applications for Community Health Nursing.* Philadelphia: Saunders.

McCormick, K. A. (1988). A unified nursing language system. In M. Ball, K. Hannah, U. Gerdin-Jelger, and H. Peterson, (Eds.), *Nursing Informatics: Where Caring and Technology Meet* (pp. 168–178). New York: Springer-Verlag.

McCormick, K. A. (1991a). Future data needs for quality of care monitoring, DRG considerations, reimbursement and outcome measurement. *Image: The Journal of Nursing Scholarship, 23*(1), 29–32.

McCormick, K. A. (1991b). The urgency of establishing international uniformity of data. In E. J. S. Hovenga, K. J. Hannah, K. A. McCormick, and J. S. Ronald (Eds.), *Nursing Informatics '91: Proceedings of the Fourth International Conference on Nursing Use of Computers and Information Science* (pp. 77–81). Berlin: Springer-Verlag.

McCormick, K. A., and Zielstorff, R. (1993). Building a unified nursing language system. In *Papers from the Nursing Minimum Data Set Conference, Edmonton, Alberta* (pp. 127–133). Ottawa, Ontario, Canada: Canadian Nurses Association.

McCormick, K. A., and Zielstorff, R. (1995). Building a unified nursing language system. In *An Emerging Framework for the Profession: Data System Advances for Clinical Practice.* Washington, DC: American Nurses Association.

McCormick, K. A., Lang, N., Zielstorff, R., et al. (1994). Toward standard classification schemes for nursing language—Recommendations of the American Nurses Association Steering Committee on Databases to Support Nursing Practice. *Journal of the American Medical Informatics Association, 1*(2), 412–427.

Miller, E. R., and Sheridan, E. A. (1992). Integrating a bedside nursing information system into a professional nursing practice model. In J. M. Arnold and G. A. Pearson, *Computer Applications in Nursing Education and Practice* (pp. 62–70, Pub. No. 14-2406). New York: National League for Nursing.

Newman, M., Lamb, G., and Michaels, C. (1991). Nursing case management: The coming togethers of theory and practice. *Nursing in Health Care, 12,* 404–408.

Newsham, D. (1991). Influencing point of care technology development: The vital edge. In E. J. S. Hovenga, K. J. Hannah, K. A. McCormick, and J. S. Ronald (Eds.), *Proceedings of the Fourth International Conference on Nursing Use of Computers and Information Science* (pp. 435–439). New York: Springer-Verlag.

Norris, J., Cuddigan, J., Foyt, M., et al. (1990). Decision support and outcomes of nurses' care planning. *Computers in Nursing, 8*(5), 192–197.

North American Nursing Diagnosis Association. (1992). *NANDA Nursing Diagnosis: Definitions and Classifications.* Philadelphia.

Ozbolt, J. (1988). Knowledge-based systems for supporting clinical nursing decision. In M. J. Ball, K. J. Hannah, U. Gerdin-Jelger, and H. Peterson (Eds.), *Nursing Informatics: Where Caring and Technology Meet* (pp. 274–285). New York: Springer-Verlag.

Perry, D. J. (1991). Using a computer database to increase efficiency in the practice setting. *Nurse Practitioners: American Journal of Primary Health Care, 16*(6), 44–47.

Probst, C. L., and Rush, J. (1990). The careplan knowledge base: A prototype expert system for post partum nursing care. *Computers in Nursing, 8*(5), 206–213.

Probst, C. L., and Rush, J. P. (1991). The careplan expert system: Information presentation preferences of novice and expert nurses. In E. J. S. Hovenga, K. J. Hannah, K. A. McCormick, and J. S. Ronald (Eds.), *Proceedings of the Fourth International Conference on Nursing Use of Computers and Information Sciences* (pp. 747–751). New York: Springer-Verlag.

Propopczak, D. (1991). The role of nursing in computer automated O.R. systems: Bridging the gap from technology to implementation. In E. J. S. Hovenga, K. J. Hannah, K. A. McCormick, and J. S. Ronald (Eds.), *Proceedings of the Fourth International Conference on Nursing Use of Computers and Information Science* (pp. 220–225). New York: Springer-Verlag.

Riopelle, L., Grondin, L., and Phaneuf, M. (1986). *Répertoir des Diagnostics Infirmiers selon le modéle conceptuel de Virginia Henderson.* Montreal, Quebec, Canada: McGraw-Hill.

Rothwell, D. J., Cote, R. A., Cordeau, J. P., and Boisvert, M. A. (1994). Developing a standard data structure for medical language—The SNOMED Proposal. In C. Safran (Ed.), *Seventeenth Annual Symposium on Computer Applications in Medical Care* (pp. 695–699). New York: McGraw-Hill.

Saba, V. K., O'Hara, P. A., Zuckerman, A. E., et al. (1991). A nursing intervention taxonomy for home health care. *Nursing and Health Care, 12,* 296–299.

Sermeus, W., and Delesie, L. (1992). Reliability of the nursing minimum data set registrations. *Acta Hospital, 32,* 39–53, 92.

Shannon, M., Dextrom, N., and Fuhrhop, M. (1989). A proactive approach to computerizing nursing process: A management perspective. *Health Care Supervisor, 7*(3), 71–81.

Sinclair, V. G. (1990). Potential effects of decision support systems on the role of the nurse. *Computers in Nursing, 8*(2), 60–65.

Tiedeken, K., Majarowitz, S. J., and Duryee, E. E. (1992). The development of a nursing information system in collaboration with two vendors. In J. M. Arnold and G. A. Pearson, *Computer Applications in Nursing Education and Practice* (pp. 71–84, Pub. No. 14-2406). New York: National League for Nursing.

Verran, J. (1986). Testing a classification instrument for the ambulatory care setting. *Research in Nursing and Health, 9*, 279–287.

Wake, M., Murphy, M., Affara, F., et al. (1993). Towards an International Classification for Nursing Practice: A Literature Review and Survey. *International Nursing Review, 40*, 77–80.

Welsh, E., and Nicholson, S. (1991). Bedside terminals: Panacea or gadget? *Nursing Economics, 9*(6), 437–441.

Werley, H. H., and Lang, N. M. (Eds.). (1988). *Identification of the Nursing Minimum Data Set.* New York: Springer.

Work Group on Computerization of Patient Records (1993). *Toward a National Health Information Infrastructure.* Washington, DC: US DHHS.

Zielstorff, R., Grobe, S., and Hudgings, C. (1992). *Nursing Information Systems: Essential Characteristics for Professional Practice.* Washington, DC: American Nurses Association.

# *11*

• • • • • • • • • • • • • • • • • • • • • •

# CRITICAL CARE APPLICATIONS
## *D. Kathy Milholland*

## OBJECTIVES

- Identify computer applications in critical care, including in the intensive care unit, emergency department, and operating rooms.
- Understand the basic elements of arrhythmia monitors and physiologic monitors.
- Describe how hemodynamic monitoring systems are used in critical care settings.
- Understand the capabilities, purposes, types, benefits, and issues of critical care information systems.
- Describe the relationship between hemodynamic monitoring systems and critical care information systems.
- Identify trends in monitoring and computerized information management.
- Identify special-purpose applications available.
- Describe computer applications in emergency departments.
- Describe computer information management technology in the operating rooms.

Critical care nursing is the nursing specialty which deals with human responses to life-threatening problems (Kinney et al., 1988). A critically ill patient is any patient with real or potential life-threatening health problems requiring constant observation and constant intervention to prevent complications and restore health (Berg, 1981). In a hospital setting, these patients are most often found and critical care nursing is most often practiced in intensive care units (ICUs), emergency departments (EDs), and operating rooms (ORs). The information management needs of critical care settings are different from those of general nursing units and outpatient areas. Nurses in critical care areas are exposed to different computer resources from those that nurses working with hospital information systems (HISs) alone would be exposed to. This chapter describes the specialized applications of computer technology currently found in critical care, as well as some trends toward new applications.

In critical care settings today, there has been an almost exponential growth in the amount of information made available to care givers. In 1986, Saba and McCormick estimated that the volume of data collected by nurses in critical care settings on a daily basis was as high as 1,500 data points. It has become increasingly difficult to manage these volumes of data, which have continued to increase. At the same time, the demand for cost-effective care has also increased (Gardner et al., 1989). Shortages of resources, both staff and time, increase the difficulty of data management. Computer technology offers solutions to these difficulties and has been increasingly employed in critical care settings.

Computer technology, especially microcomputers, is found in many patient care units in the critical care setting; this technology includes information management systems. In this chapter, arrhythmia, physiologic, and hemodynamic monitors, critical care information systems (CCISs); special-purpose systems; emergency department information systems (EDISs); and operating room information systems (ORISs) will be the focus of discussion.

## DEVELOPMENTS

Developers of automated approaches to information management in critical care settings have computerized complex physiologic formulas; stored large volumes of data that would otherwise be disorganized, lost, inaccurate, or illegible; rapidly analyzed small samples of gas or fluids; and maintained near-normal physiologic ranges with life-supporting equipment. Alarm systems have been automated so that nurses can make use of each vital second.

The advantages of these systems resemble the advantages of computerizing nursing documentation: better control of nursing observations to promote better assessment of immediate patient needs. However, these systems focus heavily on collecting, storing, and displaying physiological data. Usually, there are modules or subsystems that address the nursing process and provide care planning and nursing documentation capabilities. The functions, purposes, and benefits of these nursing process capabilities are the same as noted elsewhere in this book.

Many of the applications described in this chapter involve the use of a microprocessor, which is an integrated circuit "chip" that contains the arithmetic logic unit and the control unit of a central processing unit (CPU), the "brain" of a microcomputer. When a microprocessor is installed in a monitor or other equipment, the equipment is considered to be "microprocessed." This allows the equipment to behave like a computer, since the microprocessor allows the equipment to process data.

## COMPUTER CAPABILITIES IN CRITICAL CARE SETTINGS

Computers in ICUs, EDs, and ORs have several major capabilities:

- Microprocess physiologic data.
- File patient care documentation.
- Graph trend data.
- Regulate physiologic equipment.
- Store and process diagnostic information.
- Recognize deviations from preset ranges by an alarm.
- Comparatively evaluate patients with similar diagnoses.

## COMPUTER APPLICATIONS IN THE INTENSIVE CARE UNIT

Although many of the applications described in this chapter are also used in the ED and OR, they were often developed for the ICU and will thus be described within the ICU framework. Specifically, six types of applications will be described:

- Arrhythmia monitors
- Physiologic monitors
- Hemodynamic monitors
- Critical care information systems
- Medical information bus
- Special-purpose systems

Arrhythmia monitoring systems and special-purpose systems are usually dedicated systems; that is, the computer processes information that is used for a special purpose. Physiologic monitoring systems can be distributed or integrated. Distributed systems provide system-to-system communication; for example, these systems link the arrhythmia monitoring system with the blood pressure monitoring system. A modular system is a distributed system in which microcomputer networks that include support modules are used. Integrated data systems, often called critical care information systems (CCISs), integrate physiological data from bedside devices, data from other departments (e.g., laboratory data), and all bedside record keeping, including nursing documentation, such as nursing notes and care planning.

## Arrhythmia Monitors

The electrocardiogram (ECG) and arrhythmia monitors led computerization in the ICUs, EDs, and ORs. Computerized patient care arrhythmia monitoring systems are generally used to collect data on electrical activity of the heart, blood pressure, and heart rate. They provide continuous telemetric measurement of a patient's cardiopulmonary functions. Books have been written about the use of the computer for arrhythmia monitoring, and its use has been widely accepted since the early 1980s (Bronzino, 1982).

Computerized monitoring and analysis of cardiac rhythm has proven reliable and effective in detecting potentially lethal heart rhythms (Widman, 1992). Standards for testing and reporting the performance of arrhythmia analysis systems have been developed by the American Heart Association. A key functional element is the system's ability to detect ventricular fibrillation and respond with an alarm. However, no standards currently specify minimum accuracy for computerized detection systems (Mirvis et al., 1989).

### System Types

The basic components of arrhythmia monitors are shown in Table 11.1. There are two types of arrhythmia systems: detection surveillance and diagnostic or interpretive. In a detection system the criteria for a normal ECG are programmed into the computer. The computer might survey the ECG for wave amplitude and duration and for the intervals between waves. The program may even include an alarm response if the R-R interval is less than or equal to two-thirds of the average R-R interval. Each signal may then be analyzed to determine whether the QRS duration is greater than normal.

**TABLE 11.1**   BASIC COMPONENTS OF
ARRHYTHMIA MONITORS

- Sensor
- Signal conditioner
- Cardiograph
- Pattern recognition
- Rhythm analysis
- Diagnosis
- Written report

The next programmed search may be for the presence of a compensatory pause, that is, a prolonged R-R interval after a premature ventricular contraction (PVC). The computer may then be programmed to store the number of PVCs per minute and sound an alarm or alert the nurse visually (e.g., with a flashing red light) and audibly (a loud sound) when more than five PVCs occur within a minute. Detection systems can even store in memory the type of arrhythmia and time of occurrence so that patient's arrhythmia history can be plotted and compared to medication administration and cardiopulmonary pressures (Sorkin and Bloomfeld, 1982).

Arrhythmia systems can also be diagnostic: After the analog signals are interfaced to digital information for processing, the program analyzes and diagnoses the ECG. The computer, after processing the ECG, generates an analysis report that is confirmed by a cardiologist, usually from another site. The computers that support these types of ECGs are usually dedicated systems; that is, main memory is used only for ECG acquisition, analysis, and report generation. These systems usually communicate with the off-site cardiologist by telephone line.

Interpretive systems are beneficial because they do the following (Bronzino, 1982):

- Reduce nursing time.
- Standardize terminology.
- Can be used as teaching aids.
- Transmit information for diagnosis.
- Reduce clerical duties.
- Eliminate potential errors of interpretation.

Interpretive systems search the ECG complex for five parameters:

- Location of QRS complex
- Time from the beginning to the end of the QRS
- Comparison of amplitude, duration, and rate of the QRS complex with all limb leads
- P and T waves
- Comparison of P and T waves with all limb leads

The findings are then compared to predetermined diagnostic specifications.

## Physiologic Monitors

Most physiologic monitors consist of five basic parts, as shown in Table 11.2. The sensor is the instrument that provides information (e.g., a thermometer, an arterial pressure transducer). The signal conditioner amplifies or filters the display device (e.g., the signals, amplifier, oscilloscope, or paper record). The file holds the information (e.g., the storage files, sig-

**TABLE 11.2**   BASIC COMPONENTS OF PHYSIOLOGIC MONITORING
EQUIPMENT

- Sensors (e.g., thermometers, arterial pressure transducer)
- Signal conditioners to amplify or filter the display device (e.g., amplifier, oscilloscope, paper recorder)
- File to rank and order information (e.g., storage file, alarm signal)
- Computer processor to analyze data and direct reports (e.g., paper reports, storage for graphic files, summary reports)
- Evaluation or controlling component to regulate the equipment or alert the nurse (e.g., a notice on the display screen, alarm signal)

nals, or alarms). The computer processor analyzes the information, stores pertinent information in specific places, and controls the direction of reporting (e.g., a paper report, storage for graphic files, shift summary reports). The evaluation or controlling component either regulates the infusion pumps electromechanically or alerts the nursing personnel through a report, an alarm, or a visual notice (e.g., a notice on the display screen: "increase patient's oxygen or check for leaks"). The most used physiologic monitor in critical care is the hemodynamic monitor.

## Hemodynamic Monitors

Kenner defines patient monitoring as those protocols and devices that assess a patient's condition on a frequent or continuing basis. Information from these protocols and devices is coupled with careful clinical surveillance to provide early warnings of changes (Kenner, 1990).

Hemodynamic monitoring can be used to

- Closely examine cardiovascular function.
- Evaluate cardiac pump and volume status.
- Assess vascular system integrity.
- Evaluate the patient's physiological response to stimuli.
- Obtain estimates of cellular oxygenation (Kenner, 1990).

Today hemodynamic monitors used in patient care come in many shapes and sizes, and offer an array of monitoring functions. Advanced monitoring systems include calculation of hemodynamic indices and limited data storage. Functions of modern monitors include the following (Clochesy, 1989; Gardner et al., 1989):

- Storage of waveforms
- Measurement of hemodynamic parameters
- Continuous blood gas and electrolyte evaluation
- Continuous glucose evaluation
- Cardiac output determination

- Continuous assessment of respiratory gases (capnography)
- Pattern recognition (arrhythmia analysis)
- Feature extraction
- Automatic transmission of selected data to a computerized patient database

Hemodynamic monitoring can be invasive or noninvasive. Invasive monitoring involves the use of venous and/or arterial catheters, which have potential complications, such as infection, hemorrhage, and embolism. Frequently, invasive arterial catheters are inserted in order to monitor oxygenation (blood gases). Norman et al. (1991) write that there is a trend toward noninvasive monitoring, especially the monitoring of oxygenation using pulse oximetry technology. They believe that this will result in more dependence on indirect blood pressure measurement (noninvasive). With the sophisticated devices available today, noninvasive monitors can acquire pulse rate and systolic, diastolic, and mean blood pressure values and store those values for varying lengths of time (Mathews, 1991).

Hemodynamic monitoring can take place at the bedside or be conducted from a remote location via telemetry. Telemetry allows for the continuous monitoring of ambulatory patients. Electrodes attached to the patient are connected to a portable transmitter carried by the patient. The cardiac impulses are sent by the transmitter to antenna wires distributed around the nursing unit (usually in the ceiling) and displayed on the monitor screen at the telemetry station (Elder, 1991). A screen from a bedside hemodynamic monitoring system is shown in Fig. 11.1.

Modern technology has enabled vendors of monitoring systems to offer many features to enhance the functionality of their products. Included among these features are

- Color monitors
- Touch screens
- "Soft keys" whose functions change depending on the context
- Modules that can be added to each monitor to expand and customize the available functions
- Networks that make monitor information available in different hospital areas remote from the patient
- Portable monitors with full-size monitor functionality

A unique feature currently offered by one vendor is to allow a central station monitor to be used for educational and reference purposes (Spacelabs Medical, Inc., 1991). This feature permits the use of selected third-party software for continuing education for nurses at the central station. In addition, this feature provides access to a selected third-party database of drug interactions. If this capability proves popular, other vendors may follow suit. Care must be taken, however, to consider the ramifications of

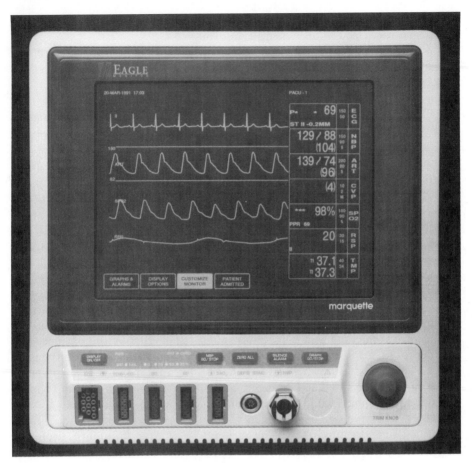

**Figure 11.1**   A bedside physiologic monitor: The Eagle Monitor System.
(Courtesy Marquette Electronics, Inc., Milwaukee, WI.)

using a central monitor for other purposes and to develop appropriate policies and procedures.

Computer-based hemodynamic monitoring offers the critical care nurse a wealth of information. However, the clinician must keep in mind that the monitor, and its information, does not replace clinical judgment or necessarily imply quality patient care (Kenner, 1990; Macy and James, 1971).

## Critical Care Information Systems

CCISs have evolved in the 1970s from the early physiological monitoring systems. These systems were called integrated patient data management systems in the 1986 Saba and McCormick text. Other names given to these are patient data management systems (PDMSs), clinical data management systems (CDMSs), or clinical information management systems

(CIMSs). In this edition, they will be called CCISs. In fact, most CCISs are intimately integrated with monitoring systems. CCISs, however, do more than acquire physiological data. These systems perform multiple functions and allow the storage of large amounts of data via a database.

A CCIS is a system designed to collect, store, organize, retrieve, and manipulate all data related to the direct care of the critically ill patient. It is focused on individual patients and the information directly related to their care. The primary purpose of a CCIS is the organization of a patient's clinical data for the clinician's use in patient care (Milholland and Cardona, 1983).

The principal goals in the early development of CCISs were to (1) accelerate the collection, processing, and presentation of data, (2) generate new data that were not usually available, and (3) reduce the workload of clinical staff. These early systems were usually called computerized monitoring systems, since their primary activity was collecting data from physiological monitors (Hilberman et al., 1975; Lewis et al., 1972; Macy and James, 1971; Manzano et al., 1980; Osborn et al., 1968).

In modern CCISs, the emphasis has changed to the information management aspects of these systems. Today, in addition to collecting physiological data, these systems focus on:

- Communicating and integrating information
- Creating and managing patient records
- Assisting in patient care decisions
- Augmenting the clinical capabilities of nurses and doctors (Alspach, 1991; Gardner et al., 1989)

A nurse using a CCIS in a patient room is depicted in Fig. 11.2.

The primary goals of CCISs have evolved from the original goals identified earlier. These goals have been described in different ways by many authors. A review of the literature revealed over 120 different statements addressing the purposes and expected benefits of CCISs. Analysis of these statements resulted in the identification of eight primary goals for CCISs. These new goals, which emphasize improving the quality of data management directed at quality patient care, are given in Table 11.3.

As CCISs have matured, the functions they offer have expanded to encompass not only data collection but also functions more commonly associated with hospital HISs, such as order entry and results reporting, care planning, and staff scheduling. Modern CCISs offer many functions to facilitate the work of critical care nurses. Clochesy (1989) describes several of these functions:

- Cardiac rhythm analysis and dysrhythmia detection
- Measurement of urine flow rate, output, and temperature
- Reporting of laboratory results
- Calculation of medication doses and fluid infusion rates

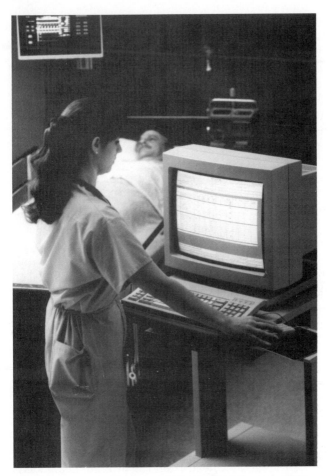

**Figure 11.2** A CCIS in the ICU: EMTEK System 2000.
(Courtesy EMTEK, Tempe, AZ.)

- Entry and transmission of physician orders
- Admission, discharge, and transfer of patients
- Organization of patient records
- Calculation of patient nutritional requirements
- Generation of a patient plan of care
- Entry and organization of care documentation

The critical care flow sheet has been the predominant display format for CCISs since their inception. As computer technology has advanced, the techniques for display of the flow sheet have been enhanced, but the flow sheet remains the major data interface. In most CCISs, the flow-sheet display is joined by a multitude of other "charts," such as lab reports, general

**TABLE 11.3**   THE NEW GOALS EMPHASIZING IMPROVING
THE QUALITY OF DATA MANAGEMENT
DIRECTED AT QUALITY PATIENT CARE

- Improve data management
- Improve data analysis
- Help staff
- Improve data quality
- Improve access to data
- Provide savings
- Improve quality of patient care
- Totally computerize patient chart

*Source:* Milholland, D. (1989). *A Measure of Patient Data Management System Effectiveness: Development and Testing.* Ann Arbor, MI: Dissertation Abstracts International.

patient assessments, specialized assessments (e.g., intravenous lines assessment), and free-text notes. A screen print of a respiratory therapy flow sheet from a CCIS is shown in Fig. 11.3.

Staff at each hospital are able to design the charts they want to use, incorporating the information structure and content with which they are most familiar. This enables each hospital and unit to tailor the systems to meet its needs. Learning the system is easier, because the learner has to learn only the technology, not the database content.

In addition to flexible charting formats and operations, current generations of CCISs offer many features to facilitate user interaction and enhance entry, retrieval, and interpretation of the clinical information within the patient database. Most of these features are available on commercial systems, although this may vary from vendor to vendor. Among the features offered by many vendors are:

- Each patient's data can be accessed from any terminal or workstation. This capability can extend across units and departments or be restricted to a single unit. In some instances, an alarm on one patient can be "forwarded" to another patient location, as determined by the nurse user.
- Admission to the CCIS database can be accomplished automatically from the HIS or as a manual operation on the clinical unit.
- Graphic displays of most data in the clinical database can be constructed. These displays may be preconfigured or may be developed dynamically as needed.
- Vital signs and other physiological data are automatically acquired from bedside instruments and incorporated into the clinical database. These data can be incorporated into flow sheets, assessments, etc.
- Fluid intake and output balances are calculated automatically as the data are entered. Hourly, daily, and shift totals are computed by the system. In addition, electrolyte and caloric balances may be routinely calculated.

EMTEK System 2000                        Fri Aug 24 11:01

Census | Utility ▼

129-23-4567      M       22      ICU7
Stanley Sokolov        45.4 kg    222222
Admit Physician: Brimm, John MD   Surgeon: Thurman, Audree MD

Sections: Flowsheet | Labs | Respiratory | Micro | Review | Notes

Forms: Ventilator

### Respiratory Therapy Flowsheet

| | | 08/24 03:00 | 04:00 | 05:00 | 06:00 | 07:00 | 08:00 | 09:00 | 10:00 | 11:00 | 12:00 |
|---|---|---|---|---|---|---|---|---|---|---|---|
| 02 FLOW | FIO2 | % | 50.00 | | 50.00 | | 50.00 | | 50.00 | | |
| 02 DEVICE | Ambu Bag/Mask in Room | | | | | | | | | | |
| MECHANICAL VENT | Ventilator Type | | Bear-I | | Bear-I | | Bear-I | | Bear-I | | |
| | Mode | | A/C | | A/C | | A/C | | A/C | | |
| | Machine Rate (AMV) | /min | 13 | | 13 | | 13 | | 10 | | |
| | Patient Rate | /min | 0 | | 0 | | 6 | | 5 | | |
| | Total Rate | /min | 13 | | 13 | | 10 | | 15 | | |
| | Pause Time | % | 15 | | 15 | | 15 | | 15 | | |
| | Flow Rate | L/min | 50.00 | | 50.00 | | 50.00 | | 50.00 | | |
| | Peak Insp Pressure | cmH2O | 20.0 | | 20.0 | | 20.0 | | 20.0 | | |
| | I:E Ratio | 1:x.x | 3.0 | | 3.0 | | 3.0 | | 3.0 | | |
| | Tidal Volume (Set) | ml | 30.0 | | 30.0 | | 30.0 | | 30.0 | | |
| | Tidal Volume (Corr) | ml | 15.0 | | 15.0 | | 15.0 | | 15.0 | | |
| | Static Compliance | L/cmH2O | | | | | | | | | |
| | Airway Temperature | C | 34.0 | | 34.4 | | 34.2 | | 33.0 | | |
| | Alarms On | | | | | | | | | | |
| | Circuit Change | | | | | | | | | | |
| PATIENT ASSESS | Breath Sounds RUL RML RLL LUL LLL | | | Clear Diminishd FineRales Crackles Crackles | | | | | | |
| | Pulse Pre Tmt During Tmt Post Tmt | | | 93 85 13 | | | | | | |
| | Resp Pre Tmt During Tmt Post Tmt | | | 13 13 | | | | | | |
| | Chest Excursion | | | N/A N/A N/A | | | | | | |
| | Cough | | | N/A | | | | | | |
| | Adverse Reaction | | | None | | | | | | |
| | Patient Tolerance | | | Fair | | | | | | |
| | Patient Position | | | Prone | | | | | | |
| | Total Time | min | | 10 | | | | | | |

Newer Data

Starting Print Screen

F1 | F3 | F5 | F7 | F9 Add Parameter | F11 Notes
F2 | F4 | F6 | F8 | F10 Add Time | F12 Print Report

**Figure 11.3**  Screen print of a respiratory therapy flow sheet from a CCIS: EMTEK System 2000. (Courtesy EMTEK, Tempe, AZ.)

- Any item entered via a flow sheet can be annotated. The annotations can be viewed via the flow sheet or as a set of notes, and they can be included with free-text notes entered separately.
- Special flow sheets incorporating required treatments and interventions may be provided. In most instances, the nurse can document the care given or not given directly on this flow sheet (on the screen). At any time, the nurse can enter an explanatory note describing the patient's response or the reasons for not delivering a specific treatment or intervention (Figs. 11.4 and 11.5).
- Assistance with many common clinical computations is provided. Intravenous medication dosage, intravenous flow rates, hyperalimentation, and aminoglycoside dose schedules are among the computations available. Depending on the system, these values may be part of the patient database or may be offered as an "off-line" calculator.
- Automatic calculation of physiological indices has been part of CCISs for many years. As selected data are entered into the patient database manually or directly from bedside devices, customer-specified algorithms are employed to calculate the cardiovascular, respiratory, neurological, and other indices.

**Figure 11.4**  An example of a flow sheet with annotations. The highlighted cell has been annotated with the comment listed in the notes cell near the base of the screen. (Courtesy Spacelabs, Inc., 1995, Redmond, WA.)

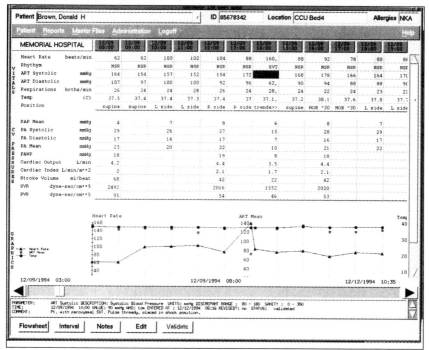

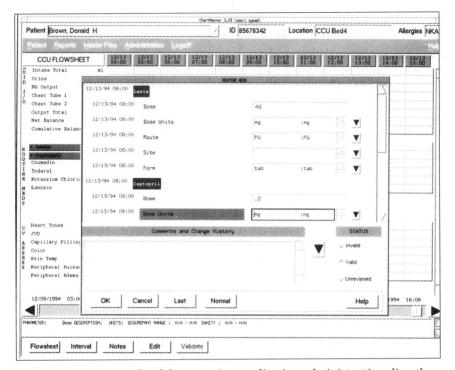

**Figure 11.5**  An example of documenting medication administration directly from the flow sheet. (Courtesy Spacelabs, Inc., 1995, Redmond, WA.)

- Automatic calculation capabilities have been extended to patient acuity, patient classification, productivity measures, and other indicators.
- Reference information is available to nurses, physicians, and other clinicians. This information may be provided by the vendor and modified by the customer, or the customer may develop all of its own materials. The information may be entered via optical scanning, direct keyboard entry, or transfer from a text file on another computer. Usually, the reference information can be printed on demand. Reference information includes specific clinical information on drugs, diseases, and patient problems, as well as policies and procedures relevant to specific units.
- Decision support features are provided, although the capabilities and operations will vary. Access to standard third-party database systems may be accomplished, and/or the vendor may supply a proprietary database management system. In all instances, these features enable the information in the CCIS to be analyzed to support research, quality improvement, outcomes, and management.

CCISs are most often used as bedside systems. That is, there is usually access to the system at every bedside in a critical care unit, as well as at the central station and various other locations. This, of course, will vary from hospital to hospital and is dependent on many factors, such as budget, space, and unit philosophy.

Initially, "dumb" terminals and keyboards were used to interact with the system. In some systems a keypad was used for bedside entry of numeric codes, supplemented by a keyboard at the central station. These terminals were connected to a computer, which provided the "brains" of the system. Now, dumb terminals have been replaced by personal computers (PCs) which are almost universally employed in CCISs. These personal computers are linked together by networks. The PCs perform data entry and screen management functions, and are frequently referred to as workstations. Figure 11.6 shows a typical CCIS workstation.

Also on the network, there may be one or two devices known as file servers that store and retrieve the patient data. Each file server supports several workstations. This use of file servers connected to several workstations is known as distributed processing. Distributed processing is currently the most prevalent approach in the architecture of CCISs.

Workstations provide users with the power traditionally found in minicomputers along with the convenience and individual use associated with personal computers. The network approach, which links the workstations together, provides several benefits:

**Figure 11.6**   A CCIS workstation: EMTEK System 2000. (Courtesy EMTEK, Tempe, AZ.)

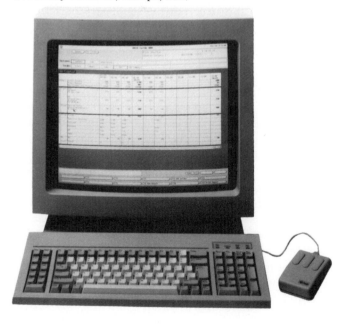

- It allows individual workstations to access a common database.
- It provides redundancy in case an individual workstation fails.
- It allows other computer devices to be shared (e.g., a printer).
- It facilitates links with other hospital computer systems (Seiver and Comerchero, 1989).

PCs also allow workstation-oriented systems to provide a graphical user interface (GUI), along with traditional keyboard interaction. The GUI allows a user to communicate with the computer system through the use of point-and-click devices such as a mouse or trackball. In addition, windows, structured lists, and icons can be used to make computer interaction easier and more meaningful to the clinical user. Seiver and Comerchero have asserted that GUIs will become standard on the CCISs of the 1990s.

Using PCs also allows access to the regular computer capabilities of the workstation. There is usually a method of exiting from the CCIS program and accessing the general computer functions of the workstation. This ability to leave the CCIS is controlled by the CCIS security system, and authorization to do so is determined by each organization. Once outside of the CCIS, the authorized user may have complete access to all computing features of the personal computer or may be restricted to a specific menu of software. Word processing, spreadsheets, and database management systems are some of the programs that could be available. In addition, if access to the full power of the computer is allowed, a user might write other programs to meet specific needs. As with central station monitors that allow the user to exit from the clinical applications, user organizations must consider the potential benefits and hazards of using this feature. Policies, procedures, and user education programs must be developed to address concerns and issues.

## Medical Information Bus

The medical information bus (MIB) is a computer-based device intended to ease the documentation workload generated by the proliferation of patient care devices (e.g., monitors, ventilators, infusion pumps) in the modern critical care setting. Most bedside devices contain built-in microprocessors for instrument control. But each manufacturer has used its own standard for defining interfaces with other devices. The proliferation of devices and standards has made integration of clinical data from different devices almost impossible, or at least prohibitively expensive. The primary purpose of the MIB is to establish a single standard that will allow a clinical user to simply "plug in" any device and achieve automatic communication of information between the device and a computer system (Nolan-Avila et al., 1988).

Unfortunately, this device probably is several years from general commercial availability. Until it is readily available, each vendor and each purchaser of systems will have to struggle with problems and issues

**TABLE 11.4**    FEATURES OF A MEDICAL INFORMATION BUS

- Automatic detection of device connection
- Notification of communications failure
- Notification of disconnect
- Identification of device for host computer
- Absence of special settings on device itself
- Automatic recovery from system failure/patient transport
- Reporting of device alarm state changes
- Remote resetting of alarms
- Large device per bedside capacity
- Clustering of device communication cables

resulting from the varying standards of patient care devices. The features of the MIB that are of most interest from a clinical user perspective are listed in Table 11.4.

CCISs provide many features and functions that assist the critical care nurse with daily patient care. Not only are documentation tasks made faster and easier, but the more important cognitive activities of assessment, diagnosis, planning, and evaluation are facilitated. CCISs facilitate the acquisition and retrieval of pertinent information organized in ways that facilitate the work of nursing. These systems help critical care nurses by managing the flood of information generated in modern critical care settings.

## Special-Purpose Systems

The following types of special-purpose systems are described in this chapter:

- Ventilator systems
- Blood gas analyzers
- Pulmonary function systems
- Intracranial pressure monitors
- Computer-processed EEG monitoring
- Drug administration systems
- Pharmacy systems
- Newborn nursery systems

### Ventilator Systems

An advantage of computer facilities in intensive care environments has been the regulation of equipment through microprocessors. Ventilators are used to deliver an adequate volume of gas to the patients' lungs and to control the pressure, volume, flow rate, inspiratory:expiratory time ratio, and oxygen concentration. The two types of ventilators, pressure-cycled and volume-cycled, have time-cycled devices that are regulated by microprocessors.

Ventilators have relied on surveillance systems by providing alarms when pulmonary function appears to be outside of a preset range or by communicating the integrity of the ventilator to the nurses' station when the patient in question is not in the intensive care environment. Computer-assisted ventilators have been developed and frequently use a micro-processor chip. Electromechanically controlled by a closed-loop feedback system, they analyze and control ventilation, blood volumes, and alveolar gases, which change as the patient's metabolic rate changes.

Processing signals by breath analysis of flow and volume has been done with various forms of microprocessors for years. The signals from respiratory pneumotachographs in association with differential pressure transducers allow on-line data collection for the inspiration and expiration phases of the respiratory cycle. Such systems were previously described by Dolcourt and Harris (1982).

Software programs specially designed for ventilation management are emerging as an important trend in ventilator management. These programs guide nurses, physicians, and respiratory therapists in analyzing the status of a ventilated patient and in making decisions about ventilator adjust-ments. An example of such a program for ventilators is described here.

One group of researchers has developed an application for ICU ven-tilator management (Tovar et al., 1991). The application appears on the computer screen as a duplicate of the ventilator control panel used in the ICU. The screen displays pulse oximeter values, arterial blood gas re-sults, cardiac output measurement, and current and recommended ven-tilator settings. The application provides four functions: an intelligent filter reduces inappropriate alarms, a monitor notes exceptional situa-tions and suggests immediate actions, a decision support tool recommends ventilatory settings based on collected data, and an interactive simula-tor allows users to experiment with different ventilator settings before actually making changes. For example, the physicians could delegate to the nurses therapeutic goals concerning maintenance of the patient's oxy-gen status. The nursing staff can use the simulator to test variations of ventilator settings before selecting the one that will best maintain that oxygen status.

### Blood Gas Analyzers

Other diagnostic or interpretive types of equipment found in critical care environments include blood gas analyzers. They are also available with microprocessor chips that are used to maintain and assist with the cali-bration of electrodes. As an analyzer system, the microprocessor automat-ically senses and calculates arterial blood gases, saturation curves, and buffer curves from normal data. These analyzers may also store data and graphically present trend analysis.

Microprocessing techniques have been used in calculations related to blood gas analysis for many years. Using a computer system can result in automation of much of the processing of calculations and reports. In blood gas testing the computer facilitates the following:

- Calculating variables
- Entering primary results as they are available
- Communicating results quickly to medical personnel
- Generating trend analysis results for patients from admission to discharge

This exceeds the usual computer adjuncts to blood gas analysis, since the standard equipment calculates variables and prints a readable report. Standard equipment, however, requires that blood gas reports be fed into a larger system, such as an HIS.

### Pulmonary Function Systems

Computer-assisted pulmonary diagnostic systems enhance spirometric testing by increasing test accuracy while decreasing test time. They automate and simplify routine lung mechanics, lung volume, diffusion capacity, and other pulmonary function tests. Specifically, a spirometric system quantifies breath-by-breath measurements of lung volume, calibrates a series of data points from the spirometer, and transmits them to the computer memory. The input represents instantaneous flow of gas volumes at each discrete interval of time, after the point recognized as the beginning of a breath or until the end of the breath. The volume input is collected with a recording device and converted to digital measurements. These measurements of the various spirometric indexes are compared with normal values, and the output is generated. Such systems can also be programmed to sequence the test procedures, store all data points during the test, calculate the results, generate a report numerically, and graphically display volume with time and flow volumes. It can also generate trend tables and graphics. The system depicts the presence and severity of expiratory and inspiratory obstructions that restrict the patient's vital capacity and is used to detect pulmonary diseases.

Spirometric systems are available as small stand-alone systems using microprocessors with dedicated software or as larger integrated systems using either a minicomputer or a mainframe. Microcomputer and minicomputer systems are usually dedicated systems with preprogrammed software packages like those made by Hewlett-Packard.

### Intracranial Pressure Monitoring

Neurosurgical nurses may use computer microprocessors in assessing intracranial pressure in patients with head injuries. The use of theoretical models for predicting the control of pressure and volume in the cerebrospinal fluid and intracranial space of head-injured patients has been tested using microprocessing techniques. A minicomputer programmed with a combination of predicted pressure curves simulating intracranial pressure and volume increases or decreases has been described. Further applications of this theoretical model with computer applications could allow intracranial pressure to be assessed and therapy introduced earlier in the course of treatment (Marmarou et al., 1981).

## Computer-Processed EEG Monitoring

Computer-processed electroencephalogram (EEG) monitoring provides a noninvasive method for continuous measurement of cerebral blood flow (CBF). EEG data from the patient are microprocessed, compressed, and displayed in a format that makes it easy to detect significant trends in the oxygenation and perfusion of the patient's brain. Printed copies of the trends shown on the screen can be obtained. Continuous EEG monitoring can be used in the critical care setting to show changes resulting from anesthetic agents, monitor brain activity during barbiturate coma, document seizure activity, and assist in determining prognosis. Decreases in high-frequency activity followed by a loss of power and amplitude in the EEG signal indicate an ischemic episode (Kinney et al., 1988).

## Drug Administration Systems

*Implantable Infusion Pumps:* Implantable infusion pumps are also regulated by microprocessors. The most developed system administers medication and stores information pertaining to equipment operation. The equipment can be programmed to deliver medication on an established, regular basis for a 24-h period. Up to six different programs, or variations in medication schedules, can be stored (Sanders and Radford, 1982).

## Pharmacy Systems

Because nursing personnel interact with several types of pharmacy systems, they may be considered a special application for nursing. Four types of pharmacy systems can be relevant to nurses:

- Unit dose order entry and supply system
- Drug interaction programs
- Medication administration systems
- Intake and output systems

*Unit Dose Order Entry:* Whether they stand alone or are a part of larger HISs, pharmacy modules are important for nursing. In one type of system, after the physician orders medication, a pharmacy computer picks up copies of the handwritten medication order form. Within 24 h, the standard orders are entered into a computer, the medications are noted, and a unit-dose cart is filled with the medication. A computerized sheet is delivered with the medications so that nursing personnel can document whether the medications were given. Medications to be given immediately are held in stock supplies on nursing units and charted manually.

More often, pharmacy modules are a part of a larger HIS. The physician writes medication orders directly at a terminal, and the orders are received in the pharmacy department. The computer establishes the time frames for each medication order and dispenses approved orders. Carts are filled with lists, and medication envelopes are prepared for unit-dose dispensing. Medication administration records are made available on-line and printed at a nursing unit at specified times. These records are used by nursing personnel to document medications given. Notification to administer a medication immediately will automatically generate a refill request. All medications about to expire are listed at the appropriate nursing unit.

In the future, these systems will change to accommodate the changes produced by health reform and outcomes management. The physician will have to justify the selection of one particular intervention rather than another, and the average costs of the different medications will be shown on the screens that the doctors are ordering from. The patient's preference will also be required in documentation systems in the future.

*Drug Interaction Programs:* Hospital formulary information is available on several HISs. Nurses may access these files to determine the usual purpose of a medication, maximum doses, side effects, and drug interactions. One reason for the number of drug interaction problems occurring in hospitals is the complexity of drug information available, the lack of time for nursing personnel to look up references, and the difficulty in finding needed references. Computerized systems facilitate access to drug interaction information (Hansten, 1983). Newer drug interaction programs are integrated with the documentation system, so that the purpose, dosage, side effects, costs, and interactions are printed at the time of order entry.

*Medication Administration Systems:* Bar code technology is being used in many pharmacy systems, including those documenting medication administration. The patient's wristband contains a bar code identifier to facilitate this type of system. Each unit dose package also has a bar code identifying the medication name, dosage, schedule, and route of administration. The nurse scans the patient's wrist bracelet using a scanner. Then the medication package is scanned. The computer system verifies that the patient, drug, dose, route, and time are correct. After administering the medication, the nurse scans his or her employee badge, which also has a bar code. Details of the medication administration are automatically stored in the computer system (Abdoo, 1992). Figure 11.7 is a printout of a medication administration report.

*Intake and Output Systems:* In intake systems, computers are linked to infusion pumps that control arterial pressure, drug therapy, fluid resuscitation, anesthesia, and serum glucose levels. They can include just the infusion system and the computer or the infusion system, the computer, and the physiologic monitors.

```
 ┌──────────────────────────────────────────────────────────────────────────────┐
 │ Rpt: Mgiven              Medical Center Hospital - SICU              Page 1     │
 │ Run: Jan 28, 91 1508                                    From: Jan 23, 91 0700  │
 │                           Medications Given             Thru: Jan 28, 91 1500  │
 └──────────────────────────────────────────────────────────────────────────────┘
  McBride,                       00022194    F 40  439 cm 112 kg          SICU 3103A
```

| Order number | Given By | When Given | Summary |
|---|---|---|---|
| 3.004 | SYSAD | Jan 23, 91 0700 | Calan Sr Caplet 240 mg TBCR PO |
| 3.002 | SYSAD | Jan 23, 91 0900 | Acyclovir (Zovirax) 100 mg CAPS PO |
| 3.003 | SYSAD | Jan 23, 91 0900 | Bactrim-DS 1 tab TABS PO |
| 3.002 | SYSAD | Jan 23, 91 2100 | Acyclovir (Zovirax) 100 mg CAPS PO |
| 3.003 | SYSAD | Jan 23, 91 2100 | Bactrim-DS 1 tab TABS PO |
| 3.004 | SYSAD | Jan 24, 91 0700 | Calan Sr Caplet 240 mg TBCR PO |
| 3.002 | SYSAD | Jan 24, 91 0846 | Acyclovir (Zovirax) 100 mg CAPS PO |
| 3.003 | SYSAD | Jan 24, 91 0846 | Bactrim-DS 1 tab TABS PO |
| 3.002 | SYSAD | Jan 24, 91 2100 | Acyclovir (Zovirax) 100 mg CAPS PO |
| 3.003 | SYSAD | Jan 24, 91 2100 | Bactrim-DS 1 tab TABS PO |
| 3.004 | SYSAD | Jan 25, 91 0700 | Calan Sr Caplet 240 mg TBCR PO |
| 3.002 | SYSAD | Jan 25, 91 0900 | Acyclovir (Zovirax) 100 mg CAPS PO |
| 3.003 | SYSAD | Jan 25, 91 0900 | Bactrim-DS 1 tab TABS PO |
| 3.002 | SYSAD | Jan 25, 91 2100 | Acyclovir (Zovirax) 100 mg CAPS PO |
| 3.003 | SYSAD | Jan 25, 91 2100 | Bactrim-DS 1 tab TABS PO |
| 3.004 | SYSAD | Jan 26, 91 0700 | Calan Sr Caplet 240 mg TBCR PO |
| 3.002 | SYSAD | Jan 26, 91 0900 | Acyclovir (Zovirax) 100 mg CAPS PO |
| 3.003 | SYSAD | Jan 26, 91 0900 | Bactrim-DS 1 tab TABS PO |
| 3.002 | SYSAD | Jan 26, 91 2100 | Acyclovir (Zovirax) 100 mg CAPS PO |
| 3.003 | SYSAD | Jan 26, 91 2100 | Bactrim-DS 1 tab TABS PO |
| 3.004 | SYSAD | Jan 27, 91 0700 | Calan Sr Caplet 240 mg TBCR PO |
| 3.002 | SYSAD | Jan 27, 91 0900 | Acyclovir (Zovirax) 100 mg CAPS PO |
| 3.003 | SYSAD | Jan 27, 91 0900 | Bactrim-DS 1 tab TABS PO |
| 3.002 | SYSAD | Jan 27, 91 2100 | Acyclovir (Zovirax) 100 mg CAPS PO |
| 3.003 | SYSAD | Jan 27, 91 2100 | Bactrim-DS 1 tab TABS PO |
| 3.004 | SYSAD | Jan 28, 91 0700 | Calan Sr Caplet 240 mg TBCR PO |
| 3.002 | SYSAD | Jan 28, 91 0900 | Acyclovir (Zovirax) 100 mg CAPS PO |
| 3.003 | SYSAD | Jan 28, 91 0900 | Bactrim-DS 1 tab TABS PO |

```
        00022194    F 40  439 cm 112 kg        SICU 3103A
```

**Figure 11.7**   Printout of a medication administration report: PC Chartmaster. (Courtesy Spacelabs, Inc., Redmond, WA.)

One of the most useful advantages of these systems for nursing is in intravenous drip rate calculation and regulation. The microprocessed infusion systems can calculate the intravenous concentrations, the body weight index, the infusion rate, and the volume (Jellife et al., 1983).

Even urine output has been microprocessed in the intensive care environment. Automated urine output systems monitor core body temperature from urinary output. The total volume in the container and the urine volume within a given time frame are measured, recorded, and shown on a digital readout.

At one hospital, an interface between the CCIS and a commercially available electronic urometer (Bard Urotrack Plus) has been developed (Nolan and Shabot, 1990). The electronic urometer automatically measures the urine volume and temperature. The interface collects the data and sends them to the CCIS, where the data are stored in the patient's record.

### Newborn Nursery System

In the newborn intensive care setting, computers are routinely used to microprocess information relative to an infant's heart and respiratory rates. In addition, systems are available to regulate the isolette temperature by sensing the infant's temperature and that of the air of the isolette. Under normal circumstances the computer automatically controls the temperature of the isolette to maintain a 36°C to 36.5°C environment. When the system is modified to store respiratory and heart rate data, the nurse has graphic data available to interpret changes in neo- nates' vital signs caused by environmental controls or physiologic function (Endo, 1981).

The nurse's role with this type of equipment in the neonatal intensive care unit has also been described. Equipment must be maintained so that the system can alert nurses by an alarm if a malfunction exists or an abnormal physiologic range is recorded. In addition, information that the computer generates must be interpreted.

A microprocessor may be used to measure the stiffness of the lung (compliance) and lung volumes in the premature infant with respiratory distress syndrome. Information on breath-by-breath regulation of lung volumes in premature infants can help prevent the development of serious lung complications and potential ventilator dependence (Dolcourt and Harris, 1982).

## EMERGENCY DEPARTMENT SYSTEMS

The ED has not benefited from computer information systems as greatly as the CCU and the OR. In most EDs, the extent of computerization is limited to the ADT application (admission, discharge, transfer) of the hospital's HIS. Order communication capabilities may be available, along with results reporting. But generally there has not been an extensive development effort toward automating the information management functions in the ED.

Conceptually, CCIS functions are applicable to the ED and may be used this way in some hospitals. However, there is a lack of information in the literature on this application of CCIS. In addition to managing specific patient information, the ED has some special information management needs which are outlined in Table 11.5 and discussed below (Brown, 1989).

**TABLE 11.5**   SPECIAL INFORMATION MANAGEMENT
                 IN EMERGENCY DEPARTMENTS

- Central register
- Triage data
- Aftercare instructions
- Post-treatment marketing
- Resource and consultation directories
- Patient location and tracking

*Source:* Brown (1989).

# Central Register

The central register is a log book, traditionally kept by hand, in which information specified by accrediting agencies is kept. The computer can make this record keeping easier by combining information from the admission database and the patient care record. The log data are used to calculate management and utilization statistics, such as patient volume, patient acuity, hourly census, etc. Cumulative log data are used in quality assurance, staffing pattern analysis, and monthly statistical reports. An example of a monthly activity report that might be generated from the central register data is shown in Figure 11.8.

# Triage Data

Automating triage data, such as the time of triage and the nurse's initial impressions and actions, can enhance initial record keeping and quality assurance efforts. Arrival and triage times can be compared with discharge ranking. Managers can assess the appropriateness of patient care prioritization and verify adherence to treatment norms and protocols. Staff productivity can be evaluated. Continuing education needs can be identified by evaluating the initial assessment with the final diagnoses.

# Aftercare Instructions

Storing patient aftercare instructions on a computer provides personalized instructions specific to the patient while eliminating the storage of large volumes of data. In addition, access to the information is easier, as is the work of updating it.

# Post-Treatment Marketing

Brown points out that automating ED data can improve a hospital's post-treatment marketing efforts (Brown, 1989). The computer can quickly gen-

MONTHLY EMERGENCY CENTER REPORT - PART 1      FEBRUARY 1990

NUMBER OF PATIENTS USING SERVICES:

| | EC PAT | OUTPAT | INPAT | TOTAL | % OF TOTAL |
|---|---|---|---|---|---|
| LAB | 1 | 0 | 0 | 1 | 33.3 |
| XRAY | 3 | 0 | 0 | 3 | 100.0 |
| EKG | 1 | 0 | 0 | 1 | 33.3 |
| RESP THERAPY | 0 | 0 | 0 | 0 | 0.0 |
| BLOOD GASES | 1 | 0 | 0 | 1 | 33.3 |
| SUTURES | 2 | 0 | 0 | 2 | 66.6 |
| BLOOD TRANS | 1 | 0 | 0 | 1 | 33.3 |
| MEDICATION | 3 | 0 | 0 | 3 | 100.0 |
| ANTIBIOTICS | 3 | 0 | 0 | 3 | 100.0 |
| IV | 2 | 0 | 0 | 2 | 66.6 |
| CAST | 2 | 0 | 0 | 2 | 66.6 |
| LBA/LEGAL EVID. | 0 | 0 | 0 | 0 | 0.0 |
| CONSULT ONLY | 0 | 0 | 0 | 0 | 0.0 |

NUMBER OF PATIENTS WHO ARRIVED:

| | | AVG/DAY |
|---|---|---|
| 0001-0200 | 0 | 0.0 |
| 0201-0400 | 0 | 0.0 |
| 0401-0600 | 0 | 0.0 |
| 0601-0800 | 0 | 0.0 |
| 0801-1000 | 0 | 0.0 |
| 1001-1200 | 1 | 0.0 |
| 1201-1400 | 1 | 0.0 |
| 1401-1600 | 1 | 0.0 |
| 1601-1800 | 0 | 0.0 |
| 1801-2000 | 0 | 0.0 |
| 2001-2200 | 0 | 0.0 |
| 2201-2400 | 0 | 0.0 |

TOTAL PATIENT CARE HOURS:   2.5

NUMBER OF PATIENTS BY PRIMARY INJURY/ILLNESS:

| | TOTAL | ADM | IFR | | TOTAL | ADM | IFR |
|---|---|---|---|---|---|---|---|
| ASSAULT | 0 | 0 | 0 | ORTHO, OTHER | 0 | 0 | 0 |
| BURN | 0 | 0 | 0 | OTHER | 0 | 0 | 0 |
| CANCER | 0 | 0 | 0 | CHILD ABUSE | 0 | 0 | 0 |
| CARDIAC | 0 | 0 | 0 | PLASTIC SURGERY | 0 | 0 | 0 |
| COMMON DISEASE | 0 | 0 | 0 | SUSPECTED VD | 0 | 0 | 0 |
| DERMATOLOGY | 0 | 0 | 0 | PSYCHIATRIC | 0 | 0 | 0 |
| SCHEDULED CASE | 0 | 0 | 0 | RENAL | 0 | 0 | 0 |
| EAR,NOSE,THROAT | 0 | 0 | 0 | RESPIRATORY | 0 | 0 | 0 |
| ENDOCRINE | 0 | 0 | 0 | RETURN VISIT | 0 | 0 | 0 |
| GASTROINTEST. | 0 | 0 | 0 | SEXUAL ASSAULT | 0 | 0 | 0 |
| GUN SHOT WOUND | 0 | 0 | 0 | SPINAL CORD | 0 | 0 | 0 |
| GYNECOLOGY | 0 | 0 | 0 | STABBING | 0 | 0 | 0 |
| HEMATOLOGY | 0 | 0 | 0 | SUBSTANCE ABUSE | 0 | 0 | 0 |
| MEDICAL | 0 | 0 | 0 | SUICIDE | 0 | 0 | 0 |
| R/O MI - MI | 0 | 0 | 0 | SURGERY | 0 | 0 | 0 |
| NEUROLOGY | 0 | 0 | 0 | TRAUMA, MINOR | 0 | 0 | 0 |
| OBSTETRICS | 0 | 0 | 0 | TRAUMA, MEDIUM | 1 | 1 | 1 |
| OPHTHALMIC | 0 | 0 | 0 | TRAUMA, MULTIPLE | 1 | 1 | 1 |
| FRACTURE/SPRAIN | 1 | 1 | 0 | UROLOGY | 0 | 0 | 0 |
| ORTHO, MV | 0 | 0 | 0 | VASCULAR | 0 | 0 | 0 |

TIME SPENT IN EMERGENCY CENTER:

| | 7-3 | 3-11 | 11-7 | TOTAL |
|---|---|---|---|---|
| 0-30 MIN | 0 | 0 | 0 | 0 |
| 31-60 MIN | 3 | 0 | 0 | 3 |
| 61-90 MIN | 0 | 0 | 0 | 0 |
| 91-120 MIN | 0 | 0 | 0 | 0 |
| 121-150 MIN | 0 | 0 | 0 | 0 |
| 151-180 MIN | 0 | 0 | 0 | 0 |
| 181-210 MIN | 0 | 0 | 0 | 0 |
| 211-240 MIN | 0 | 0 | 0 | 0 |
| 241+ MIN | 0 | 0 | 0 | 0 |

**Figure 11.8** Example of a monthly activity report for an emergency room: ER-Trak. (Courtesy Computer Support Services, Phoenix, AZ.)

erate lists of patient names and telephone numbers for post-treatment inquiries about patient satisfaction and current condition. Thank-you letters can be sent to all patients, individualized by name and date of service. Letters to physicians can be generated, informing them of the business the hospital has generated for them (e.g., the number of referrals).

## Resource and Consultation Directories

Resource and consultation directories function as on-line databases to facilitate finding the appropriate resource and/or consultant quickly and easily. Specific information about each resource or consultant, including phone numbers, address, hours of availability, specific skills, etc., is easily updated and available on a 24-h basis.

## Patient Location and Tracking

Patient location and tracking is an important application of computer technology for the ED and one that has immediate daily benefit for nurses. Unfortunately, this is an application that is just beginning to be developed. The emergence of the graphical workstation and the GUI described earlier may help in the development efforts by making the presentation and use of patient tracking information easier and faster.

One system has been developed in which the emergency room floor plan is duplicated on the workstation screen. Patients can be moved from room to room via a mouse. All active patients, the staff assigned to each patient, and a brief treatment plan for each patient can be viewed at a glance (Greenwald, 1990).

As technology continues to make programming easier and computers more inviting to use, and as EDs begin to demand solutions to their specialized information management needs, the number of computer systems for the ED will grow. Unfortunately, at this time, direct nursing involvement in these systems appears to be limited, and most systems seem primarily oriented toward physicians or administrative information management. ED nurses must become involved in system design and development if systems are to reflect nursing requirements and facilitate the nurses' work.

## OPERATING ROOM SYSTEMS

Computer systems in the OR focus on reducing the paperwork involved in managing the OR and each case. As in other areas of the modern hospital, paperwork consumes an inordinate amount of professional nursing time. Yet the paperwork is essential to a smoothly functioning and safe OR environment.

**TABLE 11.6**   TYPICAL USES OF COMPUTERS
                 IN THE OPERATING ROOM

- Staff scheduling
- Scheduling of surgeons
- Scheduling of OR
- Equipment tracking
- Intraoperative documentation
- Inventory management
- Managing staff credentialing
- Data analysis
- Preference list management

---

Typical uses of computers in the OR are listed in Table 11.6 and described in greater detail below. These uses commonly include scheduling, staff management, inventories, and data analysis.

## Data Analysis

Computerized data analysis for the OR includes identifying trends in procedures (e.g., the types of procedures done most frequently), tracking which services are growing fastest, and comparing inpatients and outpatients. Budget projections can be prepared for capital items and equipment. Analysis of trends allows the OR nurse manager to develop better, more persuasive justifications for equipment, beds, and staffing numbers (Zameska, 1991).

## Preference Lists

Computerized management of preference lists offers an excellent example of how computers can benefit staff, surgeons, ancillary departments, and patients. A preference list is a set of information used when setting up a surgical procedure for a specific surgeon (McLean, 1990). It includes information such as

- Patient positioning
- Prepping
- Draping
- Necessary equipment
- Pharmacy items and the usual doses
- The surgeon's special needs
- Explanation of the procedure

Nurses and others involved in preparing for a procedure refer to these lists frequently. In a manual system, preference lists must be periodically rewritten by hand to update them or just to obtain a clean copy. Lists can be misfiled and misplaced. Using a computer-based list eliminates these problems.

The computerized preference list in a typical OR system will go further. Once the case has been scheduled on the computer, the appropriate preference list is automatically printed. The nurse reviews the list and updates it as necessary. The updated list is sent automatically to the supply department, which uses it to collect the proper equipment and materials for the pending surgery. As items are collected, the supply department's inventories are automatically updated. When specific supplies reach a predetermined critical level, notifications are sent automatically to managers, and in some systems orders may be sent electronically to vendors (Enterprise Systems, 1991; DeRoyal Business Systems, 1991).

The OR nurse uses the same list to prepare the room and charge items. In a fully automated system, charges are automatically captured by using the computer-based preference list with verification on-line by the circulating nurse.

Using computer-based preference lists results in

- Organized lists for the supply department, including location and quantities
- Faster, more accurate billing
- Accurate, readable, accessible preference lists
- Time savings (McLean, 1990)

Figures 11.9., 11.10, and 11.11 give an example of a 3-page preference list from a computerized OR management system.

Overall benefits expected from implementation of computer systems in the OR include

- More efficient case schedules
- Maximum use of available case times
- Increased communication among staff and between departments
- Reduced room turnaround time
- Faster billing
- More accurate inventories
- Increased information for managers concerning department and employee performance
- Reduced manual paperwork (EPIC, 1991; Zameska, 1991)

All of these expected benefits are focused on helping the OR staff provide safe, effective, and efficient nursing care to their patients. OR systems have not been in widespread use, and little research has been done to examine issues, concerns, and possible negative effects of these systems. OR staff and managers must keep in mind that the systems need to be evaluated carefully for positive and negative impacts.

## COUNTY GENERAL HOSPITAL PREFERENCE LIST

Preference List:    2    DILATATION & CURETTAGE; COLD CONIZATION BIOPSY

Surgeon: ALLAND, JIM    Gloves: 8.5                                                                 Page    1

---

BEGINNING OF CASE:

TURN TABLE SO FOOT IS TOWARD STERILE CORE; MOVE TABLE HEAD PIECE TO FOOT OF

TABLE; ATTACH FAR SIDE STIRRUP; OVERHEAD LIGHT AT FOOT OF TABLE;  TABLE

ATTACHMENTS IN PLACE FOR POSITIONING TABLE SHELF; SITTING STOOL FOR SURGEON.

CHECK CHART FOR COMPLETED CONSENT FORM AND H&P.  ATTACH GROUND PAD TO UPPER

THIGH AWAY FROM PREP AREA.  DROP SUCTION AND BOVIE CORD TOWARD HEAD OF

PATIENT.

MIDDLE OF CASE:

SCRUB BE PREPARED TO ASSIST SURGEON.  CHECK WITH SURGEON FOR APPROPRIATE

LABEL IDENTIFICATION OF SPECIMEN.

---

| Item | Qty | Description |
|------|-----|-------------|
| **\*\*SHARED EQUIP NON-NEG\*\*** | | |
| 180 | 1 EA | BOVIE MACHINE 123123 |
| 216 | 2 EA | HIGH STIRRUPS 35846788 |
| | | |
| **\*\*SHARED EQUIP NEGOTIABLE\*\*** | | |
| 217 | 1 EA | SITTING STOOLS HM-123 |
| 218 | 2 EA | STIRRUP HOLDER TL-2345-SAD |
| 219 | 1 EA | FOOT EXTENSION FOR TABLE LL-PP-345 |

**\*\*POSITION\*\***

SUPINE C/ LITHOTOMY.  PT.'S

HIPS AT TABLE BREAK.  ATTACH

SECOND STIRRUP.  LEGS UP

SIMULTANEOUSLY INTO STIRRUPS

C/STOCKINETTE LEGGINGS.  LOW-

ER FOOT OF TABLE; REMOVE TABLE

EXTENSION.

| | | |
|------|-----|-------------|
| 181 | 1 PR | ARMBOARDS, DISP. PADDED COVERS 345666 |
| 220 | 2 EA | LEGGINGS, UNST 99-WTD |

| Item | Qty | Description |
|------|-----|-------------|
| **\*\*PREP\*\*** | | |

WASH PERINEUM AND UPPER INNER

THIGHS.  INTERNAL VAG. PREP AS

REQUESTED.

| | | |
|------|-----|-------------|
| 182 | 1 EA | PREP TRAY 56-345 |
| 183 | 1 BT | BETADINE SOAP 2345-23 |
| 184 | 1 BT | BETADINE PAINT SOLUTION 3245-44 |

**\*\*DRAPES & PACKS\*\***

SLIDE DRAPE SHEET UNDER HIPS.

BLOCK OFF PERINEUM C/TOWELS.

PLACE LITHOTOMY SHEET & SLIDE

LEGGINGS OVER LEGS.

| | | |
|------|-----|-------------|
| 221 | 1 EA | PACK, GYN II MM-134 |
| 189 | 1 EA | GOWN, SURG. LG. 1/PK ST.BK. 34445 |
| 187 | 1 PK | TOWELS, HEAVY 2345 |
| 188 | 1 PK | TOWELS, TINY 3455 |
| 222 | 1 EA | TOWELS, TERRY STERILE 2244 |

---

Revised:  03/09/89   By:  SMITH                                Printed JUN 01, 1989 at 1:17 PM

**Figure 11.9**   First page of a three-page printout of a typical OR preference list: ORBIT. (Courtesy Enterprise Systems, Inc., Bannockburn, IL.)

## COUNTY GENERAL HOSPITAL PREFERENCE LIST

Preference List:    2      DILATATION & CURETTAGE; COLD CONIZATION BIOPSY

Surgeon: ALLAND, JIM    Gloves: 8.5                                        Page    2

| Item | Qty | Description | Item | Qty | Description |
|------|-----|-------------|------|-----|-------------|
| | | **\*\*BASINS\*\*** | | | |
| 191 | 1 EA | BASIN GLOVE<br>CPD-400 | | | **\*\*DRESSINGS\*\*** |
| | | | 235 | 1 EA | PADS, SANITARY<br>8721 |
| | | **\*\*SURGICAL SUPPLIES\*\*** | | | |
| | | STERILE: | | | |
| 195 | 1 EA | GROUNDING PADS<br>SD-2134 | | | |
| 223 | 1 EA | CAUTERY PENCILETTE TECH-SWITCH<br>SJ0333 | | | |
| 224 | 1 EA | NEEDLE COUNTER 10/COUNT<br>455545 | | | |
| 225 | 2 EA | APPLICATOR, 6" STERILE 2/PK<br>2345 | | | |
| 226 | 1 EA | GLASS MEDICINE<br>2345-PP | | | |
| | | UNSTERILE: | | | |
| 198 | 1 EA | SUCTION CANNISTER 2000CC<br>34656-SDF | | | |
| | | **\*\*GLOVES\*\*** | | | |
| 204 | 1 PR | I CAN'T GET NO SATISFACION<br>1212-78 | | | |
| 201 | 2 PR | GLOVES, STERILE, 7.0 REG<br>1212-45 | | | |
| | | **\*\*INSTRUMENTS\*\*** | | | |
| 227 | 1 EA | SET EMERGENCY D & C<br>CS-100 | | | |
| 228 | 1 EA | MY MAIN MANAIMAL IS FAILY<br>CS-105 | | | |
| | | **\*\*SPECIAL INSTRUMENTS\*\*** | | | |
| 229 | 1 EA | CURETTE KEVORKIAN YOUNG<br>CS-67 | | | |
| 230 | 1 EA | KNIFE HANDLE #3 LONG<br>8954 | | | |
| | | **\*\*SUTURE-BLADES-NEEDLES\*\*** | | | |
| 231 | 1 EA | BLADES STERI-SHARP ASR #11<br>989-11 | | | |
| 232 | 1 EA | BLADE BEAVER NO. 91<br>566-91 | | | |
| 55 | 1 EA | SUTURE, CHROMIC 3-0 922H<br>922H | | | |
| | | **\*\*MEDS & SOLUTIONS\*\*** | | | |
| 214 | 1 EA | SOLUTION DIST WATER 1000CC<br>7865 | | | |
| 234 | 1 BT | LUGOL'S SOLUTION<br>5678 | | | |

Revised: 03/09/89  By: SMITH                                  Printed JUN 01, 1989 at 1:17 PM

**Figure 11.10**   Second page of OR preference list: ORBIT. (Courtesy Enterprise Systems, Inc., Bannockburn, IL.)

## COUNTY GENERAL HOSPITAL PREFERENCE LIST

Preference List:    2        DILATATION & CURETTAGE; COLD CONIZATION BIOPSY

Surgeon:  ALLAND, JIM    Gloves:  8.5                                      Page   3

---

END OF CASE:

LOWER LEGS FROM STIRRUPS VERY SLOWLY.  APPLY SANITARY PAD BEFORE PATIENT IS
TRANSFERRED TO PAR.  PLACE CHUCKS ON GURNEY.

---

Revised:  03/09/89  By:  SMITH                          Printed JUN 01, 1989 at  1:17 PM

**Figure 11.11**   Third page of OR preference list: ORBIT. (Courtesy Enterprise Systems, Inc., Bannockburn, IL.)

## SUMMARY

Critical care nursing has been defined as a nursing specialty dealing with human responses to life-threatening problems. Critical care nursing can be practiced in any setting, but it is most often found in CCUs, EDs, and ORs. The complexities of patient care in these settings have led to the development of technology to help nurses deliver that care. In this chapter, some of those technologies have been discussed. These include arrhythmia, physiologic, and hemodynamic monitoring systems; CCISs, special-purpose systems; and ED and OR information systems.

The basic functions of hemodynamic monitoring systems were described, as were the most common features that enhance their utilization. The trend toward noninvasive monitoring systems was discussed. Principal goals and purposes of CCISs and a history of their development were presented. The most common CCIS information management features were also covered. Modern CCISs incorporate PC technology into workstations which provide extensive computer power and many user-friendly functions. The GUI is predicted to be the primary interface for the coming decade. The MIB allows multiple patient care devices to communicate with a CCIS. Although not commercially available, the standards promulgated by the MIB effort are being incorporated by individual vendors.

ED systems are less well developed and significantly fewer in number. Patient tracking, log book maintenance, aftercare instructions, and triage data records are the primary applications. ED systems described in the literature are heavily oriented toward physician information management. ED nurses need to become involved in the systems if the systems are to help nurses in patient care.

OR systems focus on managing the case schedule, tracking equipment, providing information for case preparation, and charging supplies. Some systems support on-line entry of patient data during the operation. OR systems can relieve the nurse of much repetitious paperwork and improve the flow of activities throughout the surgical department.

Technology continues to develop at a rapid rate, and the use of computers in critical care settings will continue to expand. Not only information systems but specific patient care devices will proliferate and contribute to the information flood that has generated the need for the computer systems in the first place. Coping with technology overload is an essential skill for nurses. Learning the concepts and principles of critical care computer applications presented in this chapter can be more important than focusing on a particular system or device. Understanding the basic elements will enable nurses to more easily adapt and adopt new equipment and systems.

# REFERENCES

Abdoo, Y. (1992). Designing a patient care medication and recording system that uses bar code technology. *Computers in Nursing, 10*(3), 116–120.

Alspach, J. (1991). Computers as partners in critical care. *Critical Care Nurse, 11*(4), 7–11.

Berg, N. (Ed.). (1981). *Core Curriculum for Critical Care Nursing.* New York: Saunders.

Bronzino, J. (1982). *Computer Applications for Patient Care.* Reading, MA: Addison Wesley.

Brown, D. J. (1989) Computerization. In I. Frank (Ed.), *Managing Emergency Nursing Services.* Rockville, MD: Aspen.

Clochesy, J. M. (1989). *Advanced Technology in Critical Care Nursing.* Rockville, MD: Aspen.

DeRoyal Business Systems. (1991). *DBS O.R. Management System Product Description.* Powell, TN: DeRoyal Business Systems.

Dolcourt, J., and Harris, T. (1982). Pulmonary function in critically-ill newborn infants: Measurement by microprocessor. In B. Blum (Ed.), *Proceedings of the Sixth Annual Symposium on Computer Applications in Medical Care* (pp. 686–689). Silver Spring, MD: IEEE Computer Society Press.

Elder, A. (1991). Setting up and using a cardiac monitor. *Nursing 91, 21*(3), 58–63.

Endo, A. (1981). Using computers in newborn intensive care settings. *American Journal of Nursing*, 81, 1336–1337.

Enterprise Systems. (1991). *ORBIT Operation Room Management System.* Bannockburn, IL: Enterprise Systems.

Epic Systems. (1991). *Optime: The Operating Room Scheduling System.* Madison, WI: Epic Systems.

Gardner, R., Bradshaw, K., and Hollingsworth, K. (1989) Computerizing the intensive care unit: Current status and future directions. *Journal of Cardiovascular Nursing, 4*(1), 68–78.

Greenwald, T. (1990). An emergency department information management system. In R. A. Miller (Ed.), *Proceedings of the 14th Annual Symposium on Computer Applications in Medical Care* (pp. 943–945). Washington, DC: IEEE Computer Society Press.

Hansten, P. (1983). Utilization of drug information in pharmacy systems. In O. Fokkens et al. (Eds.), *MEDINFO '83 Seminars* (pp. 123–135). Amsterdam, Netherlands: New Holland.

Hilberman, M., Kamm, B., Tarter, M. and Osborn, J. (1975). An evaluation of computer-based patient monitoring at Pacific Medical Center. *Computers and Biomedical Research, 8,* 447–460.

Jellife, R., Shumitzky, A., D'Argenio, D., et al. (1983). Improved 2-compartment time-shared programs for adaptive control of digitoxin and digoxin therapy. In R. Dayhoff (Ed.), *Proceedings of the Seventh Annual Symposium on Computer Applications in Medical Care* (pp. 231–234). Silver Spring, MD: IEEE Computer Society Press.

Kenner, C. V. (1990). Hemodynamic monitoring. In B. Dossey, C. Guzzetta, and C. Kenner (Eds.), *Essentials of Critical Care Nursing* (pp. 206–236). Philadelphia: Lippincott.

Kinney, M. R., Pacha, D. R., and Dunbar, S. B. (1988). *AACN's Clinical Reference for Critical Care* (2d ed.). New York: McGraw-Hill.

Lewis, J., Deller, S., Quinn, M., et al. (1972). Continuous patient monitoring with a small digital computer. *Computers and Biomedical Research, 5,* 411–428.

Macy, J. and James, T. (1971). The value and limitations of computer monitoring in myocardial infarction. *Progress in Cardiovascular Diseases, 13,* 495–505.

Manzano, J. L., Villalobos, J., Church, A., and Manzano, J. J. (1980). Computerized information systems for ICU patient management. *Critical Care Medicine, 8,* 745–747.

Marmarou, A., Shapiro, K., Kosteljanetz, M., and Pasternack, D. (1981). A microprocessor based analysis of raised intracranial pressure in head injured patients. In H. Heffernan (Ed.), *Proceedings of the Fifth Annual Symposium on Computer Applications in Medical Care* (pp. 516–518). Silver Spring, MD: IEEE Computer Society Press.

Mathews, J. (1991). How to use an automated vital signs monitor. *Nursing 91, 21*(2), 60–64.

McLean, V. (1990). Computerized preference lists. *AORN Journal, 52*(3), 509–522.

Milholland, D. (1989). *A Measure of Patient Data Management System Effectiveness: Development and Testing.* Ann Arbor, MI: Dissertation Abstracts International.

Milholland, D., and Cardona, J. (1983). Computers at the bedside. *American Journal of Nursing, 83,* 1304–1307.

Mirvis, D., Benson, A., Goldberger, A., et al. (1989). Instrumentation and practice standards for electrocardiographic monitoring in special care units: A report for health professionals by a task force of the Council on Clinical Cardiology: American Heart Association. *Circulation, 79*(2), 464–471.

Nolan, L., and Shabot, M. (1990). The P1073 Medical Informatics Bus Standard: Overview and benefits for clinical users. In R. Miller (Ed.), *Fourteenth Annual Symposium on Computer Applications in Medical Care* (pp. 216–219). Silver Spring, MD: IEEE Computer Society Press.

Nolan-Avila, L., Paganelli, B., and Norden-Paul, R. (1988). The medical information bus. *Computers in Nursing, 6*(3), 115–121.

Norman, E., Gadaleta, D., and Griffen, C. (1991). An evaluation of three blood pressure methods in a stabilized trauma population. *Nursing Research, 40*(2), 86–89.

Osborn, J. J., Beaumont, J., Raison, J., et al. (1968). Measurement and monitoring of acutely ill patients by digital computer. *Surgery, 64,* 1057–1070.

Sanders, K., and Radford, W. (1982). The computer in a programmable implantable medication system (PIMS). In B. Blum (Ed.), *Proceedings of the Sixth Annual Symposium on Computer Applications in Medical Care* (pp. 682–685). Silver Spring, MD: IEEE Computer Society Press.

Seiver, A., and Comerchero, H. (1989). Clinical information management in critical care. *Intensive Care World, 6,* 4.

Sorkin, J., and Bloomfield, D. (1982). Computers of critical care. *Heart and Lung, 11,* 287–293.

Spacelabs Medical, Inc. (1991). *Spacelabs: The Informed Source for Better Patient Care.* Redmond, WA: Spacelabs Medical, Inc.

Tovar, M., Rutledge, G., Lener, L., and Fagar, L. (1991). The design of a user interface for a ventilator-management advisor. In P. Clayton (Ed.), *Fifteenth*

*Annual Symposium on Computer Applications in Medical Care* (pp. 828–832). New York: McGraw-Hill.

Widman, L. (1992). The Einthoven System: Toward an improved cardiac arrhythmia monitor. In P. Clayton (Ed.), *Fifteenth Annual Symposium on Computer Applications in Medical Care* (pp. 441–445). New York: McGraw-Hill.

Zameska, M. (1991). Computers and the future. Increasing efficiency. *Today's OR Nurse, 13*(4), 28–31.

# BIBLIOGRAPHY

Abraham, I. L., Fitzpatrick, J. J., and Jane, L. (1986). Computers in critical care nursing: Yet another technology? *Dimensions of Critical Care Nursing, 5*(6), 325–326.

Blaufuss, J. (1990). Computer technology. In J. Spicer and M. Robinson (Eds.), *Managing the Environment in Critical Care Nursing* (pp. 93–104). Baltimore, MD: Williams & Wilkins.

Brimm, J. E. (1987). Computers in critical care. *Critical Care Nursing Quarterly, 9*(4), 53–63.

Burkes, M. (1991). Identifying and relating nurses; attitudes toward computer use. *Computers in Nursing, 9*(5), 190–201.

Clochesy, J. M., and Henker, R. A. (1986). Selecting computer software applications in critical care. *Dimensions of Critical Care Nursing, 5*(3), 171–177.

Crew, A. D., and Unsworth, G. D. (1985). Does the ICU computer improve patient care? *Applied Cardiology, 131*, 9–13.

deCalonne, P. G., Hornaday, L., and Schmitt, P. (1983). Use of a microcomputer in the intensive care unit. *Heart and Lung: Journal of Critical Care, 12*(5), 516–521.

Finkelmeier, B. A., and Salinger, M. H. (1986). Dual-chamber cardiac pacing: An overview. *Critical Care Nurse, 6*(5), 12–13, 16, 18–20.

Kellogg, M. (1991, April). Technology: The future of the '90s. *Today's OR Nurse*, p. 4.

Large, W. P. (1988). Realising the potential of pocket computers for intensive care. *Intensive Care Nursing, 4*(2), 82–85.

Mann, R. E. (1992). Preserving humanity in an age of technology. *Intensive and Critical Care Nursing, 8*(1), 54–59.

McHugh, M. L. (1986). Increasing productivity through computer communications automating nursing documentation. *Dimensions of Critical Care Nursing, 5*(5), 294–302.

Muirhead, R. C. (1983). Computers in critical care nursing: The new revolution. *Dimensions of Critical Care Nursing, 2*(3), 133–134.

Murchie, C. J., and Kenny, G. N. C. (1988). Nurse attitudes to automatic computer control of arterial pressure. *Intensive Care Nursing, 4*(3), 112–117.

Replogle, K. J. (1985). Computers bring new vocabulary to critical care nurses. *Critical Care Nurse, 5*(5), 57–61.

Sabol, J., Emonds, B., Soltys, M., and Disch, J. (1993). An innovative approach to telemetry monitoring. *Medsurg Nursing, 2*(2), 99–103.

Schaefer, K. M. (1989). Retention technique. Research: Future impact on image and retention. Part 3. *Dimensions of Critical Care Nursing, 8*(1), 44–49.

Shamian, J., Hagen, B., Hu, T., and Fogarty, T. E. (1992). Nursing resource requirement and support services. *Nursing Economics, 10*(2), 110–115.

Spicer, J., and Robinson, M. (Eds.). (1990). *Managing the Environment in Critical Care Nursing*. Baltimore, MD: Williams & Wilkins.

Watt, S. (1985). Computers in intensive care nursing. *Intensive Care Nursing, 1*(1), 49–58.

# *12*

• • • • • • • • • • • • • • • • • • • • • • • • •

# COMMUNITY HEALTH APPLICATIONS

## OBJECTIVES

- Discuss the development of community health computer applications.
- Describe community health computer systems.
- Discuss state/local health department computer systems.
- Describe special-purpose computer systems.
- Discuss ambulatory care computer systems.
- Describe home health computer systems.
- Discuss classification/acuity computer systems.
- Discuss home care technology systems.

Community health focuses on the care of all people in the community. Community health nursing (CHN), earlier known as public health nursing, is a synthesis of nursing practice and public health practice concerned with promoting and preserving the health of populations. It is also concerned with care to noninstitutionalized clients in community settings where health care is provided and with the care of the sick at home.

CHN is not limited to a particular age, diagnostic group, or health care facility. It focuses on the health of the well and the care of the sick using a holistic approach to the patient/client alone and to the family, group, and community. CHN focuses not only on health promotion, maintenance, and education, but also on coordinating the continuity of care across health care settings to improve the health status of all in the community.

Computer applications and systems that have been developed to support CHN focus primarily on community health (public health) promotion and disease prevention, ambulatory care, and home health care programs. Because of the wide scope of CHN, these applications vary. They include systems designed to process information for (1) specific types of CHN agencies, e.g., state and local health departments, health maintenance organizations, or visiting nurse associations; (2) specific community health settings where services are provided, e.g., clinics, schools, or homes; and (3) specific types of programs, e.g., family planning or immunization. They also vary depending on the focus of the system, e.g., statistical reporting, billing and financial, and/or patient care. Additionally, they vary depending on the specific application being addressed, e.g., classification/acuity, the computer-based patient record, managed care, and home care and educational technologies.

This chapter provides an overview of the development of computer applications in community health as well as a description of the major types of community health computer systems, namely:

- Community health systems
- State/local health department systems
- Special-purpose systems
- Ambulatory care systems
- Home health systems
- Classification/acuity systems
- Home technology systems

## COMMUNITY HEALTH COMPUTER DEVELOPMENT PROJECTS

CHN agencies have used computers since the late 1960s, when computers were introduced into the health care industry. With the enactment of the Medicare and Medicaid legislation in 1965, reimbursement for home care services was allowed. This new legislation expanded the demand for home care services, increased the number of home health agencies (HHAs), and increased the information needs, which created the need for computer systems. As a result, as early as 1969 several commercial vendors and service bureaus developed billing and financial systems for visiting nurse associations (VNAs) and other HHAs. These systems were primarily designed to process the information, monitor the certification requirements, and manage and administer home care services as required by Medicare, Medicaid, and third-party payers.

In the 1970s and early 1980s, many state and local official health departments developed statistical reporting systems for processing information on nursing personnel, programs, and services. Many of these reporting systems are still in use. They were primarily developed to manage the information requirements of the agencies' CHN services. During the late 1980s and 1990s, as CHN came to require information not only on payment for services, but also on the quality of care, computer applications in community health advanced. Computer systems were developed to support the management and coordination of patient care data provided by clinics and/or ambulatory care settings such as health maintenance organizations (HMOs) (Saba, 1982, 1983).

During these time periods, special projects were conducted by national agencies, local CHN agencies, and/or universities that influenced the design of the community health systems. They were conducted to determine the statistical reporting requirements, management and patient information needs, reimbursement requirements, quality care indicators, and outcomes measures. Other projects led to the development of minimum data sets and/or classification systems for home care. Several of the significant projects are described below.

## National Projects

The Division of Nursing, Public Health Service, United States Department of Health and Human Services (DN, PHS, US DHHS) influenced the development of computer systems for community health and home health agencies. In the 1970s, the DN, PHS, US DHHS, supported several projects designed to develop out-of-institution computer systems and advance computer technology in the field of community health nursing (see Chap. 1).

The National League for Nursing (NLN), in collaboration with the DN, PHS, US DHHS, initiated a project designed to promote better understanding of computer-based management information systems (MISs) among public health/community health nurses and agencies. In 1973, the NLN conducted the first national conference on the use of computerized MISs for public health/CHN agencies. Between 1973 and 1976 it (1) conducted two national conferences, (2) conducted six regional workshops, and (3) published four monographs, one of which provided a compilation of selected community health computerized MISs (National League for Nursing, 1973, 1975, 1976, 1978).

The NLN also initiated a special committee to identify the content of a database to make community health agency systems operable. It identified a basic data set for CHN, a prototype for a basic minimum data set for CHN agencies. The basic data set was designed as a guide for establishing the uniform data collection needed for statistical reporting systems that could also be linked to other agencies. It also identified statistical information needed to measure and describe services related to community needs and resources, focusing on four types of data: patient, staff, agency, and community. The content was identified for computerized MISs developed for CHN agencies (National League for Nursing, 1977).

## State Projects

The DN, PHS, also supported the development of two state computerized MISs. Both systems were designed to support the computerization of state-wide CHN activities. The first was the New Jersey Home Health Care System, which focused on statewide home visiting services provided by community health nurses. The system was designed to collect and develop reports needed for the statewide statistical reporting system (New Jersey State Department of Health, 1977). The second was the Florida Client Information System, which was developed to not only register eligible residents but also collect encounter information on those residents receiving CHN services. It was the first on-line statewide computerized community health system in the country (Florida Department of Health and Rehabilitative Services, 1983).

During this time period, two surveys of state nursing and health departments were conducted by the state and territorial directors of community health nursing, one in 1974 and the other in 1985. They were conducted to determine the scope of CHN computer systems in state health departments. In both surveys, approximately half of the state and territorial directors reported that in their respective states, they had initiated some form of computer application. They reported that the applications were designed to collect statistical data on CHN programs; patient, clinic, and home visits; services by type of provider; and counts of patients by program.

## Local Projects

During this same period, several projects were also initiated by local health departments and/or VNAs. They were conducted in an effort to develop computer systems that focused on the assessment of care and the progress of patients in community health programs. However, they were generally paper-based methodologies to be used in computer systems. The major ones included: (1) Patient Progress, a methodology designed to allow community health nurses to document changes in the health status of patients, (2) a community health patient assessment tool which could be computerized; (3) a computerized model to assess, analyze, and evaluate the care of patients by community health nurses; and (4) a Patient Problem List for documenting CHN.

## Prospective Payment Projects

The Health Care Financing Administration (HCFA) funded several projects to determine the most equitable, efficient, and effective method of payment for services provided to Medicare and Medicaid patients. The Abt Project was intended to test and compare two methods of prospective payment (per visit and per episode) for home health patients. The first phase tested the per visit method of reimbursement in 10 states using HCFA Form 445. This form was specially designed to identify medical conditions and functional status, and minimized nursing care needs. The second phase of the project was to test the episode of care method of payment. This method was developed by another HCFA-funded project in which Mathematica Corp. was given a mandate to develop a prospective payment system (PPS) for HHAs. The episode of care method designed used the database from the Georgetown University Home Care Classification Project (Saba, 1991). Payment for an episode of care is based on the traditional medical model rather than on the nursing model proposed by the Georgetown project (Brown et al., 1991).

## Quality Outcomes Projects

Several quality outcomes projects have been conducted by Shaughnessy and colleagues at the University of Colorado Center for Health Policy. They have focused on developing quality indicators for long-term care, including home health. Their projects have affected the design of CHN and HHA systems by identifying the data elements which measure quality outcomes of care. One of their projects measured outcomes at time periods when changes in the health status of patients receiving home health care occurred. Another project, designed to develop a set of indicators needed to monitor quality of care based on medical outcomes, identified outcomes for specific medical conditions. The preliminary design identified a set of acute and chronic conditions as well as primary prevention screening variables that encompass broad clinical categories and varied therapies as measurements of quality outcomes (Shaughnessy et al., 1990; Shaughnessy and Kramer, 1990).

## Community Nursing Organization Demonstration Project

In 1993 the HCFA funded the Community Nursing Organization (CNO) Demonstration Project. This project was concerned with reimbursement of wellness services provided by nurse-run clinics, including home care preventive and monitoring services. Four CNOs were selected to conduct primary care demonstrations across the country: (1) Carondelet Health Services, Inc., of Tucson, Arizona, (2) Carle Clinic Association of Urbana, Illinois, (3) Visiting Nurse Service (VNS) of New York, New York, and (4) Living at Home/Block Nurse Program/Metropolitan VNA, Twin Cities, Minnesota.

A CNO is a nurse-managed operation where nurses provide primary care services to Medicare beneficiaries on a prepaid capitation basis. Services for well clients are provided not only at the clinic, but also in their homes. This project should provide not only information but also a data set on this innovative method of providing primary health care services in the community setting (Community Nursing Organizations' Consortium, 1993).

## Uniform Data Set for Home Care and Hospice Project

In 1993, the National Association for Home Care (NAHC) initiated a task force to develop a uniform data set for home care and hospice. The need for a minimum data set was determined by NAHC to be critical, and its development was considered to be the first step toward achieving standardized, comparable home care and hospice data. NAHC determined that in general, home care and hospice data are incomplete, in many instances inaccurate, and not uniform. The goal of the project is to identify the critical data elements and develop standardized definitions for a uniform minimum data set for home care and hospice programs. The initial data set is organized into two major categories, organizational- and individual-level data elements (National Organization of Home Care, 1994).

## COMMUNITY HEALTH SYSTEMS

The "community health systems" is used to connote those computerized information systems specifically developed and designed for use by community health agencies, programs, and services. Community health systems address the broad areas of health care programs, agencies, and settings. They support health promotion and disease prevention programs; statistical information required by state/local health department programs; and funding information for federal block grants, categorical programs, or other grant programs. They also assist community health agencies in the decision-making processes in the management of nursing facilities. Community health systems are also used to evaluate the impact of noninstitutional nursing services on patients, families, and community health conditions. Other systems have been developed as stand-alone/turnkey systems specifically designed for special programs, projects, and studies.

## STATE/LOCAL HEALTH DEPARTMENT SYSTEMS

The information systems for state/local health departments have traditionally been statistical reporting systems. They were specifically designed to collect the information needed to satisfy various funding sources. Other systems have been developed which have other applications and are used to support and manage nursing services. For example, a patient registration system can provide data not only on caseload and census, but also on home, clinic, and school visit services. On the other hand, personnel and management systems are used for preparing personnel payrolls and management data. The major types of systems are:

- Statistical reporting systems
- Registration systems
- Management information systems
- Personal/client management systems

## Statistical Reporting Systems

Statistical reporting systems are community health computer systems which have been developed to collect and process statistical information; they are used primarily by state and local health departments. They were developed as the need for uniform information from all official state and local health departments emerged as a national initiative. However, because the federal government has neither mandated nor provided reimbursement for health promotion and disease prevention services, it has not been able to require official state and local community health agencies to collect standardized data sets, and so these systems vary from state to state and agency to agency. As a result there is no uniform means of comparing state programs and services at a national level and no reliable method of determining trends in the effectiveness and efficiency of state and local health department programs.

Several state health departments are developing new systems for collecting community health statistics. Many states, such as Michigan, Missouri, Florida, and Kentucky, are implementing computer and communication networks that link state and local community health agencies. These are primarily statistical reporting systems designed to collect and process on-line data required for federal, state, and local community health programs. An example of a community care network is shown by the initial trial sites of the system being implemented in West Virginia (Fig. 12.1).

The Missouri Health Strategic Architectures and Information Cooperative (MOHSAIC) is an example of a state project designed to collect client-centered data, including services performed by providers. Clusters of data would also be aggregated for evaluating program-specific reporting requirements (Hoffman, 1993). Texas is linking 400 public health clinics via a new Health Integrated Client Encounter System (ICES) that was designed to meet prevention as well as outcome goals. It is used to log in all assessment data and track preventive services such as TB care, immunizations, and other preventive measures. Kansas and North Carolina are also developing similar systems that focus on community health assessment and preventive services (Clinical Data Management, 1994).

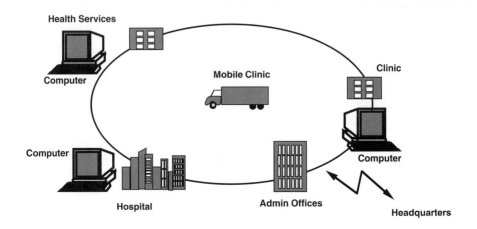

**Figure 12.1**   Community care network.

## National Information System

A national information system for collecting federal program data from state and local community health agencies is being proposed by the Center for Disease Control (CDC). CDC is the federal agency mandated to collect all state data required for statistical reporting and funding of all federal programs, such as the immunization program. In mid-1993, CDC identified not only huge data gaps but also a lack of coordination in the existing federally funded public health, surveillance, information, and other data systems. CDC proposed that these statistical reporting systems should not only use a common classification scheme but also use the same data standards. It proposed that these existing systems should be integrated into one national information system, which should collect data on all enrolled/registered state/local clients and their encounters with community health services (National Center for Health Statistics, 1994).

## Registration Systems

Client registration information systems (CISs) are systems designed to identify state/local residents/clients eligible for CHN services in clinics and homes. These systems generally consist of an on-line communication network, with terminals located in each of the local/district offices that are linked to the central computer facility and used to collect, store, and process all data. The centralized registry can then be accessed from the local/district units prior to providing services.

Many of the newer systems, such as the Michigan system and the revised Florida system, include not only a registry of eligible state residents but also encounter data on all clients receiving services from any state/local health department. Client eligibility is obtained from the client registration form, which collects baseline demographic information used to provide statistical reports on the client population being served, and the encounter data are derived from a provider activity form used to collect information on all clients receiving care from all health providers, including community health nurses. The two sets of data form the database for the system, which is used to produce statewide statistical reports needed to plan and manage health services. Many other state health departments are implementing similar statewide client registration systems in order to track client clinical data (Florida Department of Health and Rehabilitative Services, 1983; Michigan Health Department, 1988).

## Management Information Systems

Many state and local health departments have also developed MISs that focus on the management of the statistical and operational needs of the agency and the professionals. An example of a state/local health department MIS is B.E.S.T. (Barry-Eaton Software Technologies), which supports the environmental, financial and personal health activities and requirements for the Barry-Eaton Health Department, Charlotte, Michigan. This system captures a variety of professional activities focusing on patient and environmental health services. This MIS is run on a microcomputer using pull-down menus, on-line documentation, and a database management software package. This system is used to capture and query the databases, which represent a mix of computer modules and/or special subsystems (B.E.S.T., 1992).

## Personal/Client Management Systems

A personal/client management system is another type of system that provides the framework for collecting and reporting statistical and financial data needed for the management of personal/client health and programs (Michigan Health Department, 1988). The State of Michigan Personal Health: Nursing Information System (PH-NIS) is an example of such a system. It was designed to be a "road map" and not a "blueprint" for the overall management of the personal/client health program and to collect, organize, and standardize minimal statistical and financial information for the management and administration of the program activities.

This system contains two major types of data: (1) provider information and (2) client information. The provider information consists of a registry of all personnel regardless of position and/or title, including type, category, and program, e.g., staff nurse, full-time, immunization program. The personal/client health information includes demographics, patient history, and care activities.

Michigan is also a good example of a state and the local health departments using identical personal/client management systems to collect information on both the providers (personnel) and the people they serve. The state defines the minimum data that should be collected by each local health department in the state. However, the local health departments dictate and determine the data they collect. Each local agency not only has to obtain its own computer hardware (microcomputer) but also has to purchase the software from the state to implement the requirements identified in a paper-based manual.

The Michigan PH-NIS personal/client management system includes a conceptual framework to provide an overall guide for the system. It is a triangle which depicts three integrated management modules, (1) Personnel and Program Management, (2) Records Management, and (3) Financial Management, and a Report Generation Module; these are described below (see Fig. 12.2).

**Figure 12.2**   PH-NIS triangle. (Courtesy Michigan Department of Public Health, Nurse Administrator's Forum Data Committee.)

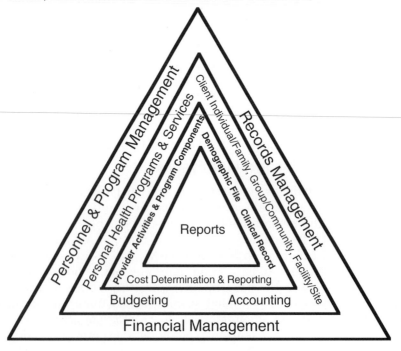

## Personal and Program Management Module

This module provides personal/client health and provider data which contribute to the delivery of an efficient and effective program as well as meet the goals of the local health department. The personal health program groupings relate to program components and provider activities.

## Records Management Module

This module documents, stores, and retrieves descriptive data about the persons/clients that are analyzed for program planning and evaluation. The client data refers to a demographic file and a clinical record in the system.

## Financial Management Module

This module is used for securing and disbursing the needed resources for the delivery of services. It also encompasses budgeting and accounting.

## Report Generation Module

The Report Generation Module allows for the retrieval of data collected using an organized format in order to provide information for internal and external reporting requirements. Reports can be structured to meet a specific purpose, provide timely data, or meet specific needs of the agency.

# SPECIAL-PURPOSE SYSTEMS

Special-purpose systems have been developed to collect statistical data not for administering the agency but for administering a specific program, regardless of what type of agency offers the program. Stand-alone systems are designed to collect and summarize management data on services in clinics, schools, and homes. These systems provide the statistics needed to obtain funds from federal, state, or local units for categorical programs and/or block grants. Programs dealing with family planning, infant immunizations, early periodic screening and testing (EPST), maternal and infant (MI), children and youth (C/Y), crippled children, tuberculosis, drug abuse, or HIV have statistical reporting requirements which can be derived from these systems.

Many other activities conducted in the field of CHN—health surveillance programs, screening clinics, immunization clinics, and special statistical studies designed to collect large databases—require special-purpose systems designed for them. The screening programs are used for early detection and prevention of diseases, epidemiological activities, and health promotion. Many such studies, programs, and projects, each of which required a computer system or application specifically designed to process the data, have been described in the literature.

The major types of computer systems developed for special programs, studies, and projects can be described as:

- Categorical program systems
- Special study systems
- Screening program systems
- Epidemiologic program systems
- School health systems

## Categorical Program Systems

Categorical program systems have been designed to support data processing and tracking for specific programs such as cancer detection, well infant clinic (WIC), maternal and child (MCH) immunization, or family planning. Other systems have been designed to collect uniform longitudinal data for a specific disease condition, such as the rheumatic diseases, which can be used as national databases. Categorical program systems generally count, track, and identify the health status of registered clients. For example, the WIC system is designed to process on-line certification and generate food vouchers. Such systems are used to prepare billing information as well as comprehensive statistical reports. They generate all data required for cost reporting and the preparation of any customized reports needed to meet a user's unique reporting requirements. An example of a computer screen from a cancer control program is illustrated in Fig. 12.3.

## Special Study Systems

Special study systems generally require a specially designed computer application. Studies that collect large volumes of data require standard statistical software programs and/or specially designed models for computer processing of these data. Generally large databases are collected for surveys, clinical trials, research studies, health policy, and other projects requiring volumes of data to resolve a problem. Many research studies analyze federal databases to develop outcomes measures. Other studies requiring special stand-alone systems are national surveys of nurses and/or CHN agencies.

One of the major obstacles in developing special study systems is that managing large databases is complex and creates time-consuming data entry tasks. The introduction of point-of-service on-line data entry terminals has replaced data collection forms, making special study systems easier to develop. With this approach, these systems can process the data in an ongoing mode, reducing the time required to process the study findings and generate reports.

Breast & Cervical Cancer Control Program
# Screening Form

Health Dept. ID └─┴─┘    Clinic ID └─┴─┘    Date of Birth └─┴─┘└─┴─┘└─┴─┘    Client Identification └─┴─┴─┴─┴─┴─┴─┴─┴─┴─┘
                                                        mo   day   yr

| Last Name | First Name | Middle Initial |
|---|---|---|

Provider Name

Type of File Maintenance Action:
1 ☐ First reporting of this screening
2 ☐ Additional data for previously reported screening
3 ☐ Delete this screening record

Which Title XV Screening Year? └─┴─┘
01 First screening by HD (Yr. 1)
02 Screening anniversary of Yr. 1 (Yr. 2)
03 Screening anniversary of Yr. 2 (Yr. 3)
etc. (NOTE: A woman may visit the HD many times for follow-up during any screening year, *but* year remains constant)

**CLINICAL BREAST EXAM:**

Date First Scheduled    Actual Date of Exam
Mo   Day   Yr           Mo   Day   Yr        Provider Notified?

___/___/___             ___/___/___          ☐ No ☐ Yes ☐ NA

Clinical Breast Exam Results: (Check all that apply)

| RIGHT | | LEFT |
|---|---|---|
| 1 ☐ | No mass present | 1 ☐ |
| 2 ☐ | Breast removed | 2 ☐ |
| 3 ☐ | Symmetrical thickening present | 3 ☐ |
| 4 ☐ | Asymmetrical thickening present | 4 ☐ |
| 5 ☐ | Smooth, mobile round/oval mass | 5 ☐ |
| 6 ☐ | Irregular, firm, mobile mass - indeterminate | 6 ☐ |
| 7 ☐ | Irregular, hard, fixed mass | 7 ☐ |
| 8 ☐ | Examination refused | 8 ☐ |
| 9 ☐ | Examination omitted | 9 ☐ |
| 10 ☐ | Other Abnormal Findings | 10 ☐ |
| | Specify _____ | |
| 11 ☐ | No change from previous exam | 11 ☐ |

Based on the Clinical Breast Exam, is Follow-up Required?    ☐ No    ☐ Yes (If yes, go to Breast Follow-up Form)

**Figure 12.3**  Cancer control program screen. (Courtesy Michigan Department of Public Health, Cancer Section.)

# Screening Program Systems

Screening programs are another type of program that requires a special-purpose computer application. Screening programs are used to detect individuals afflicted with a specific disease or predisposing health condition. Such programs generally use a computer system to collect important health information which may be mandated by federal, state, or local regulations. The computer system monitors and evaluates the results of screening tests. The data collected are transferred to a large computer facility and aggregated for program analysis. Such applications allow retrospective analysis of a large database to measure the effectiveness of the screening program. An example of a database is data for screening sickle-cell traits in the blood of children.

## Epidemiologic Program Systems

Epidemiologic program systems focus on the assessment of a population group with special health conditions. The results of such computerized assessments, such as audiovisual testing, immunization profiles, health appraisals, or dental checkups, assist in detecting health care needs. Computer applications can be customized for other epidemiological prevention programs. They can be used to conduct standardized interviews by telephone of clients who call a health care facility for assistance or information. These systems can summarize patient interviews, select care plans, and assess client problems. Other stand-alone systems include a computerized database of diabetic patients who are receiving educational services from health clinics in a specific city, such as New York. Such systems are also designed as clearinghouses for all clients enrolled in the specific program (McDonald, 1987).

Many of the newer epidemiological programs use on-line systems to collect the data that provide for early detection and prevention of diseases and for follow-up consultation services. Data on clients entered into the system at different times are used to detect high-risk individuals so that they can receive nursing care in a timely manner (Ohata, 1983).

## School Health Systems

School health systems are computerized school-based record systems designed to improve data collection and monitor and evaluate the health of students. The systems are essentially designed for school-setting clinics that not only monitor physiologic indices such as levels of fitness, e.g., blood pressure and obesity, but also track immunizations, health status, growth, and development of the students. The newer systems collect in-depth registration and encounter data. They run on a microcomputer, are menu-driven, and are used to generate statistics on school health services and facilitate follow-up of identified student health conditions.

The introduction of health care programs in schools is becoming increasingly important and provides an opportunity for collecting health-related data in schools on the student and employees in the school. These systems address the same problems as the computer-based patient record. However, they need to ensure the privacy and confidentiality of the student data before they will be implemented in all schools in the country (Basch et al., 1988).

# AMBULATORY CARE SYSTEMS

Ambulatory care is another setting where CHN is practiced. The computer systems that support ambulatory care programs vary depending on the type of ambulatory care program and setting. Ambulatory care programs are found in a variety of settings: noninstitutionalized agencies, clinics, or other affiliated units where patient services are provided. The major ones include HMOs, group practices, outpatient clinics, and freestanding community-based clinics.

Because of the wide diversity of these systems, there is an increasing need to integrate these ambulatory care systems with associated hospital departments and systems to form the computer-based patient record (CPR). However, there is no consensus on what the ambulatory patient record should contain. Ambulatory care records are generally described as containing poorly organized data and incomplete documentation. They are characterized as (1) lacking standardized content and/or format, (2) incomplete, (3) inaccurate, and (4) inaccessible. Ambulatory care systems provided in hospital-based, freestanding, and community-based clinics differ from the HMO systems (Grady and Schwartz, 1993).

## Computer-Stored Ambulatory Record System

The earliest and still the most widely used ambulatory care system is the computer-stored ambulatory record system (COSTAR). It was implemented in 1968 at Harvard Community Health Plan (HCHP). This system is used in various ambulatory care settings, including HMOs and clinical and community health settings. The system is modular and is available commercially. As a comprehensive system that documents the entire patient record, including nursing care, COSTAR is an integrated system designed to address the medical, administrative, financial, billing, and other needs of diverse ambulatory care agencies (Barnett, 1976; Saba, 1982, 1983).

COSTAR contains five functionally independent but interrelated modules based on sets of terms, words, or phrases for documenting all possible activities. A directory contains the system vocabulary, organized into coded categories for the entire system. The major categories include administrative items, diagnostic terms, medical procedures, laboratory tests, medications, therapies, and accounting terms. COSTAR is written in MUMPS, which includes a medical query language to allow users without programming knowledge to interact and search the structured database. This language uses a hierarchical database system to allow for dynamic storage. COSTAR can run on any size computer.

## Indian Health System

The Indian Health Service offers a unique example of an ambulatory care clinical information system. The original patient care information system (PCIS) was initiated in 1968 and served the Alaska natives and the Papago

Indian Reservation in Tucson, Arizona. The PCIS has evolved and continues to advance as the technology and services change. It is an on-line system located in all IHS or tribal health facilities, which are linked to each other, to the area offices, and to a main central computer facility. The major purpose of the system is to integrate patient care and cost data in a system that collects and stores a core set of health and management data. All disciplines and facilities are included. It is used to promote comprehensive care by addressing all known health problems and preventive health needs of eligible patients (Brown et al., 1971; Grady and Schwartz, 1993; Indian Health Services, 1990; Saba, 1982, 1983).

Currently, the system collects a wide range of encounter data from all settings where IHS or tribal services are provided, namely, inpatient, outpatient, and field visits. It is designed to support health care delivery, planning, management, and research for this population group. A Patient Care Component (PCC) of the IHS Resource and Patient Management System contains data on all patient health problems and preventive health needs. It is used to plan visits, aggregate data, provide system information, and conduct research. Community health nurses also enter encounter data for clients seen in the home, clinic, school, or hospital. The PCC system integrates data from a common set of files and incorporates all patient data and health information from multiple facilities into the database at each site where the patient has an active patient record. The system provides summary reports of all health care encounters at all reservation health care facilities.

## Clinical Information Systems

Some of the newer ambulatory care systems have developed clinical information systems with decision support applications that are used to monitor and track patient/client data. Generally all patient data are kept on-line regardless of where the patient in seen (office, laboratory, x-ray department) and by whom (physician, nurse, therapist). Patient data are compared with the decision support applications designed to evaluate the data. Other automated ambulatory medical record systems (AAMRS) include selected hospital data. For example, THERESA, an AAMRS at Grady Memorial Hospital, the teaching hospital for Emory Memorial Medical Center, Atlanta, Georgia, shares hospital data. It uses local area network technology to share common attributes, which include (1) data dictionaries, (2) data collected over time, (3) data retrieval, (4) selective storage of data, and (5) data security.

### Occupational Health Systems

Clinical information systems are also found in occupational settings. Occupational health systems generally provide emergency services, referring the acute care conditions to other health care facilities and providers.

Occupational health systems collect data on employee physical examinations, immunizations, and health promotion and disease prevention services. These systems are generally used to monitor and track five major areas related to occupational health: (1) employee health, (2) workplace conditions, (3) environmental agents, (4) preventive measures, and (5) regulatory, administrative, and action items. The employee health information refers to all health care data on the employee, including clinic visits and occupational injuries and/or illnesses. Information on workplace conditions refers to industrial hygiene data; information on environmental agents refers to toxicological and material safety; and information on preventive measures refers to those measures used to protect employee health and safety. The last type of information being monitored focuses on the OSHA (Occupational Safety and Health Agency) regulatory standards and action levels, as well as tracking ongoing problems and events that need follow-up and/or actions (Whyte, 1982).

## Group Practice Systems

Several of the newer ambulatory care systems support group practices in hospitals, outpatient clinics, or other clinic settings where nurse practitioners provide services. Such systems are stand-alone systems which contain broad clinical and administrative databases. They are designed to utilize all departments in the hospital for diagnostic data, which are integrated into the system. Many other hospitals have expanded their hospital information systems to encompass services provided in the ambulatory units. Generally, they are structured similarly to the hospital system but are different. Hospital systems have to capture continuous services, whereas in ambulatory care, services are episodic. Thus the systems collect data that highlight the episodes and encounters over time.

In such systems there is a common registry of patients. Terminals are usually located in every practitioner's office and examination room. This configuration allows for the acquisition of information at the point of care, making the data available on-line to all users of the system regardless of location (Grady and Schwartz, 1993).

## Health Maintenance Organization Systems

HMOs deliver comprehensive, coordinated, prepaid health care services to voluntarily enrolled members. Some HMOs also offer home care services, and many HMOs also offer preventive health care and community health nursing services. HMOs emerged as a result of legislation—HMO Act of 1973 (PL 93-222)—that promoted their development. They are increasing at an accelerated rate primarily because the focus of reform is to encourage integrated, coordinated health care services like those HMOs provide.

## HMO Systems in General

HMOs have developed different ambulatory care systems that support key features critical to the HMO. Many of the early ambulatory care computerized information systems were developed for HMOs. They were primarily designed to support the patient record systems and handle health care services and financial and administrative needs.

Integrated HMO systems process data for creating summary CPRs. They process all activities provided by the auxiliary departments such as pharmacy, laboratory, and radiology. Generally, the data are coded and defined in a time-oriented data dictionary and a system that integrates problem lists, inpatient and outpatient records, charges, visits, and all services provided to the patient. Additionally, data collected by nurses are captured by computer at the point of service. On-line queries and data retrieval are handled using a query language, and specific data for quality assurance are included. Other HMO systems provide administrative support, handling appointments, scheduling, and charge capture. And still others are used to support research and studies of effectiveness. HMOs such as the Group Health Cooperative of Puget Sound in Seattle or Kaiser Permanente have pieces of an automated medical record system.

## Community Health Plan System

One of the most sophisticated HMO systems is that of the Harvard Community Health Plan (HCHP) in Boston, Massachusetts. It consists of a health database designed to allow clients to ask a question about a specific condition and receive guidance for resolving the problem through a series of user-friendly pathways. The database uses a decision tree expert system developed by health professionals based on their practice protocols to support the client queries. A pilot project is being conducted by HCHP in order to demonstrate what can be done with direct communication linkages from the home to health care providers. Terminals have been placed in the homes of heavy users in Burlington, Massachusetts, such as families with young children, pregnant women, and the elderly in a neighboring small town. The system performs a triage of actions: (1) download hospital record to a home database; (2) answer client questions using expert system logic; and (3) provide information on self-care to assist the client to resolve the problem. The demonstration appears to have increased client satisfaction and reduce emergency room visits and "worried well" calls to physician offices. It is expected to reduce cost, improve efficiency, and improve productivity of the clinicians (Little, 1992).

## Managed Care Systems

Managed care systems emerged in the 1980s as bundled services offered by managed care organizations. Managed care systems are systems designed to monitor quality patient care, but at the same time reduce care costs. They are designed to provide a full range of health services for those requiring health care services and are characterized by several different combinations of service offerings.

With the introduction of managed care organizations, HHAs had to adjust their traditional billing systems from fee for service to calculating comprehensive health services regardless of cost. These new systems price home visits using different criteria such as patient account, procedure code or category, or payer source or plan, or based on a per diem, per case, or per capita calculation (Dodd and Coleman, 1994; Hansel, 1994).

Managed care systems are used to process resources dollars, clinical care activities, care plans, critical pathways, and outcome data. They are used to manage not only the low-volume, high-cost cases but also the large-volume, low-cost cases more efficiently and effectively. As a result, a new approach to computerizing home health care has emerged.

## HOME HEALTH SYSTEMS

Home health systems are information systems designed to support home health nursing, also called care of the sick at home. Home health systems support home care and hospice programs provided by HHAs such as VNAs, hospital-based programs, proprietary agencies, and other not-for-profit HHAs. They emerged with the enactment of the Medicare/Medicaid legislation, primarily as billing and financial systems. These systems have traditionally focused on processing billing for services provided and financial information to improve cash flow, hold down costs, and address the regulatory needs of HHAs.

Home health systems to date have been primarily designed to collect and process data in order to prepare the documents required by HCFA and third-party payers for payment for home care services. Financial, managerial, and clinical applications are used to provide efficient management of an HHA. Others offer applications which focus on scheduling, cost statistics, patient census, utilization reports, visit tracking, accounting reports, and discharge summaries. Additionally, the newer systems include applications that support patient care management and CPR systems. A recent survey of 27 home health vendors that offer HHA computer applications showed that they primarily provide financial applications, such as billing and accounts reconciliation. However, other vendors offer clinical applications such as treatment plans, patient charting, visit notes, physicians' orders, medications, test results, and/or critical pathways (Rollins, 1994).

The systems to be discussed include

- Financial and billing systems
- Scheduling systems
- Patient care management systems
- CPR systems

## Financial and Billing Systems

Financial and billing systems are found mainly in VNAs and other agencies that administer home care services. They are home health nursing information systems that were developed by commercial vendors and service bureaus. They are primarily designed to furnish information essential for reimbursement of services provided to patients eligible for Medicare, Medicaid, and other third-party payers. These systems use a variety of input forms or data entry screens—admission data, assessment data, and plan of treatment data—to collect the required information. The data are needed to obtain approval for a patient to receive reimbursable services, as well as to obtain payment for visits and services provided by all types of providers for an episode of care.

Financial and billing systems primarily prepare or provide the specific information needed for billing of services for federal and/or third-party payers. They generally include the applications listed below and an example of a vendor-advertised applications is shown in Fig. 12.4.

- General ledger
- Accounts receivable
- Accounts payable
- Billing
- Reimbursement management
- Cash management

Additionally, they generate financial reports such as

- Costs per visit
- Personnel costs
- Payroll information
- Budget projections
- Patient census
- Patient daily visits
- Patients services
- Patient supply lists

### Medicare Payment Systems

Billing and financial systems have been developed specifically for certified HHAs that provide Medicare and Medicaid program services. The systems have changed as the Medicare program payment requirements have changed. In the late 1960s, the initial Medicare program required that a Medicare Eligible Request for Payment be completed to justify care. At that time, the goal of many large HHAs was to have these new forms completed by computer in order to bring about a faster cash flow, produce detailed patient accounts receivable, and capture statistical data to meet other reporting needs (Health Care Financing Administration, 1980).

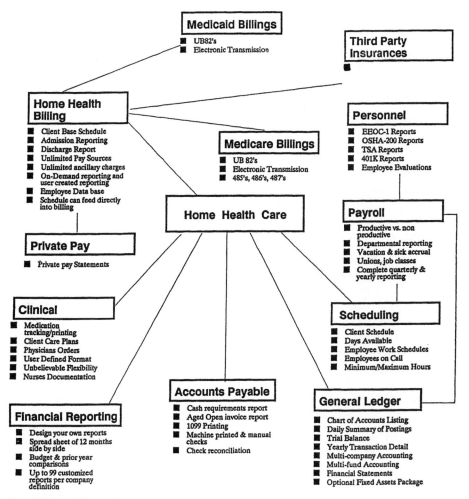

**Figure 12.4**  Home health applications. (Courtesy Advanced Information Management, Inc., Neenah, WI.)

In 1985, HCFA mandated a more comprehensive and complex method for certifying Medicare eligibility of patients, billing and payment for services, and determining the costs of care. HCFA initiated several forms for the Medicare program: HCFA Form 485, Plan of Treatment, to be completed by a physician; HCFA Form 486, Medical Update, to be completed by a nurse or therapist; and HCFA Form 487, Addendum, HCFA UB-92, Claims Form, and HCFA Form 1728, Cost Reporting (see Figs. 12.5 and 12.6.)

These forms, which are updated periodically, are required in order to collect data for Medicare claims and for third-party payers. The forms,

## HOME HEALTH CERTIFICATION AND PLAN OF TREATMENT

| 1. Patient's HI Claim No. | 2. SOC Date | 3. Certification Period | | 4. Medical Record No. | 5. Provider No. |
|---|---|---|---|---|---|
| | | From: | To: | | |

| 6. Patient's Name and Address | 7. Provider's Name and Address. |
|---|---|

| 8. Date of Birth: | 9. Sex ☐ M ☐ F | 10. Medications: Dose/Frequency/Route (N)ew (C)hanged |
|---|---|---|

| 11. ICD-9-CM | Principal Diagnosis | Date |
|---|---|---|

| 12. ICD-9-CM | Surgical Procedure | Date |
|---|---|---|

| 13. ICD-9-CM | Other Pertinent Diagnoses | Date |
|---|---|---|

| 14. DME and Supplies | 15. Safety Measures: |
|---|---|

| 16. Nutritional Req. | 17. Allergies: |
|---|---|

**18.A. Functional Limitations**

| 1 ☐ Amputation | 5 ☐ Paralysis | 9 ☐ Legally Blind |
| 2 ☐ Bowel/Bladder (Incontinence) | 6 ☐ Endurance | A ☐ Dyspnea With Minimal Exertion |
| 3 ☐ Contracture | 7 ☐ Ambulation | B ☐ Other (Specify) |
| 4 ☐ Hearing | 8 ☐ Speech | |

**18.B. Activities Permitted**

| 1 ☐ Complete Bedrest | 6 ☐ Partial Weight Bearing | A ☐ Wheelchair |
| 2 ☐ Bedrest BRP | 7 ☐ Independent At Home | B ☐ Walker |
| 3 ☐ Up As Tolerated | 8 ☐ Crutches | C ☐ No Restrictions |
| 4 ☐ Transfer Bed/Chair | 9 ☐ Cane | D ☐ Other (Specify) |
| 5 ☐ Exercises Prescribed | | |

**19. Mental Status:**

| 1 ☐ Oriented | 3 ☐ Forgetful | 5 ☐ Disoriented | 7 ☐ Agitated |
| 2 ☐ Comatose | 4 ☐ Depressed | 6 ☐ Lethargic | 8 ☐ Other |

**20. Prognosis:**

| 1 ☐ Poor | 2 ☐ Guarded | 3 ☐ Fair | 4 ☐ Good | 5 ☐ Excellent |

21. Orders for Discipline and Treatments (Specify Amount/Frequency/Duration)

22. Goals/Rehabilitation Potential/Discharge Plans

23. Verbal Start of Care and Nurse's Signature and Date Where Applicable:

| 24. Physician's Name and Address | 25. Date HHA Received Signed POT | 26. I ☐ certify ☐ recertify that the above home health services are required and are authorized by me with a written plan for treatment which will be periodically reviewed by me. This patient is under my care, is confined to his home, and is in need of intermittent skilled nursing care and/or physical or speech therapy or has been furnished home health services based on such a need and no longer has a need for such care or therapy, but continues to need occupational therapy. |
|---|---|---|
| 27. Attending Physician's Signature (Required on 485 Kept of File in Medical Records of HHA) | *Date Signed* | |

FORM HCFA-485 (C4) (4-87)

PROVIDER

**Figure 12.5** Health Care Financing Administraiton (HCFA) Form 485.

## MEDICAL UPDATE AND PATIENT INFORMATION

| 1. Patient's HI Claim No. | 2. SOC Date | 3. Certification Period | | 4. Medical Record No. | 5. Provider No. |
|---|---|---|---|---|---|
| | | From: | To: | | |

| 6. Patient's Name | 7. Provider's Name |
|---|---|
| | |

8. Medicare Covered: ☐ Y ☐ N | 9. Date Physician Last Saw Patient: | 10. Date Last Contacted Physician:

11. Is the Patient Receiving Care in an 1861 (J)(1) Skilled Nursing Facility or Equivalent? ☐ Y ☐ N ☐ Do Not Know | 12. ☐ Certification ☐ Recertification ☐ Modified

13. Specific Services and Treatments

| Discipline | Visits (This Bill) Rel. to Prior Cert. | Frequency and Duration | Treatment Codes | Total Visits Projected This Cert. |
|---|---|---|---|---|
| | | | | |
| | | | | |
| | | | | |
| | | | | |

14. Dates of Last Inpatient Stay: Admission ___ Discharge ___ | 15. Type of Facility: ___

16. Updated Information: New Orders/Treatments/Clinical Facts/Summary from Each Discipline

17. Functional Limitations (Expand From 485 and Level of ADL) Reason Homebound/Prior Functional Status

18. Supplementary Plan of Treatment on File from Physician Other than Referring Physician:
(If Yes, Please Specify Giving Goals/Rehab. Potential/Discharge Plan) ☐ Y ☐ N

19. Unusual Home/Social Environment

| 20. Indicate Any Time When the Home Health Agency Made a Visit and Patient was Not Home and Reason Why if Ascertainable | 21. Specify Any Known Medical and/or Non-Medical Reasons the Patient Regularly Leaves Home and Frequency of Occurrence |
|---|---|
| | |

| 22. Nurse or Therapist Completing or Reviewing Form | Date (Mo., Day, Yr.) |
|---|---|
| | |

Form HCFA-486 (C3) (4-87)  **PROVIDER**

**Figure 12.6**  Health Care Financing Administration (HCFA) Form 486.

once completed, are used by an HHA to obtain the certification that the patient is eligible to receive reimbursable home visits for a period of 60 days. The HCFA forms provide the basis for the HHA billing and financial computer systems. They are used to collect a variety of variables, including medical diagnoses, functional limitations, goals of care, and activities permitted. They also collect data on allowable services offered by the six types of providers—professional nurses, physical therapists, occupational therapists, speech therapists, medical social workers, and home health aides. HCFA provides reimbursement for a predetermined list of thirty nursing treatments, which are variables included in the systems (Fig. 12.7).

### Electronic Data Interchange
At this time several states have implemented laws or instituted new programs that focus on cutting administrative health care costs by using electronic data interchange (EDI) to transmit Medicare/Medicaid claims data. New York led the way, followed by Arizona, by passing a law mandating that health care providers use EDI. Iowa passed legislation for the development of a community health management information system (CHMIS) to transmit not only claims data but also clinical health care transactions data. Iowa is proposing open health information networks. Several other states involved in health care reform are also requiring the use of EDI for transmission of Medicare/Medicaid claims data (Goedert, 1994).

## Computer Systems Options

The majority of home health nursing information systems have been developed by commercial vendors, service bureaus, or computer companies. Commercial organizations contract with HHAs to handle their billing and financial record keeping. Having an outside company assume the development costs makes it possible for HHAs to reduce their administrative costs and improve the efficiency of reimbursement without having to develop or purchase their own system. With the advancement of technology, commercial companies now offer different computer configurations to enhance the capabilities of their systems. They market their home health systems as (1) timesharing systems with on-line, real-time, and/or batch processing options, (2) stand-alone/turnkey systems, or (3) some combination of the above.

### Timesharing Systems
Timesharing systems are computer-based systems developed by service bureaus which are shared by many HHAs. The service bureau purchases a mainframe computer (hardware) large enough to be shared by many HHAs, determines the hardware architecture, and develops its own proprietary computer programs (software) to process the HHA data. The service

TREATMENT CODES FOR PROFESSIONAL SERVICES REQUIRED:
SKILLED NURSING

A1    Skilled Observation and Assessment (Include Vital Signs, Response to Medications, Etc.

A2    Foley Insertion

A3    Bladder Instillation

A4    Open Wound Care/Dressing

A5    Decubitus Care (Partial tissue with signs of infection or full tissue loss etc.)

A6    Venipuncture

A7    Restorative Nursing

A8    Post Cataract Care

A9    Bowel/Bladder Training

A10   Chest Physio (Include Postural drainage)

A11   Administer Vitamin B/12

A12   Administration of Insulin

A13   Administer Other IM/Subcutaneous Injection

A14   Administer IV's/Clysis

A15   Teach Ostomy or Ileal Conduit Care

A16   Teach Nasogastric Feeding

A17   Reinsertion Nasogastric Feeding Tube

A18   Teach Gastrostomy Feeding

A19   Teach Parenteral Nutrition

A20   Teach Care of Tracheostomy

A21   Administer Care of Tracheostomy

A22   Teach Inhalation Therapy

A23   Administer Inhalation RX

A24   Teach Administration of Injection

A25   Teach Diabetic Care

A26   Disimpaction/FU Enema

A27   Other (Specify under Orders)

A28   Wound Care/Dressing - Closed Incision/Suture Line

A29   Decubitus Care (Other than A5)

A30   Teach Care of Indwelling Catheter

A31   Management and Evaluation of Patient Care Plan

A32   Teaching and Training (Specify under Orders)

**Figure 12.7**   List of Health Care Financing Administration (HCFA) approved nursing treatments.

bureau designs the data collection forms or methods for collecting data, determines the data needed for billing and financial record keeping, and develops the required reports. The bureau also develops user's manuals, provides training sessions, and supports any other technological needs for the users.

***On-Line Option*** An on-line option is a timesharing system that is offered on-line to the HHAs. The system uses an on-line communication network to link the central computer system, located in the service bureau facility, to the HHAs in other locations. Data are transmitted on-line via telephone using a computer terminal or microcomputer with a modem. In an on-line system the HHA transmits and receives data to and from the service bureau, but cannot review, manipulate, or process the data. In this type of system, the service bureau receives HHAs' data, processes the data at its own convenience at its central facility, and when completed transmits the billing and financial information on-line or forwards it in a paper format back to the HHA.

***Real-Time Option*** With the real-time option, the HHA not only transmits data on-line to the central computer, but also has direct access to and can interact in real time with the central computer's central processing unit (CPU). The data are not only transmitted on-line by a user at the remote site as the events occur but also are processed instantly in real time. With this option, the user can query, review, update the data, as well as design and generate individualized reports.

The on-line real-time option allows the user to enter visit data as they occur. The user in the HHA can review the data and make changes and adjustments as needed to assure the accuracy of billing and financial reporting. In this type of system the HHA has the computing power of the central computer while incurring the low cost of an on-line terminal.

***Batch Processing Option*** Batch processing is an option for off-line and on-line transmission of data from one site to another. In off-line transmission, paper-based data collection forms are made into batches and forwarded to the service bureau. However, in on-line batch transmission, the HHA user keys the data from paper-based or computer input forms into the computer terminal and then transmits the data set on-line in batches at a specified time, e.g., at night or on weekends.

Increasingly, HHAs are using microcomputers with fixed menus to collect, store, and batch data, then transmitting the batches on-line to the service bureau's central computer. In this instance, the agency only collects data and enters them into a computer system and does not have real-time access to patient information stored in the patient's database. On the other hand, the HHA does not have to edit the forms or enter the data into the system's database.

## Timesharing Advantages and Disadvantages

*Advantages*   The major advantage of timesharing systems is the low cost. HHAs do not have to invest in the purchase of hardware and the development of software. The service bureau generally provides all data processing needed for billing, payroll, scheduling, planning, caseload allocation, human resource management, and productivity improvement. Specifically, timesharing systems offer

- Increased billings and collections
- Greater provider productivity
- Improved efficiency of services
- Improved management of human resources
- Efficient scheduling of personnel
- Simplified payroll
- Reduced paperwork
- Improved quality of care
- Reduced costs

The service bureau is responsible for processing data, preparing patients' bills, and producing financial, statistical, and other reports for the agency. However, if a microcomputer is installed in the HHA for transmitting data on-line, then the HHA can use the microcomputer for other purposes, such as word processing.

*Disadvantages*   The major disadvantage of timesharing systems is the ownership of the data. In principle, the HHA owns the data; however, since the data are transmitted via telephone lines and are physically housed at the service bureau's facility, the responsibility for the safety and protection of the data rests with that organization. This leads to several issues which need to be considered when selecting a system, such as the following:

- What happens to the data if the company closes?
- Where are the backup files stored?
- How are discharged patients' data accessed?
- Can trend and retrospective data be generated as needed, regardless of time sequence?

## Stand-Alone Systems

Stand-alone systems (turnkey systems) are commercial systems developed for direct installation and implementation in an HHA. The HHA buys the computer system as configured by the commercial developer (hardware and software) and uses it to collect, store, process, and control its own patient and visit data. The commercial developer (vendor) provides the HHA with all the necessary equipment: the hardware (a mainframe, minicomputer, or microcomputer and any other required peripheral equipment) and software (computer programs) needed to run the system, including all forms and standardized reports used by that specific agency.

With this type of system, the commercial vendor generally maintains, updates, and supports all software programs and ensures that the software programs meet state and federal regulations. The vendor generally offers training courses on how to run the system to the HHAs. The major advantage of this option is that the agency owns its own equipment (hardware), system (software), and patient data (databases). The agency can utilize the computer system for other applications.

## Computer Network System Configurations

As a means of sharing data and communicating among users, both local area networks (LANs) and wide area networks (WANs) have been introduced. Network configurations are being introduced to efficiently utilize the latest technology as well as reduce costs. LANs are being used to link units within the HHA and remote units outside the HHAs, whereas WANs are being used to share data among agencies to establish continuity of care services across settings.

### Local Area Networks (LANs)

LANs are used to link units within an HHA and to link subunits with one another and with a central office. Many large community health agencies are using LANs to link and integrate their service units. LANs allow the HHAs to share hardware and software for their individual computer systems and also use the network to communicate with each other.

Several of these agencies have initiated LANs to link local units online with each other and their headquarters. Many large agencies have their own computer department which is responsible for integrating all the components of a network, providing support services, and generating reports and other products. It builds and coordinates the data communication network; assists in the selection, procurement and installation of appropriate equipment, initiates training of the staffs; and provides maintenance and upgrading of software and hardware for the local units.

Many agencies have linked their local units by using a dedicated LAN network linked to a central mainframe computer system. Others have developed agency-wide MISs to collect and process information from local units (Bilodeau, 1994; Custom Data Processing, 1992; Saba, 1982).

### Wide Area Networks

WANs are being implemented by state/local health departments and/or community health agencies that have their own statewide computer systems. In these instances large satellite agencies and those located in remote areas may also have a mainframe computer. In such situations, the mainframe systems are linked together so that they can share files with the other computers in the WAN. This configuration is established so that all users regardless of location can access and share data located in all computers as needed.

WANs are also used to communicate and transmit data across settings, that is, to communicate and transmit data from one system in one institution to another system in another community agency or another HHA. In this instance the WAN requires standardized data formats so that data can be communicated across settings using different brands of computers. Other WANs use dedicated communication lines to link the units in a large geographic area together. However, in the future all health agencies within communities will be networked, the information superhighway and/or the national information infrastructure (NII) will be used to link agencies across the country, and even clients will be networked to the health care facilities and to all health care providers in the community. (See the discussion of the NII in Chap. 6.)

### Laptop/Notebook Systems

The laptop/notebook systems are being designed to collect and transmit patient data as well as send and receive messages to and from the agency's main computer. Many architectural designs using this new technology are being developed to enable nurses to chart visit details, patient care services, and clinical assessment information collected at points of service such as the patient's home and downloaded them to the HHAs at a convenient time. They are portable computers which operate in a user-friendly format. The care provider can query, collect, and retrieve data from the computer system. Laptop/notebook systems generally use menu-driven software that prompt users through every step.

## Scheduling Systems

Scheduling systems are also being used to enhance home health systems. They are designed to coordinate the schedules of patients requiring visits and care givers providing services. Some systems use graphical scheduling calendars, and others provide road maps on how to travel to a location in the shortest distance. These systems can also track personnel by scheduling on- and off-duty time and generating the payroll. Since these systems are interactive, schedules can be adjusted daily and on-line as needed. They generally simplify schedules, reduce schedule conflicts, improve financial control, enhance productivity, and reduce administrative costs, as well as decrease travel time (Fig. 12.8).

## Patient Care Management Systems

Patient care management systems are generally extensions of the billing and financial systems designed for HHAs. They primarily expand patient billing and financial data to include patient care services. They focus on

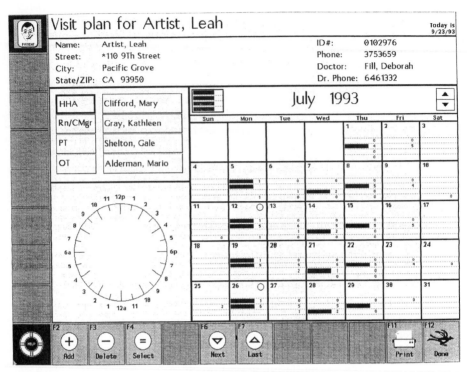

**Figure 12.8**   Home visit schedule calendar. (Courtesy Road Runner Technologies, Inc., Pleasanton, CA.)

patient/nurse encounters and episodes of care. Many of the newer systems collect information needed to document the patient care process. Such systems generally contain a patient database that includes demographic information, health history, initial nursing assessment, and patient care services information. They document and track ongoing patient care data. An example of an HHA assessment form is the innovative assessment tool that uses the 20 components of home health care developed by Saba.

In many situations the patient care systems attempt to emulate those used in hospitals. These systems include patient profiles, medical orders, care surveillance, problem lists, medication profiles, time-oriented flow-charts, care plans, care maps, patient visit reports, and treatment plans. The administrative advantages of patient care systems are many. They provide not only patient care information but also information on patient and employee satisfaction, referral sources, quality assurance, and management.

Critical pathways provide a new approach to documentation in the home care setting. The critical pathway has been defined as a diagram of the sequence of events leading to a desired outcome (Goodwin, 1992). They differ from the traditional care planning process by outlining a systematic

# NURSING CRITICAL PATHWAY FOR INSULIN DEPENDENT DIABETES MELLITUS

☐ Type I
☐ Type II

Patient's Name _____ FIRST _____ LIST _____ Pt. No. _____ Date Initiated _____

| NO. | PROBLEM LIST | WEEK 1 | WEEK 2 | WEEK 3 | WEEK 4 | WEEK 5 |
|-----|-----|-----|-----|-----|-----|-----|
| | Knowledge Deficit Re: Self-Care | | SPECIAL INSTRUCTIONS | | | |
| CONSULTS/ COORDINATION OF CARE | | Assess need for HHA, MSW, Rehab., Vol. Referrals completed as needed. | | Interdisciplinary coordination/ communication. | | |
| | | I ___ R | | R | | R |
| SKILLED EVALUATION/ TREATMENT | | Admission assessment. Assess peripheral circulation. Assess s/sx hypo/hyperglycemia. Assess diabetes complications. Glucometer testing. | | | | Blood glucose stable. No s/sx acute episode. |
| | | | | | R | |
| MEDICATION | Evaluate | Evaluate medication regime and response. Assess insulin administration skills. | | | | No medication changes within last 2 weeks. No untoward S/E's. |
| | | | | | | R |
| | | | | | | Patient/caregiver independent in medication regime. |
| | Instruct | Instruct in medication name, dose, schedule, purpose, action. Instruct in preparation and administration of insulin. Instruct in site rotation, storage of insulin and disposal of equipment. | Patient/caregiver verbalize medication name, dose, schedule, purpose. Patient/ caregiver demonstrate correct administration, site rotation, storage of insulin and equipment disposal. | Patient/caregiver verbalize action time of medication. | Continue to evaluate knowledge and teaching needs. | |
| | | I ___ | R | R | | R |
| DIET/ NUTRITION | Evaluate | Assess diet understanding and compliance. | | | | Patient follows prescribed diet. |
| | | | | | | R |
| | Instruct | Begin instruction in prescribed diet and/or food exchange system. | Instruct in meal planning. | Patient begins to follow prescribed diet. Continue instruction. | Continue to evaluate knowledge and teaching needs. | |
| | | I ___ | I | R | | |

Codes: I = Initiated   R = Resolved

©VNANV 710p1 (9/94)

DISTRIBUTION: ORIGINAL — Travel File.   YELLOW — Master File.
PINK — Home (Optional).

**Figure 12.9** Critical pathway chart. (Courtesy Visiting Nurse Association of Northern Virginia, Inc.)

# NURSING CRITICAL PATHWAY FOR INSULIN DEPENDENT DIABETES MELLITUS

Patient's Name _____ LAST ___ FIRST     Pt. No. _____     Date Initiated _____

| ACTIVITY | | WEEK 1 | WEEK 2 | WEEK 3 | WEEK 4 | WEEK 5 |
|---|---|---|---|---|---|---|
| | Evaluate | Assess level of activity. | | | Assess effects of exercise on BG levels. | |
| | Instruct | | Instruct in benefits of exercise on BG control. Instruct in interaction of activity, diet and insulin. Instruct in appropriate adjustments of each. | Instruct in safe exercise regimen. | Patient implements exercise safely. | Patient verbalizes understanding of interaction of diet, medication and exercises. Patient verbalizes benefits of exercise. |
| | | | R | | R | R |
| SYMPTOM MANAGEMENT | | Instruct in s/sx of hypoglycemia. Instruct in blood glucose testing. For Type I DM: Instruct in urine testing for ketones. | Patient/caregiver identify s/sx of hypoglycemia, means to prevent and action to take. Patient/caregiver demonstrate blood glucose monitoring and understand when to notify MD. Instruct in s/sx of hyperglycemia. Instruct in disease process and BG control goals. | Patient/caregiver identify s/sx of hyperglycemia, means to prevent and action to take. Instruct in foot/skin care. Instruct in sick day care. | Patient/caregiver demonstrate foot/skin care. Patient/caregiver verbalize understanding of sick day care. Instruct in chronic complications and prevention. | Patient/caregiver verbalize s/sx requiring medical attention. Patient/caregiver verbalize importance of dietary and exercise consistency. |
| | | I | I R | I R | I R | R |
| | | | | | | |
| | | | | | | |
| PSYCHOSOCIAL/ DISCHARGE PLANNING | | Discuss care plan, goals and discharge plans with patient/caregiver. Assess support systems. | Assess adjustment of diagnosis and treatment regimen. Patient ventilates feelings. | Instruct in need for routine medical, dental, and opthalmologic exams. Instruct in need for diabetic ID. Reinforce positive results of good DM management. | Preparation for discharge. | Patient has follow-up medical appointment. Patient has diabetic ID ordered. Patient has references for continuing education. |
| | | I | I R | I | I R | R |

Date Resolved/Initials

Codes:
I = Initiated
R = Resolved

Initials/Staff Signature and Title:

___ ___ / /

___ ___ / /

___ ___ / /

©VNANV 7/0p2 (9/94)

DISTRIBUTION: ORIGINAL — Travel File.   YELLOW — Master File.   PINK — Home (Optional).

**Figure 12.9** *Continued*

plan for interventions and teaching by diagnostic categories. An example of a critical pathway is shown in Fig. 12.9. It illustrates the pathway and provides a clear definition of patient outcomes and the time frame to meet the outcomes.

The newer systems are being configured using newer technology, such as on-line, interactive (real-time) systems using LANs to communicate and interact between users and patients' databases. Patient care systems are used by all members of the health care team to assist in delivery of patient care. They are used by (1) policy makers to assist in planning and evaluating community health status, (2) administrators to assist in establishing more efficient and effective management practices, (3) staff nurses in managing and auditing patient care, and (4) patients themselves to help understand their care. They can measure and evaluate the quality of patient care and improve and standardize the documentation of community health nursing. They document the continuity of patient care in and out of institutions and the use of health care resources. The totality of care is reflected by tracking the patient throughout the care system. Patient care information systems provide the basis for planning, administering, delivering, and evaluating patient care.

### Patient Care Management Prototype

The Information System Model developed by the Omaha VNA is a prototype patient care management system designed for administering and documenting care to clients. It contains four basic types of information: (1) client management, (2) service management, (3) personnel management, and (4) fiscal management. These four types of data provide the framework for different modules for the databases. One module is client-centered, and the remaining modules are business-centered. The client-centered module can be used to generate both patient and visit statistics as well as billing and payroll information. This module is used to collect and analyze community health nursing problems in relation to outcome criteria for the assessment of patient care. The patient data include patient/family characteristics, narrative assessment database, a list of the patient's health care problems, expected outcomes for the problems, and patient care plans or progress notes (Martin and Sheet, 1992; Saba, 1982, 1983; Simmons, 1984).

## Computer-Based Patient Record Systems

The next generation of patient care systems will be the computer-based patient record systems (CPRSs). CPRSs are envisioned as harnessing the capabilities of the computer to improve the quality and efficiency of patient care (Fig. 12.10). More complete and accurate patient information will be available across time and place for all providers. However, there is no agreement on what it should encompass and how it should be organized. The need for the CPR was identified and proposed by the Institute

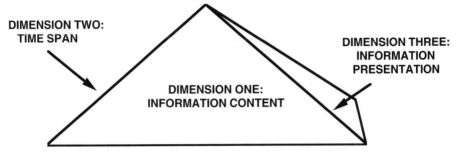

**Figure 12.10**   An example of a computer-based patient record model.

of Medicine (IOM). The IOM recommended that an organization be developed to orchestrate the development and implementation of the CPR in the health care industry (Dick and Steen, 1991).

As a result, in 1991, the Computer-Based Patient Record Institute (CPRI) was established to initiate and coordinate the activities that were urgently needed to facilitate and promote the routine use of CPRs. The CPRI defined the CPR as "an electronic patient record that resides in a system specifically designed to support users through the availability of complete and accurate data, practitioner reminders and alerts, clinical decision support systems, links to bodies of medical knowledge and other aids" (Dick and Steen, 1991, p. 167). A national information infrastructure is being developed for health and health care which is centered around the CPR (Computer-Based Patient Record Institute, 1992).

The CPRI initiated five work groups to work on CPR activities. The Codes and Structures Work Group divided its activities between two subcommittees: (1) Structures Concept Model, and (2) Codes. The Structures Concept Model subcommittee defined the CPR as "a collection of health information concerning one patient linked by a universal patient identifier." It further described the CPRS as the functions and characteristics that support the CPR, namely three dimensions: (1) information content, (2) time, and (3) information representation. The Codes subcommittee is involved with the development and use of CPR messages, communications, codes, and identifiers. The CPRS is also concerned with data security, availability, reliability, data integrity, and persistence.

The CPRSs will be designed to capture, transmit, store, manipulate, and retrieve patient-specific health care–related data. The systems will contain comprehensive longitudinal patient record data designed to provide clinical, financial, and research data. They will be linked through high-speed communication information highways capable of transmitting text, voice, and images. The CPRI is working with all the organizations involved in developing standards and is focusing on coordinating and consolidating what other groups are doing. It is not developing the data elements themselves (see Chap. 6 for descriptions of the organizations developing data standards).

# CLASSIFICATION/ACUITY SYSTEMS

Patient classification/acuity systems have been developed which provide information needed to measure care needs, predict resource use, and determine the requirements of home care. There are many reasons why a patient classification system is needed for home health nursing. In home health nursing, visits are not all equal, and patients have different care needs and require different amounts of nursing care time. A classification system designed to weight all visits by level of care could affect the practice of CHN by creating a quantifiable calculation of management and maintenance for a variable reimbursement system instead of a set cost per visit. Such a system could also be used as the basis for the productivity measurement in quality assurance programs.

Patient classification/acuity systems developed for HHAs primarily use different levels of care or client characteristics as the method for classifying patients. They are different from the acuity/classification methods, based on workload measurements, developed for predicting nurse staffing in hospitals. Generally, hospitals' methods predict hours of patient care required based on a list of patient care activities weighted by predetermined workload measures. Classification/acuity systems are being developed not only for HHAs but also for state and local health departments in order to predict resource use.

## State Health Department Classification Systems

Classification systems have been developed to allow state/local HHAs or programs to predict resource use (Alabama Home Health Branch, 1987). One classification system, developed for the State of Alabama HHA, addressed the intensity of patients' illness based on a prototype evaluation of four levels of care. The system was developed primarily because the state staff determined that the medical diagnoses were not a realistic basis for predicting care requirements. They determined that the primary medical diagnosis did not generally address the home health care needs of the patients, and that in cases with multiple medical diagnoses there was no relationship to the patient's care needs.

The Alabama State HHA's four levels of care are based on the physical or clinical assessment of the severity/intensity of the patient's condition on admission. These levels are

- Level I: Ambulatory with assistance, requiring minimal nursing care and admitted for short-term care
- Level II: Partially immobile, with an acute disease or disability

- Level III: Increased deterioration in general condition and completely immobile (bedbound)
- Level IV: Acutely ill, with major health problems requiring skilled care visits and high-tech procedures

These four levels are based on a model using 14 different variables that combine the concerns of home health nursing: (1) stage of illness, (2) level of consciousness, (3) mental status, (4) psychological state, (5) stability of disease, (6) degree of dependence, (7) supervision and observation, (8) motivation, (9) medications, (10) dressings, (11) procedure involved, (12) family status, (13) rehabilitation, and (14) teaching.

## Local Community Health Classification Systems

Many HHAs have developed classification systems. A classification system developed by the Ramsey County Public Health Nursing Service of St. Paul was designed to target the urgent needs of patients for services in order to determine who should be seen first. This unique system incorporates a measurement of patient and family functioning that provides information in three areas: services to individuals, services to families, and nursing activities. All patient/family files contain the functional status of the patient and the family. The nurse assesses the health status of each patient on admission and discharge using three functional instruments: (1) a psychosocial assessment based on a social dysfunction rating scale, (2) a functional assessment of the activities of daily living adapted from Katz's ADL scale, and (3) a family assessment based on a family coping scale. The functional assessment scores are used by nursing personnel to help establish assignment priorities by identifying which clients or patients are functioning poorly. Evaluation of services, program decisions, and financial allocations are made based on information derived from this system (O'Grady, 1984).

## Home Health Care Classification System

The Home Health Care Classification (HHCC) System was developed from the Home Health Care Classification Project conducted at Georgetown University School of Nursing. It is designed to predict home health care needs and resource use for the Medicare and elderly populations (Saba, 1991). The HHCC translates clinical nursing parameters, medical parameters, and socio-demographic data into a clinical case-mix classification for home health patients according to their expected care needs and utilization of home health resources. It predicts needs for resources in terms of home visits by nurses and all other providers for a specific time period (30 days) within an episode of home health care, and also evaluates the actual outcomes (Fig. 12.11) (Saba, 1992a, 1992b; Saba and Zuckerman, 1992).

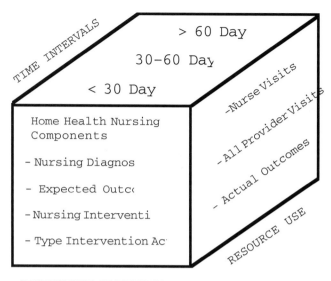

PREDICTIVE VARIABLES

**Figure 12.11**   Home Health Care Classification
(HHCC) system.


## HHCC Conceptual Framework

The HHCC system is based on a conceptual framework that uses the six
phases of the nursing process to assess patients in a holistic manner:
assessment, diagnosis, outcome identification, planning, implementation,
and evaluation (American Nurses Association, 1991). These six phases are
used by nurses to assess their patients on admission in order to classify
and predict resource use, as well as to develop a plan of care and/or care
pathways (see Fig. 12.12).

The HHCC system uses the Saba Home Health Care Classification:
Nursing Diagnoses and Interventions to code and classify the care process.
It consists of four sets of nursing parameters: (1) 145 nursing diagnoses,
(2) 3 expected outcomes ("improved," "stabilized," and "deteriorated"),
(3) 160 nursing interventions, and (4) 4 types of intervention actions
("assess," "direct care," "teach," and "manage"). The nursing diagnoses and
interventions are both classified according to 20 home health care components.
The HHCC also includes 20 medical diagnosis and surgical procedure
groups and 10 socio-demographic data elements. The Home Health Care
Classification: Nursing Diagnoses and Interventions is given in the Appendix.

Patient assessment data are correlated, using the 20 home health care
components, with the four sets of nursing parameters and the medical and
socio-demographic variables. These HHCC 20 home health care components provide the framework for assessing the functional, psychological,
physiological, and behavioral patterns of home health care, and also for

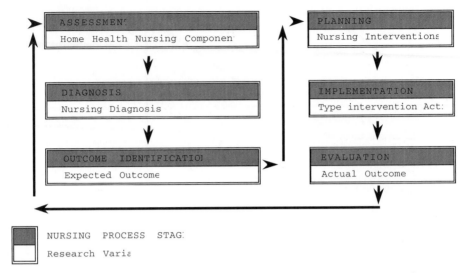

**Figure 12.12**    Home Health Care Classification (HHCC) system conceptual framework.

measuring and/or evaluating the actual outcomes. The correlations are used to derive a score which is used to predict (1) care needs in terms of home health components and their respective nursing diagnoses and interventions and (2) resource use for 30-day intervals, in terms of nursing and all provider visits (nursing, physical therapy, occupational therapy, speech therapy, medical social work, and home health aide).

The HHCC system identifies the relationships between medical and nursing diagnoses in predicting resource use. It can differentiate between short-term (30-day acute care), intermediate term (60-day intermediate care), and long-term (90-day chronic care) cases. The HHCC system 20 home health care components classify the clinical care process for an entire episode of home health care by extending the clinical assessment parameters into care pathways (Fig.12.13). The HHCC system provides HHAs with an innovative clinical classification method for predicting and allocating resources, and determining staffing needs and costs. The HHCC system can run on a microcomputer, with a portable notebook used to facilitate data collection.

## Patient Dependency Systems

This nursing project was conducted on behalf of the Australian Council of Community Nursing Service in Australia (Gliddon and Finch, 1991). Its goal was to develop a tool that could assist in the prediction and allocation of nursing resources in the community. The project demonstrated that

# Home Health Care Classification System
## Patient Assessment Form

**NOTE: DO NOT CODE a Nsg DX if a Nsg RX not identified & Vice Versa**

1.     CODE ALL Nursing Diagnoses, Use Coding Scheme, that will be addressed in the care process.
2.     ENTER Expected Outcome for Each Nursing Diagnosis as Improved, Stabilized, or Maintained.
3.     CODE ALL nursing Interventions, Use Coding Scheme, ordered by the Nurse or Physician to be provided during Episode of Care.
4.     ENTER Type of Intervention Action for Each Nursing Intervention as : Assess, Care, Teach, or Manage.

| Home Health Component | Nursing Diagnosis | Expected Outcome | | | Nursing Intervention | Type of Action | | | |
|---|---|---|---|---|---|---|---|---|---|
| | | I | S | D | | A | C | T | M |
| **BEHAVIORAL COMPONENTS** | | | | | | | | | |
| 1. Medications | | | | | | | | | |
| | | | | | | | | | |
| | | | | | | | | | |
| 2. Safety | | | | | | | | | |
| | | | | | | | | | |
| | | | | | | | | | |
| 3. Health Behavior | | | | | | | | | |
| | | | | | | | | | |
| | | | | | | | | | |
| **PSYCHOLOGICAL COMPONENTS** | | | | | | | | | |
| 4. Cognitive | | | | | | | | | |
| | | | | | | | | | |
| | | | | | | | | | |
| 5. Coping | | | | | | | | | |
| | | | | | | | | | |
| | | | | | | | | | |
| 6. Self-Concept | | | | | | | | | |
| | | | | | | | | | |
| | | | | | | | | | |
| 7. Role Relationship | | | | | | | | | |
| | | | | | | | | | |
| | | | | | | | | | |
| **PHYSIOLOGICAL COMPONENTS** | | | | | | | | | |
| 8. Cardiac | | | | | | | | | |
| | | | | | | | | | |
| | | | | | | | | | |
| 9. Respiratory | | | | | | | | | |
| | | | | | | | | | |
| | | | | | | | | | |

| I = Improved, S = Stabilized, D = Deteriorated | A = Assess, C = Care, T = Teach, M = Manage |
|---|---|

**Figure 12.13** Home Health Care Classification (HHCC) System patient assessment form.

## Home Health Care Classification System (Continued)

| Home Health Component | Nursing Diagnosis | Expected Outcome | | | Nursing Intervention | Type of Action | | | |
|---|---|---|---|---|---|---|---|---|---|
| | | I | S | D | | A | C | T | M |
| **10. Metabolic** | | | | | | | | | |
| | | | | | | | | | |
| | | | | | | | | | |
| **11. Bowel Elimination** | | | | | | | | | |
| | | | | | | | | | |
| | | | | | | | | | |
| **12. Urinary Elimination** | | | | | | | | | |
| | | | | | | | | | |
| | | | | | | | | | |
| **13. Physical Regulation** | | | | | | | | | |
| | | | | | | | | | |
| | | | | | | | | | |
| **14. Skin Integrity** | | | | | | | | | |
| | | | | | | | | | |
| | | | | | | | | | |
| **15. Tissue Perfusion** | | | | | | | | | |
| | | | | | | | | | |
| | | | | | | | | | |
| **FUNCTIONAL COMPONENTS** | | | | | | | | | |
| **16. Activity** | | | | | | | | | |
| | | | | | | | | | |
| | | | | | | | | | |
| **17. Nutrition** | | | | | | | | | |
| | | | | | | | | | |
| | | | | | | | | | |
| **18. Fluid** | | | | | | | | | |
| | | | | | | | | | |
| | | | | | | | | | |
| **19. Sensory** | | | | | | | | | |
| | | | | | | | | | |
| | | | | | | | | | |
| **20. Self-Care** | | | | | | | | | |
| | | | | | | | | | |
| | | | | | | | | | |

| I=Improved, S=Stabilized, D=Deteriorated | A=Assess, C=Care, T=Teach, M=Manage |
|---|---|

*Virginia K. Saba, 4/95

**Figure 12.13** *Continued*

468

there were many informal factors that impacted on the need for formal service; for example, the presence of an informal care giver was likely to "dilute" the nursing service requirements of high dependency patients, while the availability of a professional provider could in turn impact on its allocation. This led to the development of the Bryan Domiciliary Dependency Instrument by the Royal District Nursing Services (Melbourne, Australia). This new system incorporates four different dependency measures that allow for comparison with other health care populations. It includes activities of daily living items, health status and risk factors, and information relating to the informal care giver. It is computerized, interactive, and designed to assist nurses in decision making during the assessment and review process, but it does not predict the need for care. It can be used to monitor quality and measure resource allocation at the clinical, managerial, and funding levels.

## HOME TECHNOLOGY SYSTEMS

As home care evolved and technology advanced, innovative home technology systems emerged. The extension of technology systems into the home allows working people to save time, travel, and work days consumed by medical and other health care services. These systems maintain continuity of care from hospital to home as well as keep the family together. Technology allows the patient to view and participate interactively in his or her health care via a remote communication network.

With the introduction of on-line home-based computer terminals, communication links can bring health care information from a variety of information providers to the home. Technological applications support several innovative home technological advances:

- Home care communication systems
- Home high-tech electronic monitoring systems
- Home educational technology systems

### Home Care Communication Systems

Communication systems link patients' homes to health care facilities and health care professionals, home care workers to their supervisors, and patients and families with community resources. Communication systems make it possible for patients to communicate with providers to get health care advice, avoid inconvenient and expensive visits to health care providers, and omit unnecessary visits to health care facilities. Home health care is increasingly using devices that allow health care providers to communicate with patients in their homes.

Several projects are being supported by the High Performance Computing Communication (HPCC) program, a new federal program designed to apply high-performance computers to help solve the nation's problems, including health. Several of these projects are being conducted by university, state, and regional organizations and have been primarily initiated to address health care in rural settings using telecommunications.

The Texas Telemedicine Project in Austin, Texas, is using two-way interactive video to connect specialists in major urban centers with health professionals in rural areas for diagnosis and consultation. The communication technology is used to transmit x-rays, electrocardiograms, and other clinical data for analysis by the specialists. Electronic health care allows rural professionals to "see" more patients/clients via the two-way interactive video without having to make "home visits," thus saving travel time and ultimately cost (Preston et al., 1992).

The University of Iowa is conducting a Study of Rural Telemedicine which is designed to determine how to improve academic-rural partnerships and to increase collaboration between] the University of Iowa and community-based health care providers. Another project is being conducted by the Concurrent Engineering Research Center, West Virginia University. This project is also studying the use of real time technology for the collaboration, treatment, and longitudinal coordination of care of patients in a rural state.

## Telecommunications

Telecommunications will never replace the practitioner or direct patient-provider relationships, but it will ensure more prudent use of health care services. It is anticipated that communication networks will enhance and integrate health care services across the continuum of care from hospital to home. They will foster self-care and preventive programs by supplying extensive diagnostic and educational information to patients. Costs will be reduced as a result of the use of information-related communication via home terminals in place of home visits.

Computer terminals and/or microcomputers with a modem are used to implement communication systems (Jones, 1991). A computer terminal in a patient's home provides access to information and monitoring, which can diminish the need for routine visits with a provider, thereby improving the provider's productivity while improving the patient's health status. The terminal in a patient's home can be used to assist in self-diagnosis and preventive medicine, reduce unnecessary outpatient visits, provide self-directed triage, and eliminate the "worried well" aspects of many patient–provider interactions. This leads to the following benefits:

- Improved patient and provider satisfaction
- Patient time savings in tracking and receiving information

- Reduced need to see a health care provider
- Increased reliance on computer-based information
- Reduced information calls

While home terminals increase the productivity of home health professionals, they require that extensive diagnostic and educational information be available on-line for patients. They can, however, also streamline administrative requirements such as obtaining physician orders and confirming appointments as a result of improved communication with the physicians and other health care professionals. Queries regarding immunizations for travel, flu vaccines, side effects of medications, nonprescription medications, and school and work health forms can increase early detection and reduce visits to health professional offices and hospitals.

### Community Health Networks

A community health network is an innovative ambulatory care system specially developed to provide services by computer. Computer terminals are placed in homes of "heavy users of health care," such as families with young children, pregnant women, and the elderly. The system allows the subscribers to telephone for assistance and guidance on services offered via the terminal. The system assists in the following actions but does not necessarily provide diagnoses.

- Download the patient record from the hospital to the home database.
- Enter a series of questions about symptoms using expert system logic until the pathways are concluded.
- Track self-care or, depending on the responses to questions, call or make an appointment with a clinician.
- Provide additional information on the condition to assist the client to resolve the problem if self-care is chosen.

Community health networks appear to increase client satisfaction, and it is anticipated that they will reduce telephone calls and unnecessary trips to the emergency room or physician offices for the "worried well." The system is also expected to reduce cost and improve the efficiency and productivity of clinicians. Computer networks hold great promise for the delivery of home health care services. They are innovative, cost-effective mechanisms for providing continuity of care that uses computer technologies in the delivery of health care services (Brennan, 1993; Little, 1992).

### ComputerLink

ComputerLink is a project conducted by Case Western Reserve University (CWRU), Cleveland, Ohio, which offered programs and services to support self-care in the home. They were primarily designed to support AIDS patients and the care givers of Alzheimer's disease patients living in their homes. ComputerLink ran within the Cleveland Free Net, a public access computer network. Computer terminals were placed in the homes of the patients using standard telephone lines to allow the patients and/or their care givers to communicate with the Information Network Services staff at CWRU. ComputerLink offered home care users information, communication, and decision support to enhance self-care and promote home-based treatment of the study patients. It served as a "support group without walls" (Brennan, 1993).

## Triage Systems

Triage systems make health services more efficient. The use of triage systems that link terminals in the home to a health care triage expert system can increase self-help approaches to early detection and improved diagnoses. Their use expands patient support and fosters home-based self-care and patient education on subjects such as signs and symptoms of diseases, prevention techniques, and self-care instructions by providing nontechnical information when a client needs it. Access to care at an early and more appropriate time is improved for clients who are reluctant to see a clinician for a variety of reasons. Early intervention can help solve medical problems before they become serious and thus prevent hospitalizations and clinic visits. It is anticipated that the system will also increase prevention and improve quality.

# Home High-Tech Monitoring Systems

Home high-tech monitoring systems use computers to link patients at home to health care facilities. Monitoring devices that transmit vital signs and other critical data are used in the home to conduct, for example, post-surgical checkups. They allow health care providers to monitor the progress of their patients. Monitoring technology permits the transmission of health care information both to and from the home. Monitoring systems are being used not only for diagnosis and treatment but also for prevention. Monitoring devices will be increasingly miniaturized in size and made portable. They will be linked to home information systems and providers via cellular telephones (Little, 1992).

## Remote Defibrillator

One example of a monitoring device is a remote defibrillator that allows hospitals to diagnose and resuscitate a homebound patient who has suffered a cardiac arrest. A transtelephonic defibrillator device located in the home, called a "briefcase," is linked to a hospital base unit. When a client in the home feels that he or she is having a heart attack, he or she opens the "briefcase," activates the transmitter, and places the electrode pads on the client. An ECG is immediately transmitted to the hospital, and the interactive speakerphone is activated. If the hospital base unit determines that the client is having a heart attack, the device triggers an electronic shock to the patient to stimulate the heart.

## Electronic Devices

Communication devices are also used to relay test result information, monitor chronic illnesses, and educate clients in the home. For example, a patient can administer a home test and get feedback from a health provider without having to make a visit to the hospital to have the test administered and then to the health care provider or physician to have the test results interpreted.

Electronic devices are being used to administer dosages of drugs based on body monitoring. For example, an automated insulin pump is used to monitor the sugar levels in the blood of diabetics, and calibrate and automatically inject insulin. Many new technologies are being explored for noninvasive blood testing, and to measure changes in bodily electrical fields. Other devices are available to monitor limited body functions such as ECGs. Wristwatch devices to measure blood pressure and pulse rates are in use. Other technologies are also being offered, such as apnea monitoring, oxygen administration, and home ventilation programs (Techan, 1987).

## Telemetry Devices

Sophisticated telemetry devices such as digitized x-rays and ECGs, electronic stethoscopes, and interactive video equipment are using telecommunications technology to enable specialists at a teaching hospital to examine patients in a remote clinic. The clinicians can examine patients, hear heartbeats, study x-rays and laboratory results, and perform other critical assessments with these devices. Two monitors are used to communicate between the two locations. One monitor is used to interact with the rural physician and patient, and the other to view close up the images from cameras attached to the biomedical devices.

## Alert Systems

Alert systems are emergency systems widely used in home treatments. They are primarily communication devices that allow the homebound to signal for "help" in an emergency. A one-way signaling device that is worn around the neck allows a patient, by pressing on a button, to signal for help to a friend, hospital emergency room coordinator, fire department, etc. Another communication device being researched is a two-way communication device that allows the health care provider in a hospital to communicate with a patient in distress. Other "telemonitoring" devices have been invented that allow patients to administer tests such as measuring vital signs and transmit them to a health care provider (Little, 1992).

## Home Educational Technology Systems

Home educational technology systems require communication linkages, information access, and educational materials. These technologies permit clients to reach beyond their environment to "see" and "hear," that is, to experience, view, and visualize situations and to obtain educational information. Information access permits the network to access distant databases. There is a growing use of user-friendly technologies, making it possible to interact via on-line computer terminals using handwriting or voice (Olsen et al., 1992).

Home educational systems offer advanced learning and health promotion applications. They use technological media to enable care givers to interact with and educate patients in the home and the community. The types of learning that can be communicated into the home are still being researched. However, the developed home teaching strategies using information technologies are varied. They include active learning, personalization, individualization, cooperative learning, improving learning strategies and thinking skills, contextual learning, learning to learn, high standards for all, sophisticated evaluation strategies, and parental and community involvement.

### Educational Technologies

A critical use of home educational technologies is in the areas of effective self-care and health promotion. Home computers will offer this information as an essential commodity. New knowledge bases on treatments and on prevention and handling of chronic disabilities will meet the need for health care consumers to assume more responsibility for their own care, wellness, and prevention of disease.

Patients using communication systems will have access to health information focusing on disease prevention and health promotion activities. They will have access to clinical advice about specific diseases, information about individual health status and self-care, their own health care records, and evaluations of providers and therapies. Through interactive learning and communication technologies in the home, patients will become active participants in health care decisions.

It is anticipated that new advanced technology services for health and learning will go far beyond what can be foreseen. The benefits in health care to consumers and society will be revolutionary. Several demonstration projects are being implemented to determine the benefits of this new use of computer-based technology.

### Home Consultations and Decision-Making Systems

Consultation in the home via computer-based stand-alone software programs that do not require a communication network is now available.

Computer-assisted instruction (CAI) and interactive video (IV) programs are available for the personal computer.

### Two-Way Video Systems

Two-way video networks will enable homebound clients not only to communicate with health professionals via computer-based terminals in the home but also to participate in video conferencing. The use of two-way video systems can enhance these contacts and provide emotional support. Clinicians can provide consultation, observe their patients, and feel connected. Visual and graphic interactive communications are far more effective in educating patients than pamphlets on subjects such as nutrition. Clinicians can observe their patients and guide home health workers to use monitoring equipment, or view a specific part of the body, or teach a worker to conduct an examination for viewing. Additionally, the technology can enhance the use of electronic services to schedule health care appointments and automate insurance claims filing and information on eligibility benefits and costs.

### Self-Help Databases

Database systems are being developed whereby consumers can be linked to a "smart database" with answers and health care advice for minor problems, such as a rash or a temperature. Once the two-way video networks are in place, clients will be able to consult with health care providers without making a physical visit to a clinician.

### Videoconferencing

Videoconferencing includes the transmission of a video image with a voice in real time and visual, interactive discussion between two or more parties in different locations (Little, 1992; Preston et al., 1992). A benefit of this technology is that it can reduce health care costs in three ways, by reducing

- Time spent discussing normal test results
- Time spent monitoring chronic patients
- Time spent on information-related calls

Remote IV consultation will reduce the need for patients to travel to specialists or for specialists to travel to rural hospitals (see Fig. 12.14). Other benefits are that video consultation can

- Reduce travel time to see a specialist.
- Increase the timeliness of professional consultation.
- Improve access to care and strengthen rural hospitals.

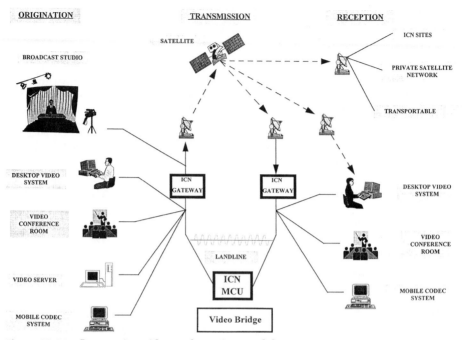

**Figure 12.14** Interactive videoconferencing model.

■ Increase patient compliance with a recommended course of treatment through increased patient convenience.

Once in place, the broadband networks can reach through existing telephone or cable TV networks into the home. They will be able to offer video consultations and video instructions, support home care services for homebound patients, and allow clinicians to provide remote diagnostic evaluations and consultations.

## FUTURE TRENDS

In home health care, nurses need to be aware of their changing responsibilities and roles. Because of the rapid growth of the use of care managers, home health care will become high-tech as well as high-touch. Community health information networks will link claims, outcomes, billing utilization reviews, and patient records on a single system. Shift claims and eligibility data will be transmitted over electronic highways and build database information to track clinical outcomes.

The technology revolution will then take place in the home as interactive voice, data, and imaging become available. The CPR will be a reality, health information consultation and monitoring systems will spread into the home, and the impact on health care and health providers will be revolutionary. These systems will put more science into the art of nursing and medicine, and will affect not only home care itself but also national health care policy. The systems as envisioned will facilitate disease prevention and health promotion, and allow outcome measures to influence effectiveness and contain health care costs (Little, 1992).

The CPR is envisioned as one lifelong health care record, incorporating every episode of health care, for each individual in the nation. It is anticipated that it will contain complete patient health care information from all sources where health care services are provided, and will be accessed regardless of where the services are offered. Health care data will be in an electronic form that can be aggregated and analyzed. The CPR will be accessed in the home via telecommunication networks and on-line computer terminals.

Through the use of telephone networks linked with broadband fiber-optic cable, such systems are possible. Implementing this technology will allow the information revolution to expand from the hospital to the home. The NII will be used to communicate among providers regardless of location and will provide "health care without walls."

## SUMMARY

This chapter described the various computer applications found in community health. It presented an overview of the beginnings and development of community health computer systems. An overview of the different types of community health systems was presented. They included systems for state/local health departments, which include statistical reporting, registration, management information, personal/client management, and school health. Special-purpose systems including those developed for categorical programs, special studies, screening programs, and epidemiological programs were also highlighted.

Ambulatory care and personal/client management systems are other types of community health systems that were described. Home health systems were also presented, including a review of LANs and WANs as the mode of communication from agencies to the commercial vendors, service bureaus, or computer companies.

The last section focused on home technology systems, which include a wide range of home communication systems, monitoring equipment, devices, and alert systems. Also a presentation was provided on the use of home educational technologies for teaching health care in the home setting.

# REFERENCES

Alabama Home Health Branch, Division of Long Term Care, Alabama Department of Public Health. (1987). *Quality assurance manual*. Montgomery, AL.

American Nurses Association. (1991). *Standards of Clinical Nursing Practice* (p. 6). Washington, DC.

Barnett, G. O. (1976). *Computer-Stored Ambulatory Record (COSTAR)* (NCHSR Research Digest Series) (DHEW Pub. No. HRA 76-3145). Rockville, MD: National Center for Health Services Research.

Basch, C. E., Gold, R. S., and Shea, S. (1988). The potential contribution of computerized school-based record systems to the monitoring of disease prevention and health promotion objectives for the nation. *Health Education Quarterly*, *15*(1), 35–51.

B.E.S.T. (1992). *Healthy People 2000*. Charlotte, MI: Barry-Eaton Software Technologies.

Bilodeau, A. (Ed.). (1994). *Clinical Data Management*. Gaithersberg, MD: Aspen.

Brennan, P. F. (1993). ComputerLink: Computer networks and community health connections. *Nursing Dynamics*, *2*(1), 9–15.

Brown, R. S., Phillips, B. R., Cheh, V. A., et al. (1991). *Case-Mix Analysis Using Georgetown Data: Home Health Prospective Payment Demonstration*. Princeton, NJ: Mathematica Policy Research.

Brown V. B., Mason W. T., and Kaczmarski, M. (1971). A computerized health information service. *Nursing Outlook*, *19*(3), 158–161.

Clinical Data Management. (1994). Texas links 400 public health clinics. *Clinical Data Management*, *1*(5), 1.

Community Nursing Organizations' Consortium. (1993). *Community Nursing Organizations National Demonstration: Mission Statement*. Millwood, VA: Project Hope.

Computer-Based Patient Record Institute. (1992). *Newsletters*. Chicago.

Custom Data Processing, Inc. (1992, draft). *On-line Software Solutions for Local Health Departments and State Government Organizations*. La Grange, IL.

Dick, R. S., and Steen, E. B. (Eds.). (1991). *The Computer-Based Patient Record: An Essential Technology for Health Care* (p. 167). Washington, DC: National Academy Press.

Dodd, K., and Coleman, J. R. (1994). Home care and managed care: Prospective partners. *Caring*, *13*(3), 68–71.

Florida Department of Health and Rehabilitative Services. (1983). *HRS Manual: System Management: Client Information System: Personal Health*. Tallahassee, FL.

Gliddon, T., and Finch, C. (1991). *Patient Dependency and Resource Allocation in Domiciliary Nursing*. Victoria, Australia: Australian Council of Community Nursing Services.

Goedert, J. (1994). More states turn to EDI as a way to cut expenses. *Health Data Management*, *2*, 35–38.

Goodwin, D. R. (1992). Critical pathways in home healthcare. *Journal of Nursing Administration*, *22*(2), 35–40.

Grady, M. L., and Schwartz, H. A. (Eds.). (1993). *Automated Data Sources for Ambulatory Care Effectiveness Research: Literature Review* (Pub. No. 93-0042). Rockville, MD: AHCPR, PHS, US DHHS.

Hansel, K. (1994, September 5). Atlanta VNHS begins test of Care 2000 seeking cost/outcomes for home health patient care and managed care (Special Report). *Home Healthline*, 1–6.

Health Care Financing Administration. (1980). *Medicare: Provider Reimbursement Manual: Part II—Provider Cost Reporting Forms and Instructions*. Baltimore, MD: HCFA (1728), DHHS.

Hoffman, N. L. (1993, December 13). *Missouri Health Strategic Architectures and Information Cooperative*. Project Report. Jefferson City, MO.

Indian Health Services, Information Systems Division. (1990). *Patient Care Component (PCC Overview)*. Tucson, AZ.

Jones, G. M. (1991). *Healthcare for an Aging America: The Role of Telecommunications*. Washington, DC: Consumer Interest Research Institute.

Little, A. D. (1992). *Telecommunications: Can It Help Solve America's Health Care Problems?* Cambridge, MA.

Martin, K. S., and Sheet, N. J. (1992). *The Omaha System: Applications for Community Health Nursing*. Philadelphia: Saunders.

McDonald, F. (1987). Computer applications in diabetes management and education. *Computers in Nursing*, 5(5), 181–185.

Michigan Health Department, Nursing Administration's Forum. (1988). *PH-NIS: Personal Health: Nursing Information System*. Lansing, MI.

National Association for Home Care. (1994). *Progress toward a Uniform Minimum Data Set for Home Care and Hospice*. Washington, DC.

National Center for Health Statistics. (1994). *Subcommittee on State and Community Health Statistics: Minutes of Meeting*. Washington, DC: NCHS, National Committee on Vital and Health Statistics.

National League for Nursing. (1973). *Management Information Systems for Public Health/Community Health Agencies*. New York.

National League for Nursing. (1975). *Management Information Systems for Public Health/Community Health Agencies: Workshop Papers*. New York.

National League for Nursing. (1976). *State of the Art in Management Information Systems for Public Health/Community Health Agencies: Report of the Conference*. New York.

National League for Nursing (1977). *Statistical Reporting in Home and Community Health Services* (Pub. No. 21-1652). New York.

National League for Nursing. (1978). *Selected Management Information Systems for Public Health/Community Health Agencies*. New York.

New Jersey State Department of Health. (1977). *Home Health Agencies Management Information System*. Washington, DC: DN, HRA, PHS, DHHS.

O'Grady, B. V. (1984). Computerized documentation of community health nursing: What shall it be? *Community Nursing*, 2(3), 98–101.

Ohata, F. (1983). PL child health care systems. In M. Scholes, Y. Bryant, B. Barber (Eds.), *The Impact of Computers on Nursing* (pp. 222–229). Amsterdam, Netherlands: North-Holland.

Olsen, R., Jones, M. G., and Bezold, C. (1992). *21st Century Learning and Health Care in the Home: Creating a National Telecommunications Network*. Alexandria, VA: Institute for Alternative Futures; Washington, DC: Consumer Interest Research Institute.

Preston, J., Brown, F., and Hartley, B. (1992). Using telemedicine to improve health care in distant areas. *Hospitals and Community Psychiatry*, 43(1), 25–32.

Rollins, S. (1994). Trends and imperatives for home healthcare IS. *Healthcare Informatics*, *11*(9), 99.40–52.

Saba, V. K. (1982). The computer in public health: Today and tomorrow. *Nursing Outlook*, *30*(9), 510–514.

Saba, V. K. (1983). How computers influence nursing activities in community health. In NIH (Ed.), *First National Conference: Computer Technology and Nursing* (pp. 7–11). (NIH Pub. No. 83-2142). Bethesda, MD: National Institutes of Health.

Saba, V. K. (1991). *Home Health Care Classification Project* (NTIS No. PB92-177013/AS). Washington, DC: Georgetown University School of Nursing.

Saba, V. K. (1992a). Home health care classification. *Caring*, *10*(5), 58–60.

Saba, V. K. (1992b). The classification of home health care nursing diagnoses and interventions. *Caring*, *10*(3), 50–57.

Saba, V. K., and Zuckerman, A. E. (1992). A new home health care classification method. *Caring*, *10*(10), 27–34.

Simmons, D. A. (1984). Computer implementation in ambulatory care: A community health model. In NIH (Ed.), *Second National Conference: Computer Technology and Nursing* (pp. 19–23) (NIH Pub. No. 84-2623). Bethesda, MD: National Institutes of Health.

Shaughnessy, P. W., Bauman, M. K., and Kramer, A. M. (1990). Measuring the quality of home health care. *Caring*, *9*(2), 4–6.

Shaughnessy, P. W., and Kramer, A. M. (1990). The increased needs of patients in nursing homes and patients receiving home health care. *New England Journal of Medicine*, *322*(1), 21–27.

Techan, C. B. (1987). Introduction. In K. Fisher and K. Gardner (Eds.), *Quality and Home Health Care: Redefining the Tradition* (pp. 5–7). Chicago: Joint Commission on Accreditation of Healthcare Organizations.

Whyte, A. A. (1982, August). Occupational health information systems. *Occupational Health and Safety*, 14–19, 36.

## BIBLIOGRAPHY

American Nurses Association. (1986). *Standards of Home Health Nursing Practice*. Kansas City, MO.

American Nurses Association. (1986). *Standards of Community Health Nursing Practice*. Kansas City, MO.

American Public Health Association. (1985). *Model Standards: A Guide for Community Preventive Health Services* (2d ed.). Washington, DC.

American Public Health Association. (1980). *The Definition and Role of Public Health Nursing in the Delivery of Health Care: A Statement of the Public Health Nursing Section*. Washington, DC.

Australian Council of Community Nursing Services Inc. (1994). *Community Nursing Minimum Data Set Australia: Version 1.0 1994: Data Dictionary and Guidelines*. Victoria, Australia.

Barnett, G. O., Justice, M. E., Somand J., et al. (1984). COSTAR system. In B. Blum (Ed.), *Information Systems for Patient Care* (pp. 270–293). New York: Springer-Verlag.

Brown, V. B., Mason, W. T., and Millman, S. (1974). The health information system—An example of a total health system. In *Management Information Systems for Public Health/Community Health Agencies: Report of the Conference* (pp. 159–161). New York: National League for Nursing.

Browne, H. (1966). A tribute to Mary Brechenridge. *Nursing Outlook, 14,* 54–55.

Buhler-Wilkerson, K. (1985). Public health nursing: In sickness or in health? *American Journal of Public Health, 75*(10), 1155–1161.

Cary, A. (1987). An assessment from the national perspective on home health care relative to nursing education. In Division of Nursing, PHS (Ed.), *Home Health Care: Issues, Trends, and Strategies* (NTIS Pub. HRP-0907168) (pp. 29–42). Rockville, MD: DN, BHP, PHS, US DHHS.

Chalmers, M., and Brady, F. (1992). Using a microcomputer program to manage contract services in a home health agency. In J. M. Arnold and G. A. Pearson (Eds.), *Computer Applications in Nursing Education and Practice* (Pub. No. 14-2406) (pp. 113–119). New York: National League for Nursing.

Collenn, M. F. (1990). Health assessment systems. In E. H. Shortliffe and L. E. Perreault (Eds.), *Medical Informatics: Computer Applications in Health Care* (pp. 562–582). Reading, MA: Addison-Wesley.

Conference of Local Health Officers. (1994). *US Local Health Officers Directory: 1994.* Washington, DC.

Davis, C. (1987). Home care and its financial support: Future directions and present policies—Impact of care. In Division of Nursing, PHS (Ed.), *Home Health Care: Issues, Trends, and Strategies* (NTIS Pub. HRP-0907168) (pp. 3–18). Rockville, MD: DN, BHP, PHS, US DHHS.

DeBack, V. (1994). Nursing practice in health promotion and disease prevention. In O. L. Strickland and D. J. Fishman (Eds.). *Nursing Issues in the 1990's.* Albany, NY: Delmar.

Division of Nursing, PHS. (1969). *Nurses in Public Health: January 1968.* Bethesda, MD: DN, BHP, PHS, DHHS.

Division of Nursing, PHS. (1978). *Survey of Community Health Nursing: 1974.* Hyattsville, MD: DN, HRSA, PHS, DHHS.

Division of Nursing, PHS. (1987). *Home Health Care: Issues, Trends, and Strategies* (NTIS Pub. HRP-0907168). Rockville, MD: DN, BHP, PHS, US DHHS.

Dolan, J. (1978). *History of Nursing* (14th ed). Philadelphia: Saunders.

Durch, J. S., and Lohr, K. N. (Eds.). (1993). *Emergency Medical Services for Children.* Washington, DC: Institute of Medicine, National Academy Press.

Ferguson, M. (1966). *How to Determine Nursing Expenditures in Small Health Agencies.* Washington, DC: DN, PHS, US DHEW.

Fiddleman, R. H. (1982). Proliferation of COSTAR: A status report. In B. Blum (Ed.), *Proceedings: The Sixth Annual Symposium on Computer Applications in Medical Care* (pp. 175–178). New York: IEEE Computer Society Press.

Florida State Department of Health and Rehabilitative Services. (1973). *Management Information Systems for Community/Public Health Nursing Services* (NO1 NU-34036). Washington, DC: US DHHS.

Freeman, R., and Heinrick, J. (1981). *Community Health Nursing Practice* (2d ed.). Philadelphia: Saunders.

Gale, B. J., and Steffl, B. M. (1992). The long-term care dilemma. *Nursing and Health Care, 13*(1), 34–41.

Halamandaris, V.J. (October). Twenty reasons for home care. *Caring, 4*(10), 8.

Harris, M. D. (1994). *Handbook of Home Health Care Administration.* Gaithersburg, MD: Aspen.

Helberg, J. L. (1989). Reliability of the nursing classification index for home healthcare. *Nursing Management, 20*(3), 48–56.

Home and Community Care Program. (1994). *Community Nursing Minimum Data Set: Australia CNMDSA, Version 1.0: Data Dictionary and Guidelines.* Victoria, Australia: Australia Council of Community Nursing Services.

Horn, S. D., Sharkey, P. D., Chambers, A. F., and Horn, R. A. (1985). Severity of illness within DRGs: Impact on prospective payment. *American Journal of Public Health, 75*(10), 1195–1199.

IHS Data Advisory Committee, Study Design Team. (1982). *Patient Care Information System (PCIS): PCIS Operations Manual.* Tucson, AZ: Indian Health Service, US DHHS.

Institute of Medicine, Committee for the Study of the Future of Public Health. (1988). *The Future of Public Health.* Washington, DC: National Academy Press.

Katz, S., Ford, A. B., Moskowitz, R. W, et al. (1963). Studies in illness in the aged: The index of ADL: A standardized measure of biological and psychosocial function. *Journal of American Medical Association, 185*, 914–919.

Kemper, P., Applebaum, R., and Harrigan, M. (1987). *A Systematic Comparison of Community Care Demonstrations.* Rockville, MD: National Center for Health Services Research, PHS, DHHS.

Kennevan, W. J. (1974). General systems theory—A logical transition. In National League for Nursing (Ed.). *Management Information Systems for Public Health/Community Health Agencies: A Report of the Conference.* New York: National League for Nursing.

Kosidlak, J. G. and Kerpelman, K. B. (1987). Managing community health nursing. *Computers in Nursing, 5*(5), 175–180.

Levenson, G. (1979). *Use of Patient Statistics for Program Planning.* New York: National League for Nursing.

Milholland, K. D. and Heller, B. R. (1992). Computer-based patient record: From pipe dream to reality. *Computers in Nursing, 10*(5), 191–192.

Moses, E. B. (1988). *The Registered Nurse Population: 1992.* Rockville, MD: DN, HRSA, PHS, DHHS.

National Association for Home Care. (1993). *Basic Statistics about Home Care 1993.* Washington, DC.

National Center for Health Statistics. (1990). *Health United States—1989* (DHHS Pub. No. 90-1232). Hyattsville, MD: NCHS, CDC, PHS, DHHS.

National League for Nursing. (1964). *Cost Analysis for Public Health Nursing Services.* New York.

National League for Nursing. (1977). *Statistical Reporting in Home and Community Health Services* (Pub. No. 21-1652). New York.

National League for Nursing. (1987). *Home Care Agencies and Community Health Services Accredited by NLN* (Pub. No. 21-1645). New York.

NYC Visiting Nurse Association. (1994). Healing at home: New York Visiting Nurse Service, 1893–1993. *Nursing and Health Care, 15*(2), 66–73.

O'Grady, B. V. (1987). The practices of home health care: Trends, issues, strategies. In Division of Nursing, PHS (Ed.), *Home Health Care: Issues, Trends, and Strategies* (NTIS Pub. HRP-0907168) (pp. 19–27). Rockville, MD: DN, BHP, PHS, DHHS.

Pender, N. J. (1982). *Health Promotion in Nursing Practice.* Norwalk, CT: Appleton-Century-Crofts.

Pender, N. J. (1987). Health and health promotion: Conceptual dilemmas. In M. E. Durfy and N. J. Pender (Eds.), *Conceptual Issues in Health Promotion: Report of Proceedings of a Wingspread Conference* (pp. 7–23). Indianapolis, IN: Sigma Theta Tau International.

Pollack, B. (1979). The evolution of an HMO. *Medical Group Management, 26*(6), 3–5.

Reitz, J. (1985). Toward a comprehensive nursing intensity index: Part I, Development. *Nursing Management, 16*(8), 22.

Rinke, L. T. (1988). *Outcome Standards in Home Health: State of the Art.* New York: National League for Nursing.

Roberts, D. E., and Heinrich, J. (1985). Public health nursing comes of age. *American Journal of Public Health, 75*(10), 1162–1172.

Saba, V. K. (1974). Basic considerations in management information systems for public health/community health agencies. In National League for Nursing (Ed.), *Management Information Systems for Public Health/Community Health Agencies: A Report of a Conference* (pp. 3–13). New York: National League for Nursing.

Saba, V. K. (1982). Computerized management information system in community health nursing. In B. Blum (Ed.), *Proceedings: The Sixth Annual Symposium on Computer Applications in Medical Care* (pp. 148–149). New York: IEEE Computer Society Press.

Saba, V. K. (1983). Computers in nursing administration: Information systems for community health nursing. *Computers in Nursing, 1*(2), 1–3.

Saba, V. K., and Levine, E. (1981). Patient care module in community health nursing. In H. H. Werley and M. Grier (Eds.), *Nursing Information Systems* (pp. 243–262). New York: Springer.

Schore, J., Brown, R. S., and Phillips, B. R. (1993, unpublished report). *Medicare Home Health Episodes 1990/1991: Distributions of Episode Length and Number of Visits Provided per Episode.* Baltimore, MD: Health Care Financing Administration, DHHS.

Simmons, D. A. (1980). *A Classification Scheme for Client Problems in Community Health Nursing* (Nurse Planning Information Series, vol. 14, NTIS No. HRP-0501501). Springfield, VA: National Technical Information Series.

Simmons, D. A. (1981). Computerized management information system in a community health nursing agency. In H. Heffernon (Ed.), *Proceedings: The Fifth Annual Symposium on Computer Applications in Medical Care* (pp. 753–754). New York: IEEE Computer Society Press.

Spradley, B. W. (1985). *Community Health Nursing: Concepts and Practices* (2d ed.). Boston: Little, Brown.

Stanhope, M., and Lancaster, J. (1992). *Community Health Nursing: Process and Practice for Promoting Health.* St Louis: Mosby.

Stienkiewicz, J. (1984). Patient classification in community health nursing. *Nursing Outlook, 32*(6), 321.

Subcommittee on State and Community Health Statistics. (1992). *The National Committee on Vital and Health Statistics, 1992* (NCVHS). Hyattsville, MD: National Center for Health Statistics, CDCP, OHS, US DHHS.

Taylor, D. B., and Johnson, O. H. (1974). *Systematic Nursing Assessment: A Step toward Automation* (DHEW Pub. No. HRA 74-17). Bethesda, MD: DN, PHS, DHHS.

Trafford, A. (1994, January 11). U.S. health costs to pass $1 trillion in 1994: Even with reform, the trend is still up. *Washington Post: Health News*, p. 7.

U.S. Department of Health, Education, and Welfare, Public Health Service, Office of Assistant Secretary for Health and Surgeon General. (1963). *Health People: The Surgeon General's Report on Health Promotion and Disease Prevention* (PHS Pub. No. 79-55071). Washington, DC: U.S. Government Printing Office.

U.S. Department of Health and Human Services, Division of Nursing. (1980). *Survey of Community Health Nursing: 1979* (NTIS No. HRP-0904449). Hyattsville, MD: DN, PHS, DHHS.

U.S. Department of Health and Human Services. (1981). *Prospectus on Health Maintenance Organizations* (DHHS Pub. No. PHS 82-50180). Rockville, MD: DHHS.

U.S. Department of Health and Human Services, Bureau of Health Professions. (1982). *Public Health Personnel in the United States* (DHHS Pub. No. HRA 82-6). Hyattsville, MD: BHP, DHHS.

U.S. Department of Health and Human Services, Division of Nursing. (1982). *Nurse Supply, Distribution and Requirements: Third Report to Congress: Nurse Training Act of 1975* (DHHS Pub. No. HRA 82-7). Hyattsville, MD: DN, PHS, DHHS.

U.S. Department of Health and Human Services, Office of Disease Prevention and Health Promotion (1982). *Prevention 1982* (DHHS Pub. No. 82-50157). Hyattsville, MD: DHHS.

U.S. Department of Health and Human Services. (1988). *Disease Prevention/ Health Promotion; The Facts*. Palo Alto, CA: Bulletin.

U.S. Department of Health and Human Services, PHS. (1990). *Healthy People 2000: National Health Promotion and Disease Prevention Objectives* (DHHS Pub. No. PHS 91-50212). Washington, DC: U.S. Government Printing Office.

United States Statutes, At Large. (1965). *89th Congress, First Session, Volume 79*. Washington, DC: U.S. Government Printing Office.

Verran, J. A. (1981). Delineation of ambulatory care nursing practice. *Journal of Ambulatory Care Management*, 4(2), 1–13.

Woerner, L., Donnelly, P., and Edwards, P. (1993). Challenges facing the home health care industry. *Nursing Dynamics*, 2(1), 5–8.

World Health Organization. (1978). *Primary Health Care: Report of the International Conference on Primary Care, Alma Ata, USSR, 6–12 September, 1978*. Geneva, Switzerland.

# *13*

• • • • • • • • • • • • • • • • • • • • • • •

# OUTCOMES AND GUIDELINES APPLICATIONS

## OBJECTIVES

- Understand outcomes and clinical guidelines applications.
- Describe the concepts of outcomes data management.
- Discuss factors influencing outcomes.
- Describe how clinical practice guidelines can be integrated into the computer-based patient record.
- Discuss advantages and disadvantages of clinical practice guidelines.
- Identify computer usage for analyzing patterns of care: critical paths and profiles of variance.
- Discuss evaluating patterns of care.
- Describe managed care and ambulatory care uses of outcome data.
- Discuss the impediments to progress in the use of outcomes and guidelines.

A shift in attention to the outcomes, effectiveness, and efficiency of care is occurring in the 1990s. And there is no more useful tool than the computer-based patient record (CPR) for managing outcomes data. Outcomes management is an integrated method of monitoring administrative, economic, and clinical variables.

Once costs have been identified, the cost-efficient method can be utilized to achieve outcomes. Unnecessary nursing actions, inefficient methods of work and care delivery, and scheduling and operational management deficiencies all add to the time required to perform work, decrease performance ratings, reduce the ability to achieve outcomes, and add to the costs of care. Underuse of needed, effective, and appropriate care also contributes to poor-quality outcomes and increased costs. Poor-quality care also results when because of lack of education, training, or skills, professional staff cannot carry out appropriate care without injuries or complications.

The focus on outcomes is moving toward transaction data-based quality measurement. All strategies for carrying out quality programs rely on better data and information systems (Institute of Medicine, 1994). This type of focus also puts an emphasis on the utilization of clinical practice guidelines.

Recently attention has been given to the possibility of using clinical practice guidelines developed by the Agency for Health Care Policy and Research (AHCPR) in the CPR (Shortliffe et al., 1992). These guidelines can be useful in managing care, since they define what are appropriate assessment and intervention procedures for achieving outcomes while reducing variability in practice. A computer with clinical practice guideline content embedded can improve the collection of accurate data to act as a decision platform upon which to guide practice.

This chapter will integrate the concepts of outcomes data management, clinical practice guidelines as content in the CPR, review criteria developed from clinical practice guidelines, and development of feedback systems to monitor critical paths, performance, and benchmarks of care, and ultimately cost out care through the CPR.

## OUTCOMES DATA MANAGEMENT

### Definition

One definition of an outcome is the "end result" of a treatment or intervention. While this definition looks and sounds simple, in practice, establishing realistic outcomes is very difficult. What is the outcome of incontinence? Dryness or the absence of wet clothes? What is the outcome of pain? Comfort or the absence of pain? What is the outcome of mobility impairment? The ability to walk, or the ability to move from wheelchair to chair? In many types of health services research, nursing research, and management literature, many types of outcomes are being discussed and described. Outcomes management examines the treatment of clinical conditions rather than individual procedures or treatments. It is the systematic assessment of clinical nursing practice, encompassing outcomes that are relevant to patients—mortality, morbidity, complications, symptom reduction, and functional status improvement. Physiologic or biologic indicators are also included (Donaldson and Capron, 1991).

## Nursing Indicators Associated with Outcomes

Table 13.1 is a partial listing of the types of indicators that might be integrated into computers to describe outcomes management. Many of the indicators listed are wrapped up in the terms "health status "and "health-related quality of life." Health status measures clinical, biological, and physiological status such as morbidity, mortality, and blood pressure, hemoglobin, or temperature. Health-related quality of life measures physical functions such as activities of daily living (ADL), instrumental ADL, emotional and psychological functions and well-being, social functioning and support, role functioning, general health perceptions, pain, vitality (energy/fatigue), and cognitive functioning. The ideal outcome documentation in the CPR would include disease-specific data elements and health-related quality of life measurements. The tools for measuring health status and health-related quality of life are described to date for one disease or condition only, and not all diseases or patient conditions have a valid identified health status tool identified with them.

Once nurse managers have a measure of health-related quality of life, these data can be correlated with age, income, geographic location of patients, severity of illness, and patient intensity of nursing index. Also, once these data are available from data management sources within a hospital for groups of patients with the same condition, or even the individual patient, there would be the capability to present longitudinal data to study health status and health-related quality of life over time. These types of systems would also help to define episodes of care, i.e., when a

**TABLE 13.1**   A PARTIAL LISTING OF THE TYPES OF INDICATORS THAT MIGHT BE INTEGRATED INTO COMPUTERS TO DESCRIBE OUTCOME MANAGEMENT

- Physiological status
- Psychosocial patterns of behavior, communications, and relationships, both interpersonal and intrapersonal
- Function measures related to activities of daily living, mobility, and communication
- Behavioral activities, skills, and actions
- Cognitive level of understanding (knowledge) about diet, medications, and treatment
- Symptom management and control such as fatigue, nausea, constipation, pain, incontinence, and diarrhea
- Quality of life measures, including life satisfaction, well-being, and standard of living
- Home functioning, including family living patterns, home environment, support and role function, and family strain
- Utilization of services like length of stay, number of clinic visits, and rehospitalizations
- Safety
- Resolution of the clinical condition
- Patient satisfaction, patient preference
- Caring and coping

patient's problem begins and when it "ends." They would make it possible to define which nursing procedures were attached to which episode or patient condition.

## Other Factors Associated with Outcome Indicators

Confounding outcomes attainment are significant risk factors. These include demographics, health status, medical severity of illness, and patient intensity of nursing; etiologic factors such as allergies and infections; intrinsic factors such as genetic predisposition, age, sex, and socioeconomic status; and environmental factors such as culture, living arrangements, and occupational exposures.

Statistical ways of tracking outcomes includes risk-adjusted probability or incidence and adjustment and standardization. In the former, the individual is given a risk factor or odds ratio of achieving an outcome. In the latter, the outcomes of a group are compared to a larger standard at the state or local level, often called a "benchmark."

Factors influencing outcomes that are not usually considered in designing a database for outcomes are (1) socioeconomic and (2) sociodemographic characteristics of patients; for example, it is difficult to cure pneumonia in older patients who are homeless, and it is difficult to cure otitis media in children who are homeless. Unless we build computer systems that can correlate the outcomes with the patient demographics, it will be difficult to determine if the outcomes are a result of nursing care or of the patient's environmental, demographic, social, or economic condition. Similarly, without demographic data it is impossible to determine the organizational characteristics of different groups of patients, e.g., illegal immigrants consuming "free" services. Demographic data are also needed to relate outcomes to the role and influence of co-morbidities, such as a history of substance abuse or the age of patient. The outcome of hip fracture surgery for an 82-year-old patient is different if the person is blind from cataracts, has diabetes, or has a history of hypertension.

Another missing component in many systems to measure outcomes is the necessity of determining who delivered the care. When multidisciplinary care is delivered in some environments, patients may see up to 100 personnel in a 24-hour period. The contributions of all those persons toward outcomes need to be clearly recorded. For example, a patient in the intensive care environment may have ventilation monitored by anesthesia, pulmonary medicine, surgery, nursing, respiratory therapy, and/or physical therapy. Contributions toward outcomes by all deliverers of patient care—medical, surgical, nursing, and allied health professionals—need to be retrievable in the automated record.

Oftentimes there is a lack of good baseline or assessment data prior to the patient's being diagnosed. For example, when tracking the outcomes of a surgical procedure, the patient's functional status before surgery is often not available in the patient record. When the outcome of surgery involves knowing if the patient's functional status has improved, the absence of baseline data is critical. If a patient has been a smoker and the pulmonary status has not been assessed prior to surgery, then postoperative pulmonary complications are more difficult to prevent or predict, the outcomes attributable to interventions are nearly impossible to describe, and the treatment of the complication is more difficult to attribute to the cause. Table 13.2 is a composite list of data required in the patient record for better integration of outcomes with patient care (Barrett, 1992, 1993; McCormick, 1991, O'Brien-Pallas et al., 1994).

## Tools to Collect Outcome Information

There are many tools described in the literature that can be automated to produce outcomes information. But what are "gold standards" for monitoring outcomes? While clinical trials and cost data may be the best gold standards to date, nursing has not had frequent access to these expensive research methodologies. Feinstein (1987) says that when gold standards are too expensive or too difficult to obtain, we need good substitutes. This section will describe some of the acceptable substitutes that nursing has already developed or tools developed by other disciplines that may have application in nursing.

## Statistical Packages

The simplest tools for collecting outcomes data are described in Chapter 15. They are the simple statistical packages that provide aggregate data and can graph trends and provide simple regression curves to determine if a patient is improving, stabilizing, or deteriorating (McCormick, 1991). Multivariate statistical models can be used to evaluate trends in large groups of patients.

### Financial Claims Data

Wennberg et al. (1987) described the use of financial claims data to examine small area analysis and variation. Using Medicare data tapes, they provided proof that the differences in utilization or differences in care provided from one geographic area to another result from decisions that providers make after their patients contact them. Variation rates in medical versus surgical procedures were studied by Cromwell and Mitchell (1988), who found that variation rates in surgery are related not only to supply and demand, but also to medical need, ability to pay, and the availability of substitute sources of care. It is not usually possible to define what causes the practice variations: cultural differences, skills, availability of services, or lack of information. Few studies of area variation, iden-

**TABLE 13.2**　　A COMPOSITE LIST OF DATA REQUIRED IN THE PATIENT
RECORD FOR BETTER INTEGRATION OF OUTCOMES WITH
PATIENT CARE

**Administrative**

- Critical pathways library
- Patient demographics
- Dates of service
- Attending physician
- Primary care nurse
- Case manager (clinical nurse specialist)

- Insurance carrier(s)/address/phone number
- Carrier contact person
- Coverage/benefits
- Living will/medical power of attorney status
- Service type

**Clinical**

- Diagnosis/DRG
- Procedures/treatments/tests
- ADL limits
- Patient history and physical/assessment
- Acuity/severity of illness
- Abnormal test results
- Nursing diagnoses/problem list
- Nursing interventions
- Progress notes for abnormal response/results
- Medications and allergies

- Variance from critical pathway
- Measurable quality outcomes
- Discharge status
- Facility transferred to
- Referrals to external providers/consultants
- Outpatient service needs
- Home health needs
- Family support
- Community services
- Risk management issues

**Profitability**

- Outstanding account balance
- Services denied by insurance

- Costs of care
- Reimbursement

**Suggested Reporting**

- Critical path variance by
  - Patient
  - Physician
  - Primary care nurse
  - DRG/diagnoses
  - Nursing diagnoses/problem list
- Concurrent resource management indicating
  - Charges to date
  - Procedures/services provided to date
  - Costs (charges) compared to expected reimbursement
  - Variances between charges and expected reimbursement

- Retrospective variation between costs and actual reimbursement by
  - Patient
  - Physician
  - Primary care nurse
  - DRG/diagnoses
  - Nursing diagnoses/problem list
  - Procedures/treatments/tests
  - Nursing interventions

*Source:* Adapted from Barrett, 1993.

tification of trends in nursing procedures, or readmission patterns have
been conducted by nurses using claims data. As more outcomes databases
are developed, more nursing variation studies should be published in the
nursing literature.

## Appropriateness Research

Appropriateness research by RAND incorporates a process beginning with the selection of procedures, then going through a literature review, clinician input, development of a list of indications for the performance of a procedure, creation of computer software, preparation of training materials, and concluding with updating standards. The extent of the appropriateness of a procedure is based on a Delphi ranking process applied by a panel of clinicians to the audit of patient records (Chassin, 1988). Measuring appropriateness, obtaining interrater reliability between panels of experts, and obtaining consensus of multidisciplinary groups remain challenges of this methodology.

## Meta-Analysis

Meta-analysis is another tool of statistical analysis that is used to synthesize the results of outcomes literature. Other methodologies to analyze outcomes and synthesize results include confidence intervals, indirect evidence, biostatistical and regulatory methods, pattern analysis, and path analysis (McCormick et al., 1994). Not all statistical tools will be valid and reliable for all patient conditions.

## WARE SF-36

The WARE SF-36 defines such domains as physical health, mental health, social and role functioning, and general perceptions of well-being, and is being used successfully with many patient groups (Ware, 1987; Ware and Berwick, 1989; Ware and Sherbournes, 1992). The Health Outcomes Institute has also developed a national study of 18 conditions and a national questionnaire of health status related to those outcomes (HSQ)(Health Outcomes Institute, 1994). The conditions that are being studied are angina, asthma, carpal tunnel, cataract, chronic sinusitis, COPD, depression, diabetes, hip fracture, hip replacement, hypertension, low back pain, osteoarthritis of the knee, panic disorder, prostatism, rheumatoid arthritis, stroke, and substance abuse with alcohol. Patterns or patient profiles of pain, mobility, or other variables are described prehospitalization, postoperatively, and for 6 to 12 months follow-up.

# Issues in Selecting Tools

There are several issues that are important in selecting tools. Most of these are research issues and are beyond the scope of this chapter. They are:

- Conceptual compatibility
- Consistency of purpose
- Sensitivity/responsiveness to change
- Approaches to data collection
- Approaches to scoring and weighting
- Metric properties of the instrument—reliability and validity

- Feasibility and practicality
  - —Different tools are needed for ambulatory care settings.
  - —Different tools are needed for measuring organizational outcomes rather than individuals alone.
  - —Relatively few scales can be used with pediatric subjects, and many scales are difficult to use with demented patients and are time-consuming.

## Issues Delaying Outcomes Data Collection

Most nursing information systems have the potential to include outcomes data, but nurses do not always document the outcomes of care. Common data limitations include the absence of core nursing data sets in many information systems (e.g., outpatient surgery and ambulatory care encounters), incomplete information on existing data sets (lack of detailed documented information), inaccurate or incomplete coding (failure to document all of the patients' problems on the discharge abstracts), and incomplete identification of the population at risk (for example, patients with co-morbidities from hypertension, asthma, or diabetes). In addition, the data tapes used to monitor trends in health care, patients' conditions, or financial uses of resources do not currently include nursing or outcomes information. Therefore, use of these tapes is often supplemented with medical record review and prospective data collection in health care facilities, which is very time-consuming. In order to manage the outcomes data in the future, several prerequisites in database management will have to be put in place. Some of these are included in Table 13.3.

**TABLE 13.3**     PREREQUISITES RELATED TO OUTCOMES DATA THAT NEED TO BE RESOLVED

- Incorporate nursing outcomes measures into existing and new health services.
- Research data sources at the hospital, local, state, HMO, and national levels.
- Develop standard data elements.
- Develop a common patient identifier.
- Develop a unique nursing identifier.
- Develop data security standards.
- Develop a standard to label health care events.
- Create longitudinal data sets.
- Utilize networks of care to provide larger sample sizes for analyses.
- Utilize managed care settings, since they represent ideal research laboratories because they are closed health care systems.
- Utilize Defense Department databases, since this department has been delivering care for several decades.

# CLINICAL PRACTICE GUIDELINES IN OUTCOMES DOCUMENTATION

## Guidelines Linked to the CPR

Why guidelines? Professional associations, academic and private institutions, insurers, hospitals, managed care associations, and even the U.S. government have been developing clinical practice guidelines during the last decade (1) because of the variability in practice, (2) because it has been difficult to define what quality of care is, and (3) because much of the information that clinicians need is not in a useful format.

Clinical practice guidelines developed by the AHCPR are defined as "systematically developed statements to assist practitioners and patients in decisions of what is appropriate in health care for specific clinical circumstances" (Institute of Medicine, 1990). Other names given to clinical practice guidelines are practice parameters (American Medical Association), guidelines, consensus conference summary reports, U.S. Preventive Task Force Statement reports, and clinical trials outcome reports. For the purpose of this chapter, the IOM definition of a clinical practice guideline will be assumed.

The methodology for developing a clinical practice guideline yields a product with broad application that can be used as content in the CPR. Developing a guideline involves nine steps: (1) multidisciplinary panel members are selected to develop the guidelines; (2) the panels conduct an extensive review of the international literature to determine what the variabilities in practice are and what outcomes for the diagnosis and treatment of conditions are currently known; (3) where there is sufficient information, summary statistics are processed on the variables and practice data, and in many data sets meta-analytic statistics can be computed; (4) where the literature is lacking, the panel develops consensus statements to fill in the missing knowledge gaps; (5) the panel invites broad national input into the guideline by hosting an open meeting to receive testimony from professional associations, activist groups, industry representatives, and research and development companies; (6) the panel invites peer review from other scientists and practitioners from throughout the United States and other foreign countries to determine the validity of the literature statements and to broaden the field of consensus where literature is lacking; (7) the panel develops algorithms based upon the logic of the practice guideline (Hadorn et al., 1992); (8) the panel conducts a cost analysis of the baseline costs and simulates the projected costs from the clinical practice guideline; and (9) the panel publishes a quick reference booklet, a guideline book with references, and a consumer version that are all in the public domain.

## Advantages of Clinical Practice Guidelines

An advantage of having clinical practice guidelines driving the content of CPRs is that the guideline content has defined outcomes that can be achieved. In addition, well-developed guidelines have scientific validity and reliability, and have had broad peer review. An alternative is to have the content of the CPR integrated with network servers to check the validity and reliability of concurrent documentation. This eliminates the need to develop "boutique" content in CPRs from state to state or even hospital to hospital. Clinical practice guidelines provide a national recommendation of what constitutes best practice patterns for assessment and interventions related to clinical conditions to achieve quality outcomes of care.

## Disadvantages of National Guidelines

A disadvantage of national guidelines is that very frequently locally adapted procedures still need to be added to the content of the guidelines, since the practitioners have developed procedures that are known to produce positive outcomes, but have not published their findings. If guidelines were pretested in CPRs at multiple clinical sites prior to release, many of the local variabilities could be predicted before issuing the clinical practice guidelines.

Another disadvantage of clinical practice guidelines is that clinical practice may ultimately have patients with 9,999 identified conditions, yet the clinical practice guidelines and practice standards released to date number only 1,500, and there is much duplication and overlap in statements. There is no clearinghouse for content where there is duplication or even contradictory recommendations from developers of different guidelines. However, although there are about 9,999 identified conditions of health care and over 100 nursing diagnoses, only 4 conditions account for one-third of the mortality in hospitals: stroke, heart attack, congestive heart failure, and pneumonia.

Guidelines are also time-consuming to write and expensive to produce. This factor would tend to discourage local development of guidelines. Also, if local development of guidelines proliferates, the "boutique" content in the CPRs will prevail. Continuation of the variability in content could be more costly than producing guidelines.

In the future, national multidisciplinary panels could be convened in order to review the best practice patterns and outcomes already in place on CPRs. If the best practice patterns vary by geographical or clinical location, the guidelines would be more flexible in describing these practice recommendations. The CPR eliminates the need for guidelines to be developed the way they currently are; however, a national structure to monitor best practices would need to be formed to conduct analyses of practice patterns, practice variability, and practice outcomes. This national effort could be a public service or remain in the private sector through hospital accrediting organizations or professional organizations.

## Guideline Updates

The usual length of life of any technology and content is at best 18 months. Therefore, the commitment to clinical practice guidelines as the content driving the content in the CPR is a commitment to updating and continually improving these guidelines. For example, for the first three guidelines released by AHCPR in the spring of 1992, thousands of journal articles and other literature sources were reviewed. By the spring of 1994, each multidisciplinary panel was reviewing hundreds to thousands of new pieces of evidence, new devices, new drugs, and new procedures that had been described in the literature. If the guideline content is to remain current to influence best practice, most guidelines need to be updated and a new product released at least every 24 months. An exception to this involves guidelines in areas that generate less literature and where there are few research breakthroughs or new technologies discovered. For the most part, however, guideline update is a commitment of time and money that most local hospitals and managed care associations cannot make. It requires continuous monitoring of the Food and Drug Administration's new releases, the Center for Disease Control's new recommendations, and the National Institutes of Health advances in clinical and biological science, in addition to the extensive amount of published literature and consensus of opinion.

## Guidelines Linked to Quality Management

Translation of clinical practice guidelines into review criteria is also a mandate of the AHCPR clinical practice guideline program. The translation into review criteria is the link between guidelines and the development of quality review programs. A recent paper provides constructive recommendations and a model for translating clinical practice guidelines into products to be used in quality programs (Kibbe et al., 1994). It assumes that health care is provided in complex organizations, with many multidisciplinary professionals delivering care. It assumes that organizational components that lead to quality include availability and timeliness of service, adequate staffing and training for skill mix, and the achievement of acceptable cost levels. Outcomes can be the result of multiple subsystems functioning to support patient care. The stages the authors propose for adoption of guidelines in an organizational quality program are described below.

### Recognition

The first stage is recognition that the organization is not fully meeting the expectations for outcomes identified in the guideline, or is not within the boundaries of acceptable procedures, treatments, or outcomes for the specific condition. This stage involves collecting baseline information to determine what the procedures to resolve a clinical problem currently are, what the interventions are, and what outcomes are being achieved. Feedback to health provider staff that inappropriate procedures are being used or outcomes are not being achieved provides background information to discuss possible solutions, including guidelines.

## Identification

Identification that the guidelines can be used to improve the outcomes of care given is the next step. At this stage actual steps in the organization to solve problems need to be identified. Panels of hospital experts and personnel knowledgeable about quality measurement may be convened to determine alternative methods for solving organizational problems. National guidelines may be one tool to adapt for local use.

## Implementation

The next stage is implementation of the guideline by the relevant groups within the organization. Just like any educational improvement, implementation does not occur by itself. Intervention programs facilitate the utilization of guidelines in clinical settings (Soumerai et al., 1993). This often involves in-service education about the content of the guideline and a description of the hospital's current performance related to the condition. The provision of feedback to the clinical groups who have been implementing the guidelines to determine if the guidelines are in fact improving the attainment of outcomes in clinical care is important in the implementation stage. Feedback that outcomes are being achieved is a very important facilitator of the next stage.

## Institutionalization

Institutionalization involves use of the guideline by the relevant clinical groups in the organization. Critical paths and other methods of managing the process of information are useful tools for integrating guidelines into quality programs. Identifying clinical indicators and review criteria are other measures of assuring the integration of guideline content into quality programs. Current research efforts are evaluating the advantages of using clinical practice guidelines to determine their utility in establishing quality review criteria.

These stages are congruent with the process of outcomes management identified by others (Bachrach et al., 1988; Crede and Hierholzer, 1988). It makes the concept of outcomes management broader than monitoring individual provider performance and patient response. Included in the broader process of outcomes management are (1) data elements considered for outcomes monitoring, (2) issues associated with data reliability and validity, (3) issues associated with identifying severity of illness (and patient intensity of nursing index) and the link between severity, complexity, and risk adjustments, (4) issues associated with measuring nursing resource inputs linked to outcomes, and (5) methods of including risk-adjusted outcomes in the analysis (Shamian et al., 1994).

## Issues Related to Implementing Clinical Practice Guidelines

There has been a great deal published in the nursing and medical literature about methods of disseminating best practice ideas and implementing them. Several principles are consistent between models and need consideration. An automated system with the best practice patterns can remain unused if nursing administrators fail to consider several issues related to implementation:

- Models are needed to define dissemination practices to different audiences.
- Models of how consumer and provider behavior can be effectively and efficiently changed need to be developed (e.g., feedback, surveillance, administrative regulation, financial incentives, behavioral management, peer pressure, penalties).
- Mechanisms need to be developed to resolve the issue of conflicts among different practice guidelines recommended by different groups, e.g., there are about 70 guidelines on HIV.
- Strategies are needed to monitor trends in practice patterns and identify changes in these patterns over time.
- The development and use of information management systems and their influence on studying patient outcomes needs to be determined.

Of paramount importance for the decade ahead is the ability to capture "patient preferences" for diagnostic procedures and treatments on the patient documentation systems. When the nurse knows that procedures a, b, and c produce outcomes of 79 percent, 83.2 percent, and 84 percent, respectively, but the complication rates are 20 percent, 40 percent, and 90 percent, the patient will be asked to enter into the decision about treatments to attain the outcomes. Systems for the 1990s and into the twenty-first century will have to capture the patients' preferences for outcomes. When the nurse can offer the incontinent patient cure or complete dryness, but the patient's preferred outcome is just to have dry clothes and no visible wetness, the documentation of the patient's decision needs to be recorded.

Of equal importance will be the necessity to capture the patient's or family's "satisfaction" with care. Oftentimes, even if the outcome is death, the family or significant others will be very satisfied with the nursing care. To capture these data in the new outcomes, databases will be critical.

# Clinical Practice Guidelines Translated to Review Criteria

When clinical practice guidelines are linked to quality assurance and accrediting standards, the retrieval of information should be computerized. Inherent in accomplishing this is the ability to translate the clinical practice guideline into criteria that can be used to review whether clinical practice guidelines have been followed in delivering care (Beavert and Magoffin, 1993; Schoenbaum, et al., 1995).

### Review Criteria

Review criteria are defined as systematically developed statements that can be used to assess the appropriateness of specific health care decisions, services, and outcomes, whereas standards of quality are authoritative statements of (1) minimum levels of acceptable performance or results, (2) excellent levels of performance or results, or (3) the range of acceptable performance or results (Institute of Medicine, 1992).

Performance measures are methods or instruments to estimate or monitor the extent to which the actions of a health care practitioner or provider conform to practice guidelines, medical review criteria, or standards of quality. Standards can be set by the hospital, by a professional group, or for specific clinical conditions (Institute of Medicine, 1992; Duggar and Palmer, 1995).

A professional association or private-sector accrediting association needs to set the rate at which it will consider selective practices a standard. Current standards of practice can be better defined in terms of best practice when the CPR is utilized to provide such data on large local, state, or national groups. For example, if the guideline on urinary incontinence states that the patient should have behavioral intervention to become 100 percent dry, the nursing profession can establish a rate of 85 percent performance as a national standard. By monitoring patient documentation throughout the country to determine if the nursing profession is using behavioral interventions to attain 100 percent dryness, the rate of 85 percent could be published as a national professional standard.

While many hospitals have used continuous quality improvement (CQI) or total quality management (TQM) to improve areas such as billing, purchasing, and departmental management, they have only just begun to use them to reduce unnecessary variation in procedures and outcomes. Models integrating the guidelines into quality assurance programs are being developed to determine if the natural variations in patients and conditions can allow this industrial model to work in health care.

Regardless of the type of quality assurance program that the nursing profession uses, some type of review criteria needs to be developed. Part of the uncertainty of clinicians in practice today arises because they are unaware of the over 1500 review criteria that are in place to review care for patients with the same condition. The review criteria are imposed by hospital accrediting organizations, private insurers, federal payers and providers, entitlement programs, HMOs, managed care sites, and others.

If CPRs with clinical practice guidelines embedded have one set of review criteria to make a determination if quality of care is delivered, this simplifies clinical practice. An example of a match between recommendations from a guideline and review criteria developed to match those recommendations is given in Table 13.4. A nursing example of urinary incontinence is used because both the clinical practice guidelines and the review criteria have been developed by national committees with funding from the AHCPR (Urinary Incontinence Guideline Panel, 1992).

## Translating Guidelines
One of the steps in translating guidelines to review criteria is the development of algorithms for scoring the criteria developed from each guideline. These algorithms help to reveal the logic in the written criteria and can also be computerized (Schoenbaum, et al., 1995).

**TABLE 13.4**   GUIDELINE AND REVIEW CRITERIA FOR NURSING HISTORY

**Guideline—Patient History**

- Patient identification
- Person's sex
- Age
- Frequency of incontinent episodes
- Volume of incontinent episodes (small or large)
- Patient's use of protection pads, briefs, etc.
- Number of pads, briefs, etc., used per day/per week
- Length of time the patient has had this problem
- Medications patient is currently taking
- Type of situations that precipitate incontinence (key in the door, cold water, cold air, a cough, a sneeze, aerobic exercise, standing from a sitting position)
- Presence of other urinary tract symptoms (nocturia, dysuria, hesitancy, straining, interrupted stream, hematuria, pain, frequency, urgency, increased leakage)
- Other medical or neurologic conditions
- Fluid intake pattern
- Routine bowel and bladder habits
- Sexual function
- Social/environmental factors

**Review Criteria—History**

- HX:1   A focused history was done.
- HX:2   A history of urinary symptoms was taken.
- HX:3   A history of neurological problems was taken.
- HX:4   A history of gyn or urinary problems was taken.
- HX:5   A treatment history was taken.
- HX:6   If patient is dependent, a social/environmental history was taken.

The translation of guidelines into review criteria is important to nursing because (1) review criteria are the basic structure for evidence-based performance measurement in nursing practice, (2) review criteria provide explicit statements that clinicians, health care organizations, payers, and quality and utilization reviewers can use to determine if the process of care conforms with guideline content, (3) review criteria offer a means to improve the value and credibility of oversight from federal payers, certification agencies, licensure, malpractice, workers' compensation, and regulation of utilization review, and (4) review criteria inform state efforts in profiling health care costs and utilization data.

## Quality Assurance

Quality assurance computerized systems focus on research to describe, measure, and deliver quality care to patient. Quality of care models, nursing standards, and compliance requirements have been recommended by the Joint Commission on Accreditation of Health Care Organizations (JCAHO). Quality assurance systems have many benefits. Data must be reliable and the quality of the data must be analyzed. Donabedian distinguished between the definition and measurement of health and the definition and measurement of quality. Quality of care measurements need to be both applied to the study of quality of care and included in the quality assurance information systems (Donabedian, 1966; Hegyvary, 1991).

## Guidelines Linked to Malpractice Protection

According to Shortliffe et al. (1992), much of health care is practiced defensively; thus the use of unnecessary or duplicate practices could be monitored if clinical practice guidelines were incorporated into the computerized documentation (Shortliffe et al., 1992). Recent malpractice reductions in the state of Massachusetts of as much as 20 percent from monitoring practice for completeness with machine-readable formats to chart patient encounters are encouraging. Several other authors in health care are describing the positive influence guidelines could have on malpractice protection (Garnick et al., 1991; Hirshfield, 1991).

## CPR Scenario Linked to Clinical Practice Guidelines

This section provides a scenario of a nurse encounter with the documentation in a CPR in which clinical practice guideline data are embedded. The guidelines now become available at the point of service; they are an integral part of the documentation, rather than a book on a shelf, a policy document, or another part of the information system. The documentation is now based upon current science and the best practices known within the past 2 years, rather than on research that might be 5 to 10 years old. Since this is just a scenario, many of the technical details and capabilities of systems have been left out. However, many microcomputer vendors already have integrated guidelines into the content of their systems.

Upon admission, the nurse sees a patient, using a hand-held computer or a notebook. On the computer the nurse types the cause of admission, or the patient's major condition. In our example, the patient will be seen for urinary incontinence. The nurse is prompted by the computer to ask a series of history and physical questions. They include, for example,

- Patient identification
- Sex
- Age
- Frequency of incontinent episodes
- Volume of incontinent episodes (small or large)
- Types of protection (pads, briefs, etc.) the patient uses
- Number of pads, briefs, etc., used per day or per week
- Length of time the patient has had this problem
- Medications the patient is currently taking
- Type of situations that precipitate incontinence (key in the door, cold water, cold air, a cough, a sneeze, aerobic exercise, standing from a sitting position)
- The presence of other urinary tract symptoms (nocturia, dysuria, hesitancy, straining, interrupted stream, hematuria, pain, frequency, urgency, increased leakage)
- Other medical or neurologic conditions
- Fluid intake pattern
- Routine bowel and bladder habits
- Sexual function
- Social/environmental factors

After this brief history, the nurse is asked to fill in the descriptors after looking at the genitourinary area, abdominal area, pelvic area, and rectal area, and doing a general exam (a cognitive exam for dependent patients) to identify co-morbidities. They include

- Skin integrity
- Color
- Presence of a full bladder (estimated post-void residual volume)
- Presence of a full rectum
- Amount of strength during squeeze (internal muscle sphincter, external muscle sphincter)
- Voiding diary

In all incontinent persons, identified transient causes of incontinence need to be documented. They are known as the DIAPPERS characteristics for this condition. They represent the following characteristics:

- **D**elirium
- **I**nfection (symptomatic urinary tract infection)
- **A**trophic vaginitis
- **P**harmaceuticals that affect continence (sedative hypnotics, diuretics, anticholinergic agents, alpha-adrenergic agents, calcium-channel blockers)
- **P**sychological factors (especially depression)
- **E**xcessive urine production
- **R**estricted mobility
- **S**tool impaction

This example is based on the logic contained in a small laptop computer designed to validate the urinary incontinence guideline (Dufresne et al., 1994).

After sending the urine for urinalysis and entering the results, the nurse is given the following probable nursing diagnoses of the patient's condition: stress urinary incontinence, urge urinary incontinence, combined stress and urge incontinence, or neurogenic incontinence secondary to another condition. This is a decision support system that includes diagnosis and treatment decisions. Even after being given these options, however, the nurse must use professional judgment to determine if the condition suggested by the computerized system is probable and likely.

The next selection that the computer generates is probable nursing interventions for this patient. They include

- Patient education
- A two-hour toileting schedule
- Pelvic muscle exercises
- Medication (local or systemic)
- Biofeedback
- Vaginal cones
- A recommendation to send the patient to an obstetrician/gynecologist or urologist for a consultation
- Electrical stimulation

If the team is using a critical path approach, a computer-generated critical path can be printed to plan interventions, visits, monitoring points, potential outcomes, and review criteria for quality assurance for the patient for the next 6 to 8 weeks.

Information about the costs of the history, physical, urinalysis, and any other interventions can be embedded in the guidelines. When the decision to select different medications is presented to the nurse, the average costs of those medications can be shown. The comparative costs of alternative treatments can also be shown, e.g., the costs of behavioral intervention compared to vaginal cones compared to biofeedback. Thus, after the nurse documents the care provided, the documentation can be used directly by the financial department or the budget manager to capture costs, estimate expected reimbursement, and determine actual expenses compared to patient or reimbursement payment. This concept is covered in more depth in Chap. 9.

## Data Needs of Health Providers

Different health providers require different data for different purposes. For example, the nurse administrator may desire patient classification data to determine the type and amount of nursing resources required, whereas the clinician is interested in determining if outcomes are met and how care can improve outcomes in future patients, labeling health care episodes by interventions that affect outcomes, and determining what influences the choice of diagnostic and therapeutic procedures. The hospital administrator, on the other hand, usually wants to identify the total resources needed to meet requirements of each patient episode and produce patient satisfaction in order to market the hospital to future patients. The same set of outcomes and cost data may not be useful to all persons for all purposes in health care.

As follow-up, the nurse can enter into the computer the number of episodes of incontinence per day/per week/per month and establish a baseline. Each time the patient is seen, the patient should be put on a regular toileting schedule and the results entered into the computer. An example of the results over 7 weeks to determine progress is shown in Fig. 13.1. The planned outcome is 100 percent dry; and this figure shows a patient with a remarkable improvement during just 7 weeks of behavioral treatment. By following the episodes of incontinence per day, the nurse can see the improvement in the patient at weekly intervals. If the patient is not improving, treatment can be stopped or changed to another intervention, or the patient can be maintained on the program for up to 8 weeks (in an outpatient setting) before determining if there will be improvement.

If the patient is being seen as an outpatient, he or she keeps daily records and brings them into the clinic during routine follow-up. Before the patient is examined, the data are entered into the computer, so that the clinician can see the patient's level of improvement, stabilization, or deterioration before examining the patient. In the example, the review criteria stated that within 72 hours of admission, the hospitalized patient should have a history, physical, and urinalysis. The documentation demonstrates that these were done, and the questions match those that should be asked of all incontinent patients. Similarly, the review criteria examine the recommended intervention procedures, determine the effectiveness of the intervention, and provide follow-up on the patient's outcome over time. The outcome becomes broader than mortality and morbidity, because the

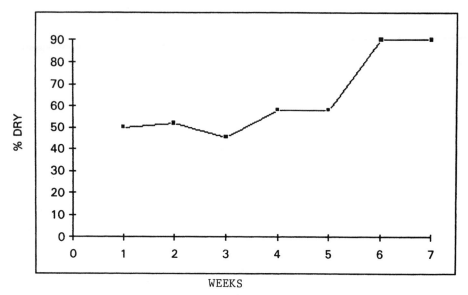

**Figure 13.1**  Outcomes of a patient showing improvement over 7 weeks. (Adapted from P. Spath, *Succeeding with Critical Paths,* Brown-Spath & Associates, Forest Grove, OR, 1993.)

actual outcome for this patient's condition is documented. These same criteria will suffice for hospital accreditation documentation without additional documentation as the JCAHO Agenda for Change becomes implemented.

With the guidelines driving the content for documentation and the review criteria driving the assurance of quality, the well-designed computer of the next decade will simply need "review criteria-enter" typed in, and all variances from quality assurance will be printed out. This is the same function that discharge planning moved to when computerized discharge planning was defined. Upon discharge, typing in "discharge plan" automatically prints all remaining unfilled orders and goals in patient care. The corollary can now exist with review criteria for quality assurance.

In the past, quality assurance has focused on structure and process; only recently has it begun to focus on outcomes. With that change, there has now been a shift to focus on the behavior changes in the physician and nurse providers of care (Donabedian, 1991). Nursing behavior change is currently an area requiring new nursing research.

## Guidelines Linked to Decision Analysis in Tracking Outcomes

Computerized documentation allows clinical practice guidelines in tracking outcomes at the point of service to be used for decision making to improve clinical care. Oftentimes, intervention and outcome information is not available from the literature. The decision analysis model provides a mechanism for linking interventions to outcomes when the evidence is not available (Owens and Nease, 1993). Although several approaches are useful in guideline development, influence diagrams to make the choices between length of life, quality of life, and costs when looking at the overall value of an intervention related to a condition have been described in the literature. Each of these methods helps to delineate the explicit links between interventions and outcomes, whether they are literature-based or consensus-based.

### Nursing Decision Support Systems

Nursing decision support systems encompass the results of decision analysis studies. Such studies generally focus on the development of nurses' skills in decision making, analysis strategies, clinical reasoning, and theories of skill acquisition. Decision analysis theories use patient care data to study nurses' cognitive processes, problem-solving techniques, and clinical simulation criteria. Case simulations, knowledge engineering, and protocol analysis studies have been used to describe problem-solving techniques. They provide the basis for expert systems and artificial intelligence (AI) models that are being developed (Brennan and McHugh, 1988).

Nurses use these modeling systems to solve a decision problem when more analysis is needed instead of more data. Modeling is one approach to providing decision support. There are several software packages that build models to provide nurses with decision support capabilities. Decision support systems generally use one of two models to construct their decision problem, from which a course of action to achieve a specific outcome is determined.

The decision-analytic model in nursing relies on rules to determine the outcome with the greatest probability of achievement, whereas the multiple criteria model dictates the best course of action based on choices. A computerized decision support system developed by Brennan links computer technology with decision-making algorithms to support decisions made by nurses providing clinical care.

### Expert Systems

Chang has developed an expert system model that outlines the components of an expert system. An expert system is a computer program that uses AI technology to represent human logic, knowledge, experience, and judgment for a specific domain. Chang's expert system model illustrates the relationships between three modules: (1) the factual data or knowledge base, (2) the influence engine controlling the rules of the knowledge base, and (3) the user interface which allows the nurse to communicate with the expert system. Expert systems are used in health care to address a clinical, educational, or research problem (Chang, 1988).

An expert system for nursing diagnosis based on nurses' orientation to patients, setting, health status, and nursing actions was also developed by Chang. She used three models for the rules to determine the level of dependency, using a different approach to weighting the conditions; namely: Model I, Critical Element Approach; Model II, Score-Averaging Approach; and Model III, Arbitrary Weighting. This approach provided the conditions for collecting and analyzing patient data. Chang used a commercially available software package to serve as the building tools or shell for the development of the expert system. It facilitated the three approaches used in the model.

In a review of most decision support systems that can be used to attain medical and nursing outcomes, a nursing system that met all of the criteria of decision support to attain outcomes was found to have been developed on the nursing diagnosis of urinary incontinence (Johnston et al., 1994; Petrucci et al., 1992). More decision support systems to support achieving health outcomes need to be developed by nursing professionals.

## Guidelines on Networks

The content of a guideline on the Internet or other international networks or servers can be used by any clinician in the United States or other countries. Thus the guideline helps to break down the cultural barriers in health care by providing a framework for a clinical condition based upon the international literature and consensus opinion. Electronic on-line communication systems are used to disseminate information and offer communication between persons. As well as on-line communication, the major types of systems include electronic teleconference networks, electronic bulletin boards, and electronic mail.

Communication network systems used for the on-line transmission of computer-based databases are also used to access and transmit on-line the results of bibliographic literature searches and information from knowledge bases. The electronic teleconference networks, bulletin boards, and E-mail are used to disseminate the synthesis of research through guidelines, research findings, conclusions, and results from the researchers to the users.

## PATTERNS OF CARE

In evaluating care, the CPR documentation is used to understand the logic of diagnosis, planning, interventions, and outcomes achieved. Trends toward prospective management or point-of-service management are emerging, since retrospective management offers less opportunity to rationally manage care.

For identification of patterns of care, and of providers who are high performers or low performers, data are needed over time and in relation to the outcomes of care achieved. The patient record becomes the site for placing clinically relevant events into units of analysis, describing the persons served, and summarizing these events. This type of analysis is becoming especially important to clinical nurse specialists who serve as profile managers or case managers.

The data elements required for such evaluations need to be stored in such a way that the data managers do not have to peruse the entire patient record. The important input data in the patient record need to be identified so that the output criteria can be matched to them, in order to determine if adequate care was delivered. Clinical practice guidelines can be used to provide the input into documentation systems. The review criteria from these guidelines can then be used to monitor if the data elements relevant to the review of the case were present (Silva and Zawilski, 1992).

The utility of collecting information in administration is that the information can be managed to support the evaluation of quality of care, patterns of variation in services, utilization, and outcomes achieved (Davies, 1992). Quality of care can be expanded to include studies of clinical competence (decision making, accuracy of diagnosis, recording behavior), the appropriateness of the diagnosis and therapeutic interventions and procedures used, and the effectiveness of treatment procedures, drugs, and technology. Patterns of variation include providers, resources, procedures, tests, drugs, treatments, geographic area, patient type, specialty or provider type, and location of care.

Utilization includes the definition of the episode of care and a calculation of the advantages of preventive versus palliative services.

As mentioned earlier in this chapter, outcomes include broader concepts than morbidity and mortality, and are extended to include case mix, severity, co-morbidities, adverse events, health status, functional status, and patient satisfaction.

## Critical Paths

A critical path (critical pathway) is "a description of key events in the process of patient care, that if performed as described, is expected to produce the most desirable outcomes. The critical path is a case management tool that helps the patient care team to reach a defined goal for a particular patient in the most efficient, effective manner" (Spath, 1993). According to Spath, this stop-and-think type of planning reminds clinicians to consider the recommendations made in clinical practice guidelines during their process of delivering care.

In 1988, Zander began writing about the New England Medical Center Hospital's critical path management of patient care (Zander, 1988). People who write about the use of critical paths describe more effective patient outcomes, reductions in system inefficiencies, and improved team-work among care givers. In case after case, where critical paths have been implemented, hospitals boast of decreased length of stays, decreased patient complications, decreased total costs, increased patient satisfaction, and decreased mortality. The reason for the supposed successes can be attributed to successful management of (1) system breakdown, (2) communication breakdown, and (3) variations in practice patterns (Spath, 1993).

A critical path is built by identifying the major functions of a care process and the critical elements necessary to complete these major functions. In clinical practice these processes and elements are endless unless boundaries are placed on the critical elements. The clinical practice guidelines are tools that can be used to begin to define the team's approach to a patient condition.

Critical paths can be step-oriented, time-oriented to the hours or days the patient is being seen, or oriented to levels of care such as movement from the ER, to the ICU, to the Step-Down Unit, to Home; or from the Labor Suite to the Delivery Suite, first 4 h, next 12 h, 20 h, and discharge. In ambulatory care settings, critical paths may use visits as the intervals of time, e.g., first admission, visit 2, visit 3, visit 4, visit 5, visit 6, discharge.

Some organizations have developed patient-oriented versions of the critical path so that the patient understands the path he or she will go through, e.g., the preadmission tests, treatment, medications, pain control, diet, and activity, and the path for the day of surgery.

Critical paths are best used for patients of low nursing intensity because the care is less complex, in patients where there is agreement on the assessment and treatment regimes, and where new advances in treatment need to be implemented in patient care. They can be most helpful when they integrate patient data on continuity of care issues, resource use, utilization management, and payer issues.

Data elements that might be employed in using critical paths include those listed in Table 13.5. This extensive list identifies some of the data that can be used to produce aggregate data and provide profiles or benchmarks of care.

Critical paths need to be updated by the team as new information becomes available, new guidelines are released, or feedback from aggregate patient groups indicates that care is ineffective or inefficient.

## Profiles of Variance

Variance from the critical path is documented with a date and time. This can be done manually or in the CPR with individual patient data, provider data, or aggregate patient data. When an organization attempts to compare its results with those from other organizations who are getting better results and modifying their practices accordingly, this is called "benchmarking." An example of benchmarking comes from severity of illness

**TABLE 13.5**   ELEMENTS FOR CONSIDERATION IN A CRITICAL PATH

1. Overall length of stay
2. Overall costs
3. Costs and charges by department
4. Timing of surgery
5. Number of operating room minutes
6. Number of postoperative recovery room minutes
7. Selection and use of supplies
8. Use of critical care days
9. Use of monitored beds
10. Use of appropriate laboratory tests
11. Use of appropriate radiology exams
12. Appropriate timing of tests
13. Use of appropriate medications, dosage, and route
14. Timing of key events during recovery, such as smoking cessation, dietary instructions, catheter removal, exercise rehabilitation, vaccination
15. Timing of nonphysician interventions
16. Recognition of delayed or missed services
17. Recognition of errors, incidents, iatrogenic events, complications, or other risks
18. Recognition of redundant testing
19. Recognition of inappropriate communication
20. Recognition in achieving outcomes of care
21. Quality of discharge planning
22. Failure to issue stop orders
23. Timing of STAT orders
24. Failure of preparing patients for radiology exams
25. Failure to treat patients with allied health services such as rehabilitation, speech therapy, physical therapy, respiratory therapy
26. Failure to follow clinical practice guidelines
27. Length of time on a specialty service
28. Failure to request/provide specialty consultation in hospital
29. Blood loss from surgery
30. Failure to assess preoperatively for postoperative complications, e.g., pulmonary function in smokers, ADL prior to eye, or hip surgery, continence prior to hip replacement
31. Variability in delivery of procedures
32. Failure of patient compliance within the care setting
33. Failure to write patient orders as required
34. Recognition of patient co-morbidities that take patient out of the critical path plan
35. Recognition of patient mix into nonhomogenous groups
36. Recognition of delays in placing patients in skilled nursing home facilities after discharge
37. Recognition of other delays in patient discharge
38. Inappropriate discharge planning
39. Failure to report communicable diseases
40. Failure to sign and date orders
41. Acknowledge rehospitalizations
42. Functional and health status at time of discharge
43. Identification of length of episodes of care, including readmissions
44. Recognition of time for patient to return to work
45. Recognition of goals not met or unattainable
46. Failure to identify allergies
47. Inappropriate acuity classification/severity of illness
48. Failure to plan/refer to home care
49. Failure to plan/refer to outpatient visits/consultations
50. Failure to plan/refer to community services

*Source:* Adapted from P. Spath, *Succeeding with Critical Paths*, Brown-Spath & Associates, Forest Grove, OR, 1993.

software vendor Mediqual, who has looked at profiles of variance for pneumonia, coronary artery bypass graft, heart failure, and shock using low mortality as the outcome criterion.

Outcomes achieved need to be documented either manually or in the CPR. Ways to present variances are shown in Figs. 13.2 to 13.5. The way that the data are presented is merely related to how the team prefers to look at its successes and variances. In the first figure, a scatter diagram presents patients' lengths of stay as a function of numbers of co-morbidities. Graphs to show changes in patient days and charges with and without case management are presented in Fig. 13.3. Figure 13.4 reports frequencies or cumulative summaries of reasons for variance. In Fig. 13.5 a control chart summarizes mean data over time and the outliers (positive or negative) by department.

Profiles are cumulative reports that can be prepared reflecting patient, nurse provider, physician provider, department, or condition variances within a care facility. Profiles can be generated between hospitals in a chain, they can be generated for multiple sites for local or state reporting purposes, and they can be summarized by region to enter into even larger databases for national aggregate data. These data can then be used to show regional or statewide variation by facility type or other trends. An example of profile data pooled from several sites is shown in Fig. 13.6. The outputs can document the average length of stay (or length of treatment for outpatients), procedures used, medications used, side effects, complications, or other outcomes achieved. The outcomes achieved can be used for quality management; the costs and length of stay used for financial management; the procedures and medications used for resource management; complications, medication errors, incident reports, and extended lengths of

**Figure 13.2**  A scatter diagram of length of stay varying by patient co-morbidities. (Adapted from P. Spath, *Succeeding with Critical Paths,* Brown-Spath & Associates, Forest Grove, OR, 1993.)

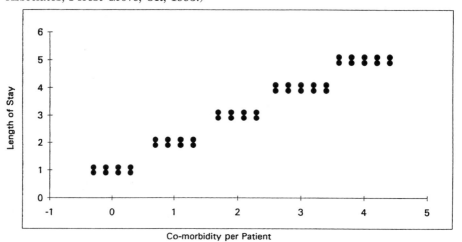

Co-morbidity per Patient

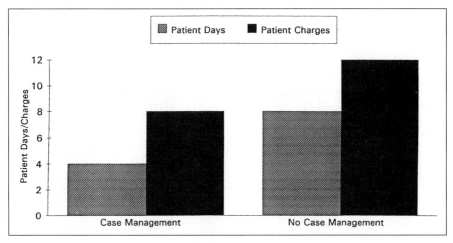

**Figure 13.3**    Variations in patient days and charges with and without case management for the same conditions (TURPS). (Adapted from P. Spath, *Succeeding with Critical Paths,* Brown-Spath & Associates, Forest Grove, OR, 1993.)

stay used for risk management; and the professional practice used for level of care management.

Large national groups like the Voluntary Hospitals of America, Sun-Health, the University Hospital Consortium, the Minnesota Clinical Comparison and Assessment Project, and the Maryland Quality Indicator Project offer members the ability to benchmark and compare themselves to one another. State data from about 30 states can be obtained from the National Association of Health Data Organizations. The Commission on

**Figure 13.4**    Frequencies of causes of variance. (Adapted from P. Spath, *Succeeding with Critical Paths,* Brown-Spath & Associates, Forest Grove, OR, 1993.)

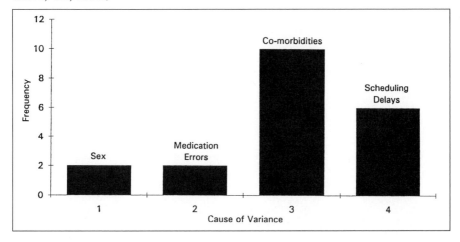

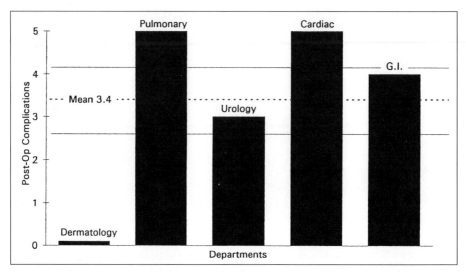

**Figure 13.5**   Outliers per department of frequency of postoperative complications. (Adapted from P. Spath, *Succeeding with Critical Paths,* Brown-Spath & Associates, Forest Grove, OR, 1993.)

Professional and Hospital Activities is another source of national association data. Companies that are available to analyze data include HCIA in Baltimore, Systemetrics, Fu and Associates in Virginia, and Health Care Investment Analysts in Baltimore. The Chicago-based Lexecon Health

**Figure 13.6**   Profile data on mortality pooled from several hospital sites for patients with ARDS. (Adapted from P. Spath, *Succeeding with Critical Paths,* Brown-Spath & Associates, Forest Grove, OR, 1993.)

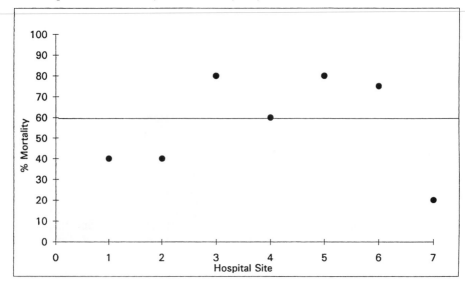

Services designs custom analyses using public Medicare data and private data sources. Since the sources of most of these data are billing forms and discharge abstracts, outcome data are scant to nonexistent. The challenge to the large groups in the future is to provide more outcomes than mortality and morbidity. Also missing from most of today's computerized patient profiles is the ability to document patient preference and patient and employee satisfaction, and to determine profiles of provider and patient groups.

## Large National Databases to Determine Profiles of Variance

Another way to obtain profiles in the interim, until the infrastructure for the CPR is in place, is to use already established databases (McCormick, 1993). Table 13.6 is a summary of available federal and public tapes, Department of Veteran Affairs tapes, and private/public national and state tapes that require purchase or licensing agreements to access data. These databases are described in an article by Paul et al. (1993).

## Profiles for Achieving Positive Outcomes

Focused examples of profiles for achieving positive outcomes are becoming popular as a way to describe automation efforts that have improved outcomes of care. To date there are few examples of nursing interventions that have improved outcomes and therefore reduced costs. Studies of nursing interventions have been done relating pain management, incontinence management and cure, and pressure ulcer prevention, treatment, and cure to the outcomes and the costs. More examples exist in medical literature, but they need replication using nursing information systems to achieve outcomes. In one study, use of a workstation resulted in reduction in charges per patient admission of almost $900 and reduction in length of stay of almost 1 day (Tierney et al., 1993). At the Latter-Day Saints Hospital in Salt Lake City, several studies of automation have described reductions in antibiotic usage 94 percent of the time with a consultant support system. This computer system was also to demonstrate that the use of antibiotics prior to surgery reduces postsurgical infection (Evans et al., 1987).

## MANAGED CARE USE OF OUTCOME DATA

In the decade ahead, managed care may shift the focus of computerized systems from managing revenues to managing resources. Specific managed care uses of such data might include charges to date for patients with specific conditions, types and numbers of procedures used, number of consultations with specialty practices requested, costs (or charges) com-

**TABLE 13.6**    TAXONOMY OF LARGE DATABASES WITH SPECIFIC
EXAMPLES

I. Administrative databases
  A. Claims/utilization data
    1. Federal-level data
      a. HCFA Medicare Statistical System
        (1) Payment databases and bill records
        (2) Financial databases: PPS, HCRIS
        (3) Research databases for Medicare Parts A and B: MEDPAR, BMAD, MADRS
        (4) Special program databases: ESRD
        (5) National claims history
      b. Medicaid data (federal level)
        (1) Medicaid statistical information
        (2) Tape-to-tape project date
      c. Department of Veteran Affairs (VA) data
        (1) Patient treatment file (PTF)
        (2) Outpatient file (OPF)
      d. Department of Defense data
        (1) AQCESS in patient data form
        (2) CHAMPUS health care data for dependents
    2. State-level data
      a. Medicaid management information system data
      b. State hospital discharge data systems
      c. State divisions of health statistics special studies and databases
    3. Private/proprietary databases
      a. Blue Cross/Blue Shield data
      b. Other provider/insurer and HMO data
        (1) United HealthCare
        (2) Kaiser Permanente
      c. Contracter databases
        (1) Commission on Professional and Hospital Activities (CPHA)
        (2) MEDSTAT/SysteMetrices, Inc.
        (3) Shared Medical Systems, Inc.
  B. Data on individual providers
    1. Uniform Physician Identification Number (UPIN) data (federal level)
    2. American Medical Association MasterFile database
    3. State licensing boards

  C. Hospital certification and survey data
    1. Medicare provider of service (POS) file (federal)
    2. American Hospital Association (AHA)
II. Clinical/epidemiological and health survey databases
  A. Disease registries
    1. National Cancer Institute (NCI) SEER data
    2. Centers for Disease Control (CDC) communicable disease registries
    3. CDC Birth Defects Monitoring Program
  B. Epidemiological studies
    1. U.S.-based
      a. Framingham Study
      b. Baltimore Longitudinal Study on Aging
    2. International
      a. Oxford Medical Record Linkage Study
      b. British Regional Heart Study
      c. Manitoba health database
  C. Health survey data
    1. National Health Interview Survey (HIS)
    2. National Health and Nutrition Examination Survey (NHANES)
    3. National Medical Expenditure Survey (NMES)
    4. Medicare Health Status Registry
    5. Current Beneficiary Survey
III. Socio-demographic/socioeconomic data
  A. Census data
  B. Health resource and manpower data
    1. Area Resource File (ARF)
  C. Vital and health statistics databases
    1. National Death Index (NDI) (federal level)
    2. Birth and death certificate data (state level)
  D. Other (non–health care) program data
    1. Supplemental Nutrition Program for Women, Infants, and Children (WIC) data
    2. Food stamps data

Taxonomy adapted and modified from Agency for Health Care Policy and Research. (1991) Report to Congress: The feasibility of linking research-related databases to federal and non-federal medical administrative databases (Pub. No. 91-0003). Rockville, MD: Agency for Health Care Policy and Research.

*Source:* Paul et al., 1993.

pared to expected reimbursement, variance between costs and actual reimbursed dollars by patient or by provider, differences between nurse and physician providers, differences between general physician and specialty physician providers, and differences between conditions (e.g., management of stress incontinence versus urge incontinence or both). Kaiser-Permanente, Puget Sound, the New England Medical Center, the Harvard Community Health Plan, and other large managed care groups have been developing automated monitoring systems to determine areas of variance, profiles, and benchmarks in care. The use of comparisons in data sets gives the health plans an opportunity to work together to develop better outcome measures, benchmark their performance, and exchange information on best practices.

## Health Plan Employer Data and Information Set

A consortium of managed care leaders, under the direction of the National Committee for Quality Assurance (NCQA), has developed a standard framework for information management in managed care associations. In November 1993, the NCQA released the Health Plan Employer Data and Information Set Version 2.0 (HEDIS 2.0) (Corrigan and Nielsen, 1993). This is a core set of health plan performance measures that seek to improve patient care quality in partnership with managed care plans, purchasers, consumers, and the public sector. It is the intent of this project to develop report cards on health plans. Included in HEDIS 2.0 are measurements of quality, access, patients' satisfaction, membership and utilization, and finance. The output of HEDIS is designed to enable managed care plans to accurately report trends in performance. Much of the content in HEDIS is based on public health priorities from Healthy People 2000, such as compliance with national guidelines on vaccination schedules, cholesterol screening, mammography screening, prenatal care and outcomes, management of asthma, and diabetic eye care. Priorities were given to areas where there is evidence of the relationship between process and outcome. Table 13.7 shows the HEDIS 2.0 list of quality measures. Although this system has been developed for managed care, it can be adapted to include Medicare and other private payer data.

## AMBULATORY CARE USE OF OUTCOMES DATA

Hayward et al. (1993) developed a guideline application program (GAP) to facilitate the design and implementation of guideline-based, computerized, patient-administered questionnaires, and the preparation of feedback reports and suggestions for patients in the ambulatory care setting. The three applications include a preventive health screening system, a preop-

**TABLE 13.7**     HEDIS LIST OF QUALITY MEASURES

| Administrative (Transaction) Measure | Data Specification | Medical Record Review Specification |
|---|---|---|
| I. Preventive services | | |
| 1. Childhood immunization | Yes | Yes |
| 2. Cholesterol screening | Yes | Yes |
| 3. Mammography screening | Yes | Yes |
| 4. Pap smears for cervical cancer | Yes | Yes |
| II. Prenatal care | | |
| 5. Low-birthweight rates | Yes | No |
| 6. Prenatal care in first trimester | Yes | Yes |
| III. Acute and chronic illness | | |
| 7. Asthma inpatient admission rate | Yes | No |
| 8. Diabetic eye care | Yes | Yes |
| IV. Mental health | | |
| 9. Ambulatory follow-up after hospitalization for major affective disorders | Yes | Yes |

*Source*: Corrigan and Nielsen, 1993.

erative test selection program, and a geriatric functional status assessment instrument.

This system is not interactive, but the guideline content includes questionnaires written to solicit pertinent information from patients. In the system, algorithms are generated, feedback is used to prepare messages that appear on a printout for clinicians and/or patients, and draft applications are tested using simulator functions.

## IMPEDIMENTS TO PROGRESS

Nurses will have to commit to using the CPR in order to receive the advantages that it offers. CPRs offer more efficient, effective documentation. They offer assisted decision making, with access to information not presently available at the point of service. They offer feedback on decisions that have been made, patients' progress, and quality. They offer simplification of the review process that currently is burdening the nurse with paperwork.

Without national standards for the CPR, these systems will remain useful at local levels only. Additionally, without changes in nurse behavior to value this type of documentation system, more guidelines to provide the data elements for computers, the infrastructure to share data nationally, and the establishment of security measures to assure confidentiality and privacy of information, these systems will remain available for use only in managed care, local hospitals, or facility chains (Donaldson, 1994).

Value added in this model is the ability to extend the resources in health care beyond single sites to multiple sites for national or regional profiles. Only then will the data gathered be useful in providing feedback to national monitoring organizations so that guidelines can be developed from clinical practice experience rather than literature and expert opinion.

The nursing profession has to assure that unified data exist. A more thorough description of nursing involvement in the achievement of unified data was given in Chap. 10. Minimum data requirements are assured, and nursing outcomes are covered in databases measuring outcomes of care. Since nurses currently are the utilization and review criteria surveyors, this group needs to accept the challenge to look for the review of nursing documentation that demonstrates nursing influences on patient outcomes.

## SUMMARY

New tools exist for more efficient and effective management in the health care arena of the 1990s and beyond. This chapter discussed how outcomes can be effectively managed in computerized databases, and the development and potential use of clinical practice guidelines as content in the CPR. The expansion of medical decision-making methods will be greatly enhanced by the content in clinical practice guidelines. The critical path model of establishing outcomes linked to guidelines and monitoring the variances from interventions and outcomes was described. All of these methods are made more efficient by computerized information systems. The availability of these systems through nursing networks to describe profiles and benchmarks of care were further described. Examples of computerized decision support systems, expert systems, managed care systems, and ambulatory care systems were also provided.

## REFERENCES

Bachrach, M. K., Ballesteros, P., Black, A. N., et al. (1988). Using patient outcomes to define nursing practice. *Nursing Administration Quarterly, 12*(2), 45–51.

Barrett, M. J. (1992). Is your organization ready for total quality management? *American Journal of Medical Quality, 7*(4), 106–110.

Barrett, M. J. (1993, June). Case management a must to survive managed care. *Computers in Healthcare,* 22–25.

Beavert, C. S., Magoffin, C. H. (1993). Medical review criteria: A tool for quality management. *Group Practice Medical, 42*(4), 53–57.

Brennan, P. F., and McHugh, M. (1988). Clinical decision-making and computer support. *Applied Nursing Research, 1*(2), 89–93.

Chang, B. L., Roth, K., Gonzales, E., et al. (1988). CANDI: A knowledge-based system for nursing diagnosis. *Computers in Nursing, 6*(1), 13–21.

Chassin, M. R. (1988). Standards of care in medicine. *Inquiry, 25*(4), 437–453.

Corrigan, J. M., and Nielsen, D. M. (1993). Toward the development of uniform reporting standards for managed care organization: The health plan employer data and information set (Version 2.0). *The Journal of Quality Improvement, 19*(12), 566–575.

Crede, W. B., and Hierholzer, W. J. (1988). Mortality rates as quality indicator: A simple answer to a complex question. *Infection Control Hospital Epidemiology, 9*(7), 330–332.

Cromwell, J., and Mitchell, J. B. (1988). Physician-induced demand for surgery. *Journal of Health Economics, 5*(4), 293–313.

Davies, A. R. (1992). Health care researchers' needs for computer-based patient records. In M. J. Ball and M. F. Collen (Eds.), *Aspects of the Computer-Based Patient Record* (pp. 46–56). New York: Springer-Verlag.

Donabedian, A. (1966). Evaluating the quality of medical care. *Milbank Memorial Fund Quarterly.* 44 (Supplement), 166–206.

Donabedian, A. (1991). Reflections on the effectiveness of quality assurance. In R. H. Palmer, A. Donabedian, and G. Povar (Eds.), *Striving for Quality in Health Care: An Inquiry into Policy and Practice* (pp. 59–128). Ann Arbor, MI: Health Administration Press.

Donaldson, M. S. (1994). Gearing up for health data in the information age. *Journal of Quality Improvement, 20*(4), 202–214.

Donaldson, M., and Capron, A. (Eds.) (1991). *Patient Outcomes Research Teams: Managing Conflict of Interest.* Washington, DC: National Academy Press.

Dufresne, A., Berlinguet, M., McCormick, K.A., et al. (1994). Verification and validation of the AHCPR urinary incontinence clinical practice guideline using an expert system and review of medical records. Unpublished manuscript.

Duggar, B., and Palmer, H. (1995). *Understanding and Choosing Clinical Performance Measures for Quality Improvement: Development of a Typology and Attachments.* AHCPR Contract, Pub. Nos.: 95-N001 and 95-N002.

Evans, R. S., Reed, M. G., Burke, J. P., et al. (1987). A computerized approach to monitor prophylactic antibiotics. In W. E. Stead (Ed.), *Proceedings of the Eleventh Annual Symposium on Computer Applications in Medicine Care* (pp. 241–245). Silver Spring, MD: IEEE Computer Society Press.

Feinstein, A. (1987). *Clinimetrics.* New Haven, CT: Yale University Press.

Garnick, D. W., Hendricks, A. M., and Brennan, T. A. (1991). Can practice guidelines reduce the number and costs of malpractice claims? *Journal of the American Medical Association, 266*(20), 2856–2860.

Hadorn, D. C., McCormick, K. A., and Diokno, A. (1992). An annotated algorithm approach to clinical guideline development. *Journal of the American Medical Association, 267*(24), 3311–3314.

Hayward, R. S., Langton, K. B., Roizen, M.F., et al. (1993). A clinical information tool for preventive care. In C. Safran (Ed.), *Proceedings of the Seventeenth Annual Symposium on Computer Applications in Medical Care* (p. 943). New York: McGraw-Hill.

Health Outcomes Institute. (1994). *Update: The Newsletter of the Health Outcomes Institute.* Bloomington, MN.

Hegyvary, S. T. (1991). Issues in outcomes research. *Journal of Nursing Quality Assurance, 5*(2), 1–6.

Hirshfield, E. B. (1991). Should practice parameters be the standard of care in malpractice litigation. *Journal of the American Medical Association, 266*(29), 2886–2891.

Institute of Medicine. (1990). *Clinical Practice Guidelines: Directions for a New Program*. Washington, DC: National Academy Press.

Institute of Medicine. (1992). *Guidelines for Clinical Practice: From Development to Use*. Washington, DC: National Academy Press.

Institute of Medicine (1994). *America's Health in Transition: Protecting and Improving Quality*. Washington, DC: National Academy Press.

Johnston, M. E., Langton, K. B., Haynes, R. B., and Mathieu, A. (1994). Effects of computer-based clinical decision support systems on clinician performance and patient outcomes. *Annals of Internal Medicine, 120*, 135–142.

Kibbe, D. C., Kaluzny, A. D., and McLaughlin, C. P. (1994). Integrating guidelines with continuous quality improvement: Doing the right thing the right way to achieve the right goals. *Journal of Quality Improvement, 20*(4), 181–191.

McCormick, K. A. (1991). Future data needs for quality of care monitoring, DRG considerations, reimbursement and outcome measurement. *Image: The Journal of Scholarship, 23*, 4–7.

McCormick, K. A. (1993). Nursing effectiveness research using existing databases. In *Patient Outcomes Research: Examining the Effectiveness of Nursing Practice: Proceedings of the State of the Science Conference* (NIH Pub. No. 93-3411) (pp. 203–209). Bethesda, MD: NIH, PHS, US DHHS.

McCormick, K., Moore, S., and Siegel, R. (1994). *Methodologic Perspectives of Clinical Practice Guidelines*. Pub. No. 95-0009. Rockville, MD: AHCPR, PHS, US DHHS.

O'Brien-Pallas, L. L., Irvine, D., Murray, M., and Cockerill, R. (June 1994). *Factors Which Influence Variability in Nursing Workload and Outcomes of Care in Community Health Nursing*. Personal communication.

Owens, D. K., and Nease, R. B. (1993). Development of outcome-based guidelines: A method for structuring problems and synthesizing evidence. *Journal of Quality Improvement, 19*(7), 248–264.

Paul, J. E., Weis, K. A., and Epstein, R.A. (1993). Data bases for variations research. *Medical Care*, 31(5), S96–102.

Petrucci, K. M., Jacox, A., McCormick, K. A., et al. (1992). Evaluating appropriate use of a nurse expert system's patient assessment. Urological Nursing Information System (UNIS). *Computers in Nursing, 10*(6), 243–249.

Schoenbaum, S. C., Sundwall, D. N., Bergman, D., et al. (1995). *Using Clinical Practice Guidelines to Evaluate Quality of Care. Volume I: Issues; Volume II: Methods*. (Pub. Nos. 95-0045 and 95-0046). Rockville, MD: US DHHS, PHS, AHCPR.

Shamian, J., Petryshen, P., and O'Brien-Pallas, L. L. (1994). *Outcomes Monitoring: Adjusting for Risk Factors and Severity of Illness when Determining Outcomes*. Paper presented at Post Conference on Informatics: The Infrastructure for Quality Assessment and Improvement in Nursing, Austin, TX.

Shortliffe, E. H., Tang, P. C., Amatayakul, M. K., et al. (1992). Future vision and dissemination of computer-based patient records. In M. J. Ball and M. F. Collen (Eds.), *Aspects of the Computer-Based Patient Record* (pp. 273–293). New York: Springer-Verlag.

Silva, J. S. and Zawilski, A. J. (1992). The health care professional's workstation: Its functional components and user impact. In M. J. Ball and M. F. Collen (Eds.), *Aspects of the Computer-Based Patient Record* (pp. 102–124). New York: Springer-Verlag.

Soumerai, S. B., Salem-Schatz, S., Avorn, J., et al. (1993). A controlled trial of education outreach to improve blood transfusion practice. *Journal of the American Medical Association, 270*(8), 961–966.

Spath, P. (1993). *Succeeding with Critical Paths (p. 1).* Forest Grove, OR: Brown-Spath & Associates.

Tierney, W. M., Miller, M. E., Overhage, J. M., and McDonald, C. M. (1993). Physician inpatient order writing on microcomputer workstations: Effects on resource utilization. *Journal of the American Medical Association, 269*(3), 379–383.

Urinary Incontinence Guideline Panel. (1992). *Urinary Incontinence in Adults: Clinical Practice Guideline* (Number 2, Quick Reference, and Consumer Guide. AHCPR Pub. No. 92-0038,0041,0040). Rockville, MD: AHCPR, PHS, DHHS.

Ware, J. E. (1987). Standards for validating health status measures: Definition and content. *Journal of Chronic Diseases, 40*(6), 473–480.

Ware, J. E., and Berwick, D. M. (1989). Patient judgements of hospital quality: Conclusions and recommendations. *Medical Care Review, 28*(9), S39–42.

Ware, J. E., and Sherbournes, C. (1992). The MOS 36-item short-form health survey (SF-36). *Medical Care, 30*, 473–483.

Wennberg, J., Freeman, J. L., and Culp, W. J. (1987). Are hospital services rationed in New Haven or over-utilized in Boston? *Lancet, 1*(8543), 1185–1189.

Zander, K. (1988). Nursing case management. Strategic management of cost and quality outcomes. *Journal of Nursing Administration, 18*, 23–30.

## BIBLIOGRAPHY

Abramowitz, J. M., Cote, A. A., and Berry, E. (1987). Analyzing patient satisfaction: A multidimensional approach. *Quality Review Bulletin*, 13, 122–130.

Acute Pain Management Guideline Panel. (1992). *Acute Pain Management: Operative or Medical Procedures and Trauma.* Clinical Practice Guideline (Number 1, Quick Reference for Adults, Quick Reference for Infants, and Consumer Guide. AHCPR Pub. No. 92-0032,0020,0019,0021). Rockville, MD: AHCPR, PHS, US DHHS.

Agency for Health Care Policy and Research. (1991). *Interim Manual for Clinical Practice Guideline Development.* Rockville, MD.

Agency for Health Care Policy and Research. (1992). *Annotated Bibliography Information Dissemination to Health Care Practitioners and Policymakers.* Rockville, MD.

Agency for Health Care Policy and Research. (1993). *Program Note. Clinical Practice Guideline Development.* Rockville, MD.

Anderson, G. F., Hall, M. A., and Steinberg, E. P. (1993). Medical technology assessment and practice guidelines: Their day in court. *American Journal of Public Health, 83*(11), 1635–1639.

Audet, A. M., Greenfield, S., and Field, M. (1990). Medical practice guidelines: Current activities and future directions. *Annals of Internal Medicine, 113*(9), 709–714.

Ayello, E. A. (1993). A critique of the AHCPR's "Preventing Pressure Ulcers—A Patient's Guide" as a written instructional tool. *Decubitus, 6*(3), 44–50.

Battista, R. N., and Fletcher, S. W. (1988). Making recommendations on preventive practice: methodological issues. *American Journal of Preventive Medicine, 4,* S53–67.

Battista, R. N., and Hodge, M. J. (1993). Clinical practice guidelines: Between science and art. *Canadian Medical Association Journal, 148*(3), 385–389.

Bergener, M. (1989). Quality of life, health status, and clinical research. *Medical Care, 27*(3), S148–156.

Bergener, M., Bobbitt, R. A., Carter, W. B., and Bigson, B. S. (1981). The Sickness Impact Profile: Development and final revision of a health status measure. *Medical Care, 19,* 787–804.

Bernstein, I. L., Blassing-Moore, J., Fineman, S., et al. (1993). Establishing practice parameters: Parameters for the diagnosis and treatment of asthma. *Annals of Allergy, 71*(3), 197–199.

Burns, L. R., Denton, M., Goldfein, S., et al. (1992). The use of continuous quality improvement methods in the development and dissemination of medical practice guidelines. *Quality Review Bulletin, 18*(122), 434–439.

Bush, J. W. (1984). *Quality of Well-Being Scale. Function Status Profile and Symptom/Problem Complex Questionnaire.* San Diego, CA: Health Policy Project, University of California.

Cataract Management Guideline Panel. (1993). *Cataract in Adults: Management of Functional Impairment* (Clinical Practice Guideline Number 4, Quick Reference, and Consumer Guide. AHCPR Pub. No. 93-0542,0543,0544). Rockville, MD: AHCPR, PHS, DHHS.

Chalmers, I., Enkin, M., and Keirse, M. J. (1993). Preparing and updating systematic reviews of randomized controlled trials of health care. *Milbank Quarterly, 71*(3), 411–437.

Coffey, R. J., Richards, J. S., Remmert, C. S., et al. (1992). An introduction to critical paths. *Quality Management in Health Care, 1*(1), 45–54.

Department of Health Care and Promotion, Canadian Medical Association. (1993). Workshop on clinical practice guidelines: Summary of proceedings. *Canadian Medical Association Journal, 148*(9), 14359–14362.

Depression Guideline Panel. (1993). *Depression in Primary Care: Volume 1. Detection and Diagnosis. Volume 2. Treatment of Major Depression* (Clinical Practice Guideline Number 5, Quick Reference, and Consumer Guide. AHCPR Pub. No. 93-0550, 0551, 0552, 0553). Rockville, MD: AHCPR, PHS, DHHS.

Dixon, A. S. (1990). The evolution of clinical policies. *Medical Care, 28*(3), 201–220.

Dolan, J. C., and Bordley, D. R. (1992). Using the analytic hierarchy process to develop and disseminate guidelines. *Quality Review Bulletin, 18*(12), 440–447.

Donabedian, A. (1980). *Explorations in Quality Assessment and Monitoring* (Volume I). Ann Arbor, MI: Health Administration Press.

Durand-Zaleski, I., Bonnet, F., Rochant, H., et al. (1992). Usefulness of consensus conferences: The case of albumin. *Lancet, 340*(8832), 1388–1390.

Eddy, D. M. (1990). The challenge. *Journal of the American Medical Association, 263*(2), 287–290.

Eddy, D. M. (1990). Comparing benefits and harms: The balance sheet. *Journal of the American Medical Association, 263*(18), 2493, 2494, 2501, passim.

Eddy, D. M. (1990). Designing a practice policy: Standards, guidelines, and options. *Journal of the American Medical Association, 263*(22), 3077, 3081, 3084.

Eddy, D. M. (1990). Guidelines for policy statements: The explicit approach. *Journal of the American Medical Association, 263*(16), 2239–2240, 2243.

Eddy, D. M. (1990). Practice policies: Guidelines for methods. *Journal of the American Medical Association, 263*(13), 1839–1841.

Eddy, D. M. (1990). Resolving conflicts in practice policies. *Journal of the American Medical Association, 264*(3), 389–391.

Eddy, D. M. (1991). What care is "essential"? What services are "basic"? *Journal of the American Medical Association, 265*(6), 782, 786–788.

Eddy, D. M. (1991). *A Manual for Assessing Health Practices and Designing Practice Policies: The Explicit Approach*. Philadelphia: American College of Physicians.

Ellwood, P. M. (1988). Outcomes management: A technology of patient experience. *New England Journal of Medicine, 318*(23), 1549–1556.

El-Sadr, W., Oleske, J. M., Agins, B. D., et al. (1994). *Evaluation and Management of Early HIV Infection* (Clinical Practice Guideline. No. 7. AHCPR Pub. No. 94-0572). Rockville, MD: AHCPR, PHS, US DHHS.

Evans, R. S., Pestotnik, S. L., Classen, D. C., and Burke, J. P. (1993). Development of an automated antibiotic consultant. *M.D. Computing, 10*, 17–22.

Gardner, E. (1992, September). Putting guidelines into practice. *Modern Healthcare*, 24–26.

Grol, R. (1993). Development of guidelines for general practice care. *British Journal of General Practice, 43*(369), 146–151.

Grudick, G. (1991). The critical path system: The road toward an efficient OR. *American Operating Room Nursing Journal, 53*, 705–714.

Hansen, D. T., Adams, A. H., Meeker, W. C., and Phillips, R. B. (1992). Proposal for establishing structure and process in the development of implicit chiropractic standards of care and practice guidelines. *Journal Manipulative Physiologic Therapy, 15*(7), 430–438.

Havinghurst, C. C. (1990). Practice guidelines for medical care: The policy rationale. *St. Louis University Law Journal, 34*(4), 777–819.

Hayward, R. S., and Laupacis, A. (1993). Initiating, conducting and maintaining guidelines development programs. *Canadian Medical Association Journal, 148*(4), 507–512.

Hayward, R. S., Steinberg, E. P., Ford, D. E., et al. (1991). Preventive care guidelines. *Annals of Internal Medicine, 114*, 758–783.

Hayward, R. S., Wilson, M. C., Tunis, S. R., et al. (1993). More informative abstracts of articles describing clinical practice guidelines. *Annals of Internal Medicine, 118*, 731–737.

Hicks, W. E. (1993). Development of ASHP practice standards. *American Journal of Hospital Pharmacists, 50*(5), 878, 880.

Hoffman, P. A. (1993). Critical path method: An important tool for coordinating clinical care. *Journal of Quality Improvement, 19*(7), 235–246.

Hollenberg, N. K., Testa, M., and Williams, G. H. (1991). Quality of life as a therapeutic end-point. *Drug Safety, 6*(2), 83–93.

Hutchinson, B. G. (1993). Critical appraisal of review articles. *Canadian Family Physician, 39*, 1097–1102.

Jacox, A. (1993). Developing clinical practice guidelines: An interview with Ada Jacox [Interview by Barbara Bednar]. *American Nephrology Nurses' Association Journal, 20*(2), 121–126.

Johnson, M., and McCloskey, J. C. (1992). Quality in the nineties. *Series on Nursing Administration, 3,* 59–68.

Kane, R. A., and Kane, R. L. (1981). *Assessing the Elderly: a Practical Guide to Measurement.* Lexington, MA: Lexington Books.

Karnowsky, D. A., Abdelmann, W. H., Craver, L. F., and Burchenal, J. H. (1948). The use of nitrogen mustard in the palliative treatment of carcinoma. *Cancer, I,* 634–656.

Kelly, J. T., and Swartwout, J. E. (1990). Development of practice parameters by physician organizations. *Quality Review Bulletin, 16*(2), 54–57.

Kelly, J. T., and Toepp, M. C. (1992). Practice parameters: Development, evaluation, dissemination, and implementation. *Quality Review Bulletin, 18*(12), 405–409.

Koepke, M. D., Cronin, C. A., and Lazar, A. (1992). How insurers, purchasers, and employers view their need for guidelines: Report of the Washington Business Group on Health: AHCPR Focus Groups. *Quality Review Bulletin, 18*(12), 480–482.

Lawrence, R. S., and Mickalike, A. D. (1987). Preventive services in clinical practice: Designing the periodic health examination. *Journal of the American Medical Association, 257*(16), 2205–2207.

Lawton, M., and Brody, E. (1969). Assessment of older people: Self-maintaining and instrumental activities of daily living. *Gerontologist, 9,* 179–186.

Lomas, J. (1993). Making clinical policy explicit. Legislative policy making and lessons for developing practice guidelines. *International Journal of Technology Assessment in Health Care, 9*(1), 11–25.

Lomas, J., Anderson, G. M., Domnick-Pierre, K., et al. (1989). Do practice guidelines guide practice? The effect of a consensus statement on the practice of physicians. *New England Journal of Medicine, 321*(19), 1306–1311.

Lomas, J., Sisk, J. E., and Stocking, B. (1993). From evidence to practice in the United States, and United Kingdom, and Canada. *Milbank Quarterly, 71*(3), 405–410.

McConnell, J. D., Barry, M. J., Bruskewitz, R. C., et al. (1994). *Benign Prostatic Hyperplasia: Diagnosis and Treatment* (Clinical Practice Guideline, Number 8, AHCPR Pub. No. 94-0582). Rockville, MD: AHCPR, PHS, US DHHS.

McCormick, K. A. (1992). Areas of outcome research for nursing. *Journal of Professional Nursing, 8*(2), 71.

McCormick, K. A., and Fleming, B. (1992, December). Clinical Practice Guidelines. *Health Progress,* 30–34.

McGuire, L. B. (1990). A long run for a short jump: Understanding clinical guidelines. *Annals of Internal Medicine, 113*(9), 705–708.

McIntyre, J. (1990). Developing practice parameters: An interview with John McIntyre [interview by John A. Talbott]. *Hospital Community Psychiatry, 41*(10), 1103–1105.

Meeker, C. I. (1992). A consensus-based approach to practice parameters. *Obstetrics & Gynecology, 79*(5), 790–793.

Mitchell, J. B., and Cromwell, J. (1981). *Physician-Induced Demand for Surgical Operations* (DHHS Pub. No. HCFA 81-03086). Washington, DC.

Naylor, C. D., Sibbald, W. J., Sprung, C. L., et al. (1993). Pulmonary artery catheterization. Can there be an integrated strategy for guideline development and research promotions. *Journal of the American Medical Association, 269*(18), 2407–2411.

Office of Science and Technology Policy. (1994). *High Performance Computing and Communications: Toward a National Information Infrastructure* (pp. 1–176).

Oxman, A. D. (1993). Coordination of guidelines development. *Canadian Medical Association Journal, 148*(8), 1285–1288.

Padilla, G., Ferrell, B., Grant, M. M., and Rhiner, M. (1990). Defining the content domain of quality of life for cancer patients with pain. *Cancer Nursing, 13*(2), 108–115.

Panel for the Prediction and Prevention of Pressure Ulcers in Adults. (1992). *Pressure Ulcers in Adults: Prediction and Prevention* (Clinical Practice Guideline, Number 3, Quick Reference, and Consumer Guide. AHCPR Pub. No. 92-0047,0050,0048). Rockville, MD: AHCPR, PHS, DHHS.

Perry, S., and Wilkinson, S. L. (1990). The technology assessment and practice guidelines forum: A modified group judgement method. *International Journal of Technology Assessment in Health Care, 8*(2), 289–300.

Phelps, C. E. (1993). The methodologic foundations of studies of the appropriateness of medical care. *Journal of the American Medical Association, 329*(17), 1241–1245.

Pierce, E. D. (1990). The development of anesthesia guidelines and standards. *Quality Review Bulletin, 16,* 65–70.

Roper, W. L., Winkenwerder, W., Hackbarth, G. M., and Krakauer, H. (1988). Effectiveness in health care: An initiative to evaluate and improve medical practice. *New England Journal of Medicine, 319*(18), 1197–1202.

Safran, C. (1993). Using information technology to fight AIDS. *MD Computing, 10*(5), 292–293.

Safran, C., Rind, D. M., Davies, R. M., et al. (1993). An electronic medical record that helps care for patients with HIV infection. In C. Safran (Ed.). *Proceedings of the Seventeenth Annual Symposium on Computer Applications in Medical Care* (pp. 224–228). New York: McGraw-Hill.

Selker, H. P. (1993). Criteria for adoption in practice of medical practice guidelines. *American Journal of Cardiology, 71,* 339-341.

Sickle Cell Disease Guideline Panel. (1993). *Sickle Cell Disease: Screening, Diagnosis, Management, and Counseling in Newborns and Infants* (Clinical Practice Guideline Number 6, Quick Reference, and Consumer Guide. AHCPR Pub. No. 93-0562, 0563, 0564). Rockville, MD: AHCPR, PHS, DHHS.

Simpson, R. L. (1994). How technology enhances total quality improvement. *Nursing Management, 25*(6), 40–41.

Sisk, J. (1993). Improving the use of research-based evidence in policy making: Effective care in pregnancy and childbirth in the United States. *Milbank Quarterly, 71*(3), 477–496.

Siu, A. L., McGlynn, E. A., Morgenstern, H., et al. (1992). Choosing quality of care measures based on the expected impact of improved care on health. *Health Services Research, 27*(5), 619–650.

Sox, H. C., Jr., and Woolf, S. H. (1993). Evidence-based practice guidelines from the US Preventive Health Services Task Force [editorial]. *Journal of the American Medical Association, 269*(20), 2678.

Tancredi, L. R., and Bovbjerg, R. R. (1992). Creating outcomes-based systems for quality and malpractice reform: Methodology of accelerated compensation events. *Milbank Quarterly, 70*(1), 183–216.

Thompson, K. S., Caddick, K., Mathie, J., et al. (1991). Building a critical path for ventilator patients. *American Journal of Nursing, 91*(7), 28–31.

U.S. Preventive Services Task Force. (1989). *Guide to Clinical Preventive Services: An Assessment of the Effectiveness of 169 Interventions.* Baltimore, MD: Williams & Wilkins.

U.S. Preventive Services Task Force Policy Statement (1993). Screening for adolescent idiopathy scoliosis. *Journal of the American Medical Association, 269*(20), 2667–2672.

Weinert, C. (1988). Measuring social support: Revision and further development of the Personal Resource Questionnaire. In C. Waltz and O. Strickland (Eds.), *Measurement of Nursing Outcomes* (pp. 309–327). New York: Springer.

Wennberg, J., Freeman, J. L., Shelton, R. M., and Bulbolz, T. A. (1989). Hospital use and mortality among Medicare beneficiaries in Boston and New Haven. *New England Journal of Medicine, 321*(17), 1168–1173.

Woolf, S. H. (1990). Practice guidelines, a new reality in medicine: I. Recent Development. *Archives of Internal Medicine, 150*(9), 1811–1818.

Woolf, S. H. (1992). Practice guidelines, a new reality in medicine: II. Methods of developing guidelines. *Archives of Internal Medicine, 152*(5), 946–952.

Wortman, P. M., Vinokur, A., and Sechrest, L. (1988). Do consensus conferences work? A process evaluation of the NIH consensus development program. *Journal of Health Politics, Policy & Law, 13*(3), 469–498.

Zander, K. (1992). Focusing on patient outcome: Case management in the 90s. *Dimensions of Critical Care Nursing, 3,* 127–129.

# 14

# EDUCATIONAL APPLICATIONS
*Joan Burggraf Riley*

## OBJECTIVES

- Describe the uses of computers in the educational process.
- Describe the uses of computers in the management of nursing education.
- Describe the computer resources needed for nursing education.
- Discuss the integration of computer technology into a nursing curriculum.
- Discuss computer applications for staff education, nurse extenders, and patient education.

Computer technology is developing at a rapid pace—a far more rapid pace than the incorporation of computer technology into nursing education and practice. The use of computers in nursing education has escalated, as it has in the health care industry generally. Nurse educators must prepare tomorrow's nurses to meet the challenges imposed by computer technology. Nurses at all levels and in all roles must have the knowledge and skill to interact with computers. They must be "computer literate" to utilize computer technology effectively.

The use of computers to support nursing education has traditionally been referred to as computer-based education (CBE), which encompasses computer-assisted instruction (CAI) and computer-managed instruction (CMI). However, computer technology in nursing education encompasses all educational activities that require and involve the use of the computer. It includes the use of computers to support (1) the educational process, including instruction and evaluation, (2) the administration of nursing educational programs, and (3) the integration of computer technology into the nursing curriculum.

Computer resources must also be available to students and faculty to support and address educational applications. Without the proper computer equipment, including hardware, software, and technological tools for implementation, computer applications in nursing education are not possible. This chapter describes the major concepts of computer technology in nursing education:

- Educational process
- Management of education
- Computer resources
- Curriculum integration

## BACKGROUND

Educational applications emerged and evolved with the development and advances of computer technology in general and in the health care industry. These applications emerged to meet the needs of developers of hospital information systems who needed computer-literate nurses to assist in the design and implementation of information systems in health care facilities.

In early 1980s, with the introduction of the microcomputer, the personal computer (PC), another computer revolution occurred that created an increased need for computer technology in education. Microcomputers made it possible for nurses to use user-friendly generic software packages, such as word-processing programs, to perform their educational and administrative activities. Microcomputers created a new group of nurses who were knowledgeable about the uses of the PC. However, they did not understand the capabilities of mainframe computers and how they were used in the emerging hospital and nursing information systems. Also, they did not understand how computers were used in nursing education, research, administration, and clinical nursing practice.

Computer applications in nursing education also developed as collegiate nursing education changed from passive to active teaching. The emergence of individualized and self-paced learning also promoted the use of computer applications in nursing education. Distance learning programs, schools without walls, and education in the workplace require that computer technology be used to communicate and to network remote students with the university facility and faculty.

# Early Educational Resources

## PLATO

During the period before the introduction of microcomputers, PLATO (Programmed Logic for Automatic Teaching Operations) was developed at the University of Illinois as a nationwide network set up by Control Data Corporation (CDC). The on-line network of terminals communicated via telephone with a CDC mainframe computer (Tymchyshyn, 1982).

PLATO provided a computer-based educational system that offered individualized student instruction (CAI). It not only offered nursing educational information but also tracked students' progress and stored their responses as they were made. In the early 1980s, CDC began to offer PLATO using microcomputers in place of the on-line terminals.

## COMMES

COMMES (Creighton On-line Multiple Medical Education Services) is another computer-based educational system; it was developed as an artificial intelligence system for nursing. COMMES serves as an educational consultant and provides information such as plans of care for a specific disease condition. It requires its own hardware and software, which was created by the faculty at Creighton University. COMMES has gone through several generations as the technology has advanced (Ryan, 1985).

# Workshops and Conferences

In the late 1970s and early 1980s, many workshops, conferences, and educational institutions were conducted to introduce computer applications for nursing to nursing professionals seeking information on this new specialty. For example, in 1981, more than 700 nurses attended one of the first conferences on computer technology and nursing, held at the National Institutes of Health, Bethesda, Maryland.

In the 1980s, because of continued demand for information about this new specialty, several educational institutions conducted summer institutes or initiated graduate courses in nursing educational programs on computer applications in nursing. Two such institutes are conducted annually, the HealthQuest/HBO Nurse Scholars Program and an institute conducted by the University of Maryland; both provide a comprehensive overview of computer applications in nursing (Skiba et al., 1992). By the 1990s, several universities had instituted master's and doctoral programs in computer applications in nursing and/or nursing informatics. Other educational institutions offered post-doctoral fellowships in informatics. This increase in academic endeavors, including courses in graduate nursing education, not only increased the level of qualifications of nurses who were "computer-literate" but also created a critical mass of nurses with information management and science expertise.

In 1989, the University of Maryland became one of the first to introduce graduate-level study in nursing informatics. Its major objective is to educate professionals to provide leadership in the application and management of information technology in nursing and health care (Heller et al., 1989). Other universities, such as the University of Utah and Case Western Reserve, have also established graduate nursing informatics education, and others offered academic courses (see Chap. 1).

## National Nursing Organizations

The two national nursing organizations—the American Nurses Association (ANA) and the National League for Nursing (NLN)—also became involved with nursing informatics. In 1984, the ANA created the Council on Computer Applications in Nursing, and at subsequent biannual conventions it adopted several resolutions that promoted the introduction of computer technology into nursing practice and recommended that nursing informatics be integrated into nursing practice at all levels. In 1992, the ANA designated nursing informatics as a new nursing specialty (see Chaps. 1 and 7).

In 1985, the NLN created a Council on Nursing Informatics, originally called the National Forum on Computers in Health Care in Nursing. The NLN subsequently passed two critical resolutions. The first, in 1987, focused on the need to include computer technology in nursing education. Then, in 1991, the NLN passed a second resolution which recommended that computer technology be included in the nursing curricula of educational institutions and that it become an integral part of accreditation criteria for educational institutions.

## EDUCATIONAL PROCESS

The use of computer technology in nursing education, or CBE, encompasses all activities that involve instruction and evaluation of student learning. CBE focuses on educational applications and more specifically CAI and interactive video (IAV) (Sparks, 1990). Computer applications that support other aspects of the educational process, such as testing and evaluation, have been also developed. This section will discuss the following:

- Computer-assisted instruction
- Interactive video instruction
- Testing systems
- Authoring systems
- Distance learning systems

## Scope of Educational Process

Computer-based educational applications need to be an integral part of nursing education rather than an "add-on," or "homework." The use of CAI and IAV instructional media helps carry out many of the teaching strategies that lead to success. They support the needs of students by allowing them to work at a time that meets their needs, at their own pace, with immediate feedback about their progress.

The use of CAI and/or IAV provides students with a systematic way to form their thinking. Educational computer applications train students to be careful, deliberate, and goal-directed in their thinking without the risk to patient care. The use of computers as instructional tools provides students the opportunity to make nursing decisions and to receive feedback on their actions.

When these educational technologies are used by individual students or small groups, each student must make his or her own decisions, and each student receives immediate feedback about the consequences of those decisions. In a large group class, one member of the class makes the decision, and a passive experience ensues for others in the class.

In the typical classroom situation, faculty must create a mental image of a patient situation for teaching purposes. Computers have turned the mental image into patient simulations which are usable both in the classroom and by individual students. The success of a classroom experience depends on a variety of factors, including the emotional status of the teacher and student, the time of day, the environment, and the material being taught (McGuiness, 1991). These educational technologies do provide for active learning.

## Computer-Assisted Instruction

CAI uses the computer for the purpose of instruction or teaching. It is an educational technique that involves two-way interaction between a computer and a learner. The objective is to achieve greater learning and retention than is possible with didactic instruction, since the computer allows the learner to interact at his or her own pace, and as many times as needed to master content.

CAI software allows a student or user to interact with a single microcomputer or with a microcomputer linked via a network to a file server in a learning resource center. Some CAI includes illustrations and minimal visual graphics of a procedure, but CAI does not have the sound and motion characteristics of IAV, which is described later in this chapter. In general, software for either type of computer program responds to a variety of user needs in order to achieve educational outcomes. Computer software therefore needs to be evaluated to determine its usefulness. An example of a computer software evaluation form is shown in Fig. 14.1.

---

## COMPUTER SOFTWARE EVALUATION

*Quality software is a computer program which provides a purposeful, valued, well-designed, interactive, content-accurate, motivational learning experience that capitalizes on the potentials of the computer, responds to a variety of user input, and facilitates the achievement of desirable predetermined outcomes by a target population efficiently, effectively, and creatively.*

Title of program: _____

Source: _____  Address: _____

Date produced: _____  Cost: _____  Program version: _____

Suggested running time: _____  Type of computer: _____

DOS[ ]   OS2[ ]   Other [ ]                Memory: _____K  Number disk drives required: 1[ ]  2[ ]

Hard disk: Required [ ]  Preferred [ ]  Monitor/Display: Mono [ ]  Color [ ]  [Required Adapter: _____]  Printer: Yes [ ]  No [ ]

Videodisc: [ ]   Video Interface [Manufacturer]: _____  Videotape player: [ ]  Other equipment required: _____

Additional instructional materials required: _____

Program copyrighted: Yes [ ]  No [ ]   Back-up copy: Yes [ ]  No [ ]

### COMMENTS OF REVIEWER

Program type (i.e., tutorial, drill, and practice): _____

Student Level: AD [ ]  BS [ ]  Higher Degree [ ]  Other [ ]

Program runs with minimal difficulty: Yes [ ]  No [ ]

Appropriate use of computer: Yes [ ]  No [ ]

Problems encountered: _____

Comments: _____

Recommend to others: Yes [ ]  No [ ]

Reviewed by: _____  Date: _____

Institution: _____

### A. CONTENT

Please circle either Y (Yes), N (No) or NA (Not Applicable).

1. Key concepts defined                                        Y   N   NA
2. Learning objectives clearly stated                          Y   N   NA
3. Content accurate and current                                Y   N   NA
4. Content relevant                                            Y   N   NA
5. Content free of stereotypes and cultural bias               Y   N   NA
6. Content organized and clearly presented                     Y   N   NA
7. Scope and depth of content appropriate for intended use     Y   N   NA

Comments:

### B. SUPPORT OF THE LEARNING PROCESS

1. Consistent with curriculum              Y   N   NA
2. Instructional design evident            Y   N   NA
3. Instructional design achieves purpose   Y   N   NA
4. Student participation promoted          Y   N   NA

**Figure 14.1**   Computer software evaluation. (Courtesy SREB: A product of a regional seminar funded by a nursing special projects grant and sponsored by the Southern Council on Collegiate Education for Nursing in affiliation with the Southern Regional Education Board.)

## Types of CAI

There are several types of CAI software available. The major ones are listed below:

5. Evaluation provided:
   Formative                                                    Y   N   NA
   Summative                                                    Y   N   NA
6. Feedback:
   Objective                                                    Y   N   NA
   Helpful                                                      Y   N   NA
   Varies with user imput                                       Y   N   NA

Comments:

---

### C. USER APPEAL

1. Captures and sustains user interest                          Y   N   NA
2. Can be used independently with minimal instruction           Y   N   NA
3. Adapts to user input                                         Y   N   NA
4. Speed of presentation under control of user                  Y   N   NA
5. Is efficient of user time                                    Y   N   NA
6. Protects privacy of user responses                           Y   N   NA

Comments:

---

### D. TECHNICAL ASPECTS

1. Program runs smoothly without glitches and blind loops       Y   N   NA
2. Screen display is clear with consistent format               Y   N   NA
3. Color/sound/animation/video/graphics used appropriately      Y   N   NA
4. Capable of producing hardcopy, if needed                     Y   N   NA
5. Able to enter and exit program as needed                     Y   N   NA
6. Able to make minor modifications in content to match curriculum  Y   N   NA
7. Able to adapt hardware/software to make program operational  Y   N   NA
8. Record keeping capacity adequate to meet future needs        Y   N   NA
9. Documentation is clear and complete                          Y   N   NA

Comments:

---

### E. PURCHASE CONSIDERATIONS

1. Benefits/frequency of use worth cost now and in future       Y   N   NA
2. Duplicates existing materials available (i.e., filmstrip)    Y   N   NA
3. Has mechanism for keeping content updated as needed          Y   N   NA
4. Requires additional instructional materials (i.e., workbooks)  Y   N   NA
5. Vendor support available                                     Y   N   NA
6. Purchase options:
   sale                                          [  ]
   lease                                         [  ]
   site license/network                          [  ]
   discount on multiple copies                   [  ]
7. List institutions currently using: _____

---

**ADDITIONAL COMMENTS:**

Revised 1988

---

**Note:** This Software Evaluation Tool was developed by: **Linda Speranza** (seminar leader), Valencia Community College, Orlando, Florida; **Kathleen C. Brown,** University of Alabama at Birmingham; **Frances C. Henderson,** Alcorn State University, Natchez, Mississippi; **Kathleen J. Mikan,** University of Alabama at Birmingham; **Marilyn Ann Murphy,** University of Texas Health Science Center, San Antonio; **Rose Marie Norris,** Georgia State University; **Maribeth K. Traer,** Lynchburg College, Lynchburg, Virginia; **Carol M. Wiggs,** Baylor University, Dallas, Texas.

**Figure 14.1** *Continued*

- Drill and practice
- Tutorials
- Simulations

These terms have traditionally been used to describe CAI; however, some experts indicate that they can also be used to describe different aspects of IAV software.

***Drill and Practice***  Drill and practice routines allow the student to practice previously learned material. The typical format consists of questions with multiple answers. Generally, well-designed CAI will not only indicate if the answer is correct or incorrect, but also provide explanations about the content. It will score and track the student's progress and provide feedback to the student when the program is completed.

Students may spend as much time in practice as desired. Many drill and practice CAI programs are available for standard nursing education content such as dosage calculations. Other CAI programs are also available, such as NCLEX to review for state board examinations.

***Tutorials***  Tutorials or remedial instruction is CAI software that provides didactic information and uses branching technique. This technique enables the student to move from easier to more advanced levels of learning. Tutorials use text, and in many cases include illustrations and diagrams. They can include drill exercises that provide feedback that helps the student determine if he or she can move forward to new material. Tutorials are utilized to provide instruction on a specific content area, usually in place of classroom or textbook coverage.

***Simulations***  Simulations are case studies and/or models written to provide the student with individualized experiences. They are designed to provide opportunities to deal with realistic clinical or administrative problems. The learner can attempt to solve problems before entering the clinical environment, thus reducing the risks of decision making while practicing clinical skills, and can make mistakes without affecting a patient's well-being. Simulations allow students to work through assessment and nursing actions for patients with, for example, pediatric oncology and medical-surgical conditions. Some nursing education programs even allow students to enter its hospital information system (HIS) to document patient care through simulation programs.

Simulations have also been developed for the training laboratories of most HISs to teach prospective users how the system functions. Academic computer laboratories are gaining access to these hospital systems to provide learning experiences for students. Such access extends the capabilities of computer-assisted software for assessment and decision-making skills and shows students the actual content of nursing information systems in use to document patient care (Holzemer et al., 1983).

### Characteristics of CAI

CAI must be stimulating and motivating to provide for optimal learning. The four instructional design features that make CAI interesting are (1) objectives, (2) attentiveness, (3) individual control, and (4) reinforcement (Farabaugh, 1990). Numerous studies have been reported on the effects of CAI on concept acquisition in nursing. While no significant differences have been found between computer and other strategies on immediate recall, intermediate retention, or long-term retention, others report a decrease in instructional time and the development of positive attitudes toward computers (Belfry and Winnie, 1988; Murphy, 1991; Rizzolo, 1994; Thiele and Holloway, 1992).

Nursing skills are subjects with significant software development potential. Other areas of software development include classic scientific principles and specialized nursing practice simulations. Areas currently lacking software development are OSHA standards on protection from bloodborne pathogens and TB precautions and JCAHO topics such as fire safety. These areas require annual review by both staff nurses and student nurses.

Developers of CAI caution that quality programs require computer screens that are specifically designed to be instructionally sound, aesthetically pleasing, and comfortable for student use. CAI must be stimulating and motivating to promote optimal learning (Farabaugh, 1990).

## Advantages of CAI

CAI has been in existence long enough for significant studies to have been done to evaluate its impact on nursing education. Some of its main advantages are as follows (Norman, 1982). CAI provides immediate feedback to the student, indicating whether answers are correct or incorrect, whether the process followed was appropriate or inappropriate, and, over time, whether the student's ability to reach correct decisions has improved. CAI allows the student to respond to the computer program as it is received by analyzing graphics, manipulating animated forms, or answering questions.

The CAI programs are designed to respond to the student with endless patience, repeating information and offering guidance indefinitely. CAI also offers individualized instruction because many of the software programs allow the student to create scenarios or structure models or frameworks for study. Additionally, CAI programs make learning available when the student has the time and interest to learn. This enables CAI to supplement the classroom content. CAI programs lay the groundwork for computer literacy as the student creates or uses the programs. Students become more comfortable using computers when they are familiar with their specific instructions. Finally, CAI as a learning medium can be artful and imaginative.

Other advantages of CAI have been cited by other experts: (1) computer laboratories help reduce the number of large lecture classes and provide for smaller instructional groups with seminar atmospheres, (2) students can proceed at a pace determined by their own capacity and motivation and not at the pace of the academic schedule, (3) skills can be updated through simulation programs, and (4) continuing education can emanate from the academic community to professionals in practice throughout the country.

## Evaluation of CAI

Nursing educators must be involved in the selection of CAI. They must review and evaluate the programs for their specific course content. There are several evaluation tools that can be used to review, score, and determine the usefulness of the CAI programs. One short form is shown in Fig. 14.2.

Faculty must also evaluate the use of CAI as a teaching methodology. This will require postgraduation evaluation by employers to determine preparedness in the clinical setting, evaluation by administrators for ongoing support and resources, evaluation by students for satisfaction and learning, and evaluation of CAI as a teaching methodology by faculty. The availability and usability of CAI software programs must also be evaluated.

# Interactive Videodisc Instruction

IAV software programs, also called IVD, combine the CAI interaction made possible by the microcomputer with the motion and sound stored on a videodisc or laser disc. IAV uses a touch-screen monitor to activate the sequences, and a laser videodisc player which integrates and runs the motion and sound of the software program. IAV integrates computers with video systems, providing students with live tapes of learning activities and allowing them to interact with a motion picture or graphic video system under computer control.

## Characteristics of IAV

IAV uses a computer monitor with a touch-screen feature, which provides for ease of use even for the computer novice. It also allows the student to branch off into related and supporting content areas as the individual users' needs require. Students enjoy the "real-life" simulations IAV provides. Instead of seeing a simple videotape of a nursing skill, students are able to have decision-making opportunities by utilizing IAV (Ullmer, 1989, 1990). There are three levels of videodisc players and systems:

- Level I: Videodisc player and monitor. A player is used to access individual frames or full motion on a videodisc.
- Level II: Videodisc player, monitor, microprocessor, and control device. A videodisc player with a built-in microprocessor is programmed to respond to a decision frame and branch to another section of the videodisc.
- Level III: Videodisc player, monitor, microcomputer, control device, and program control information. In Level III, the newest and most common IAV, an interactive video system combines a videodisc player with a microcomputer. It allows for a blend of video, audio, and computer. It is programmed to branch using complex sequences, respond with educational information, and keep records (Rizzolo, 1994).

## Guidelines for CAI Review

CAI Title: _____

Publisher: _____

|  | Low | | | High |
|---|---|---|---|---|
| **1. Ease of Use** | 1 | 2 | 3 | 4 |

Easy to begin program
User controls pace and sequence
Instructions easy to follow
Comments:

|  |  |  |  |  |
|---|---|---|---|---|
| **2. Maximizes Microcomputer Attributes** | 1 | 2 | 3 | 4 |

Interaction is frequent and varied
Immediate and satisfying feedback
Uses graphics and/or animation
Uses rapid calculations
Comments:

|  |  |  |  |  |
|---|---|---|---|---|
| **3. Interest Level** | 1 | 2 | 3 | 4 |

Holds attention
Motivating
Personalized
Individualized by use of branching
Individualized by use of varied feedback
Comments:

**I would give this program a rating of:**  (Please circle)

| * | ** | *** | **** |
|---|---|---|---|
| 1 | 2 | 3 | 4 |

This program could be used for:
1.

2.

© Diskovery, 1985

**Figure 14.2**  Guidelines for CAI review. (Courtesy C. Bolwell, *Directory of Educational Software for Nursing*, 5th ed., New York: NLN.)

The microcomputer allows the expansion of these two technologies so that students can have individualized, user-controlled, user-paced instruction with the potential for immediate remediation and feedback during testing. After information is provided to the student through video systems, the computer controls the learning objectives, content, and test questions. If the student does not answer a question correctly, the section of tape that provided the correct answer can be replayed. Each student's experience with an IAV program will be different. The student's responses and decisions will affect the instructional experience. The ability to participate in the assessment, implementation, and evaluation of nursing care in a very thoughtful and deliberate manner contributes significantly to the goal of developing critical thinkers.

The computer augments the video display in several ways: (1) it provides interaction between the student and the computer so that difficult material can be clarified, (2) it points out the mechanism or exception to the current educational setting, (3) it provides drill and practice in content areas, (4) it provides a self-assessment posttest, and (5) it tracks student progress through study modules (Tymchyshyn, 1983).

Utilizing IAV for teaching psychomotor skills in a student technologies laboratory has been very successful. Students work through the IAV program at their own pace with the relevant patient care equipment next to the IAV equipment. Skills such as medication administration, intravenous (IV) therapy, or wound care can be mastered by students with the use of IAV at the bedside in the technologies laboratory. For example, the student reviews the IAV intravenous therapy program, then demonstrates mastery of the skill during the same class period.

### Advantages of IAV

IAV can be a useful teaching tool in the skills laboratory, particularly because students must practice skills prior to implementing them in the clinical setting. IAV allows the student to see and perform the skill simultaneously under various scenarios. Such practice provides an easier transition of skill from the laboratory to client care, something that simple video or lecture teaching cannot provide. It reduces learning time, provides flexibility in access time, is self-directed, allows for individual involvement, and can be repeated as needed (Bolwell, 1993b).

As nursing education programs stress the development of critical thinking skills over simple memorization of recipes for skill performance (such as suctioning), nursing education has turned to problem-based learning, which utilizes few or no lecture-style classes. The role of IAV in this process has been to provide more stimulating and challenging instruction. Many advantages have been reported by educators using IAV. Students are less anxious about performing skills after the realistic practice experience presented with IAV, and they enjoy the exciting, complex situations that IAV provides without risk to patient safety.

Students have been found to meet therapeutic communication course objectives more efficiently when they use IAV. In one study, students in both the control and IAV groups were able to meet the communication objectives, but the students utilizing IAV were able to achieve these objectives at a higher level within the first month of the semester. The benefit of this achievement is that students can better meet patient communication needs earlier in their clinical experiences. However, additional research about IAV's impact on learning is required (Napholz and McCanse, 1994).

### Evaluation of IAV

Like CAI, IAV needs to be evaluated prior to selection. Evaluation of this type of instructional software should not only include instructional design features and operational features, but also the IAV features. IAV should be reviewed before purchase, since IAV programs are expensive. An example of an IAV evaluation form is shown in Fig. 14.3. This tool has been found to be both comprehensive and easy to use, according to the University of Cincinnati and the University of Texas Medical Branch.

## Testing Systems

Testing systems are software programs designed by developers or teachers as computerized evaluations or programmed tests. Computerized test banks in the areas of dosage calculation and NCLEX review are extremely helpful and widely utilized. Computerized tests for testing students on, for example, the physical assessment skills course have been implemented in many of the newly initiated Advanced Practice Nurse curricula. These tests include objective questions as well as diagrams, which are imported into the tests via scanning hardware.

Students' reactions to the computerized testing methodology are generally positive. Students like the fact that they can receive grades and information about incorrect answers immediately. They also prefer the flexibility of being able to take a particular test when convenient during a week's time frame rather than at a specified class time. Testing programs are often structured in such a way that students are unable to return to previously asked test questions. This is probably the one disadvantage to testing systems, even though it is identical to the way the new on-line NCLEX examination is provided. Students do grow accustomed to this format in time.

Effective April 1994, the National Council Licensure Examinations for Registered Nurses (NCLEX-RN) changed from paper-and-pencil, twice yearly administration to year-round administration via on-line computer-based testing in selected locations in every state and United States territories. Familiarity with computer testing is not essential, as the NCLEX test utilizes two keys on the computer keyboard. Nevertheless, many educators want their students to be exposed to computer adaptive testing

# Interactive Videodisc Program Evaluation Form
University of Cincinnati and University of Texas Medical Branch Version

Title of Program _____

Please check the box for each item that best descibes your rating of the interactive video disk program.

| Instructional Design Features | Not Applicable | Poor | Fair | Average | Above Average | Excellent | Comments |
|---|---|---|---|---|---|---|---|
| 1 Accurate and clear content? | ☐ | ☐ | ☐ | ☐ | ☐ | ☐ | _____ |
| 2 Correct spelling, grammar, & punctuation? | ☐ | ☐ | ☐ | ☐ | ☐ | ☐ | _____ |
| 3 Screen displays aesthetic? | ☐ | ☐ | ☐ | ☐ | ☐ | ☐ | _____ |
| 4 Effective branching? | ☐ | ☐ | ☐ | ☐ | ☐ | ☐ | _____ |
| 5 Multiple paths or levels provided? | ☐ | ☐ | ☐ | ☐ | ☐ | ☐ | _____ |
| 6 Feedback supports learning objectives? | ☐ | ☐ | ☐ | ☐ | ☐ | ☐ | _____ |
| 7 Free from stereotypes? | ☐ | ☐ | ☐ | ☐ | ☐ | ☐ | _____ |
| 8 Creative design? | ☐ | ☐ | ☐ | ☐ | ☐ | ☐ | _____ |
| 9 Effectively captures user's attention? | ☐ | ☐ | ☐ | ☐ | ☐ | ☐ | _____ |
| 10 Reading level appropriate? | ☐ | ☐ | ☐ | ☐ | ☐ | ☐ | _____ |
| 11 Objectives of program met? | ☐ | ☐ | ☐ | ☐ | ☐ | ☐ | _____ |
| 12 Effective cues for knowledge retention? | ☐ | ☐ | ☐ | ☐ | ☐ | ☐ | _____ |
| 13 Size and style of text easy to read? | ☐ | ☐ | ☐ | ☐ | ☐ | ☐ | _____ |
| **Operational Features** | | | | | | | |
| 14 Clear instructions? | ☐ | ☐ | ☐ | ☐ | ☐ | ☐ | _____ |
| 15 Free of programming errors? | ☐ | ☐ | ☐ | ☐ | ☐ | ☐ | _____ |
| 16 Able to identify where you are in program? | ☐ | ☐ | ☐ | ☐ | ☐ | ☐ | _____ |

**Figure 14.3** Interactive videodisc program evaluation form. (Courtesy B. Weiner, University of Cincinnati, OH/AJN CO.)

(CAT) prior to licensure examination. The one feature of CAT that initial users have difficulty with is the inability to skip questions and go back to them or to review answers to previous questions. Students exposed to this testing format in their nursing education program will have less difficulty with NCLEX.

| | Not Applicable | Poor | Fair | Average | Above Average | Excellent | Comments |
|---|---|---|---|---|---|---|---|
| 17 User can control order of presentation? | ☐ | ☐ | ☐ | ☐ | ☐ | ☐ | _____ |
| 18 Can review previous screens? | ☐ | ☐ | ☐ | ☐ | ☐ | ☐ | _____ |
| 19 Touch panels clearly indentified? | ☐ | ☐ | ☐ | ☐ | ☐ | ☐ | _____ |
| 20 Able to distinguish choice you made? | ☐ | ☐ | ☐ | ☐ | ☐ | ☐ | _____ |
| 21 Screen transitions smooth? | ☐ | ☐ | ☐ | ☐ | ☐ | ☐ | _____ |
| 22 Control amount of time on each screen? | ☐ | ☐ | ☐ | ☐ | ☐ | ☐ | _____ |
| 23 Easily exit to various areas of the program? | ☐ | ☐ | ☐ | ☐ | ☐ | ☐ | _____ |
| 24 Easily exit program? | ☐ | ☐ | ☐ | ☐ | ☐ | ☐ | _____ |

### Interactive Videodisc (IVD) Features

| | Not Applicable | Poor | Fair | Average | Above Average | Excellent | Comments |
|---|---|---|---|---|---|---|---|
| 25 Content presented effectively using IVD? | ☐ | ☐ | ☐ | ☐ | ☐ | ☐ | _____ |
| 26 IVD format enhances learning? | ☐ | ☐ | ☐ | ☐ | ☐ | ☐ | _____ |
| 27 Effective use of color? | ☐ | ☐ | ☐ | ☐ | ☐ | ☐ | _____ |
| 28 Effective use of graphics? | ☐ | ☐ | ☐ | ☐ | ☐ | ☐ | _____ |
| 29 Effective use of sound? | ☐ | ☐ | ☐ | ☐ | ☐ | ☐ | _____ |
| 30 Effective use of touch screen? | ☐ | ☐ | ☐ | ☐ | ☐ | ☐ | _____ |
| 31 Effective use of video vs. computer to present content? | ☐ | ☐ | ☐ | ☐ | ☐ | ☐ | _____ |
| 32 Quality of Video? | ☐ | ☐ | ☐ | ☐ | ☐ | ☐ | _____ |
| 33 Length of Video segments? | ☐ | ☐ | ☐ | ☐ | ☐ | ☐ | _____ |
| 34 Authenticity of on-screen characters? | ☐ | ☐ | ☐ | ☐ | ☐ | ☐ | _____ |
| 35 Quality of narration? | ☐ | ☐ | ☐ | ☐ | ☐ | ☐ | _____ |
| 36 Your OVERALL rating of the program? | ☐ | ☐ | ☐ | ☐ | ☐ | ☐ | _____ |

Length of Time Spent Reviewing Program_____Modules Covered_____

Date_____Reviewer_____Institution_____

Reprinted With Permission

**Figure 14.3**   *Continued*

## Authoring Systems

Authoring systems are computer programs that allow educators or nurses to create instructional tools or evaluation materials for the computer without having to prepare a computer program. Authoring software does not require the user to have any previous programming experience in order to develop courseware. These systems provide on-screen tools (menus, prompts, icons) to help users enter text, prepare graphics, or prescribe branching (Locatis, 1992).

Numerous authoring software programs with differing complexities are available. Finding the appropriate authoring system for different courses is important (Christensen and Murphy, 1990). General-purpose authoring software is designed for development of materials for use by the purchaser only, not for distribution or sale (Pogue, 1985).

## Distance Learning Systems

Computer technology allows students in different locations to attend and participate in the same class simultaneously. Many institutions are creating electronic classrooms. These electronic classrooms use cable television, telephone lines, and computers with modems to provide opportunities for participation by students located at various remote sites. Homework assignments are delivered by fax/digital transmission, and students' computer terminals serve as blackboards and notebooks by which the teacher in the classroom communicates with the students.

Faculty participating in such programs try to liven up their classes to help maintain interest among those participating via video monitors. Faculty also express concern about students turning into passive viewers. Cooperative learning activities can help to prevent passive learning. Administrators hope that cable television or computer-based courses will cut costs while at the same time allowing them to serve more students. However, multimedia resource centers, computer laboratories, software programs, and technical support are still expensive to establish and to operate, especially because technology is changing so rapidly.

## MANAGEMENT OF NURSING EDUCATION

The management of nursing education, sometimes referred to as CMI, is defined as the use of computer systems to support the administration and management of nursing education programs. These computer applications support the management of all paperwork and records required by nursing education programs. They include the storage and retrieval of information required by the nursing education program, including the evaluation of student progress, courses in the curriculum, and faculty.

Many mundane functions, such as record keeping, are required in education. As a result, computer systems have been developed to collect, store, and process information about students, staff, and curricula. Such systems provide student and program record keeping and thus serve to monitor students' progress. One such system designed to evaluate students and educational programs was a curriculum model developed by the Boston College School of Nursing. It was one of the first models which identified a framework for collecting information about nursing students, courses, clinical patient care experiences, and postgraduate work experience. It also offered a method for evaluating decision-making procedures relative to program effectiveness (Sweeney et al., 1980).

## Advantages of Management Applications

Computer applications for the administration and management of records to support nursing education have several advantages, the most important being the saving in time. Secondary benefits, also important, include the following: (1) enhanced communication between faculty and nurse supervisors regarding student rotations, (2) planned curriculum experiences for students, (3) advanced monitoring of students' health, grade, and attendance records, (4) appropriate clinical experiences matched to students' learning objectives, (5) resource allocation, (6) cost reduction, and (7) ability of faculty to provide efficient programs while having time to teach.

## Types of Management Applications

Types of administration systems utilized in nursing education include the following:

- Student records
- Student rotations
- Course evaluations
- Educational reports

### Student Records

Innovative education directors have used management systems to create educational records that serve as documentation for outside accrediting agencies. CMI records provide tools for monitoring students' progress through the curricula and monitoring program effectiveness. As the requirements for documentation increase, computerized records are essential to keep track of each student's compliance with curricula criteria. CMI allows the tracking of student requirements such as CPR certification, passed prerequisite courses, or the required yearly tuberculin skin test. Easy access to this information by clinical agencies, faculty, advisers, and students themselves is essential.

Student files provide an enormous amount of demographic data, information about career training, health records, and program flow (Fig. 14.4). Using computers, student records can be profiled, criteria for admission to certain programs can be reviewed or established, reasons for leaving school can be analyzed, and students can be compared (Davis and Williams, 1980).

## Student Rotations

Just as staff scheduling can be computerized, so can student rotations and schedules. An important part of student nurse curricula is balancing course preparation with clinical rotations. Certain obligatory training must be acquired at specific times. The advanced practice nursing students that major in a clinical nursing specialty must have a variety of clinical experiences in their respective specialties. Computerized scheduling systems are being implemented to schedule the appropriate experiences for them. Computerized rotation records allow an easy and comprehensive

**Figure 14.4**   Student records database. (Courtesy Georgetown University School of Nursing, Office of Student Affairs, Washington, DC.)

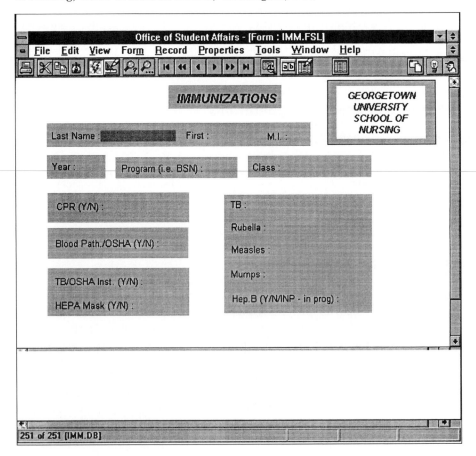

method of keeping records about each student's experience to allow faculty to identify their further clinical placements.

Computer systems are also used in other countries, such as Canada, North Wales, and the Netherlands, for allocating student rotation, allowing for vacation leave, and tracking information on absences due to sickness. The allocation and tracking of students become complex when multiple hospitals are used as rotation sites, when nurse supervisors must be informed of the number of students they will have before assigning staff nurses, when variable training blocks are scheduled, and when flexibility of training must be considered. These functions are facilitated by computers (Ellis, 1981; Pluyter-Wenting, 1983; Pritchard, 1982).

Use of the storage and retrieval capabilities of computers has been maximized by the General Nursing Council (GNC) for England and Wales, which maintains a registry of student nurses. One such system is being used in the United Kingdom and the European Union to monitor nursing training and the movement of qualified persons based on skill levels (Collins, 1983).

## Course Evaluations

Course and clinical evaluation analysis and summaries can be produced to assess educational activities. This is an effective utilization of technology to provide curricula evaluation. Scanned and computer-processed course evaluations provide faculty feedback on courses. An example of a specially designed form used at Georgetown University is shown in Fig. 14.5. It allows the student to evaluate three different areas of the course. The first covers the characteristics of students in the course, such as attendance or amount of time spent studying for the class. The second addresses whether the stated objectives were met, whether course requirements were helpful in meeting objectives, the fairness of exams and grading, and the students' rating of the quality and extent of their learning. The third area is the students' evaluation of the instructor, including faculty preparation for class, the quality of classroom presentation, availability of the faculty, and the ability of the faculty to challenge and encourage learning.

Computer scanning of these evaluations provide comprehensive and rapid feedback to faculty regarding course successes and failures. The system also provides a cumulative summary sheet of the course evaluations to date. This allows faculty to demonstrate progress and growth in their teaching skills and course development.

## Educational Reports

Computers are used for storing other student information, such as test items, for analysis of test results for individual students and groups of students, and for generating test questions from test pools. Many computer systems exist that document nurse licensure and continuing education experience. These systems were developed when continuing education became mandatory in many states in order for nurses to qualify for

Graduate School of Nursing
Uniformed Services University of the Health Sciences
Course Evaluation

DO NOT WRITE IN THIS BOX

INSTRUCTOR:
COURSE #:
COURSE TITLE:
SEMESTER:

To the student:
Your response to this form provides not only an opportunity to reflect on your experience in this course, but also to be helpful to faculty in teaching and planning for the future. Your answers, which are confidential, will be most helpful if they are as accurate and complete as possible. Besides filling in the "objective" sections, you are asked to give special attention to the sections on the back of this form for written comments. Use a #2 pencil for shading in your responses to each question.

I.   **STUDENT**    Please provide the following information about yourself:
Mark the space to the right which corresponds to the letter of your answer.

1. Your graduating year:    a. 1995    b. 1996    c. 1997    d. Other

2. In what program are you enrolled:    a. FNP    b. NA    c. Other

3. During the semester did you miss any classes?    a. None    b. A few    c. Many

4. Approximately how many hours did you spend studying for this class in a typical week?
     a. More than 10    b. 6-10    c. 3-5    d. Less than 3

5. Please use the space on the back for additional comments on your preparation for or involvement in this course.

II.   **COURSE**    Please rate the specific aspects of the course using a scale of 5
(high, outstanding) to 1 (low, poor); 0 = not applicable.

HIGH OUTSTANDING   LOW/POOR   NOT APPLICABLE

1. To what degree were the stated objectives of the course met?

2. How effective were the readings, research, and other requirements in helping you to meet these objectives?

3. Did the exams or other graded material fairly represent the content and skills taught in the course?

4. Do you believe that exams and other work were graded fairly?

5. To what degree do specialized forms of study (labs, language drills, field trips, e.g.) contribute to the value of the course?

6. How much have you learned in the course? (Your assessment of the quality and extent of that learning)

7. Please use the space on the back of this page to explain your ratings or to comment further on any aspect of the course.

III.   **INSTRUCTOR**    Please comment on the instructor's handling of this class, keeping in mind that we recognize the importance of a variety of teaching styles and approaches. Again the scale is 5 (high, outstanding) to 1 (low, poor) and 0 for not applicable. If the course had more than one instructor please fill out a separate sheet for each one. The name of the instructor is shown on the top of this form.

1. Did the instructor seem consistently well prepared for class?

2. Was the quality of classroom presentation stimulating (consider effectiveness of discussions, demonstrations and lectures)?

3. How available, willing and helpful was the instructor in advising and assisting students outside of class?

4. Did the instructor establish high standards, challenge you, and encourage you to do your best work?

5. What is your overall evaluation of the instructor?

6. Please use the space on the back of this page to explain or comment on your evaluation. (You might wish to take into account such factors as the size of the class, the inherent difficulty or complexity of the material, availability of resources for study, or any other factors you consider relevant.)

SCANTRON   FORM NO. F-7218-USU   © SCANTRON CORPORATION 1994 ALL RIGHTS RESERVED   Scantron asks that you please RECYCLE this product.   M10.3594-C   F0105-12 11 10 9 8 7 6 5 4 3 2 1

**Figure 14.5**    Course evaluation form. (Courtesy GSN/USUHS.)

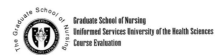

Graduate School of Nursing
Uniformed Services University of the Health Sciences
Course Evaluation

COMMENTS: Please use the spaces below for comments about this course, the instructor, or your involvement in the class that might not be covered adequately by the questions on the front of this sheet. Thank you for taking the time to work on this evaluation.

I.    COMMENTS on your involvement in this course.

II.   COMMENTS on your evaluations of the course.

III.  COMMENTS on your evaluations of the instructor.

**Figure 14.5**   *Continued*

relicensure. Currently, the presentation of continuing education credits is not monitored nationally; however, systems that have been designed for awarding continuing education credits at state levels could be expanded to include such quality monitoring controls.

## COMPUTER RESOURCES

Computer resources for nursing education must be available to faculty and students to enable them to utilize educational applications of computer technology. Students must have access to state-of-the-art equipment in order to be efficient and effective in their role as students and to be prepared to utilize computer technology in their role as professional nurses.

### Planning for Computer Applications

Planning is essential for successful computer implementation and must take into account the mission and goals of the nursing education program. Successful implementation of computer technology into educational institutions requires more than the acquisition of computer equipment and resources (Arnold, 1992; Mikan, 1992).

A computer resources committee should be established as a permanent standing school committee. Such a committee should have representatives who use computers for various purposes. They should include (1) faculty members representing the different types of teaching programs, such as basic clinical courses, graduate courses, or specialty courses such as midwifery, (2) researchers and/or research staff involved in individual and school research studies, (3) administrative staff involved in the maintenance of student records and databases, and (4) representatives from other university departments that affect the school of nursing, such as the library.

Collectively, the committee needs to develop a plan, strategy, and budget for the development, maintenance, and upgrading of computer resources for the entire educational institution. The committee should evaluate the nature of the students, identify their needs, and determine the nature of educational technology in the institution. The full range of possible applications of computer technology should be explored during this planning phase (Larson, 1985; Perciful, 1992).

The computer resources committee should identify and develop short- and long-range goals with milestones and a budget needed to support computer applications that address the need to

- Integrate computer technology into the undergraduate and graduate education.
- Enhance faculty knowledge of computer applications in nursing education.
- Support nursing research and administrative activities.

- Coordinate and collaborate with other departments that affect student education.
- Develop tools to determine the level of need, educational requirements, and evaluation of the applications.
- Develop teaching strategies to make all students and faculty computer-literate.
- Establish a learning resources center (LRC) with appropriate staff, equipment, and other materials.
- Establish an organizational structure to administer the computer applications in the institution, including the LRC (see Fig. 14.6).

## Learning Resource Center

An LRC with a computer laboratory enables faculty to function effectively in their roles as educators, researchers, administrators, and practitioners. Such a center must be available to students for access to CAI and IAV instruction, review of course materials, and preparation of school papers. Sophisticated LRCs are only as useful as the skill levels of the faculty and students who use them, and as the technical support for and resources available to them. The basic requirements for an LRC include

- Hardware
- Software
- Technical support
- Supporting materials.

**Figure 14.6**   Computers in the curriculum model.

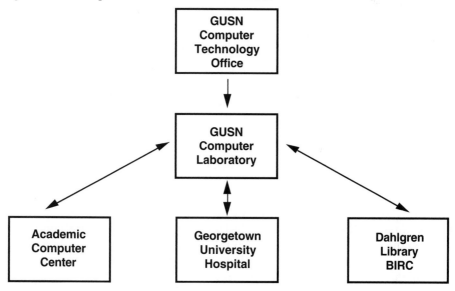

## Hardware

Hardware should be chosen for its suitability for the priority tasks to be performed. Generally LRCs will have state-of-the-art equipment: (1) microcomputers with different size disk drives, (2) keyboards, (3) mouses, (4) compatible printers with graphics capability (laser printers can be linked to multiple computers), and (5) IAV computer units. The IAV computer units include not only a microcomputer with a touch-screen monitor, but also a laser disc player for the visual and sound clips.

*Local Area Network*   An important consideration when selecting computers is the need for a local area network (LAN) to link the computers. An LAN links individual computer units to a file server (dedicated computer), which is used for storing all available software. This feature allows for teaching of students using identical software programs. Operating an LAN offers a facility many advantages. Computers accessible to students should also be networked with computers in faculty and administrative offices for efficient use of the resources.

*On-Line and/or Facsimile (Fax) Capabilities*   A fax modem is needed to provide on-line communication to other departments, such as the library's on-line knowledge databases, hospital information systems, and other external computer systems. The modem is also needed to link to the Internet via a "node," which is generally available in most educational institutions. Internet offers several functions, such as E-mail, bulletin boards, and services like Gopher, MOSAIC, and World Wide Web (WWB). Other on-line nursing resources are also available via communication networks and/or the Internet, such as (1) Sigma Theta Tau, which provides its electronic library and journal, (2) FITNET ON-LINE, which provides information on software, hardware, interactive video, CAI, and other materials requested by users, (3) E.T. Net, which provides information on interactive educational materials, and (4) AJN Network, ANA* NET, and several on-line networks which provide other educational information services and resources to the nursing community (see Chap. 7.)

Fax hardware allows the transmission of written documents. These two communication modes provide a valuable link for scholars to work together in different locations.

*Projection Equipment and Portable Classrooms*   Other equipment needed in an LRC includes a computer projector for hands-on demonstrations of computer applications in the center and/or classroom. Many LRCs are now offering portable computers for faculty and students to check out on weekends. Other centers are initiating portable notebook computer classrooms, which convert traditional classrooms into computer classrooms. This innovative strategy allows for versatile, instead of dedicated, classroom space for student education.

*Ergonomics*   Another major factor to consider when selecting LRC resources is the ergonomics of the facility. Computer furniture must be selected to support the hardware equipment in a user-comfortable environment. Many LRCs with space limitations use computer buddies, tables designed to stack hardware efficiently in small spaces. It is important that computer chairs be height adjustable in order to minimize users' back strain.

## Software

The careful selection of software computer programs is essential when planning for the integration of computer technology into nursing education. Computer software should include generic software packages, including (1) word processing, (2) spreadsheets, (3) database management systems, (4) statistical analysis, (5) graphics, (6) communication, (7) authoring systems, and (8) testing systems. The selection of CAI and IAV programs is also critical to the introduction of computer technology into the classroom, curricula, and educational process. When the basic software packages and programs are purchased, site licenses should be obtained so that these programs can be loaded on all computers, not only in the computer laboratory but also in the entire educational institution.

*Authoring and Testing Software*   Authoring and/or testing software can be purchased and ready to use on installation or can be designed specifically for a course. A new type of authoring software allows a developer to create a specific program with graphics for a specific application, such as how to use the mouse. This new software, which uses the graphical capability of the Windows operating system, makes it possible for an instructor to load all the slides for a specific topic and/or course. For example, the slides for the cell biology or human anatomy course are loaded onto a software program that students can access for review. This type of software supplements the classroom presentations of didactic information.

*Special Software Programs*   Still other specific software programs can be developed to assist users to (1) communicate with bibliographic retrieval systems, (2) format a disk, (3) prepare a term paper using American Psychological Association (APA) guidelines, and/or (4) format specific CAI care protocols such as "care of chest tube." Icons representing different CAI and generic software programs are illustrated on the screen in Fig. 14.7.

## Technical Support

Technical support for an LRC can take various forms, depending on the goals of the laboratory. Generally, the LRC needs a computer specialist who (1) maintains and repairs the hardware and software, (2) assists users, and (3) prepares teacher-made programs using educational software. The computer specialist should have student assistants to staff the LRC during the day, in the evenings, and on weekends, when student

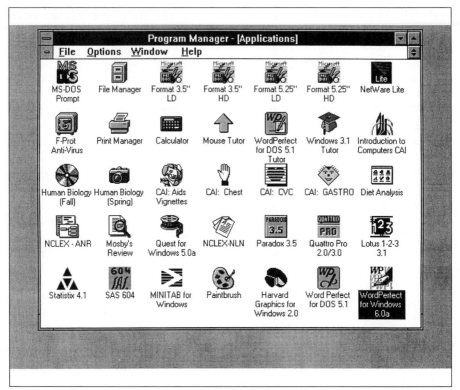

**Figure 14.7**   Icons used by Georgetown University School of Nursing: Microsoft Windows, Program Manager.

use is heavy. The computer specialist should also supervise student assistants in the computer coding, input, and basic analysis of surveys and/or research studies.

## Supporting Materials

Resource materials are essential for the LRC. It is recommended that supporting manuals for the hardware and software be available. Other materials which enhance their use can be obtained. The amount of software has expanded so significantly that a text of educational software programs is prepared annually by Bolwell and published by the NLN (Bolwell, 1993a). This book provides an unbiased description and evaluation of CAI and IAV programs for nursing. Each software program is evaluated for ease of use, interest, micro attributes, and overall rating (Fig. 14.8). The rating indicates the value other educators have placed on the program. The text also includes the educators' comments.

Resources for the LRC users should also include computer books, journals, newsletters, directories, conference proceedings, directories of computer systems and software, and other supporting materials (Nelson and

Joos, 1992). Information about computer communication sources and Internet services and resources must be developed and kept current. Additionally, sources of hardware and software should be available for review.

## Educational Staffing

Generally, the computer technology applications in an educational institution should be administered as a separate department of the institution. That department should be directed by a computer-literate faculty member who

- Is responsible for being knowledgeable and current about the state of the art in the field of nursing informatics.
- Surveys student and faculty needs for computer-based education.
- Oversees the integration of computer technology into the curriculum.
- Teaches computer applications in nursing to students, faculty, and staff.
- Oversees the LRC, including the selection of computer resources: hardware, software, and other materials.
- Prepares a budget for the entire department.
- Conducts and supports research activities.

## External Financial Support

Several organizations provide software programs needed to help nursing education programs to integrate computer technology. The Helene Fuld Health Trust and the Fuld Institute in Nursing Education (FITNE) are nonprofit membership organizations that assist basic nursing education programs in the implementation and integration of multimedia technol-

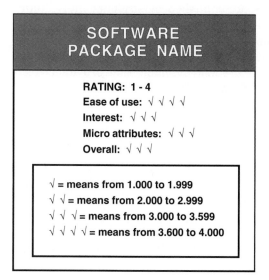

**Figure 14.8**   Bolwell evaluation score box with ratings. (Courtesy C. Bolwell, *Directory of Educational Software for Nursing,* 5th ed. New York: NLN.)

ogy, including CAI and IAV. FITNE conducts educational seminars, offers demonstrations, provides consultation, and evaluates different IAV programs. FITNE also develops IAV instructional programs for the nursing field (McAffoes, 1994). Another organization that is developing IAV is the American Journal of Nursing Company. It has developed several IAV software programs that have set the standards, along with FITNE, for this educational medium.

Many educational institutions have begun their use of computers in nursing education using grant funds. These grants have been awarded for the purpose of establishing computer laboratories or to finance the purchase of hardware and/or software to accomplish a goal that requires the use of computers.

## Teaching Strategies

Teaching students to use microcomputers most effectively requires an organized approach to the introduction and orientation of students to computer technology (Arnold, 1992). All incoming students should be given a short computer survey to determine their level of competency and to identify their specific computer technology knowledge. This survey is a useful tool for identifying the experiences and types of equipment with which students have competencies. An example of a computer survey is shown in Fig. 14.9, and an informatics questionnaire is shown in Fig. 14.10.

As computer technology programs are being introduced in primary and secondary schools, an increasing number of students entering college are computer-literate. Challenge exams can be utilized to exempt such students from classes that introduce computer content in which they are already proficient. Software programs must be available that provide CAI on the use of computer hardware and software. This instruction can also take place in formal classes or be accomplished by students individually.

Guidelines for implementation of computer applications have been developed for nursing education. Some guideline software packages are available commercially. These guidelines contain exercises for students to use to master competencies. Others are also available that provide criteria to evaluate student competencies (Bolwell, 1990).

## CURRICULUM INTEGRATION

In many educational institutions, "computer literacy" has become a goal and computer systems have been introduced to support the integration of technology into the curricula of nursing education programs. Educational frameworks have also been developed to guide the integration of computer technology in academic institutions. These frameworks provide the philosophies and methodologies to direct the integration of nursing informatics into nursing education.

---

**Georgetown University School of Nursing
Computer Literacy Survey**

I.  **DEMOGRAPHIC STATUS**

A.  Student Name:_____    Course Number: _____

B.  Class: (Circle one)
    a.  Freshman          e.  ACC Program
    b.  Sophomore         f.  RN to BSN Program
    c.  Junior            g.  Graduate Program
    d.  Senior                (Any Major)

II.  **COMPUTER STATUS**

1.  Own Microcomputer/Personal Computer (PC): Yes / No

2.  If YES: Circle one
    a.  Apple MacIntosh
    b.  IBM/IBM Clone
    c.  Other (Specify): _____

III.  **COMPUTER COMPETENCIES**

A.  PC Experience: (Circle one)
    1.  Can Operate PC Efficiently
    2.  Can Operate PC Minimally
    3.  Cannot Operate PC

B.  Computer Skills:
    1.  USE Keyboard                        Yes / No
    2.  USE Mouse                           Yes / No
    3.  Can FORMAT Disk                     Yes / No
    4.  Can LOAD Program onto Hard Disk     Yes / No
    5.  Can RUN Software Package            Yes / No
    6.  Can NAME File                       Yes / No
    7.  Can SAVE/RETRIEVE File              Yes / No

C.  Computer Software: (Circle all that apply)
    1.  Word Processing
        a.  Word Perfect/DOS
        b.  Word Perfect/Windows
        c.  Word/Windows
        d.  Other Word Processing (Specify): _____

---

**Figure 14.9**  Computer literacy survey form.

C.     Computer Software (Continued):  (Circle all that apply)
   2.     Spreadsheet
       a.     Lotus 1-2-3
       b.     Quattro Pro
       c.     Other Spreadsheet (Specify): _____

   3.     Database
       a.     DBase IV
       b.     PARADOX
       c.     Other (Specify): _____

   4.     Statistics
       a.     SAS
       b.     SPSS
       c.     Other (Specify): _____

   5.     Communications
       a.     E-Mail
       b.     Internet
       c.     Other (Specify): _____

D.     Computer-Based Instruction: (Circle one)
   1.     Computer-Assisted Instruction (CAI)
       a.     Familiar
       b.     Minimal Exposure
       c.     Not Familiar

   2.     Interactive Video (IAV)
       a.     Familiar
       b.     Minimal Exposure
       c.     Not Familiar

E.     Searching Nursing Literature Databases:
   1.     Can Search:
       a.     MEDLINE                    Yes / No
       b.     Grateful Med              Yes / No
       c.     CINAHL                        Yes / No

   2.     Can use Boolean Logic Operations:
       a.     AND Operation           Yes / No
       b.     OR Operation              Yes / No
       c.     NOT Operation           Yes / No

F.     Can use American Psychological Association (APA)
   Format for Student Papers?                Yes / No

**Figure 14.9**   *Continued*

INFORMATICS QUESTIONNAIRE

| | Check (✓) to indicate area of interest | Indicate level of expertise: 1: Beginner 2:Intermediate 3:Advanced | | |
|---|---|---|---|---|
| | | User | Manager | Developer |
| **Administration:** | | | | |
| Budgeting | | | | |
| Forecasting/Strategic Planning | | | | |
| Staff Evaluation | | | | |
| Staffing/Scheduling | | | | |
| Decision Support | | | | |
| Other | | | | |
| **Clinical Systems:** | | | | |
| Nursing Documentation | | | | |
| Order Entry | | | | |
| Ancillary Systems | | | | |
| Other | | | | |
| **Education:** | | | | |
| CD-ROM | | | | |
| CAI | | | | |
| Interactive Video Disk | | | | |
| Distance Learning | | | | |
| Other | | | | |
| **General:** | | | | |
| Data Base | | | | |
| Desk-Top Publisher | | | | |
| Spreadsheet | | | | |
| Word Processor | | | | |
| Other | | | | |
| **Research:** | | | | |
| Data Collection | | | | |
| Data Analysis | | | | |
| Other | | | | |
| **Telecommunication:** | | | | |
| E-mail | | | | |
| Computer Conferencing | | | | |
| Bulletin Boards | | | | |
| Other | | | | |

**Figure 14.10** Informatics questionnaire. (Council of Nursing Informatics / NLN, Nursing Informatics Application.)

The integration of computers into educational institutions has taken various forms. Many institutions have introduced separate academic courses at the undergraduate and graduate levels to teach computer technology in nursing. Other educational institutions have attempted to integrate the content into the existing courses of study. Still others require students to participate in workshops to learn essential computer technology content. Additionally, some educational institutions develop self-paced computer modules that provide students with guidelines for developing knowledge and competency in nursing technology and becoming computer-literate. However, the most successful integration occurs when an educational institution has the following characteristics: (1) faculty convinced of the importance of computer technology in nursing, (2) a computer resource center with not only hardware, but also appropriate CAI, IAV, and other software programs necessary for teaching the content, and (3) an educational framework and plan that assist faculty in the implementation of nursing informatics in the school and the curricula.

One such successful program is that developed at Georgetown University School of Nursing. A description of its model, used as a framework for integrating computer technology into the school of nursing, is described below.

## Nursing Informatics Education Model

The Nursing Informatics Education Model (NIEM) was developed by Riley and Saba at Georgetown University School of Nursing (Fig. 14.11). The NIEM focuses on the identification of three dimensions of content that comprise nursing informatics as defined in earlier chapters, namely com-

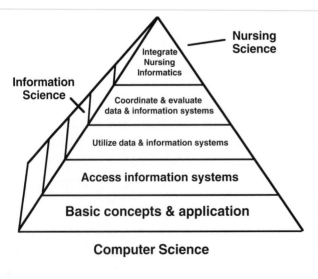

**Figure 14.11** Nursing Informatics Education Model (NIEM). (Courtesy Riley and Saba.)

puter science, information science, and nursing science. The NIEM focuses on the educational outcomes which must be addressed in all three domains of learning: cognitive, affective, and psychomotor.

By achieving objectives in each domain of learning, students can fully integrate nursing informatics into their nursing roles. This integration of knowledge and competence in nursing education requires that programs include both content, "hands on" application, and attitude. This model supports the integration of computer technology into nursing education to enhance the critical thinking skills of students of nursing and provides an active learning experience.

Computer application in nursing education allows students to make decisions in simulated case studies without risk to patients. Confidence level (Weiner et al., 1993), psychomotor skill level, and knowledge attainment are all enhanced when computer technology is used in the educational process. The integration of technology into nursing education was introduced at the School of Nursing several years ago. After much experimentation, the NIEM framework was selected and developed to provide an organized and systematic method of introducing computer technology into the curriculum.

### Undergraduate Nursing Education

NIEM provides a "road map" for the implementation and integration of computer technology at the undergraduate level. Using this model, a computer technology thread is introduced throughout the curriculum. The terminal objective for NIEM for the undergraduate curriculum has been identified as

> The development of the knowledge and competencies necessary to apply and manage nursing informatics, computer technology, and data management.

There are four steps in integrating computer concepts into the undergraduate curriculum.

*First Step*  Students are first introduced to the role of computer technology as nursing students. In this first step, students are given the knowledge and technical skills to function as efficient and effective students. Computers and networks are required as standard media for educational and scholarly activities.

The computer science content for beginning students includes the concepts of computer hardware, computer software, and computer system components. Students are oriented to the computer resource center that is available to them. The computer application content includes the use of a word-processing software package to prepare written assignments and the format and preparation requirements for scholarly papers using APA. The information science content includes the use of the computerized library system for on-line searching of the card catalogue for nursing books and of bibliographic databases for nursing journal articles.

Students are introduced to the many uses of the computer by nurses in all settings: practice, administration, education, and research. By introducing the student during this first step to computer technology, the playing field is leveled so that all the nursing students will learn how to use these media and can use them effortlessly.

*Second Step*  In the second step, students begin to apply computer technology to document and access health information for purposes of patient assessment. They are oriented to the HIS. In addition, they begin to use the School of Nursing's newly developed nursing assessment and data collection tool based on the school's conceptual framework.

This computerized assessment tool utilizes the Saba Home Health Care Classification (HHCC) of Nursing Diagnosis and Interventions, including an adapted version of the 20 home health care components with questions and cues, to guide the student's assessment of a patient. The student's response to cues allows the computer to branch if a need for nursing is identified to link the student to the critical path based on the nursing process. This computerized assessment tool is utilized in the classroom to develop patient care plans. The tool is also emulated in the hospital patient information system for recording patient care.

*Third Step*  In the third step, students are introduced to advanced concepts. They utilize the information systems to plan and implement patient care. Specifically, they utilize technology systems available in clinical agencies to administer medications, provide physiological monitoring, utilize data available in information systems, and enter documentation of patient care in the patient record through the HIS.

*Fourth Step*  In the last step, students are able to integrate the technology into their patient care. This includes evaluating patient care, participating in quality improvement (QI), collaborating with members of the health care team, and utilizing available resources within the technology. At all levels students must examine the social, legal, and ethical issues that they encounter as a result of their use of technology. This model follows the level objectives common in many nursing programs related to the nursing process: assessment, outcome identification, diagnosis, planning, implementation, and evaluation. Activities for each level of student are identified in Table 14.1.

### Graduate Nursing Education

The terminal objective for graduate students is that at the completion of their graduate education they will be able to utilize advanced nursing informatics in the role of the advanced practice nurse as a practitioner, administrator, researcher, and educator.

**TABLE 14.1**     BASIC COMPUTER CONTENT FOR UNDERGRADUATE
                STUDENTS

**First Step**
- Computer overview
- Computer components
  - Hardware
  - Software
- Word processing software
  - Computer-based papers
- Bibliographic retrieval systems
  - Conduct literature searches

**Second Step**
- Overview of information systems
- Patient care documentation
- Social/legal/ethical issues
  - Computer-based patient record
- Educational applications
  - Computer-assisted instruction (CAI)
  - Interactive videodisc instruction (IAV)

**Third Step**
- Use advanced software programs
- Implement nursing care documentation
  - Drug administration systems
  - Physiological monitoring
- Care planning documentation
- Patient instruction
- Evaluation of instruction

**Fourth Step**
- Coordinate patient care data
- Analyze databases
- Quality assurance program
- Utilize computer networks
- Evaluate computer hardware
- Evaluate computer software
- Assure ethical standards

Advanced practice nurses must be knowledgeable about the full range of activities that provide for information handling for nursing practice. That is, they must be able to (1) document nursing practice, (2) access, use, and coordinate the flow of data and information, and (3) communicate with the multidisciplinary team using computer-based patient/clinical information systems. To meet this objective, students must learn computer concepts (computer science), information processing (information science), and data management, focusing on nursing practice data (nursing science). Students must also have the ability to use computer applications to document care and make decisions.

Health care reform initiatives now being considered promote the advanced practice nurse as a primary care provider. The advanced practice nurse, who is educated at the graduate level, must be adept at technological applications in order to collaborate and to interact effectively with other members of the multidisciplinary team. Care will be provided both in traditional care facilities and in diverse community-based facilities. Computer technology plays an important role in providing efficient and effective communication, which in turn improves care.

Graduate nursing education must include content and opportunities to develop the knowledge, skill, and attitude of students in nursing informatics. Nursing informatics concepts that should be included in graduate nursing education are shown in Table 14.2. In addition to concepts, all advanced practice nurses require competencies or skills in computer applications. These computer competencies are identified in Table 14.3.

## OTHER EDUCATIONAL APPLICATIONS

Specifically, the following will be discussed:

- Educational models
- Staff education and inservice
- Nurse extenders
- Patient education

## Educational Models

### General Curriculum Development Model

The general curriculum development model was developed by Ronald and Skiba (1987) as a framework for basic computer education. They set forth assumptions and guidelines that could serve as the basis for the computer educational curriculum framework. Their framework serves to introduce computer concepts to educators. They also advocated a continuum of learning experiences with both cognitive and interactive components that encompasses the informed user, the proficient user, and the developer (Fig. 14.12).

The cognitive component relates to basic computer concepts and applications that nurses need to function effectively in the health care delivery system. The interactive component refers to the skills necessary for operating computer hardware, managing computer software, and using the computer as a problem-solving tool. This framework identifies a continuum that extends from informed user to developer. Expectations for the learner at the points on the Ronald and Skiba computer education continuum are shown in Table 14.4.

**TABLE 14.2**    ADVANCED COMPUTER CONTENT FOR GRADUATE
STUDENTS

**Hardware**
- Hardware architecture
- Workstations
- Communication networks
  - Internet services and resources

**Software**
- Nursing information systems
- Expert systems
- Knowledge databases
- Decision support systems

**Data**
- Data, data management, and data processing
- What is data: data elements, records, files, and databases
- How to code, edit, and verify data
- How to design data files and databases
- How to program data analysis
- Nursing data

**Nursing information systems**
- Nursing informatics concepts
- Nursing data standards
  - Coding strategies
- Nursing classifications, taxonomies, and vocabularies
- Computer applications in nursing practice
  - Nursing process
- Computer applications in nursing administration
- Computer applications in nursing education
- Computer applications in nursing research
- Computer-based patient record (CPR) systems
- Life cycle of information systems
- Privacy, confidentiality and security issues

## Collaborative Education Model

This recent model was developed by Ronald at the University of New York
at Buffalo. There, all graduate and undergraduate nursing students are
required to achieve basic concepts and skills in nursing informatics. The
students are required to use computers in the academic and practice
aspects of their educations. In addition, all graduate students are required
to use the computer for data analysis (Ronald, 1991).

The Collaborative Education Model is essentially a collaboration between the School of Nursing and the School of Management to offer a
major in informatics. It gives doctoral students in nursing administration
the opportunity to specialize in management of information systems, an
informatics subspecialty. This collaboration between departments makes

**TABLE 14.3**   UNDERGRADUATE AND GRADUATE COMPUTER
COMPETENCIES

**Hardware skills**
- Understand computer configurations

**Software packages skills**
- Word processing
- Spreadsheets
- Database management programs
- Statistical analysis
- Graphic
  - Poster presentation

**Databases**
- Bibliographic retrieval systems
  - Knowledge of databases for nursing
- Develop databases
  - Design, code, and edit data forms
  - Prepare, manage, and process data
  - Conduct analysis

**Communication**
- Understand LANs and WANS
- Understand and use Internet
- Know nursing networks
- Travel on information highway
  - Nursing resources

such specialization possible without the need to introduce a new specialty program in the School of Nursing.

Several other educational models have been introduced into nursing education at all levels and need to be researched when determining how and what level of computer technology should be introduced into the educational institution.

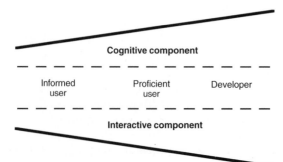

**Figure 14.12**  Computer education continuum model. (Courtesy Ronald and Skiba, 1987.)

**TABLE 14.4**   BASIC COMPUTER EDUCATION CONTINUUM

| Points on Continuum | Cognitive Components | | Interactive Components |
|---|---|---|---|
| | **Basic Concepts** | **Applications** | |
| Informed user | Be familiar with computer terminology | Identify common applications in nursing | Operate a computer system |
| Proficient user | Understand basic computer concepts | Assess the relative value of existing computer systems and communicate nursing needs for the development of future systems | Use the computer as a tool to solve nursing problems |
| Developer | Have in-depth knowledge of computer concepts and information management | Apply systems analysis and design concepts to the development of computer applications for nursing | Use programming skills to maximize the potential of software to solve nursing problems |

*Source:* Ronald and Skiba, 1987.

## Staff Education and Inservice

CAI has also been developed for the nurse practicing in a hospital setting. One such CAI system that is particularly useful for newly employed nurses is an authoring program on drug therapy developed by Pogue (1982). This program was developed on two Apple microcomputers and programmed with PASCAL. This CAI replaces a quarterly lecture series consisting of 2-h classes twice weekly over a 6-week period. The system was designed to provide multiple-choice formats for drill and practice and simulations of patient management problems to permit the development of more complex strategies.

Programs to provide instruction, simulation, and testing in CPR are also available. These programs decrease instructor time needed for CPR certification. They have also been found to provide consistent course content from class to class.

Advantages of computerized inservice education are as follows: (1) staff nurses are free to use the system when they have time, (2) the program reduces the preparation time of nurse educators, (3) each lesson has been reviewed for quality control, (4) the systems are interactive with the users and provide immediate feedback for correct or incorrect answers, (5) the user can repeat information not learned from a single trial, which makes the system self-directing as well as self-pacing, (6) classes need not be scheduled, and (7) the dialogues are user-friendly.

Computer-assisted programs have also been developed for use by staff nurses in primary health areas. One such program is a computer simulation program using a pediatric minor illness encounter (Woodbury, 1982). This program evaluates nurses' problem-solving skills in clinical practice. The program is divided into four problem-solving areas: (1) subjective or historical data about a patient, (2) objective data collection (e.g., a physical assessment, laboratory test results), (3) a potential or actual diagnosis, and (4) a plan of care, with educational needs for the patient and the need for follow-up treatment.

Staff selections are evaluated by the supervisor. Using a medical diagnosis model and incorporating appropriate nursing diagnosis selections based on assessment data integrated with objective test results, this program has many potentials for nursing education.

## Nurse Extenders

When not enough nurses are available to structure patient education programs, computers can serve as nurse extenders by providing educational materials for patients. One creative way in which computers can be used for patient education is as a consultant for patient inquiries. For example, computers have been used by nurses to provide a training program for persons with diabetes. The training program involves two parts: health facts, which include content on the symptoms of hypoglycemia and hyperglycemia, insulin administration, foot care, and urine testing; and diet management. After preliminary information is entered, this program calculates appropriate caloric intakes for a patient, who receives individualized information from the printer.

A nurse shows the patient how to use the computer. Thereafter, the patient answers several questions, including the type of instruction that is needed. The flow or sequence of the program is then based on the patient's responses. In this way, patients control the flow of information that they receive by answering yes or no to selected questions. Patients can return to the computer later to continue instruction where they left off.

The main advantage of this system is that patients documented improved learning. The computer supplements the teaching provided by staff nurses.

## Patient Education

Computers have been used in several hospitals to identify and solve problems in patient education. Some of these problems relate to the number of staff available to teach patients and meet patients' educational needs. Others involve the continuing change in patients' diagnoses and educational needs. Computers facilitate patient education by providing a database that tracks patients who are eligible for education, identifies patients who have received education, highlights patients who have not participated in educational programs, identifies staff educational needs, and provides data on the costs of such a program. Some systems also provide the patient with an educational plan at the time of discharge.

CAI for patient education has been developed on mainframes, mini-computers, and microcomputers. These systems are mostly used in outpatient facilities or in areas where large numbers of persons are screened each day. The advantages include the following (Donovan et al., 1983): (1) patients feel more comfortable responding to the computer than to a nurse or physician, (2) patients spend more time on content they do not understand by reviewing material as many times as necessary, (3) information is printed and given to patients to review at home, and (4) patients feel that use of the computer results in more time being spent by the biomedical staff on their problems.

In the climate of health promotion and disease prevention, consumers are seeking more knowledge and resources in areas such as diet, exercise, smoking cessation, and stress management to assist them in staying well. Technology-based patient education is an accessible, private, and efficient means to provide health promotion teaching (Sweeney, 1994).

## SUMMARY

Computer applications for nursing education have been available for several decades. Many nursing education programs, however, do not use computers at all, and many others use computers merely for word processing. Students entering nursing education programs from secondary schools have varying levels of computer experience and skills. Their roles as nursing students and as future health care providers require that they interact with and exploit available technology.

The use of technology in the educational process was described as a powerful tool to provide instruction and evaluation. The uses of CAI and IAV to provide active learning and to enhance critical thinking skills were also presented. Computer management of student records and curricula data, providing the means for collection, storage, processing, and retrieval of information about students, faculty, staff, and curricula, was highlighted. Developments in data management are occuring rapidly. The NLN is now testing software to facilitate the process for accreditation of nursing programs.

Computer resources were presented. In order for students, faculty, and administrators to interact with technology, they must have resources, and the types of hardware, software, and other equipment needed were identified in this chapter. Nursing education programs must formulate plans based on their individual needs. Experts are needed and available to assist in this process. Finally, other educational applications of technology which are emerging as the technology finds its way into the health care system were described. These applications present many opportunities for staff and patient education. As nurses move into the community setting in greater numbers, scheduling staff meetings becomes more difficult. Patients are also seeking care in the community, closer to home. Both groups benefit from computer-assisted learning.

In order to derive maximum benefits, students should become familiar with and utilize computers effectively from the beginning of their nursing education. NIEM, which establishes an integration formula that provides nursing students with the necessary tools to use computers and related technology efficiently and effectively in their nursing education, was described in detail. This chapter demonstrated how NIEM is used to prepare nurses for careers in which their professional development will be influenced by their ability to exploit new technology.

Integration of computer technology into nursing education is no longer a luxury. Students must be able to interact with technology in order to function in health care systems. Technology opens doors so that nurses in all settings can access the latest knowledge.

## REFERENCES

Arnold, J. A. (1992). How to use microcomputer simulations in academic and staff development settings. In J. M. Arnold and G. A. Pearson (Eds.), *Computer Applications in Nursing Education and Practice* (pp. 183–190). New York: National League for Nursing.

Belfry, M. J., and Winnie, P. (1988). A review of the effectiveness of computer assisted instruction in nursing education. *Computers in Nursing, 6*(2), 77–85.

Bolwell, C. (1990). *Diskovery: Computer-Integrated Learning Series for Nursing Education: Nursing Educators Microworld.* Saratoga, CA: Microworld.

Bolwell, C. (1993a). *Directory of Educational Software for Nursing. (5th ed.).* New York: National League for Nursing.

Bolwell, C. (1993b). Using interactive video: Integration into the curriculum. In M. A. Rizzolo (Ed.), *Interactive Video: Expanding Horizons in Nursing* (pp. 97–116). New York: American Journal of Nursing Company.

Christensen, M. N. and Murphy, M. A. (1990). Authoring systems: Finding the right tool for your courseware development project. *Computers in Nursing, 8*(2), 73–78.

Collins, S. (1983). Computer based systems for professional education and training. In M. Scholes, Y. Bryant, and B. Barber (Eds.), *The Impact of Computers in Nursing* (pp. 350–355). Amsterdam, Netherlands: North-Holland.

Davis, J., and Williams, D. (1980). Learning for mastery: Individualized testing through computer managed evaluation. *Nurse Educator, 5*(1), 9.

Donovan, M., Zielstorff, R., Mauldin, T., et al. (1983). Using COSTAR to assist nurses in hypertension screening and education. In R. Dayhoff (Ed.), *Proceedings of the Seventh Annual Symposium on Computer Applications in Medical Care* (pp. 487–490). Silver Spring, MD: IEEE Computer Society Press.

Ellis, L. (1981). Computer based education: Problems and opportunities. In H. Heffernan (Ed.), *Proceedings of the Fifth Annual Symposium on Computer Appli-*

*cations in Medical Care* (p. 196). Silver Spring, Maryland: IEEE Computer Society Press.

Farabaugh, N. (1990). Maintaining student interest in CAI. *Computers in Nursing*, *8*(6), 249–253.

Heller, B. R., Damrosch, S., Romano, C., and McCarthy, M. (1989). Graduate specialization in nursing informatics. *Computers in Nursing*, *7*(2), 68–77.

Holzemer, W., Slichter, M., Slaughter, R. and Stotts, N. (1983). Development of the University of California, San Francisco microcomputer facility for nursing research and development. In R. Dayhoff (Ed.), *Proceedings of the Seventh Annual Symposium on Computer Applications in Medical Care* (pp. 484–486). Silver Spring, MD: IEEE Computer Society Press.

Larson, D. (1985). Cost-effectiveness of educational computing in nursing education. In K. Hannah, E. Guillemin, and D. Conklin (Eds.), *Proceeding of the IFIP-IMIA International Symposium on Nursing Uses of Computers and Information Science* (pp. 217–221). Amsterdam, Netherlands: North-Holland.

Locatis, C. (1992). *Authoring Systems*. Bethesda, MD: National Library of Medicine, NIH, US DHHS.

McAfooes, J. (1994). The Helene Fuld Health Trust and FITNE: Helping nurse educators implement technology. In M. A. Rizzolo (Ed.), *Interactive Video: Expanding Horizons in Nursing* (pp. 137–150). New York: American Journal of Nursing Company.

McGuiness, B. (1991). Using computers in nurse education, staff development and patient education. In J. Turley, and S. Newbold (Eds.), *Proceeding of the Nursing Informatics Pre-Conference*. New York: Springer-Verlag.

Mikan, K. J. (1992). Computer use in undergraduate nursing. In J. M. Arnold and G. A. Pearson (Eds.), *Computer Applications in Nursing Education and Practice* (pp. 346–350). New York: National League for Nursing.

Murphy, M. A. (1991). Effects of a computer based adaptive instructional lesson on concept acquisition in nursing. In E. Hovenga, K. Hannah, K. McCormick, and J. Ronald (Eds.), *Proceedings of the Fourth International Conference on Nursing Use of Computers and Information Science* (pp. 607–611). New York: Springer-Verlag.

Napholz, L. and McCanse, R. (1994). Interactive video instruction increases efficiency in cognitive learning in a baccalaureate nursing education program. *Computers in Nursing*, *12*(3), 149–153.

Nelson, R., and Joos, I. (1992). Strategies and resources for self-education in nursing informatics. In J. M. Arnold and G. A. Pearson (Eds.), *Computer Applications in Nursing Education and Practice* (pp. 9–19). New York: National League for Nursing.

Norman, S. (1982). Computer assisted learning—Its potential in nursing education. *Nursing Times*, *78*, 1467–1468.

Perciful, E. G. (1992). The relationship between planned change and successful implementation of computer assisted instruction. *Computers in Nursing*, *10*(2), 85–90.

Pluyter-Wenting, E. (1983). Computerized student-nurse training and allocation system. In O. Fokkens et al. (Eds.), *Medinfo 83* (pp. 322–326). Amsterdam, Netherlands: North-Holland.

Pogue, L. (1982). Computer-assisted instruction in the continuing education process. *Topics in Clinical Nursing*, *4*, 41–50.

Pogue, L. (1985). Authoring systems: A key to efficient production of computer-based nursing learning materials. In K. Hannah, E. Guillemin, and D. Conklin (Eds.). *Proceeding of the IFIP-IMIA International Symposium on Nursing Uses of Computers and Information Science* (pp. 229–233). Amsterdam, Netherlands: North-Holland.

Pritchard, K. (1982). Computers. III. Possible applications in nursing. *Nursing Times, 78,* 465–466.

Rizzolo, M. A. (1994). Interactive video: Evolution, issues effecting development, current status in nursing. In M. A. Rizzolo (Ed.), *Interactive Video: Expanding Horizons in Nursing* (pp. 7–30). New York: American Journal of Nursing Company.

Ronald, J. S. (1991). A collaborative model for specializing in nursing informatics. In E. V. Hovenga, K. J. Hannah, K. A. McCormick, and J. S. Ronald (Eds.), *Nursing Informatics '91* (pp. 662–666). New York: Springer-Verlag.

Ronald, J. S., and Skiba, D. J. (1987). *Guidelines for Basic Computer Education in Nursing.* New York: National League for Nursing.

Ryan, S. (1985). An expert system for nursing practice. *Computers in Nursing,* 77–84.

Skiba, D. J., Ronald, J. S., and Simpson, R. L. (1992). HealthQuest/HBO nurse scholars program: A corporate partnership with nursing education. In J. M. Arnold, and G. A. Pearson (Eds.), *Computer Applications in Nursing Education and Practice* (pp. 224–235). New York: National League for Nursing.

Sparks, S. M. (1990). *Computer-Based Education in Nursing.* Bethesda, MD: National Library of Medicine, NIH, US DHHS.

Sweeney, M. A. (1994). Technology-based patient education. In M. A. Rizzolo (Ed.), *Interactive Video: Expanding Horizons in Nursing* (pp. 117–128). New York: American Journal of Nursing Company.

Sweeney, M. A., Regan, P., O'Malley, M., and Hedstrom, B. (1980). Essential skills for baccalaureate graduates: Perspectives of education and service. *Journal of Nursing Administration, 10,* 37–40.

Thiele, J. E., and Holloway, J. R. (1992). Development of a taxonomy of decision-making properties of computerized clinical simulations. In J. M. Arnold and G. A. Pearson (Eds.), *Computer Applications in Nursing Education and Practice* (pp. 351–362). New York: National League for Nursing.

Tymchyshyn, P. (1982). An evaluation of the adoption of CAI in a nursing program. In B. Blum (Ed.), *Proceedings of the Sixth Annual Symposium on Computer Applications in Medical Care* (pp. 543–548). Silver Spring, MD: IEEE Computer Society Press.

Tymchyshyn, P. (1983). New tricks for an old game: Teaching. In J. Van Bemmel, M. J. Ball, and O. Wigertz (Eds.). *Medinfo 83* (pp. 190–193). Amsterdam, Netherlands: North-Holland.

Ullmer, E. (1989). *Videodisc Technology.* Bethesda, MD: National Library of Medicine, NIH, US DHHS.

Ullmer, E. (1990). *Interactive Technology.* Bethesda, MD: National Library of Medicine, NIH, US DHHS.

Weiner, E. E., Gordon, J. S. and Gilman, B. R. (1993). Evaluation of a labor and delivery videodisc simulation. *Computers in Nursing, 11*(4), 191–196.

Woodbury, P. (1982). Computer assisted evaluations of problem solving skills of primary health care providers using a case management simulation model. In

B. Blum (Ed.), *Proceedings of the Sixth Annual Symposium on Computer Applications in Medical Care* (pp. 539–542). Silver Spring, MD: IEEE Computer Society Press.

# BIBLIOGRAPHY

Aiken, E. (1988). *Moving into the Age of Computer-Supported Education: A Regional Experience in Education*. Atlanta: Southern Regional Education Board.

Aiken, E. (1989). *Computer Use in 513 Undergraduate Nursing Programs*. Atlanta: Southern Regional Education Board.

Aiken, E. (1990). *Continuing Nursing Education in Computer Technology: A Regional Experience*. Atlanta: Southern Regional Education Board.

Alpert, D., and Bitzer, D. (1970). Advances in computer-based education. *Science, 167,* 1582–1590.

American Nurses Association. (1987). *Computers in Nursing Education*. Kansas City, MO.

Armstrong, M. A. (1986). Computer competence for nurse educators. *Image, 18*(4) 155–160.

Arnold, J., and Pearson, G. (1992). *Computer Applications in Nursing Education and Practice*. New York: National League for Nursing.

Association of American Medical Colleges. (1986). *Medical Education in the Information Age*. Washington, DC.

Billings, D. (1984). Evaluating computer assisted instruction. *Nursing Outlook, 32,* 50–53.

Bolte, I. and Denman, L. (1977). We are ready for ANA's continuing education data bank. *Journal of Continuing Education in Nursing, 8*(5), 5.

Cambre, M. A., and Castner, L. J. (1991). *The Status of Interactive Video Technology in Nursing Education Environments*. Athens, OH: Fuld Institute for Technology in Nursing Education.

Clark, C. E. (1991). Interactive videodisc: Its place in today's nursing curricula. *Computers in Nursing, 9*(6), 210–214.

Dixon, J., Gouyd, N., and Varricchio, D. (1975). A computerized education and training record. *Journal of Continuing Education in Nursing, 6,* 20–23

Dorken, S., Tait, G. and Brophy, J. (1991). Computerized testing for intensive care unit cardiopulmonary resuscitation recertification. In E. Hovenga, K. Hannah, K. McCormick, and J. Ronald (Eds.), *Proceedings of the Fourth International Conference on Nursing Use of Computers and Information Science* (pp. 740–744). New York: Springer-Verlag.

Gaston, S. (1988). Knowledge, retention, and attitude effects of computer-assisted instruction. *Journal of Nursing Education, 27*(1), 30–34.

Gothler, A. (1985). Nursing education update: Computer technology. *Nursing and Healthcare, 6,* 509–510.

Grobe, S. (1984). *Computer Primer and Resource Guide for Nursing*. Philadelphia: Lippincott.

Grosso, C. (1988). Knowledge and knowledge acquisition for the development of expert systems for nursing. In N. Daly and K. Hannah (Eds.), *Proceeding of the Third International Symposium on Nursing Use of Computer and Information Science* (pp. 422–430). St. Louis: Mosby.

Hannah, K. J., Ball, M. J., and Edwards, M. J. A. (1994). *Introduction to Nursing Informatics*. New York: Springer-Verlag.

Happ, B. (1988). The management of artificial intelligence/expert systems in nursing and health care. In N. Daly and K. Hannah (Eds.), *Proceeding of the Third International Symposium on Nursing Use of Computer and Information Science* (pp. 506–517). St. Louis: Mosby.

Hebda, T. (1988). A profile of the use of computer assisted instruction within baccalaureate nursing education. *Computers in Nursing, 6*(1), 22–29.

Heller, B., Romano, C., Damrorsch, S., and Parks, P. (1985). Computer applications in nursing: Implications for the curriculum. *Computers in Nursing, 3*(1), 14–22.

Heller, B., Romano, C., Moray, L. and Gassert, C. (1989). The implementation of the first graduate program in nursing informatics. *Computers in Nursing, 7*(5), 209–213.

Hoffer, E. P., and Barnett, G. O. (1990). Computers in medical education. In E. H. Shorliffe and L. M. Fagan (Eds.), *Medical Informatics: Computer Applications in Health Care* (pp. 535–561). Reading, MA: Addison-Wesley.

Howard, E. P. (1987). Use of a computer simulation for the continuing education of registered nurses. *Computers in Nursing, 5*(6), 208–213.

Howse, E., Smith, B., and Perkins, C. A. (1994). Difference between manual and computer-based methods for clinical learning assignments. *Computers in Nursing, 12*(6), 280–288.

Joos, I., Whitman, N., Smith, M., and Nelson, R. (1992). *Computers in Small Bytes: The Computer Workbook*. New York: National League for Nursing.

Koch, E. W., Rankin, J. A., and Stewart, R. (1990). Nursing students' preferences in the use of computer assisted learning. *Journal of Nursing Education, 29*, 122–126.

Kruckenberg Schofer, K. K., and Ward, C. J. (1990). The computerization of the patient education process. *Computers in Nursing, 8*(3), 116–122.

Laborde, J. (1984). Expert systems for nursing. *Computers in Nursing, 2*(4), 130–135.

Larson, D. (1987). A day in the life of a computer-using nursing instructor, 1990. *Computers in Nursing, 5*(2), 78–80.

Locatis, C. (1989). *Videodisc Repurposing*. Bethesda, MD: National Library of Medicine, NIH, US DHHS.

Mikan, K. J. (1984). Computer integration: A challenge for nursing education. *Nursing Outlook, 32*(1), 6–8.

National League for Nursing. (1988). *Preparing Nurses for Using Information Systems: Recommended Informatics Competencies*. New York: National League for Nursing.

Nursing Educators MicroWorld. (1994). NCLEX Information from National Council. *Nursing Educators MicroWorld, 8*(2), 12.

O'Neil, D. H. (1993). *Health Professions Education for the Future: Schools in Service to the Nation*. San Francisco: PEW Health Professions Commission.

Peterson, H., and Gerdin-Jelger, U. (Eds.). (1988). *Preparing Nurses for Using Information Systems: Recommended Informatics Competencies*. New York: National League for Nursing.

Pinheiro, E. (1994). *Introduction to Multimedia*. Arlington, VA: Stewart.

Preparing for the next 5 years of instructional technology. (1992). *Nursing Educators Microworld*, *6*(2), 9, 11.

Reynolds, A., and Pontious, S. (1986). CAI enhances the medication dosage calculation competency of nursing students. *Computers in Nursing*, *4*(4), 158–165.

Rizzolo, M. A. (1994). Interactive video: A technological solution for some educational problems in nursing. In M. A. Rizzolo (Ed.), *Interactive Video: Expanding Horizons in Nursing* (pp. 1–6). New York: American Journal of Nursing Company.

Rizzolo, M. A. (Ed.). (1994). *Interactive Video: Expanding Horizons in Nursing*. New York: American Journal of Nursing Company.

Schare, B., Dunn, S., Clark, H., et al. (1991). The effects of interactive video on cognitive achievement and attitude toward learning. *Journal of Nursing Education*, *30*(3), 109–113.

Schwirian, P. M. (1987). Evaluation research in computer-based instruction. *Computers in Nursing*, *5*(4), 128–131.

Sweeney, M. A. (1985). *The Nurse's Guide to Computers*. New York: Macmillan.

Thiele, J. (1988). There's a computer in the curriculum. *Computers in Nursing*, *6*(1), 37–40.

Thomas, B. (1985). A survey study of computers in nursing education. *Computers in Nursing*, *3*(4), 173–179.

Ullmer, E. (1990). *Optical Disc Technology*. Bethesda, MD: National Library of Medicine, NIH, US DHHS

Valish, A., and Boyd, J. (1975). The role of computer-assisted instruction in continuing education of registered nurses: An experimental study. *Journal of Continuing Education in Nursing*, *6*, 13–32.

Vanderbeek, J., Ulrich, D., Jaworski, R., et al. (1994). Bringing nursing informatics into the undergraduate classroom. *Computers in Nursing*, *12*(5), 227–231.

Van Dover, L., and Boblin, S. (1991). Student nurse computer experience and preferences for learning. *Computers in Nursing*, *9*(2), 75–79.

Warnock-Matheron, A. (1988). Expert systems: Automated decision support for clinical nursing practice. In N. Daly and K. Hannah (Eds.), *Proceeding of the Third International Symposium on Nursing Use of Computer and Information Science* (pp. 492–497). St. Louis: Mosby.

Where in the hospital is the best place to use CAI? (1990). *Nursing Educators Microworld*, *5*(1), 4.

Wong, J., Wong, S. and Richard, J. (1992). Implementing computer simulations as a strategy for evaluating decision-making skills of nursing students. *Computers in Nursing*, *10*(6), 264–269.

Yoder, M. E., and Heilman, T. (1985). The use of computer assisted instruction to teach nursing diagnosis. *Computers in Nursing*, *3*, 262–265.

# *15*

● ● ● ● ● ● ● ● ● ● ● ● ● ● ● ● ● ● ● ● ● ● ●

# RESEARCH APPLICATIONS

## OBJECTIVES

- Understand computer applications in nursing research.
- Discuss the use of computers in the nursing research process.
- Discuss searching the literature.
- Identify bibliographic retrieval systems.
- Describe informational databases.
- Describe research methods.
- Discuss processing of research data.
- Describe research databases.
- Discuss statistical analyses.
- Identify research conclusions.
- Describe dissemination of research results.

For many years, computers have supported the nursing research process. Computer applications provide ways to facilitate research and the scientific method. More recently, because of the advancement and implementation of computerized information systems in health care facilities, computers are increasingly being used for clinical nursing research. The introduction of the microcomputer made it easier to collect patient care data for research purposes. The information explosion has made possible nursing research which would have been prohibitive in past decades. With the computer, millions of variables can be processed for a single research study. More than ever before, through computers, millions of data elements can be collected, stored, processed, and analyzed, to produce information and ultimately knowledge.

This chapter describes the research process as background for discussion of the uses of the computer and computer applications in nursing research. Generally, research attempts to discover new facts or assess new relationships among facts. There are a wide range of research approaches, however, regardless of the topic to be studied or the problem to be solved, the use of the computer is critical for conducting research. Moreover, there are primarily four major uses of computers in the nursing research process: information retrieval, data processing, computerized databases, and statistical analysis.

## RESEARCH PROCESS

The research process consists of a series of progressive steps that provide the framework for conducting research regardless of specialty or type. The research process is based on the scientific method and is the recognized way to construct and develop scientific hypotheses and theories in order to develop scientific knowledge. The uses of the computer are discussed in detail in the context of the major areas of the research process, and the computer hardware, computer software, computer databases, and electronic communication systems that are employed are identified. The computer encompasses multiple applications that vary but are specific to the research process (Abdellah and Levine, 1986, 1994; American Nurses Association Task Force, 1992; Sweeney, 1985).

The nursing research process can be described in several major areas, each of which encompasses at least one or more computer application. They include the following:

- Research problem
- Research literature
- Research method
- Data processing
- Statistical analysis
- Research conclusions

There are many steps or activities to be accomplished in each of these major areas, as shown in Table 15.1 and discussed below.

**TABLE 15.1**    COMPUTERS IN NURSING RESEARCH PROCESS

**Research Problem**
- Define the problem

**Research Literature**
- Search the literature
- Review bibliographic retrieval systems
- Review informational sources and databases

**Research Method**
- Identify research methodology
- Determine nursing framework
- Define study population and sample
- Define variables/data elements

**Data Processing**
- Design data collection forms
- Develop data files and databases
- Review database types

**Statistical Analysis**
- Summarize/reduce data
- Conduct statistical tests
- Select statistical software
- Develop analytical models

**Research Conclusions**
- Describe findings
- Determine conclusions
- Disseminate results
- Identify electronic systems

*Source:* Adapted from Abdellah and Levine, 1986.

# RESEARCH PROBLEM

## Define Problem

The first step of the research process is selecting the topic and formulating the problem. This includes conducting a review of the relevant literature and information sources on the topic to formulate the research problem. The advent of computerized bibliographic, informational, and knowledge-based systems permits the retrieval of data on the topic from extensive sources and facilitates the literature search.

# RESEARCH LITERATURE

## Search the Literature

The literature search is based on and involves the development of a search strategy. Traditionally, conducting a search of the literature consisted of manually searching the pertinent nursing indexes, using knowledge of the field to identify the critical literature that would affect the research problem. Today, computerized bibliographic retrieval systems are used to search the nursing literature.

Computer searching of the literature requires knowledge of the computerized bibliographic retrieval system's database and its indexing terminology and characteristics. Further, by using Boolean logic, combinations of key words or concepts can be used to retrieve more precise information on a specific topic. Boolean logic consists primarily of three basic operations, "AND," "OR," and "AND NOT," or combinations of these operations. These logical operations are based on the algebraic rules of George Boole, known as the Boolean theory (see also Chap. 4).

Computer searching facilitates broader coverage of the literature, is cost-effective, and saves time. Searching of the on-line bibliographic retrieval systems makes the nursing information in those databases available. However, at this time, there is no one database that contains all nursing literature, and searching several databases that include nursing literature is necessary for a comprehensive search or to obtain broad coverage of a topic (Sinclair, 1987; Smith, 1988; Sparks, 1986).

### Search Strategy

The development of the search strategy is critical to assure retrieval of relevant citations, references, and/or abstracts on a topic. Subject searching is the most common design for a search strategy. A subject can be selected from the list of indexed keyword headings, subheadings, or key concepts (words) from the titles of the indexed articles. Other methods of searching include using the names of journals, authors, publishers, or organizations. There are several points that should be considered when formulating a search strategy.

***State the Problem*** Specify the purpose of the information and reason it is needed.

***Analyze the Problem*** Restate the problem succinctly to include all facets and concepts. For example, for a study of a specific cancer protocol, the search should not be for all literature on cancer protocols but should be limited to the specific type of cancer. The search statement must be in terms that conform with the indexing scheme, vocabulary, and search capabilities of the selected bibliographic database. A list of synonyms, variant spellings, scientific terms, and technical terms will provide added precision for the search statements.

***Determine the Limitations*** Limit the scope of the search strategy by defining age, population group, geographic location, ethnic group, language, publication years, and any other characteristics that could improve the precision of the search.

***Design Strategy Steps*** Use Boolean logic to design the strategy steps. Boolean operators are used to restrict and develop efficient searches. The commonest Boolean operators or operations are "AND," "OR," and "AND NOT." They are used to combine the results of two or more subject searches. They differ as follows:

## AND

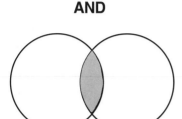

**Figure 15.1** Venn diagram with operator "AND."

**AND:** Concept 1 "AND" Concept 2 = This means that only articles with both concept 1 and concept 2 are searched for (Fig. 15.1).

## OR

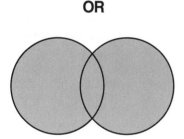

**Figure 15.2** Venn diagram with operator "OR."

**OR:** Concept 1 "OR" Concept 2 = This means that only articles with either concept 1 or concept 2 are searched for (Fig. 15.2).

## AND NOT

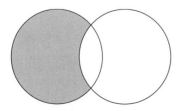

**Figure 15.3** Venn diagram with operator "AND NOT."

**AND NOT:** Concept 1 "AND NOT" Concept 2 = This means that only articles with concept 1 that do not include concept 2 are searched for (Fig. 15.3).

## Review Bibliographic Retrieval Systems

Bibliographic retrieval systems which contain citations to the relevant nursing literature need to be reviewed to determine which systems should be searched. Bibliographic retrieval systems vary according to scope and content of their databases. Generally, they contain citations or references to the paper-based nursing literature. Primarily they are databases that consist of indexed citations with or without an abstract of the journal articles, letters, and editorials focusing on a specific topic.

Most bibliographic retrieval systems can be searched on-line, which is an electronic alternative to searching manually through a card catalog, an index, or any other traditional information access tool. On-line searching involves gaining access, by use of a computer, to the bibliographic or informational databases stored in a computerized bibliographic retrieval or information system, in order to identify articles or documents on a particular subject, by a particular author, in a specific journal, or with some other defining characteristic.

However, since there is no one system that contains all citations for the entire spectrum of the nursing literature, several relevant bibliographic systems need to be reviewed to obtain all the articles and/or other literature on the topic. Knowledge of the specific database in the bibliographic retrieval system lessens the chance of making common searching mistakes, such as errors in using Boolean logic, inappropriate keyword selection, or incomplete vocabulary (Saba et al., 1989).

There are several computerized bibliographic retrieval systems relevant for research that yield references and/or citations to the nursing literature. The major ones are

- MEDLARS (Medical Literature Analysis and Retrieval System)
- CINAHL (Cumulative Index to Nursing and Allied Health Literature)
- ERIC (Educational Resources Information Center)
- SOCIAL SCISEARCH (Social Sciences Citation Index)
- PsycINFO (Psychological Abstracts)
- DISSERTATION ABSTRACTS ON LINE (Dissertation Abstracts)
- EMBASE (Excerpta Medica)
- AGELINE (American Association of Retired Persons)
- NTIS (National Technical Information Service)

### MEDLARS

MEDLARS (Medical Literature Analysis and Retrieval System) is the National Library of Medicine's (NLM's) computerized bibliographic retrieval system. The NLM is the world's largest research library in a single scientific and professional field and serves as a national resource for all U.S. health science libraries. MEDLARS was established in the early 1960s to achieve rapid bibliographic access to the NLM's vast store of biomedical information. It was a pioneering effort to use computer technology. MEDLARS was designed and continues to be used for preparing and photocomposing three of its bibliographic publications: *Index Medicus* (IM), *International Nursing Index* (INI), and *Index to Dental Literature*.

MEDLARS represents a family of databases, of which MEDLINE is the best known. In 1972, MEDLARS advanced to an on-line system, and MEDlars onLINE emerged as MEDLINE, the first of several MEDLARS databases. Since then, at least 40 other databases have been developed which cover biomedical literature from 3,900 journals, audio-visual materials, and information on acquired immunodeficiency syndrome (AIDS), toxicology, cancer, and other specialized areas of health and disease. The MEDLARS databases are given in Table 15.2. They are available on-line to individuals and institutions throughout the world (MEDLARS, 1991; Sparks, 1986).

***MEDLINE***   MEDLINE (Medical Literature Analysis and Retrieval System onLINE) is the largest bibliographic database system in the world. In 1992, MEDLINE contained 6.6 million references to articles from approximately 3,900 biomedical journals published in over 70 countries, and to nursing literature and books for twenty years beginning in 1966. There are over 100,000 articles being written each month, and of those, the NLM currently indexes approximately 33,000 per month, or 400,000 articles, letters, and editorials per year from selected medical, nursing, and health care journals, in MEDLINE (MEDLARS, 1991; MEDLINE, 1992; National Library of Medicine, 1992).

MEDLINE consists of bibliographic references to the journal articles in the system. Each reference which is indexed includes the author, title, date, source publication, and, if available, an abstract (Fig. 15.4). MEDLINE searches have also been made more accessible through an on-line service using a user-friendly IBM PC or Apple Mac microcomputer search software package named Grateful Med, which was released in 1986. New coded search strategies have also been developed to assist in searching the nursing literature. MEDLINE is also offered in a compact disc read-only memory (CD-ROM) format. It contains citations from MEDLINE's three major indexes, as well as the thesaurus from MeSH. MEDLINE also offers on-line computer searches for a fee to most libraries or individuals who have access to the MEDLINE database. It is available on the Internet and can be accessed through basic Internet processes such as Telnet and File Transfer Protocol (FTP), or through software clients such as Gopher for Gopher servers and Mosaic for World Wide Web servers.

***MeSH***   The databases within MEDLARS use a controlled vocabulary thesaurus (indexing terminology) called MeSH (Medical Subject Headings). MeSH is the language used to access the 3,900 biomedical journals. It is the foundation of the NLM's IM, the monthly and annual, subject/author guide to articles published in journals. MeSH is a set of terms or subject headings, categories, subcategories and cross references to other headings using

**TABLE 15.2**    LIST OF MAJOR MEDLARS DATABASES

## MEDLARS Databases

| Database | Subject | Type |
|---|---|---|
| AIDSDRUGS | ∏ Substances being tested in AIDS-related clinical trials | Factual |
| AIDSLINE (AIDS information onLINE) | Acquired immune deficiency syndrome (AIDS) and related topics | Bibliographic citations |
| AIDSTRIALS (AIDS Clinical TRIALS) | Clinical trials of substances being tested for use against AIDS, AIDS-related complex (ARC), AIDS-related opportunistic diseases, and HIV infection | Factual and referral |
| AVLINE (Audiovisuals onLINE) | Biomedical audiovisual materials and computer software | Bibliographic citations |
| BIOETHICSLINE (BIOETHICS onLINE) | Ethics and related public policy issues in health care and biomedical research | Bibliographic citations |
| CANCERLIT (CANCER LITerature) | Major cancer topics | Bibliographic citations |
| CATLINE (CATalog onLINE) | Bibliographic records covering the biomedical sciences | Bibliographic citations |
| CCRIS (Chemical Carcinogenesis Research Information System) | Chemical carcinogens, mutagens, and tumor promoters | Factual |
| ChemID (CHEMical IDentification) | Dictionary of chemicals | Factual |
| CHEMLINE (CHEMical dictionary onLINE) | Dictionary of chemicals | Factual |
| CLINPROT (CLINical cancer PROTocols) | Clinical investigations of new anticancer agents and treatment modalities | Factual and referral |
| DBIR (Director of Biotechnology Information Resources) | Biotechnology information resources | Referral |
| DENTALPROJ (Dental Projects) | Ongoing dental research projects | Factual and referral |
| DIRLINE (Directory of Information Resources onLINE) | Directory of organizations providing information services | Referral |
| DOCUSER (DOCument delivery USER) | Directory of libraries and other information-related organizations that use NLM's interlibrary loan (ILL) services or are a part of the National Network of Medical Libraries | Referral |
| ETICBAK (Environmental Teratology Information Center BACKfile) | Teratology and developmental and reproductive toxicology | Bibliographic citations |
| HEALTH (HEALTH planning and administration) | Nonclinical aspects of health care delivery | Bibliographic citations |

**582**

**TABLE 15.2** *Continued*

## MEDLARS Databases

| Database | Subject | Type |
|---|---|---|
| HISTLINE<br>(HISTory of medicine onLINE) | History of medicine and related sciences | Bibliographic citations |
| HSDB<br>(Hazardous Substances Data Bank) | Hazardous chemicals; toxic effects, environmental fate, and safety and handling | Factual |
| HSTAR<br>(Health Services Technology Assessment Research) | Health Services Research | Bibliographic citations |
| HSTAT*<br>(Health Services Technology Assessment Text) | AHCPR Clinical Practice Guidelines, NIH consensus reports, and U.S. preventive services and task force reports | Full text |
| IRIS<br>(Integrated Risk Information System) | Potentially toxic chemicals | Factual |
| MEDLINE<br>(MEDlars onLINE) | Biomedicine | Bibliographic citations |
| MeSH VOCABULARY FILE | Thesaurus of biomedicine-related terms | Factual |
| NAME AUTHORITY FILE (NAF) | Authority list for names, series, and uniform titles used as headings in bibliographic records resident in CATLINE and AVLINE | Factual |
| PDQ<br>(Physician Data Query) | Advances in cancer treatment and clinical trials | Factual and referral |
| POPLINE<br>(POpulation information onLINE) | Populations, demographics, and family planning | Bibliographic citations |
| RTECS<br>(Registry of Toxic Effects of Chemical Substances) | Potentially toxic chemicals | Factual |
| SDILINE<br>(Selective Dissemination of Information onLINE | Biomedicine | Bibliographic citations |
| TOXLINE<br>(TOXicology information onLINE) | Toxicological, pharmacological, biochemical, and physiological effects of drugs and other chemicals | Bibliographic citations |
| TOXLIT<br>(TOXicology LITerature from special sources) | Toxicological, pharmacological, biochemical, and physiological effects of drugs and other chemicals | Bibliographic citations |
| TRI<br>(Toxic [Chemical] Release Inventory) | Annual estimated releases of toxic chemicals to the environment | Factual |

*Source:* NLM OnLine Databases and Databanks Factsheet, National Library of Medicine, January 1993.
*HSTAT Factsheet, National Library of Medicine, April 1995.

```
                          (TM)
                  The mini-MEDLINE SYSTEM

      Set A - SABA VK   (2)

      SEARCH OPTIONS:
        1 Author
        2 Title Word
        3 Journal
        4 Subject
      DISPLAY OPTIONS:
        5 References from a single Set
        6 All References from more than one Set (Boolean OR)
        7 Combine References Common to two or more Sets (Boolean AND)
        8 Print or Download an Entire Set
      OTHER OPTIONS:
        9 Delete one or more sets
        10 Set Display and Print Preferences
        11 Quit
      CHOICE? 5
```

```
      Set A - SABA VK   (2)
                        (enter letter of set)
      Display Set: A

      REFERENCES SELECTED FOR PRINTING WILL BE SAVED AND
      PRINTED AT THE END OF THE SEARCH SORTED BY JOURNAL
      Reference 1 of 2

      UI  - 91239104
      AU  - Saba VK
      AU  - O'Hare PA
      AU  - Zuckerman AE
      AU  - Boondas J
      AU  - Levine E
      AU  - Oatway DM
      TI  - A Nursing Intervention Taxonomy for home health care.
      MH  - Automatic Data Processing
      MH  - Home Care Services/*classification/economics
      MH  - Human
      MH  - *Nomenclature
      MH  - Nursing Care/*classification
      MH  - Nursing Theory
      MH  - Reimbursement Mechanisms/economics
      SO  - Nurs Health Care 1991 Jun;12(6):296-9
      Enter RETURN to continue, B to go back, Number of reference to display
       P to print, D to deliver document, Q to quit, S to select for a new set
       [RETURN/B/NUMBER/P/D/Q/S] ?
```

**Figure 15.4**  Example of a mini-MEDLINE system main menu and citation from the Georgetown University Library Information System.

**584**

related terms. There are approximately 16,000 main headings in MeSH and 59,000 in a special chemical thesaurus (Medical Subject Headings, 1993).

Separate category codes in MeSH address the nursing literature. The "N" category codes in a special chapter are used to identify health care activities and personnel types that apply to nursing. For example, conditions that focus on patient care such as "postnatal care," population groups such as "mental health," and/or personnel types such as "nurse midwives" are listed, and these categories and terms can be used to search for the selected nursing topics.

A new value has been added to the nursing journals indexed in MED-LINE. A Journal Subset (SB) label using the letter "N" has been added to tag all nursing journals. This new label not only is added to all new articles indexed for MEDLINE, but also has been added retrospectively to all previously indexed nursing articles. This feature makes it possible to limit any MEDLINE search to articles from nursing journals by adding to the search strategy the letter "N." This is in addition to a more restrictive Special List Indicator (LI). A value of "N" (SB) in the "LI" field of MED-LINE records indicates that the article comes from a non–Index Medicus journal in the field of nursing or from one of the approximately 300 nursing journals indexed in *Index Medicus*. Other letters with "SB" allow the search to be more inclusive and allow retrieval of any nursing journal (International Nursing Index, 1993).

***Grateful Med***   Grateful Med is a front-end microcomputer software program of the NLM that makes searching the literature easier and provides a user-friendly way to access the MEDLARS databases. Using Grateful Med nurses can easily locate literature via a microcomputer with a compatible modem, through appropriate communication software, or through direct access to a communication Internet server. Over 100,000 copies of the Grateful Med software have been sold since 1986.

The Grateful Med software is obtained by applying to the NLM for a user program, code, and password. Each time a new version of Grateful Med is released, the original purchasers are provided with a free upgrade of both the software and the manual. Many nursing educational institutions have introduced instructions on Grateful Med into the nursing research, informatics, and graduate courses. The NLM also provides access to Grateful Med to students at reduced rates and to professional organizations (Grateful Med, 1992).

Most of the MEDLARS databases can be searched through Grateful Med. The searcher can begin with his or her own key words or select from over 16,000 MeSH categories which are accessible in the Grateful Med software program. The search can be constructed using the software program on a microcomputer before it is run via on-line connection to the NLM computer. This strategy tends to define the search more effectively, and keep the costs of the search to a minimum. The citation includes the same information retrieved from a MEDLINE search citation—author's name, title of the article, information on the source of the article, an abstract if available, and the MeSH subject headings. Once a search is completed, the user can print or save the search strategy and retrieved citations on a designated file.

***Loansome Doc*** Grateful Med has a document-ordering feature that permits users to order full-text articles for the references retrieved in the search, called Loansome Doc. This feature is available when users make an arrangement with their medical library in their region which sets up this service. The local medical library needs to have access to DOCLINE to utilize this feature. The feature allows articles to be delivered by mail, fax, or through pick-up at the local library (DOCLINE, 1991; Loansome Doc, 1991).

***Special List Nursing*** The Special List Nursing is a separate file in the MEDLINE database. It represents the *International Nursing Index (INI)*, which is one of the three files in the MEDLINE database. (The other two are *Index Medicus* and *Index to Dental Literature*). This file, "Special List Nursing," covers the INI, which is published quarterly by the NLM in cooperation with the American Journal of Nursing Company, New York, using the computer processing capability of MEDLARS. INI is the basis for the nursing literature found in the MEDLINE and can be specially searched (International Nursing Index, 1993).

The INI cites references to over 300 nursing journals in all languages throughout the world. Approximately half of these journals are sponsored by national and state nurses' associations. Foreign countries account for the other half. Also included in the INI are nursing articles from the approximately 3,700 allied health and biomedical journals currently indexed for the IM, its recurring bibliographies, and MEDLARS' Health (Planning and Administration) Database.

The INI lists the indexed nursing periodicals and serials, current nursing publications of organizations and agencies, and published nursing documents. It also lists a thesaurus of the subject categories and an alphabetic listing of articles and authors, including a list of the country of origin. The INI index has its own thesaurus which is specific for nursing. This classification scheme of approximately 750 subject categories is mapped to the appropriate MeSH terms. Most articles are indexed under three or more subject categories, whereas each article indexed in MEDLINE has its full bibliographic description, as well as 10 to 20 key words that describe the contents of the articles (Index Medicus, 1992).

### Other Bibliographic Retrieval Systems

There are several other computerized bibliographic databases or retrieval systems that contain nursing references and should be searched on-line when conducting nursing research. Generally, they cover databases that are not found in MEDLINE and are offered via the commercial vendors of databases such as BRS (Bibliographic Retrieval Services) and DIALOG. They include CINAHL (Cumulative Index to Nursing and Allied Health Literature), ERIC (Educational Resources Information Center), SOCIAL SciSEARCH (Social Science Search), PsycINFO (Psychological Abstracts), DISSERTATION ABSTRACTS (Dissertation Abstracts), EMBASE (Excerpta Medica), and AGELINE (American Association of Retired Persons); as well as the NTIS (National Technical Information Service), which provides other references to nursing (Bibliographic Retrieval Services, 1991; CINAHL, 1991, 1992; DIALOG, 1991).

***CINAHL***  CINAHL is the on-line version of the *Cumulative Index to Nursing and Allied Health Literature*, often referred to as the "Red Index." This bibliographic retrieval system provides authoritative coverage of the literature in nursing and allied health. Almost all English-language nursing journals are indexed along with publications from the American Nurses Association and the National League for Nursing. In total more than 550 English-language publications, 50 of which are nursing journals, are regularly indexed. Abstracts are included for over 300 journals beginning in 1986 to the present. CINAHL also provides access to selected health care documents, doctoral dissertations, selected conference proceedings, and standards of professional practice (Fig. 15.5).

The terminology used in CINAHL is specific to the nursing and allied health fields with over 6,400 subject headings, 2,000 of which are unique to CINAHL. The terminology is modeled after MeSH; however, it includes related terms and cross references and scope notes making searching easier and more user-friendly. CINAHL not only provides on-line searching of the nursing literature using magnetic tapes, but also is offered as a CD-ROM (Fried et al., 1988; Kilby et al., 1989; Saba et al., 1989).

***ERIC***  ERIC (Educational Resources Information Center) is a bibliographic retrieval system developed by the U.S. Department of Education. The ERIC database contains over 700,000 citations covering many document types: research reports, evaluation studies, curriculum guides, lesson plans, bibliographies, course descriptions, theses, journal articles, pamphlets, and other "fugitive" materials.

ERIC is one of the most comprehensive sources for information relating to the field of education. It consists of two databases: one covers the 700 periodicals indexed in the *Current Index to Journals in Education*, and the other, *Resources in Education*. The databases include other printed documents on education, providing complete coverage of all educational literature concerned with the most significant timely education research reports, including nursing education.

The vocabulary, or indexing language, of ERIC is a controlled vocabulary of educational terms. It uses a subject focus for indexing ERIC documents. Each document is indexed using the thesaurus and abstracted with a 20- to

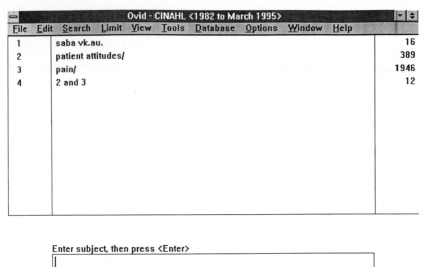

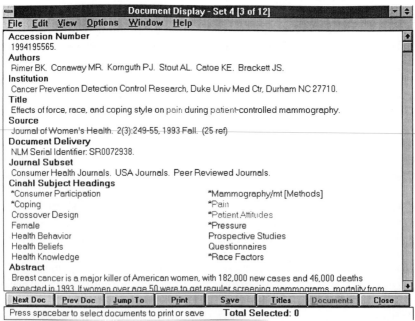

**Figure 15.5** Example of CINAHL screens. Permission by CINAHL. Database Copyright © 1995, CINAHL Information Systems, California. Screen Copyright © 1995, CDP Technologies, Inc.

50-word summary. Each ERIC bibliographic reference that is retrieved from on-line searches contains a complete bibliographic citation, the descriptors from the ERIC thesaurus, and its abstracted annotation (ERIC, 1990).

*SOCIAL SCISEARCH* SOCIAL SCISEARCH is a bibliographic retrieval system and database prepared from the Social Sciences Citation Index (SSCI) by the Institute for Scientific Information, established by Eugene Garfield in 1963. The SOCIAL SCISEARCH database is an international multidisciplinary index to 1,500 social, behavioral, and related science journals. Also, articles relevant to the social sciences are selected from over 2,400 journals in the natural, physical, and biomedical sciences.

The SOCIAL SCISEARCH index contains all natural language words of subject importance that are meaningful and found in the title of the cited article. The information retrieval techniques are unique in this system because the citations are also indexed. It differs from other computerized databases in that it offers two different means of searching the database: (1) source searching of bibliographic references to journal literature, or the traditional bibliographic reference, and (2) citation searching, which lists the author's cited references (citations listed at the end of the article). By using citation analysis and networks, scientific topics can be analyzed, traced historically, and used as a predictor for scientific topics (SOCIAL SCISEARCH, 1991).

*PsycINFO* The PsycINFO (Psychological Abstracts) database provides access to the international literature in psychology and related behavioral and social sciences in over 20 languages. It is produced by the American Psychological Association and covers over 800,000 literature sources as of 1992, including over 1,300 journals from experimental psychology, communications, psychometrics, social processes, personality studies, developmental psychology, physical and psychological disorders, substance abuse, sex roles, treatment and prevention of psychological disorders, personnel evaluation and performance issues, educational psychology, special and remedial education, applied psychology, military psychology, and sport psychology in a database dating from 1967 forward. Records of virtually all journal articles are accompanied by abstracts, and all records are indexed using the controlled vocabulary from the *Thesaurus of Psychological Index Terms* (PsycINFO, 1990).

*DISSERTATION ABSTRACTS* DISSERTATION ABSTRACTS ON LINE is a definitive subject, title, and author guide to virtually every American dissertation granted at an accredited North American university since 1861. It contains more than 1,000,000 citations to U.S. and Canadian dissertations. These dissertations can be accessed through a series of printed indexes: *Dissertation Abstracts International* and *Masters Abstracts International*. Since 1980, each dissertation is accompanied not only by a citation, but also by an abstract which is included in the database. The citations and abstracts index offers references to nursing dissertations (Dissertation Abstracts, 1989).

***EMBASE (Excerpta Medica)*** EMBASE (Excerpta Medica) has long been recognized as an important, comprehensive index of the world's literature on human medicine and related disciplines. EMBASE, an international database, is less frequently used in this country, but is available as an on-line service. This service includes articles referenced from 2,900 primary journals from 110 countries and an additional 600 journals that are screened for drug articles. About 35,000 records are added annually, of which 75 percent contain abstracts. In 1988 15 drug-linking descriptors and 12 disease-linking descriptors were added to improve searching by directly linking drug and disease descriptors. The EMBASE database produces 46 printed abstract bulletins and two printed drug literature bibliographies. Although this service does not include nursing terms, it does include several sections important to nursing research (EMBASE, 1991).

***AGELINE*** The AGELINE database is produced by the American Association of Retired Persons (AARP) and provides bibliographic coverage of social gerontology—the study of aging in social, psychological, health-related, and economic contexts. The delivery of health care to the older population and its associated costs and policies is particularly well covered, as are public policy, employment, and consumer issues. The literature covered is of interest to researchers, health professionals, service planners, policy makers, employers, older adults and their families, and consumer advocates. Journal citations compose roughly two-thirds of the database, with the rest devoted to citations from books, book chapters, and reports. An original informative abstract accompanies each citation. Documents are indexed using the *Thesaurus of Aging Terminology*. There is no printed equivalent of the database. AGELINE is built primarily on the library collection of AARP's National Gerontology Resource Center, which acquires a wide array of aging-related publications from both trade publishers and organizational sources. It contains over 28,000 records, and about 500 journal articles are scanned routinely, with new titles added continually (AGELINE, 1990).

***NTIS*** NTIS is produced by the National Technical Information Service (NTIS) of the U.S. Department of Commerce, the central source for the public sale and dissemination of U.S. government-sponsored research. The database consists of unclassified government-sponsored research, development, and engineering reports, as well as other analyses prepared by government agencies, their contractors, or grantees. Included in this coverage are federally generated machine-readable data files and software. The NTIS database includes material from both the "hard" and "soft" sciences, including health planning, social problems, and nursing (NTIS, 1992).

## Bibliographic Database Vendors

There are several vendors that offer searching and retrieval services to the major bibliographic databases relevant to nursing. Other than the National Library of Medicine, which offers the MEDLARS databases on-line, two private vendors, BRS and DIALOG, offer the majority of databases found in health science, medical, and nursing school libraries. They utilize the major commercial telecommunication networks for on-line access and communication (DIALOG, 1991).

***BRS***   BRS (Bibliographic Retrieval Services) Information Technologies has three product lines, the most significant being BRS/SEARCH. BRS/SEARCH delivers a complete electronic library, with databases covering virtually every discipline including health, medicine, pharmacology, the biosciences, science and technology, education, business and finance, the social sciences, and the humanities. Databases include current and historical information from journal articles, books, dissertations, and government reports. Many databases are a comprehensive index to available literature, while others include abstracts and complete text.

***DIALOG***   DIALOG Information Retrieval Service is offered by Dialog Information Services, Inc. and has been serving users since 1972. DIALOG offers over 400 databases composed of thousands of resources. They include reports, periodicals, publications, corporate directories, news services, and bibliographic and information resources. It offers unequaled subject balance, a variety of disciplines, and is the most complete and useful on-line information system available anywhere in the world. The coverage, combined with the DIALOG searching capabilities, make it one of the most important on-line commercial systems of its type.

The bibliographic retrieval systems described above—MEDLINE, CINAHL, ERIC, SOCIAL SCISEARCH, PsycINFO, and NTIS—are available on-line and can be accessed through either of the two commercial vendors, Dialog and BRS/SEARCH. Many of these systems are also available in CD-ROM format from commercial companies such as SilverPlatter. For example, MEDLINE and CINAHL are available as a CD-ROM–based information retrieval system offering unlimited searching at fixed costs and containing the same information that is available on-line.

## Review Informational Sources and Databases

There are other information retrieval sources that contain nurse-related data and other health-related data that may be relevant to nursing research. They include computerized databases derived from surveys, studies, or specific computer applications, and are not necessarily developed for general usage. They may also be derived from synthesis of research results.

These sources contain administrative, clinical, disease, and death information. Many of these databases are now available on-line from the organizations to users.

Some sources and/or databases are called public use tapes and are offered by several federal agencies, such as the Health Care Financing Administration (HCFA), National Center for Health Statistics (NCHS), Agency for Health Care Policy (AHCPR), or National Institutes of Health (NIH). They are also available from private sources—professional associations, e.g., the American Hospital Association (AHA); insurance companies, e.g., Blue Cross; or research corporations, e.g., Rand Corporation. Many of these computerized databases are not user-friendly and are not easily accessed. However, the databases that can be reviewed as part of a data search when conducting nursing research are described below (McCormick, 1981; Saba et al., 1989).

### Nurse-Related Databases

The nurse-related databases consist of data from major surveys, studies, and other research directly related to nursing or health-related resources. They are derived from studies conducted periodically and/or one-time studies whose findings are considered germane. They include national surveys conducted by federal and/or private nonprofit organizations which include nurse-related data such as number of nurses employed, number of schools of nursing, or number of nurses in hospitals. For example, the National Sample Survey of Registered Nurses, the Annual Survey of Schools of Nursing, and the Annual Survey of Hospitals generate relevant databases with nursing data.

### Health-Related Databases

The health-related informational databases are similar; however, they do not include nursing data. Such surveys contain relevant data from which nursing implications can be derived. For example, the Uniform Clinical Data Set (UCDS) collected by HCFA contains hospital patient care data that can be used to identify nursing care. Several of the HCFA databases contain data collected for other purposes, such as reimbursement of Medicare and Medicaid services, which have implications for nursing.

### Knowledge-Based Databases

There are several knowledge databases that consist of specific biomedical information exclusive of literature. These databases contain information on the specific focus of the database, such as drugs, poisons, diseases, diagnostic protocols, or other research. They provide factual information on the subject, are generally developed specifically for computer use, and can be searched by users. Generally, they are on-line, and are available to nurse researchers on public terminals through dial-up access using commercial vendors such as BRS and DIALOG. Knowledge databases are also included in knowledge-based networks which are emerging in health center libraries and are being offered to researchers.

The knowledge databases are categorized by the type of information in their database and not by nursing per se; however, they may have implications for nursing research. They are generally described as systems that focus on (1) factual topics, (2) diagnostic protocols, or (3) research in progress. These types of informational databases have implications for nursing research and could be of interest to other researchers.

***Factual Databases*** Factual databases are systems that contain information for a specific topic or subject. These on-line knowledge informational databases are developed as discrete databases which can be used and/or communicated to other researchers. Generally, they focus on one complete topic in the health science field. They cover all the pertinent facts, and resemble a reference book on the topic. For example, there are several knowledge databases that focus on only drug information.

***Diagnostic Protocols*** Diagnostic protocols provide another type of knowledge database that can be used by students and researchers. RECONSIDER and Dxplain are two databases which provide criteria and protocols for differential medical diagnoses. RECONSIDER is a medical diagnostic prompting program which uses the text of *Current Medical Information and Terminology* as its knowledge base. It is used as an educational tool for clinical problem solving. Dxplain offers external access to the diagnostic decision support system based at Massachusetts General Hospital, Harvard Medical School. The database contains thousands of relationships between diseases and clinical manifestations. They provide clinical protocols that may have implications for nursing research.

***Research in Progress*** Still another type of knowledge database contains information on ongoing research efforts. There are several research-in-progress systems which are being used by researchers. Such systems are used to share research in progress and are being built as the research progresses. The major ones include the international sequence databases of EMBL (European Molecular Biology Laboratory), Protein Information resource, GENEBANK (Gene Databases), and the GCG (Genetics Computer Group) sequence analysis software.

## Knowledge-Based Networks

Through research efforts, knowledge-based networks are emerging in health science centers as part of Integrated Academic Information Centers (IAIMS) and are offering on-line computerized knowledge databases. BioSYNTHESIS was developed by an IAIMS project in 1987, and is an example of a knowledge network. It was developed at Georgetown University, Medical Center Dahlgren Library (Broering and Bagdoyan, 1992; Broering et al., 1991).

**TABLE 15.3**   KNOWLEDGE NETWORK IAIMS AND LIS DATABASES

**Bibliographic Databases**

- Online Catalog (Medical Center Library)
- miniMEDLINE SYSTEM
- Alerts/Current Contents
- Bioethicsline
- CINAHL
- EMBASE
- NLM AIDS
- Grateful Med
- George (Catalog Main Campus Library)
- GULLiver (Catalog Law Center Library)

**Information Databases**

- Drug and Poison Information (MICROMEDEX)
- Drug Interactions (MediSpan DTSS)
- PDQ (Cancer Protocols)
- Medical Facts File
- Clinical Alerts

**Diagnostic Databases**

- Reconsider
- DXplain

**Research Databases**

- Molecular Biology (DNA Sequences)
- Genome Database (OMIM/GDB)
- NIH Guide

**Communication**

- Electronic News
- E-Mail
- Gopher
- Internet Access (UNIX)
- World Wide Web (Lynx)

*Source:* Adapted from Broering and Bagdoyan, 1992.

*BioSYNTHESIS* BioSYNTHESIS is a gateway system that provides transparent access not only to bibliographic retrieval systems, but also to several knowledge-based databases—factual, diagnostic, and research-in-progress systems which reside on other diverse computers. Through Bio-SYNTHESIS users have access to multiple in-house and external databases from a single point of entry. It provides a network which links the Medical Center users in the hospital, medical, and nursing school. The network also links to other campus libraries, external institutions, physician offices, and the residences of users who have access to the network. It offers an array of databases for researchers.

Each of the databases in the IAIMS knowledge-based network is user-friendly, and the user is unaware of how it is accessed. Dial-up access is available via a local area network (LAN) and an electronic gateway to the Internet controlled by the computer network "server" at the library. Some of the databases are loaded onto the computer, and others are linked via the Internet (a communication network). The system provides a direct connection from the user to any target database by passing direct dial-up and logon protocols for each. Table 15.3 provides a list of the major IAIMS databases offered as part of the BioSYNTHESIS knowledge-based network.

As technology advances, knowledge-based networks will improve information access and information management and will enhance the reference resource capabilities for researchers. New knowledge-based databases will be developed, and other knowledge resources, such as graphical interfaces, will enhance these networks.

## Nursing Networks

Nursing networks are emerging, several of which are available sources of nursing research resources. They are available to the nursing community and more specifically to nursing researchers via the Internet and/or on-line communication networks. Several are described below.

***Electronic Library*** The Virginia Henderson International Nursing Library of Sigma Theta Tau International Nursing Library has initiated an Electronic Library which can be accessed on-line or through the Internet. This new communication network supports the mission of Sigma Theta Tau International and offers knowledge resources and library services as well as disseminating nursing information and knowledge to its members. The Electronic Library offers primarily two types of information. The first is the dissemination of databases from the Registry of Nursing Knowledge, which includes a Directory of Nurse Researchers, Research Conference Abstracts, Sigma Theta Tau Grant Recipients, Projects, and other similar databases. The second provides access to the on-line *Journal of Knowledge Synthesis for Nursing*, which is offering a full-text electronic version of the journal (Graves, 1994).

***AJN Network*** American Journal of Nursing Company (AJN) is developing a new national computer network, an on-line service called AJN Network. This network will be offered on the Internet and become a high-performance computing and communication (HPCC) initiative for implementing the NII. It will provide information to nurses in medically underserved communities. It will offer the following services: (1) a nurse consultant service to which nurses can pose questions, (2) a bulletin board where nurses can post problems for discussion, (3) CAI programs that can be used for continuing education (CE) credit, (4) patient information on various topics, (5) nursing-related national and international news, and (6) other resource databases of nursing interest.

***ANA\*NET*** The American Nurses Association (ANA) is developing ANA\*NET, a combination of public and private databases compiled to assist and support ANA staff and state nursing associations by communicating and offering instant access for their information needs. ANA\*NET not only provides essential national policy information to the state organizations, but also offers numerous nursing and health care databases, resources and services, including bibliographic, nursing practice, economic, and general welfare databases, such as Grateful Med and CINAHL (American Journal of Nursing, 1993).

***E.T. Net*** The Educational Technology Network (E.T. Net) is an on-line computer conference network offered by NLM. E.T. Net is a bulletin board system which is designed to electronically link developers and users of interactive technology in health care education and interactive educational materials. E.T. Net provides the opportunity via Internet for the users and developers to share reviews, as well as view new applications of interactive hardware and/or software (Sparks, 1993).

## RESEARCH METHOD

The second step in the nursing research process is to determine the research method. The major activities include the following steps: (1) identifying the research methodologies, (2) determining the study population and sample, and (3) identifying the variables and/or the data elements to be researched.

### Identify Research Methodology

The determination of the research methodology depends on how the hypothesis is stated, the assumptions made, limitations of the research area scope, and identification of variables to be studied. The perimeters provide the basis for the research method selected—explanatory, descriptive, experimental, or nonexperimental—which determines the computer requirements (Abdellah and Levine, 1986).

### Define Nursing Framework

Nursing science provides the basis for the nursing profession and uses the nursing process as its conceptual framework. A conceptual framework is generally needed to provide a model for the research. There are primarily four types of clinical research which require a conceptual framework. They focus on (1) nursing data type including the vocabularies which provide the basis for the framework of patient care, (2) nursing strategies that provide the foundation for identifying and solving patient problems, (3) nursing service delivery patterns that concentrate on the organization, and (4) specific types of nursing service patterns. Nursing science is being advanced through clinical nursing research. The major conceptual frameworks are

- Nursing data
- Nursing strategies
- Nursing services
- Nursing practice

#### Nursing Data
Nursing data form the basis for documenting nursing and patient care. Nursing data need a language—vocabularies, terminologies, and taxon-

omies—to document the nursing process: assessment, diagnosis, outcome identification, planning, implementation, and evaluation. Nursing data dictionaries are required for the computer systems used to document patient care. Nursing data have to be defined and coded for computer applications.

***Taxonomies*** Nursing terminologies, vocabularies, and taxonomies are needed to define, categorize, and code nursing data sets for computer systems. Standardized nomenclatures are essential for computer systems that utilize nursing data. The nursing minimum data set (NMDS) encompasses 16 data elements that include nursing diagnoses, nursing interventions, nursing outcome, and intensity of nursing care. The data set and data elements were described earlier in the book.

At this time the ANA has recognized four nursing vocabularies, which are also described in Chap. 7: (1) NANDA Taxonomy I; (2) Saba Home Health Care Classifications (HHCC) of Nursing Diagnoses and Interventions, (3) the Omaha System, and (4) Nursing Intervention Classification (NIC) (Lang et al., 1995; McCormick et al., 1994).

Other taxonomies that affect patient care have been identified and include: the *International Classification of Diseases* (ICD), which is used to code medical diagnoses for inpatient conditions and is the basis for the diagnosis-related groups (DRGs), and *Current Procedure Terminology* (CPT), which codes medical treatments and surgical procedures outside hospitals.

## Nursing Strategies

Nursing strategies for solving patient problems focus primarily on the nursing information systems (NISs) which computerize protocols of nursing care of patients. For research purposes, the NISs need to encompass a range of nursing applications which include (1) skill acquisition, (2) clinical simulations, and (3) decision support. Systems need to encompass the strategies used by nurses to acquire nursing skills, which include understanding of the cognitive processes. Clinical simulations require analysis of actual clinical cases which have been effective. Decision support systems need to include problem-solving techniques as well as the principles of knowledge engineering, expert systems, and artificial intelligence (AI). They are needed to provide the basis for the models and systems being developed such as the following examples.

## Nursing Services

Nursing service applications focus on systems that can plan, forecast, and model nursing resources. The systems need to be consistent with other systems in similar facilities across categories, settings, and regions. Nursing resources include measurements of facility size, organizational structure, staffing size, nursing services, and cost. Nursing administration models have been used to outline the design specification of administration of nursing services systems.

## Nursing Practice

Nursing practice focuses on the actual process of delivering patient care. JCAHO has recommended adherence to the nursing process as the method for documenting patient care. Several research tools and/or instruments have been selected as a means of studying clinical nursing and are also described below. Several research models have been developed as frameworks for nursing practice. They generally focus on patient care and the nursing care planning process. They reflect the nursing theory that provides the basis for the care philosophy in a given hospital. For example, a model that bases patient care on the Orem theory will structure its computer-based system differently from one that is based on Maslow's hierarchy of needs.

## Define Study Population and Sample

The selection of the study population and sample is generally derived from existing statistical survey findings or databases. The conceptual framework and methodological approach provides the determination of the sample. It is critical that power statistics (size of sample needed to be significant) be used to ascertain an adequate sample size to make reliable interpretations of the data (Saba, 1991).

Many national surveys that relate to the use of nursing resources contain raw data that have been summarized for statistical analysis and that can be made available on a machine-readable medium. Such databases are excellent sources for the selection of a sample. For example, Medicare and Medicaid Automated Classification System (MMACS) computer tape contains information on approximately 5,880 certified agencies and their employed personnel. Computer selection of the research sample from such existing survey off-line informational databases provides for an innovative approach to the research design.

## Define Variables/Data Elements

The defining of the research variables and/or data elements requires outlining the conceptual framework that focuses on the areas to be addressed by the research. Conceptual issues generally include the structure and content of the tools to be developed. The type, size, scope, extent, and structure of the variables and data elements require a knowledge of computer systems. Several tools for collecting data as well as methods which can be used for generating databases and considered to be critical are

- Scales/indexes/scores
- Observations and interviews

### Scales/Indexes/Scores

Scales, indexes, and scores are tools which provide meaningful characteristics for collecting patient care data. They can be designed for both quantitative and qualitative research. Scales, indexes, or scores need to be developed to provide computable measures for computer systems. They enhance the structure and organization of the systems. Used to determine the normal ranges of physical measurements, physiological monitoring systems, for example, highlight normal values for an event, and the APGAR scores the health status of the newborn in a delivery room.

Other scales, such as nominal scales, can also be developed to provide baseline data for patient care systems. Such data are developed by counting the number of subjects, called frequency or summary data. Ordinal scales are used to rank according to some sequence. Other scales can be used to measure qualitative opinions on a continuum, rate quantitative values, or evaluate a series of statements which can provide a criterion measure for a variable. These tools provide the parameters for patient care measurements and the criteria for the normal values for a patient care system (Abdellah and Levine, 1986).

### Observations and Interviews

Observational tools are used to collect direct observations for clinical nursing research. Observational tools are needed to determine the data for a specific computer system. For example, the design of acuity classification systems is generally based on workload measures of patient care. Actual observations of activities performed by the nurses in caring for patients are collected.

Observational tools can also be used for other clinical computer research, such as determining how often the computer terminal is used and by what level personnel when evaluating a computer system. Observational tools can highlight the scope of use of computer systems. Other tools can be used to collect data at the source of the research, such as interview schedules and/or questionnaires. Interview schedules can cover the complexities of the problem under investigation. Open-ended and closed-ended questions coded and effectively used can provide clear descriptive information. Questionnaires, on the other hand, can be administered without an interviewer. All of these instruments are critical to the research process.

## DATA PROCESSING

Data processing, the third area of the research process, includes specifying the data collection method, outlining the strategy for coding the data, and specifying the method to input the data into data files and databases. Today, data are processed via computer systems. The design of the data collection method and forms, the strategy for coding the data and the structure of the files and databases must be adapted to computerized systems. Consideration must also be given to the capabilities of the computer hardware and computer software that are available for the research.

## Design Data Collection Forms

The design of the data collection forms involves several steps which are critical and constitute a major effort in any research study. They include coding, reviewing, and editing of data elements for input into a computerized database.

Research data are processed by computer, and therefore the data collection forms need to be precoded and ready for data processing. Data are generally collected on forms such as questionnaires, abstract forms, and a wide assortment of paper forms. The data elements on these forms need to be entered into a computerized database and will dictate (1) the size of the computer (mainframe, minicomputer, or microcomputer) and the memory needed to store the data elements, (2) the design of the file structures for dealing with the single and multiple variables, (3) the selection of software computer programs or packages, and (4) the database management system to organize the database.

As computer technology has advanced, several methods have emerged which can improve the data collection activities. The major ones include (1) computer-readable forms such as mark sense or optical scan forms which can be scanned directly into a computer database, (2) psychometric software that records observations through sensors which can transpose data directly into a database, or (3) computer notebooks which allow for data entry at the point of collection. They can be used to collect data with modems, on-line, or for direct entry by "downloading" into a computerized database. These examples of computer technology applications increase the accuracy of the research process, decrease the data processing time, increase efficiency, minimize errors, and allow nursing research to be cost-effective and ultimately more productive (American Nurses Association Task Force, 1992).

## Develop Data Files and Databases

### Create Data Files

File creation is another essential requirement for the design of the research database. A file is a collection of records considered to be one unit of related information. Files need to be designed to store like data elements together, making it easier to manipulate and process the data. Once the data have been entered into a computer system, they have to be edited, corrected, and prepared for statistical analysis. Data editing requires several tasks, such as identifying the disqualifies, reviewing each data element for completeness, identifying unacceptable responses, managing missing data, verifying precoded data, and validating the coded data.

Computer programs can be specially designed to generate error listings of data that need to be corrected, and in many instances other programs can be designed to correct the data.

## Create Databases

The data files, once edited and corrected, are ready for analysis. They need to be converted into a computerized database which can be transferred to a mainframe computer, minicomputer, or microcomputer for statistical analysis. Databases can be designed so that different statistical analyses and/or statistical models can be run for different statistical methods using different software programs and different computers. The size of the database will have to be matched with the size of memory in order to determine which statistical software package is the most appropriate to run on what size computer (Saba, 1991).

Database design is critical. Using database management systems, which are described in Chap. 5 emphasizes the need to group logical sets of data into tables and data sets. The databases should not store redundant data, and the data in a database should include only the critical variables needed to research the problem being studied (Hettinger and Brazile, 1992).

# Review Database Types

There are several types of databases that affect nursing research. They include aggregated databases and nursing information system databases.

## Aggregated Databases

Aggregate data derived from new clinical research or research on an existing computer system provide the baseline for another generation of the system. Such data provide new norms based on fact instead of interpretations derived from a sample population. Aggregated data can be obtained from any computer system used to document patient care. For example, a nursing care planning system that documents nursing diagnoses can be "downloaded" as a separate data set for analysis. The nursing diagnoses can then be compared with the most effective outcomes as a result of specific nursing interventions. Such a strategy could enhance the care protocols and form the basis for a decision support system. New protocols can provide the data needed to validate nursing science.

Aggregated data can provide the basis for determining norms, updating a system, and forecasting projections for planning. These data can also provide the normal baseline information for developing nursing care protocols as well as for designing nursing decision support systems.

## Meta-Analysis

Meta-analysis is a methodology for integrating and evaluating the research results using statistical techniques. Meta-analysis focuses on a different type of database. Generally it is a technique used to analyze "like" raw data aggregated from multiple sources. The aggregated data are analyzed to test a hypothesis based on existing data. Meta-analysis follows the same steps as those identified for the research process.

This new method has emerged because large volumes of data are available that can be used to make inferences from "what is" in order to predict "what can be." Aggregated data are also used in the clinical trials being conducted to study the cause of specific diseases such as AIDS or to study health conditions such as smoking and health, pregnancy, and premature infants. Clinical trials have been conducted with funding from the National Institutes of Health for several decades and have contributed to many advances in health promotion and disease prevention (Abdellah and Levine, 1994).

## Nursing Information System Databases

Nursing information system databases can be used as sources of aggregated databases which are critical to nursing and nursing research. As information systems are being implemented and used for nursing research, databases are being developed that aggregate nursing practice, nursing delivery, and nursing personnel data. Generally, data elements collected for a specific nursing information system application can be aggregated for planning, forecasting, and research purposes. Aggregated data from nurse classification systems can provide trend databases which can be used specifically for the hospital concerned or compared with other hospitals using the same system. Aggregating the NMDS on hospital discharge for specific types of patient, disease, or condition can provide valuable data for conducting research on nursing practice.

With the development and implementation of nursing information systems, these computer systems are increasingly becoming the major sources of aggregated data. They will provide the basis for the design of knowledge-based databases that focus on nursing, nursing practice, and the outcomes of care.

## Outcomes Databases

The clinical practice research tools influence the outcomes of care. Outcomes of care focus on the results of nursing practice—patient care process and decision-making skills of nurses. Computer applications have emerged as a result of research studies which have influenced several different systems, namely (1) decision support systems, (2) quality assurance systems, (3) effectiveness systems, and (4) cost containment systems.

*Decision Support Systems* Decision support systems encompass the results of decision analysis studies. Such studies generally focus on the development of nurses' skills in decision making, analysis strategies, clinical reasoning, and theories of skills acquisition. Decision analysis theories use patient care data to study nurses' cognitive processes, problem-solving techniques, and clinical simulation criteria. Case simulations, knowledge engineering, and protocol analysis studies have been used to describe problem-solving techniques. They provide the basis for expert systems and AI models being developed (Abraham et al., 1990; Shortliffe, 1990).

***Quality Assurance Systems***   Quality assurance systems focus on research that describes, measures, and delivers quality care to patients. Quality of care models, nursing standards, and compliance requirements have been recommended by JCAHO. Quality assurance systems have many benefits. Data must be reliable, and quality data must be analyzed. Donabedian distinguished between the definition and measurement of health and the definition and measurement of quality. Quality of care measurements need to be used to study the quality of care and be included in the quality assurance information systems (Donabedian, 1966; Hegyvary, 1991).

***Effectiveness Systems***   Today, the use of information systems and documentation systems has been described frequently in relation to outcomes as effectiveness research (Agency for Health Care Policy and Research, 1990). Basic issues in the evaluation of patient care outcomes are the end results of treatments and care. Outcome assessment focuses on four categories: clinical, functional, financial, and perceptual (Hegyvary, 1991).

***Cost Containment Systems***   Cost containment systems are also critical to the information systems being developed that focus on clinical nursing practice. They are being used to measure the cost of nursing care and become the basis for prospective payment systems for patient care (Prescott and Phillips, 1988).

## STATISTICAL ANALYSIS

Statistical analysis is critical to the research process.

Statistical analysis is the fundamental component in the research process. The major phases of statistical analysis include

- Summarize/reduce data
- Conduct statistical tests
- Select statistical software
- Develop analytical models

How data are analyzed will depend on the size and complexity of the database. The statistical units will vary depending on whether the quantity of study data is small or large. It is critical that the method of analysis be designed prior to data collection. Statistical software packages make it possible to process data easily without having to prepare the specific computations to analyze the data.

## Summarize/Reduce Data

As noted, a major activity in computer analysis is to summarize and/or reduce raw data into a "digestible" body of knowledge. Initially the statistical analysis of any data set should be computer-generated as descriptive analysis. Each data element should be processed as a numeric frequency in order to categorize and group them for statistical analyses. For example, the age distributions for 1,000 cases could have as many as 100 cells; however, in reviewing the frequencies, we can collapse them into four or five unique groups.

The commonest summary statistics include summary tables of descriptive statistics for the variables; frequency tabulations of discrete or continuous data, including histograms with bar graph frequency distributions; percentiles which compute the percents for a list of variables; cross tabulations of the variables; and a breakdown of the sums, means, and standard deviations. Summarized data should also provide descriptive statistics on the sample population and/or provide descriptive inferences describing the relationships between two or more variables.

## Conduct Statistical Tests

After the data are summarized, the next critical step in the statistical analysis process is to conduct statistical techniques or tests to produce research findings. The selection of the technique will depend on the data being analyzed and the techniques required to classify the data, categorize them into groups, and validate the findings. A broad array of statistical tests can provide techniques for analyzing single and multiple variables such as $t$ tests, one-way analysis of variance (IOV), and partial or complete correlations. Advanced techniques include such tests as multiple regression, basic and advanced multivariate analysis of variance (ANOVA), linear regression, clustering analyses, and stepwise regression. And still other tests can provide complex mathematical formulas to manipulate large databases, in order to test statistical hypotheses or determine population parameters (Statistix, 1992).

## Select Statistical Software

Statistical software packages have evolved from the simple descriptive and statistical computer programs that appeared in the late 1950s, to more recent customized models. A large number of statistical software packages are now available for use on the three sizes of computers—mainframe computers, minicomputers, and microcomputers. Generally, the more complex analytical methods require large memory capacity for processing.

There are several statistical software packages available which can run on any size computer. Depending on the size of the database, the selection of the computer to process the data is critical. Generally, vendors of a statistical package offer several versions, making it available for processing data on a mainframe, minicomputer, and microcomputer. However, because of the evolving technology, microcomputers and computer workstations are now replacing the need for mainframe or minicomputer processing, making it possible to process all research data by a single computer workstation.

Several new statistical packages have been developed which run on Microsoft Windows. This new graphical interface operating system makes the computer software user-friendly. As a result, several statistical packages that run on Windows make statistics "fun." Even the traditional statistical packages which use Microsoft Disk Operating System (MS DOS) and are described below are also available using Microsoft Windows. The majority of the software packages are used for analyzing quantitative research data; however, there are several new software packages for analyzing qualitative research data. They are packages that have (1) tools specifically designed for word processing, (2) word retrievers that are designed to retrieve instances of words and/or phrases, (3) text base managers that are designed to organize text systematically for search and retrieval, (4) code and retrieve programs that are designed to divide text into segments and/or chunks as well as code to the chunks, (5) theory builders that are designed to connect categories of information, and (6) conceptual network builders that are designed to build and test a theory (Miles and Weitzman, 1992).

### SAS and SPSS

The major statistical packages are primarily used for nursing research and biomedical research. They are SAS (Statistical Analysis System), SPSS (Statistical Package for the Social Sciences), and Biomedical Statistical Software Package (BMDP). There are several other packages emerging that are user-friendly and use the Windows operating system. These packages make it possible for staff and students to conduct their own research and analyze their own data.

*SAS*  SAS software packages continue to be enhanced as the technology advances. They are available for statistical analyses using a mainframe computer, minicomputer, and/or microcomputer. The most recent versions make it possible to store data values and retrieve them, modify data, compute simple statistics, and create reports all in one session. SAS packages can also provide graphics, forecasting, data entry, and sophisticated statistics.

The SAS software packages are grouped by the type of statistical method to be performed. The major ones used are data description, frequency tables, regression analysis, analysis of variance, multivariant analysis, life and survival tables, nonparametric, cluster analysis, and time series analyses (SAS, 1988).

*SPSS* SPSS also offers powerful statistical and information analysis computer programs that can run on a wide selection of computers. The newest versions offer new capabilities and enhanced flexibility in choosing portions of the data that meet the research requirements. They use menus for building commands and for contextual help as well as command-line and batch operation modes. Procedures such as factor analysis, cluster analysis, quick cluster analysis, and reliability analysis enhance their usability (Norasis, 1990).

BMDP is another package of statistical programs used in biomedical research. This software, available since 1961, contains statistical programs ranging from simple descriptive statistics to advanced statistical techniques.

## Develop Analytical Models

Statistical packages can also be customized to develop analytical models that can be used for the analysis of large databases and multiple variables. Many classes of models exist. Models can be designed for forecasting univariate and bivariate spectral analysis of parametric models. Other models can be classed into time series or regression (parametric) time series models which are used for decision making or testing theories. The building of statistical models consists of several stages which influence the research process: (1) identification and selection of a tentative model, (2) estimation of the model parameters, (3) testing the fit, (4) forecasting the future observations, and (5) selection of the linear model procedures.

### Correlations and Comparisons

Correlations and comparative data add statistical significance to clinical nursing research. Data interpreted as correlations and comparisons can provide new information and findings needed to develop, revise, or enhance a computer system. For example, correlations and/or comparisons between nursing and medical data, nursing and medical department personnel data, or physiologic and psychologic data can provide new information and influence the decision making of the users. They can be used to highlight different theoretical frameworks, care protocols, and models.

### Models and Forecasts

Models are abstractions of analytical methods for decision making. Modeling of the research content can provide predictions of nursing protocols. Computer modeling techniques consist of statistical procedures and tests or mathematical measurements which are determined to be clinically significant. They emulate real-life situations and are used for forecasting, planning, and decision making. Models can be used to predict care requirements, staffing, effective nursing actions, and patient outcomes.

## Linear Profiles

Linear profiles and longitudinal data track patient care over time. Profiles can be used to track a hospital, home health, or chronic ambulatory patient episode from admission to discharge. Linear profiles can be used to identify outcomes of care and patient responses to care. Clinical data sets can highlight the care requirements, including the costs of care. With a longitudinal health record, lifelong profiles can be used to predict and perhaps prevent medical events from occurring. For example, if a child has been diagnosed as having a genetic defect, the implications for lifelong health and nursing care requirements, including the cost, can be predicted and planned. Also, genetic counseling for pregnancy can be anticipated and outlined.

## RESEARCH CONCLUSIONS

The last step of the research process focuses on the research conclusions. It includes (1) describing the findings of the research, (2) determining the conclusions and their implications, (3) developing a strategy for disseminating the results, and (4) using the electronic communication systems.

## Describe Findings

The interpretation of the data consists of relating the problem being researched with the hypothesis, and determining whether the problem was solved by the research study variables. It consists of interpreting the meaning of the data, the significance and importance of the findings and results. It is also critical to link the findings to the existing scientific knowledge. The interpretation of the findings includes the discussion of the research findings and their implications. The interpretation of the results needs to integrate all the findings and be discussed in terms of the original hypothesis. The statistical findings need to have clinical significance as well as relevance to nursing and implications for nursing practice. Tables should present the implications for nursing practice, patient care, and/or nursing science.

### Computer Programs

Several computer applications are used to describe the research findings. They include software packages that have been described in Chap. 4.

***Word Processing***   Word-processing packages are primarily used to prepare all documentation for the research study. Word-processing capabilities can create, manipulate, revise, edit, and print a document. Word-processing packages have streamlined communicating via typewriter and the typewritten page.

***Spreadsheets*** These packages are used to present research tables that depict numbers, i.e., budget or accounting requirements. Spreadsheets are used in several research applications such as preparing the budget, presenting tables and graphs, preparing projections of time, making cost and personnel forecasts, and outlining milestone tasks and charts.

***Graphics*** They are used to display graphs depicting the research data. A graphic display is a useful way to describe data and reveal trends, unusual values, or relationships between variables. Graphic packages are available for all types of data presentations, such as pie charts, line and bar graphs, and cluster maps, as well as a variety of color schemes. Frequency tables summarize results from surveys, clinical studies, and experiments when data are qualitative or categorical, e.g., sex, or an answer to a multiple-choice question; discrete but ordered, e.g., education preparation; or continuous but grouped intervals, e.g., height and weight.

Data can be plotted as a histogram of a frequency distribution or the cumulative distribution (histograms and univariate plots), or as a graph of the data values in a normal or half-normal probability plot (bivariate scatter plots). Also, data from one variable can be plotted against the data for another variable. For example, if time is in column one and blood pressure is in column two, a graph representing those data can be plotted (Statistix, 1992).

***Graphics Data Show*** Graphical data show packages also provide an innovative means of displaying and communicating research findings. This type of software allows the data screens to be sequentially prepared and displayed via computer projector in any environment. Such a method allows electronic poster sessions to be prepared and presented instead of paper poster sessions which are developed using the same screen displays.

***Desktop Publishing Packages*** As part of the preparation of final reports and manuscripts, text editing and desktop publishing are available. Text editing software packages make project documentation easier and information dissemination timely. Desktop publishing software also allows for the direct publication of articles via electronic dissemination to research journals. Manuscripts can be transmitted to publisher, library, or vendor via a communication network system with a computer modem.

## Determine Conclusions

Determining the conclusions of the statistical analyses requires statistical and clinical knowledge. The interpretations of the statistical findings should focus on the practical meaning of the data. Statistical tests of significance in research studies are frequently misused and should be reviewed in relation to the purpose of the research. The misuses of the tests of significance are numerous and depend upon the quality of the measurements of the variables of the study. The data should be presented in tables that reveal answers to the research questions (Abdellah and Levine, 1986).

## Disseminate Results

Dissemination of research results includes not only the sharing of information with other researchers and users, but also the preparation of a final report, article, and paper. The electronic communication systems provide the means for the sharing of research findings. They can be used to communicate the findings to libraries, publishers, and bibliographic system databases.

Traditionally, the preparation of a final report is usually a requirement of the funding source. For example, all government grantees and contractors of nursing research must submit a final report, which is submitted to NTIS for indexing, abstracting, and reproduction. The report is indexed as a reference in the on-line health information database and is available for on-line searching. The scholarly article, which is generally the professional responsibility of the principal investigator, should be published in a refereed professional or scientific journal. Once published, it will be indexed and incorporated into one or several on-line bibliographic retrieval systems which can be accessed and searched and the article retrieved. Also, research results should be presented as papers at research conferences which may be a part of a teleconference network.

Another step in the dissemination process is the implementation of the procedures, methods, or protocols which have been developed into a health care facility or nursing practice. If they become the basis for a new information system or become integrated into a computerized information system, they should be evaluated after 6 months or sufficient time to test their usability.

## Identify Electronic Systems

Electronic on-line communication systems are used to disseminate research results and offer communication between researchers. The communication systems provide the means of transmitting on-line information. The major types provide not only on-line communication but also electronic teleconference networks, electronic bulletin boards, and electronic mail.

Communication network systems used for the on-line transmission of computerized databases are also used to access and transmit on-line bibliographic literature searches, and information from knowledge databases. The electronic teleconference networks, bulletin boards, and mail are used to disseminate research findings, conclusions, and results from the researchers to the users.

## Electronic Teleconference Networks

The electronic teleconference networks, such as those of health care educational media, link developers and users together. They allow researchers to share available information as if they were all located at the same site.

## Internet

The Internet has emerged as a network of networks. Internet has emerged as the preferred method of communicating and transmitting digital data from one researcher to another. It is used not only to provide different services, such as E-mail and bulletin boards, but also different tools and protocols such as Gopher and World Wide Web (WWW) to access nursing resources around the world. The Internet is also used to share and communicate findings, exchange databases, using the file transfer protocols (FTP), to disseminate research findings to other researchers and interested users. Telnet is a program/command that allows users to link remotely via a telephone line to another Internet server and/or "node."

## Other Communication Networks

There are other electronic communication networks used for communicating on-line information that are connected to Internet. The major ones include TELENET, BITNET, CompuServe, and America OnLine. These networks are used to transmit and communicate data primarily via telephone lines. They are also being used to transmit messages and electronic mail, as well as to transfer documents if connected to the Internet.

***TELENET*** is a public commercial network used primarily by vendors to communicate on-line databases to users. This dial-in service provides a gateway to a variety of commercial services such as America OnLine or CompuServe. These dial-in services are available throughout the world via local telephone lines. It requires a computer, modem, and computer communication software.

***BITNET*** This communication network has primarily been used to link institutions of higher education and research centers. It has been designed to facilitate communications among supercomputers in universities. BITNET users share information via real-time terminal messages and electronic mail transfer of documents, programs, and data.

***CompuServe*** This communication network is used by professional organizations to communicate with their members. It not only acts as a bulletin board but also provides its users with an array of services, including product information, publications, more research materials, computer files, and so forth.

***America OnLine*** This popular communication network is smaller but more user-friendly than the other on-line services and designed to make computing "fun." It offers similar services such as E-mail, news services and magazines, computer software, and games shopping.

## SUMMARY

This chapter provided an overview on how the computer supports and facilitates research in every phase of the process. Applications of the computer in nursing research were discussed from the document retrieval to manuscript preparation. Bibliographic retrieval systems that have replaced manual searching and periodic broad coverage of the available literature on a research topic were identified. Discussion of the MEDLARS databases and others with nurse-related data, how they are structured and how they can be searched, is comprehensive. How the computer assists in determining the research design and methodology was described.

Nursing data are the basis for documenting research. The language and vocabularies of nursing data and the coding required for computer systems were explained. Selecting the study population and sample, defining the variables, and identifying the tools for collecting data were also described. Included was a discussion of how computerized tools—scales, indexes, and scores—influence the measures of quantitative and qualitative research. The capabilities and limitations of available hardware and software for data processing and statistical analysis, including databases, were made explicitly clear. In conclusion, computer applications for the last step of the research process were presented. This included describing the findings, determining the conclusions, and developing a strategy for documenting the results. The essential knowledge and understanding of the use of the computer for conducting nursing research was contained in this chapter.

## REFERENCES

Abdellah, F. G., and Levine, E. (1986). *Better Patient Care through Nursing Research* (3d Ed.). New York: Macmillan.

Abdellah, F. G., and Levine, E. (1994). *Preparing Nursing Research for the 21st Century: Evolution, Methodologies, Challenges.* New York: Springer.

Abraham, I., Backer, A., DeBeckers, P., et al. (1990). Decision support for nursing research. In J. Ozbolt, D. Vanderwal, and K. Hannah (Eds.). *Decision Support Systems for Nursing.* St. Louis: Mosby.

*AGELINE File Description* (163). (1990). Palo Alto, CA: DIALOG Information Retrieval Services.

Agency for Health Care Policy and Research. (1990). *AHCPR: Purpose and Programs.* Rockville, MD: AHCPR, PHS, US DHHS.

American Journal of Nursing. (1993). *Nursing Education Computer Network to Be Developed.* New York: AJN Press Release.

American Nurses Association, Task Force on Computers in Nursing Research: Abraham, I., Schroeder, M. A., and Schwirian, P. M. (1992). *Computers in Nursing Research: A Theoretical Perspective.* Washington, DC.

Bibliographic Retrieval Services (BRS). (1991). *BRS Colleague: The Immediate Consult.* New York: BRS Information Technologies.

Broering, N. C., and Bagdoyan, H. E. (1992). The impact of IAIMS at Georgetown: Strategies and outcomes. *Bulletin of the Medical Library Association, 80*(3), 263–275.

Broering, N. C., Hylton, J. S., Guttman, R., and Eskridge, D. (1991). BioSYNTHE-SIS: Access to a knowledge network of health sciences databases. *Journal of Medical Systems, 15*(2), 139–153.

CINAHL. (1991). *Nursing & Allied Health (CINAHL) ONLINE Search Guide: Online Files.* Glendale, CA: Glendale Adventist Medical Center.

CINAHL Information Systems. (1992). *Nursing and Allied Health (CINAHL) 1992 Subject Heading List: Alphabetic List, Tree Structures, and Permuted List (Volume 37).* Glendale, CA: Glendale Adventist Medical Center.

*DIALOG Service.* (1991). Palo Alto, CA: DIALOG Information Retrieval Services.

*DISSERTATION ABSTRACTS ONLINE File Description* (35). (1989). Palo Alto, CA: Dialog Information Retrieval Services.

*DOCLINE Fact Sheet.* (1991). Bethesda, MD: National Library of Medicine, NIH, PHS, US DHHS.

Donabedian, A. (1966). Evaluating the quality of medical care. *Millbank Memorial Fund Quarterly,* 44 (Supplement), pp. 166–206.

*EMBASE (Excerpta Medica).* (1991). *ONTAP EMBASE File Description* (File 272). Palo Alto, CA: Dialog Information Retrieval Services.

*ERIC File Description* (1). (1990) Palo Alto, CA: DIALOG Information Retrieval Services. *E.T. Net (Educational Technology Network Fact Sheet.* (1991, March). Bethesda, MD: National Library of Medicine, NIH, PHS, US DHHS.

Fried, A. K., Killion, V. J., and Schick, L. C. (1988). Computerized databases in nursing: Information at your fingertips. *Computers in Nursing, 6*(6), 244–252.

*Grateful Med Fact Sheet.* (1992, August). Bethesda, MD: National Library of Medicine, NIH, PHS, US DHHS.

Graves, J. R. (1994). Updates; Virginia Henderson International Nursing Library. *Reflections, 20*(3), p. 39.

Hegyvary, S. T. (1991). Issues in outcomes research. *Journal of Nursing Quality Assurance, 5*(2), 1–6.

Hettinger, B. J., and Brazile, R. P. (1992). A database design for community health data. *Computers in Nursing, 10*(3), 109–114.

*Index Medicus.* (1993). Bethesda, MD: National Library of Medicine.

*International Nursing Index.* (1993). New York: American Journal of Nursing Company.

*HSTAT Fact Sheet.* (1995). Bethesda, MD: National Library of Medicine, NIH, PHS, US DHHS.

Kilby, S. A., Fishel, C. C., and Gupta, A. D. (1989). Access to nursing information resources. *IMAGE, 21*(1), 26–30.

Lang, N. M, Hudgings, C., Jacox, A., et al. (1995). Toward a national database for nursing practice. In *An Emerging Framework for the Profession: Data System*

*Advances for Clinical Nursing Practice.* Washington, DC: American Nurses Association.

*Loansome Doc Fact Sheet.* (1991). Bethesda, MD: National Library of Medicine.

McCormick, K. A. (1981). Nursing research using computerized data bases. In H. Heffernan (Ed.), *Proceedings of the Fifth Annual Symposium on Computer Applications in Medical Care* (pp. 738–743). New York: IEEE Computer Society Press.

McCormick, K. A., Lang, N., Zielstorff, R., et al. (1994). Toward standard classification schemes for nursing language: Recommendations of the American Nurses Association Steering Committee on Databases to Support Clinical Nursing Practice. *Journal of the American Medical Informatics Association, 1*(6), 421–427.

*Medical Subject Headings (MeSH) Fact Sheet.* (1993). Bethesda, MD: National Library of Medicine, NIH, PHS, US DHHS.

*MEDLARS: The World of Medicine at Your Fingertips.* (1991). Bethesda, MD: National Library of Medicine, NIH, PHS, US DHHS.

*MEDLINE Fact Sheet.* (1992). Bethesda, MD: National Library of Medicine, NIH, PHS, US DHHS.

Miles, M. B., and Weitzman, E. A. (1992). Appendix: Choosing computer programs for qualitative data analysis. In M. B. Miles and A. M. Huberman, *Qualitative Data Analysis: An Expanded Sourcebook* (pp. 311–317). London: Sage.

National League for Nursing. (1993). NLN recipient of Internet grant. *Connections,* p. 3.

*National Library of Medicine Fact Sheet.* (1992). Bethesda, MD: National Library of Medicine, NIH, PHS, US DHHS.

*NTIS File Description.* (1992). Palo Alto, CA: Dialog Information Retrieval Services.

Norasis, J. M. (1990). *SPSS/PC+4.0 Base Manual for the IBM PC/XT/AT and PS/2.* Chicago: SPSS.

Prescott, P. A., and Phillips, C. V. (1988). Gauging nursing intensity to bring costs to light. *Nursing and Health Care, 9*(1), 17–22.

*PsycINFO: ONTAP PsycINFO File Description.* (1990). Palo Alto, CA: Dialog Information Retrieval Services.

Saba, V. K. (1991). *Home Health Care Classification Project.* (NTIS Pub. No. PB92-177013/AS). Washington, DC: Georgetown University.

Saba, V. S., Reider, K. A., and Oatway, D. (1989). How to use nursing information sources. *Nursing Outlook, 37*(4), 189–195.

*SAS Introductory Guide for Personal Computers: Release 6.03 Edition.* (1988). Cary, NC: SAS Institute.

Schneider, D. (1993). Internet: Linking nurses, scholars, libraries. *Reflections, 19*(1), 9.

Shortliffe, E. H. (1990). Clinical decision-support systems. In E. H. Shortliffe and L. E. Perreault (Eds.), *Medical Informatics: Computer Applications in Health Care* (pp. 466–502). Reading, MA: Addison-Wesley.

Sinclair, V. G. (1987). Literature searches by computer. *IMAGE, 19*(1), 35–37.

Smith, L. (1988). Microcomputer-based bibliographic searching. *Nursing Outlook, 37*(2), 125–127.

*SOCIAL SCISEARCH: ONTAP SOCIAL SCISEARCH File Description.* (1991). Palo Alto, CA: Dialog Retrieval Information Services.

Sparks, S. M. (1986). The U.S. National Library of Medicine: A worldwide nursing resource. *International Nursing Review, 33*(2), 47–49.

Sparks, S. M. (1993). National Library of Medicine offers nursing resources. *Reflections 19*(1), 7.

*Statistix: Version 4.0: User's Manual.* (1992). St. Paul, MN: Analytical Software Corp.

Sweeney, M. A. (1985). *The Nurse's Guide to Computers.* New York: Macmillan.


# BIBLIOGRAPHY

Abdellah, F. G., and Levine, E. (1966). Future direction of research in nursing. *American Journal of Nursing, 66,* 112–116.

Broering, N. C. and Cannard, B. (1988). Building Bridges: LIS-IAIMS-BioSYN-THESIS, *Special Libraries, 79*(4), 302–309.

Degner, L. (1985). Computers in Clinical Nursing Research. In K. Hannah, E. Guillemin, and D. Conklin (Eds). *Nursing Uses of Computers and Information Science* (pp. 279–283). New York: Elsevier North-Holland.

Gortner, S. (1980). Nursing research: Out of the past and into the future. *Nursing Research, 29,* 204–207.

Hadorn, D. C., McCormick, K. A., and Diokno, A. (1992). An annotated algorithm approach to clinical guideline development. *Journal of the American Medical Association, 267*(24), 3311–3314.

Hirsch, R. R., and Riegelman, R. K. (1992). *Statistical First Aid: Interpretation of Health Research Data.* Boston: Blackwell Scientific.

Holzemer, W. L. (Ed.). (1989). *Review of Research in Nursing Education: Volume II.* New York: National League for Nursing.

Holzemer, W. L., Slaughter, R. E., Chambers, D. B., and Dulock, H. L. (1989). The development of a computer-based tutorial for an introductory course to nursing research. *Computers in Nursing, 7*(6), 258–265.

Jane, L. H. (1989). On statistical expert systems. In I. Abraham, D. Nadzam, and J. Fitzpatrick (Eds), *Statistics and Quantitative Methods in Nursing: Issues and Strategies for Research and Education* (pp. 37–39). Philadelphia: Saunders.

Joos, I., Whitman, N. I., Smith, M. J., and Nelson, R. (1992). *Computers in Small Bytes: The Computer Workbook.* New York: National League for Nursing.

Kilby, S. A., and McLindon, M. N. (1992). Searching the literature yourself: Why, how, and what to search. In J. M. Arnold, and G. A. Pearson (Eds.), *Computer Applications in Nursing Education and Practice* (pp. 23–34). New York: National League for Nursing.

Lancaster, F. (1978). *Information Retrieval Systems: Characteristics, Testing and Evaluation* (2d ed). New York: John Wiley.

Marek, K. D. (1989). Outcome measurement in nursing. *Journal of Nursing Quality Assurance, 4*(1), 1–9.

McCormick, K. A. (1983). Data capture: Use of statistical packages and computer literature searches. In O. Fokkens et al. (Eds.), *Medinfo 83 Seminars* (pp. 343–347). Amsterdam, Netherlands: North-Holland.

McCormick, K. A. (1988). Accessing clinical data. In J. S. Shockley (Ed), *Information Sources for Nursing: A Guide* (pp. 87–102). New York: National League for Nursing.

McCormick, K. A. (1988). Conceptual considerations, decision critical, and guidelines for development of the nursing minimum data set from a research perspective. In H. H. Werley and N. M. Lang (Eds.), *Identification of the Nursing Minimum Data Set* (pp. 34–47). New York: Springer.

McCormick, K. A. (1991). Future data needs for quality of care monitoring, DRG considerations, reimbursement and outcome measurement. *IMAGE, 23*(1), 29–32.

McCormick, K. A., and McQueen, L. (1986). The development and use of a database management system for clinical geriatric research. In R. Salamon, B. Blum, and M. Jorgensen (Eds.), *MEDINFO '86* (pp. 527–531). New York: Elsevier.

Miles, M. B., and Weitzman, E. A. (1994). Appendix: Choosing computer programs for qualitative data analysis In M. B. Miles and A. M. Huberman (Eds.), *Qualitative Data Analysis: An Expanded Sourcebook* (pp. 311–317). London: Sage.

Miluleky, M. P., and Ledford, C. (1987). *Computers in Nursing: Hospital and Clinical Applications*. Menlo Park, CA: Addison-Wesley.

Naisbitt, J. (1982). *Megetrends: Ten Directions Transforming Our Lives*. New York: Warner Books.

Palmer, M. H., McCormick, K. A., and Langford, A. (1989). Do nurses consistently document incontinence? *Journal of Gerontological Nursing, 15*(12), 11–16.

Palmer, M. H., McCormick, K. A., Langford, A., et al. (1992). Continence outcomes: Documentation on medical records in the nursing home environment. *Journal of Nursing Care Quality, 6*(3), 36–43.

Petrucci, K., McCormick, K., and Scheve, A. (1987). Documenting patient care needs: Do nurses do it? *Journal of Gerontological Nursing, 13*(11), 34–38.

Popyk, M. K. (1988). *Up and Running: Microcomputer Applications*. New York: Addison-Wesley.

Saba, V. (1981). *A Comparative Study of Document Retrieval Systems of Nursing Interest*. Washington, DC: American University.

Saba, V. K., and Skapik, K. (1979). Nursing information center. *American Journal of Nursing, 79*, 86–87.

Schwirian, P. (1983). The comparative utility of a file cabinet program vs. a general statistical program in micro-computer management and analysis of clinical nursing data. In R. Dayhoff (Ed.), *Proceedings of the Seventh Annual Symposium on Computer Applications in Medical Care* (pp. 565–567). Silver Spring, MD: IEEE Computer Science Press.

Schwirian, P. (1983). Schwirian's cube: The research dimension. *Computers in Nursing, 1*(1), 5–8.

Schwirian, P. (1985). Manifest and latent functions of microcomputer use in clinical nursing research. In K. Hannah, E. Guillemin, and D. Conklin (Eds), *Nursing Uses of Computers and Information Science* (pp. 303–307). Amsterdam, Netherlands: Elsevier, North-Holland.

Schwirian, P. (1986). The NI pyramid: A model for research for nursing informatics. *Computers in Nursing, 4*(3), 134–136.

Schwirian, P., and Byers, S. (1982). The microcomputer in the clinical nursing research unit. In B. Blum (ed.), *Proceedings of the Sixth Annual Symposium on Computer Applications in Medical Care* (pp. 658–661). Silver Spring, MD: IEEE Computer Society Press.

Shockley, J. S. (1988). *Information Sources for Nursing: A Guide*. New York: National League for Nursing.

Siegel, E. R., Cummings, M. M., and Woodsmall, R. M. (1990). Bibliographic-retrieval systems. In E. H. Shortliffe and L. E. Perreault (Eds.), *Medical Infor-*

*matics: Computer Applications in Health Care* (pp. 434–465). Reading, MA: Addison-Wesley.

Smith, J. T. (1993). Assessing information: It's easier than you think. *Nursing Dynamics, 2*(1) 15–19.

Study Group Nursing Information Systems. (1983). Special report: Computerized nursing information systems: An urgent need. (1983). *Research in Nursing and Health, 6,* 101–105.

Sweeney, M. A., and Olivieri, P. (1981). *An Introduction to Nursing Research.* Philadelphia: Lippincott.

Werley, H. (1981). Impact of computers on nursing research. In H. Heffernan (Ed.), *Proceedings of the Fifth Annual Symposium on Computer Applications in Medical Care* (pp. 728–729). Silver Spring, MD: IEEE Computer Society Press.

Werley, H., and Grier, M. (1981). *Nursing Information Systems.* New York: Springer.

Wiederhold, G., and Perreault, L. E. (1990). Clinical research systems. In E. H. Shortliffe and L. E. Perreault (Eds.), *Medical Informatics: Computer Applications in Health Care* (pp. 503–521). Reading, MA: Addison-Wesley.

Zielstorff, R. (1980). *Computers in Nursing.* Wakefield, MA: Nursing Resources.

# APPENDIX

# HOME HEALTH CARE CLASSIFICATION (HHCC)


Nursing Diagnoses and Nursing Interventions

By

Virginia K. Saba, Ed.D., R.N., F.A.A.N., F.A.C.M.I.

Terminology modifications and definitions made in collaboration with Sheila M. Sparks, D.N.Sc., R.N., C.S. Assistant Professor, Georgetown University.


©V.K. Saba, April 1994
HHCC Project funded by HCFA No: 17C-98983/3

**Table 1. Home Health Care Classification: 20 Nursing Components: Alphabetic Index with Codes**

A ACTIVITY COMPONENT

B BOWEL ELIMINATION COMPONENT

C CARDIAC COMPONENT

D COGNITIVE COMPONENT

E COPING COMPONENT

F FLUID VOLUME COMPONENT

G HEALTH BEHAVIOR COMPONENT

H MEDICATION COMPONENT

I METABOLIC COMPONENT

J NUTRITIONAL COMPONENT

K PHYSICAL REGULATION COMPONENT

L RESPIRATORY COMPONENT

M ROLE RELATIONSHIP COMPONENT

N SAFETY COMPONENT

O SELF-CARE COMPONENT

P SELF-CONCEPT COMPONENT

Q SENSORY COMPONENT

R SKIN INTEGRITY COMPONENT

S TISSUE PERFUSION COMPONENT

T URINARY ELIMINATION COMPONENT

# HOME HEALTH CARE CLASSIFICATION:
## NURSING DIAGNOSES
### with
## EXPECTED OUTCOMES/GOALS
### and
## CODING STRUCTURE

The coding structure for the Home Health Care Classification of Nursing Diagnoses is described below. The structure is used when coding home health nursing diagnoses including an expected outcome/goal. The coding structure consists of five alphanumeric characters; the first character is an alphabetic character representing the Home Health Care Component; the second and third characters are numeric digits representing the major Home Health Nursing Diagnoses; a fourth digit is blank or a decimal digit representing a diagnostic subcategory; and the fifth character is a decimal digit (1,2,or 3) representing the expected outcome/goal, modifier.

---

## CODING STRUCTURE

- HOME HEALTH CARE COMPONENT: 1st Alpha Code A to T
- NURSING DIAGNOSIS MAJOR CATEGORY: 2nd/3rd Digit: 01 to 50
- NURSING DIAGNOSIS SUBCATEGORY: 4th Decimal Digit:1 to 9
- DISCHARGE STATUS/GOAL: 5th Digit: 1 to 3 (Use Only One)
  1=Improved, 2=Stabilized, 3=Deteriorated

---

Table 2: Home Health Care Classification: Nursing Diagnoses and Coding Scheme: 50 Major Categories and 95 Subcategories[1]

## I. 50 NURSING DIAGNOSIS MAJOR CATEGORIES & 95 SUBCATEGORIES

**A - ACTIVITY COMPONENT**

    **01 Activity Alteration**
        01.1 Activity Intolerance
        01.2 Activity Intolerance Risk
        01.3 Diversional Activity Deficit
        01.4 Fatigue
        01.5 Physical Mobility Impairment
        01.6 Sleep Pattern Disturbance

    **02 Musculoskeletal Alteration**

**B - BOWEL ELIMINATION COMPONENT**

    **03 Bowel Elimination Alteration**
        03.1 Bowel Incontinence
        03.2 Colonic Constipation
        03.3 Diarrhea
        03.4 Fecal Impaction
        03.5 Perceived Constipation
        03.6 Unspecified Constipation

    **04 Gastrointestinal Alteration**

**C - CARDIAC COMPONENT**

    **05 Cardiac Output Alteration**

    **06 Cardiovascular Alteration**
        06.1 Blood Pressure Alteration

**D - COGNITIVE COMPONENT**

    **07 Cerebral Alteration**

08     Knowledge Deficit
       08.1   Knowledge Deficit of Diagnostic Test
       08.2   Knowledge Deficit of Dietary Regimen
       08.3   Knowledge Deficit of Disease Process
       08.4   Knowledge Deficit of Fluid Volume
       08.5   Knowledge Deficit of Medication Regimen
       08.6   Knowledge Deficit of Safety Precautions
       08.7   Knowledge Deficit of Therapeutic Regimen

09     Thought Processes Alteration

E  -    COPING COMPONENT

10     Dying Process

11     Family Coping Impairment
       11.1   Compromised Family Coping
       11.2   Disabled Family Coping

12     Individual Coping Impairment
       12.1   Adjustment Impairment
       12.2   Decisional Conflict
       12.3   Defensive Coping
       12.4   Denial

13     Post-Trauma Response
       13.1   Rape Trauma Syndrome

14     Spiritual State Alteration
       14.1   Spiritual Distress

F  -    FLUID VOLUME COMPONENT

15     Fluid Volume Alteration
       15.1   Fluid Volume Deficit
       15.2   Fluid Volume Deficit Risk
       15.3   Fluid Volume Excess
       15.4   Fluid Volume Excess Risk

G  -    HEALTH BEHAVIOR COMPONENT

16     Growth and Development Alteration

17     Health Maintenance Alteration

18     Health Seeking Behavior Alteration

19     Home Maintenance Alteration

20     Noncompliance

        20.1    Noncompliance of Diagnostic Test
        20.2    Noncompliance of Dietary Regimen
        20.3    Noncompliance of Fluid Volume
        20.4    Noncompliance of Medication Regimen
        20.5    Noncompliance of Safety Precautions
        20.6    Noncompliance of Therapeutic Regimen

**H   -    MEDICATION COMPONENT**

21     Medication Risk
        21.1    Polypharmacy

**I   -    METABOLIC COMPONENT**

22     Endocrine Alteration

23     Immunologic Alteration
        23.1    Protection Alteration

**J   -    NUTRITIONAL COMPONENT**

24     Nutrition Alteration
        24.1    Body Nutrition Deficit
        24.2    Body Nutrition Deficit Risk
        24.3    Body Nutrition Excess
        24.4    Body Nutrition Excess Risk

**K   -    PHYSICAL REGULATION COMPONENT**

25     Physical Regulation Alteration
        25.1    Dysreflexia
        25.2    Hyperthermia
        25.3    Hypothermia
        25.4    Thermoregulation Impairment
        25.5    Infection Risk

25.6   Infection Unspecified

**L  -   RESPIRATORY COMPONENT**

26   Respiration Alteration
  26.1   Airway Clearance Impairment
  26.2   Breathing Pattern Impairment
  26.3   Gas Exchange Impairment

**M  -   ROLE RELATIONSHIP COMPONENT**

27   Role Performance Alteration
  27.1   Parental Role Conflict
  27.2   Parenting Alteration
  27.3   Sexual Dysfunction

28   Communication Impairment
  28.1   Verbal Impairment

29   Family Processes Alteration

30   Grieving
  30.1   Anticipatory Grieving
  30.2   Dysfunctional Grieving

31   Sexuality Patterns Alteration

32   Socialization Alteration
  32.1   Social Interaction Alteration
  32.2   Social Isolation

**N  -   SAFETY COMPONENT**

33   Injury Risk
  33.1   Aspiration Risk
  33.2   Disuse Syndrome
  33.3   Poisoning Risk
  33.4   Suffocation Risk
  33.5   Trauma Risk

34   Violence Risk

**Nursing Diagnoses Cont.**

**O  -  SELF-CARE COMPONENT**

35  Bathing/Hygiene Deficit

36  Dressing/Grooming Deficit

37  Feeding Deficit
 37.1  Breastfeeding Impairment
 37.2  Swallowing Impairment

38  Self Care Deficit
 38.1  Activities of Daily Living (ADLs) Alteration
 38.2  Instrumental Activities of Daily Living (IADLs) Alteration

39  Toileting Deficit

**P  -  SELF-CONCEPT COMPONENT**

40  Anxiety

41  Fear

42  Meaningfulness Alteration
 42.1  Hopelessness
 42.2  Powerlessness

43  Self Concept Alteration
 43.1  Body Image Disturbance
 43.2  Personal Identity Disturbance
 43.3  Chronic Low Self-Esteem Disturbance
 43.4  Situational Self-Esteem Disturbance

**Q  -  SENSORY COMPONENT**

44  Sensory Perceptual Alteration
 44.1  Auditory Alteration
 44.2  Gustatory Alteration
 44.3  Kinesthetic Alteration
 44.4  Olfactory Alteration
 44.5  Tactile Alteration
 44.6  Unilateral Neglect
 44.7  Visual Alteration

**Nursing Diagnoses Cont.**

45      Comfort Alteration
     45.1    Acute Pain
     45.2    Chronic Pain
     45.3    Unspecified Pain

**R**    -     **SKIN INTEGRITY COMPONENT**

46      Skin Integrity Alteration
     46.1    Oral Mucous Membranes Impairment
     46.2    Skin Integrity Impairment
     46.3    Skin Integrity Impairment Risk
     46.4    Skin Incision

47      Peripheral Alteration

**S**    -     **TISSUE PERFUSION COMPONENT**

48      Tissue Perfusion Alteration

**T**    -     **URINARY ELIMINATION COMPONENT**

49      Urinary Elimination Alteration
     49.1    Functional Urinary Incontinence
     49.2    Reflex Urinary Incontinence
     49.3    Stress Urinary Incontinence
     49.4    Total Urinary Incontinence
     49.5    Urge Urinary Incontinence
     49.6    Urinary Retention

50      Renal Alteration

## HOME HEALTH CARE CLASSIFICATION:
### NURSING INTERVENTIONS
#### with
### TYPE OF INTERVENTION ACTION
#### and
### CODING STRUCTURE

The coding structure for the Home Health Care Classification of Nursing Interventions is described below. The structure is used when coding home health nursing interventions including type of intervention action. The coding structure consists of five alphanumeric characters; the first character is an alphabetic character representing the Home Health Care Component; the second and third characters are numeric digits representing the major Home Health Nursing Interventions; a fourth digit is blank or a decimal digit representing an Intervention subcategory; and the fifth character is a decimal digit (1, 2, 3, or 4) representing the Type of Intervention Action, modifier.

---

## CODING STRUCTURE

- **HOME HEALTH CARE COMPONENT  1st Alpha Code A to T**
- **NURSING DIAGNOSIS MAJOR CATEGORY: 2nd/3rd Digit: 01 to 50**
- **NURSING DIAGNOSIS SUBCATEGORY: 4th Decimal Digit:1 to 9**
- **DISCHARGE STATUS/GOAL: 5th Digit: 1 to 4 (Use Only One)**

     **1=Assess, 2=Care, 3=Teach, 4=Manage**

---

# I. 60 NURSING INTERVENTION MAJOR CATEGORIES & 100 SUBCATEGORIES

## A. ACTIVITY COMPONENT

01  Activity Care
01.1 Cardiac Rehabilitation
01.2 Energy Conservation

02  Fracture Care
02.1    Cast Care
02.2    Immobilizer Care

03  Mobility Therapy
03.1    Ambulation Therapy
03.2    Assistive Device Therapy
03.3    Transfer Care

04  Sleep Pattern Control

05  Rehabilitation Care
05.1    Range of Motion
05.2    Rehabilitation Exercise

## B. BOWEL ELIMINATION COMPONENT

06  Bowel Care
06.1    Bowel Training
06.2    Disimpaction
06.3    Enema

07  Ostomy Care
07.1    Ostomy Irrigation

## C. CARDIAC COMPONENT

08  Cardiac Care

**Nursing Interventions Cont.**

    46  Violence Control

**Q.**   **SENSORY COMPONENT**

    47  Pain Control

    48  Comfort Care

    49  Ear Care
        49.1    Hearing Aid Care
        49.2    Wax Removal

    50  Eye Care
        50.1    Cataract Care

**R.**   **SKIN INTEGRITY COMPONENT**

    51  Decubitus Care
        51.1    Decubitus Stage 1
        51.2    Decubitus Stage 2
        51.3    Decubitus Stage 3
        51.4    Decubitus Stage 4

    52  Edema Control

    53  Mouth Care
        53.1    Denture Care

    54  Skin Care
        54.1    Skin Breakdown Control

    55  Wound Care
        55.1    Drainage Tube Care
        55.2    Dressing Change
        55.3    Incision Care

**S.**   **TISSUE PERFUSION COMPONENT**

    56  Foot Care

    57  Perineal Care

T.     **URINARY ELIMINATION COMPONENT**

# INDEX
●●●●●●●●●●●●●●●●●●●●●●●●●●

Page numbers in italics indicate figures; page numbers followed by *t* indicate tables.

ISBN 0-07-105418-9

9 780071 054188

90000>

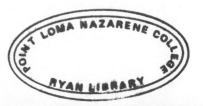